Therapeutic Modalities

Fifth Edition

••••••••

Therapeutic Modalities

For Sports Medicine and Athletic Training

••••••••••••••••••••••••••

William E. Prentice, Ph.D., P.T., A.T.C.

Professor, Coordinator of Sports Medicine Specialization,
Department of Exercise and Sport Science
Clinical Professor, Division of Physical Therapy,
Department of Medical Allied Health Professions,
Associate Professor, Department of Orthopaedics
School of Medicine
The University of North Carolina,
Chapel Hill, North Carolina

Boston   Burr Ridge, IL   Dubuque, IA   Madison, WI   New York   San Francisco   St. Louis
Bangkok   Bogotá   Caracas   Kuala Lumpur   Lisbon   London   Madrid   Mexico City
Milan   Montreal   New Delhi   Santiago   Seoul   Singapore   Sydney   Taipei   Toronto

McGraw-Hill Higher Education ℘

*A Division of The **McGraw-Hill** Companies*

THERAPEUTIC MODALITIES: FOR SPORTS MEDICINE AND ATHLETIC TRAINING
FIFTH EDITION

Published by McGraw-Hill, a business unit of The McGraw-Hill Companies, Inc., 1221
Avenue of the Americas, New York, NY 10020. Copyright © 2003, 1999, 1994, 1990, 1986
by The McGraw-Hill Companies, Inc. All rights reserved. No part of this publication may be
reproduced or distributed in any form or by any means, or stored in a database or retrieval
system, without the prior written consent of The McGraw-Hill Companies, Inc., including,
but not limited to, in any network or other electronic storage or transmission, or broadcast
for distance learning.

Some ancillaries, including electronic and print components, may not be available to customers outside the United States.

This book is printed on acid-free paper.

2 3 4 5 6 7 8 9 0 QPF/QPF 0 9 8 7 6 5 4 3

ISBN 0–07–246211–6

Vice president and editor-in-chief: *Thalia Dorwick*
Publisher: *Jane E. Karpacz*
Executive editor: *Vicki Malinee*
Senior developmental editor: *Michelle Turenne*
Senior marketing manager: *Pamela S. Cooper*
Project manager: *Mary Lee Harms*
Production supervisor: *Enboge Chong*
Freelance design coordinator: *Gino Cieslik*
Supplement producer: *David A. Welsh*
Media technology producer: *Lance Gerhart*
Compositor: *Shepherd, Inc.*
Typeface: *10/12 Photina*
Printer: *Quebecor World Fairfield, PA*

Library of Congress Cataloging-in-Publication Data

Therapeutic modalities : for sports medicine and athletic training / [edited by] William E.
Prentice. —— 5th ed.
    p.   cm.
    Rev. ed. of: Therapeutic modalities in sports medicine. 4th ed. ©1999.
    Includes bibliographical references and index.
    ISBN 0–07–246211–6 (alk. paper)
    1. Sports injuries—Treatments. 2. Sports physical therapy. I. Prentice, William E.
II. Therapeutic modalities in sports medicine.
    [DNLM: 1. Athletic Injuries—therapy. 2. Athletic Injuries—rehabilitation. 3. Physical
Therapy Techniques—methods. QT 261 T398 2003]
RD97 .T484 2003
617.1'027—dc21   2002016618
                                    CIP

This text was based on the most up-to-date research and suggestions made by individuals
knowledgeable in the field of athletic training. The authors and publisher disclaim any
responsibility for any adverse effects or consequences from the misapplication or injudicious
use of information contained within this text. It is also accepted as judicious that the coach
and/or athletic trainer performing his or her duties is, at all times, working under the guidance
of a licensed physician.

www.mhhe.com

Brief Contents

Contents

PART TWO   Thermal Modalities

PART THREE   Electrical Modalities

PART FOUR   # Mechanical Modalities

10   Therapeutic Sports Massage   256

William E. Prentice and Clairbeth Lehn

11   Intermittent Compression Devices   282

Daniel N. Hooker

12   Spinal Traction   297

Daniel N. Hooker

Preface

HOW DO ATHLETIC TRAINERS USE THERAPEUTIC MODALITIES?

There is little argument that athletic trainers use a wide variety of therapeutic techniques in the treatment and rehabilitation of sports-related injuries. One of the more important aspects of a thorough treatment regimen often involves the use of therapeutic modalities. At one time or another, virtually all athletic trainers make use of some type of therapeutic modality. This may involve a relatively simple technique such as using an ice pack as a first aid treatment for an acute injury or more complex techniques such as the stimulation of nerve and muscle tissue by electrical currents. There is no question that therapeutic modalities are useful tools in injury rehabilitation. When used appropriately, these modalities can greatly enhance the athlete's chances for a safe and rapid return to athletic competition. For the athletic trainer, it is essential to possess knowledge regarding the scientific basis and the physiologic effects of the various modalities on a specific injury. When this theoretical basis is applied to practical experience, it has the potential to become an extremely effective clinical method.

What Role Should a Modality Play in Injury Rehabilitation?

An effective treatment program includes three primary objectives: (1) management or reduction of pain associated with an injury, (2) return of full nonrestricted range of movement to an injured part, and (3) maintenance or perhaps impvement of strength through the full range. Modalities, though important, are by no means the single most critical factor in accomplishing these objectives. Therapeutic exercise that forces the injured anatomic structure to perform its normal function is the key to successful rehabilitation; however, therapeutic modalities certainly play an important role in reducing pain and are extremely useful as an adjunct to therapeutic exercise.

It must be emphasized that the use of therapeutic modalities in any treatment program is an inexact science. If you were to ask ten different athletic trainers what combination of modalities and therapeutic exercise they use in a given treatment program, you would probably get ten different responses. There is no way to "cookbook" a treatment plan that involves the use of therapeutic modalities. Thus, what this book will attempt to do is to present the basis for use of each different type of modality and allow the individual athletic trainer to make his or her own decisions as to which will be most effective in a given clinical situation. Some recommended protocols developed through the experiences of the contributing authors will be presented.

Formal Instruction in the Use of Therapeutic Modalities

The athletic trainer continues to gain acceptance in the medical community as a highly qualified and well-educated allied health professional concerned with the treatment and rehabilitation of injuries to athletes. It is essential for the programs educating student athletic trainers to provide classroom instruction in a wide range of specialty areas including injury prevention, care and management, injury evaluation, and therapeutic treatment and rehabilitation techniques. Formal classroom instruction in the use of therapeutic modalities is required in all educational programs for student athletic trainers who intend to pursue a career in sports medicine, regardless of whether the program is accredited by the Committee on Accreditation of Allied Health Education Programs (CAAHEP), approved as a Graduate Athletic Training Education Program by the NATA, or in exisiting internship programs. In fact, instruction in the use of therapeutic modalities has been specifically identified and mandated in the *Athletic Training Educational Competencies,* which was prepared by the National Athletic Trainers' Association.

Legal Issues in Using Therapeutic Modalities

The use of therapeutic modalities in the treatment of athletic injuries by individuals with various combinations of educational background, certification, and licensure is currently a controversial issue. Specific laws governing the use of therapeutic modalities by athletic trainers vary considerably from state to state. Many states have specific guidelines in the Licensure Act that dictate how the athletic trainer may incorporate therapeutic modalities into the treatment regimen. Each athletic trainer should be careful that any use he or she makes of a modality is within the limits allowed by the law of his or her particular state. I do not intend for the athletic trainer to interpret anything in this book as encouraging him or her to act outside the scope of the laws of his or her state.

Why Should This Text Be Used to Teach the Student Athletic Trainer About Therapeutic Modalities?

It is hoped that this fifth edition will continue to be a useful tool in the ongoing growth and professional development of the athletic trainer concerned with and interested in the field of sports injury rehabilitation. The following are a umber of reasons why this text should be adopted for use.

New to This Edition. Based on the helpful input we have received from users of the text, you will find the following features in this fifth edition:

- Self-quizzes included in every chapter to assess student comprehension. Answers are provided in Appendix D.
- New content is provided on frostbite, electromyography, and biofeedback.
- Images from the text will be available on the Image Presentation CD-ROM that accompanies *Arnheim's Principles of Athletic Training,* eleventh edition, also by William E. Prentice.

Comprehensive Coverage of Therapeutic Modalities in a Sports Medicine Setting. The purpose of this text, as in past editions, is to provide a theoretically based but practically oriented guide to the use of therapeutic modalities for the athletic trainer who routinely treats sports-related injury. It is intended for use in advanced courses in athletic training and sports medicine where various clinically oriented techniques and methods are presented.

The sequencing of the chapters in this fifth edition has been reorganized to place emphasis on those modalities most often used by athletic trainers by presenting those chapters earlier in the text (i.e., infrared modalities, therapeutic ultrasound, and shortwave and microwave diathermy). In addition, each chapter has been expanded and updated to include the latest available research that has been published in related professional journals since the last edition was published.

This edition is divided into five parts. Part One, *Foundations of Therapeutic Modalities,* begins with Chapter 1 discussing the scientific basis for using various therapeutic modalities in athletics and classifying the modalities in a logical order in relation to the electromagnetic and acoustic spectra. Chapter 2 establishes guidelines for selecting the most appropriate modalities for use in different phases of the healing process. In Chapter 3, pain is discussed in terms of neurophysiologic mechanisms of pain and the role of therapeutic modalities in pain management. Part Two, *Thermal Modalities*, begins with a discussion of the infrared modalities, including thermotherapy and cryotheraphy in Chapter 4. Therapeutic ultrasound is covered in Chapter 5, followed by shortwave and microwave diathermy in Chapter 6. Part Three, *Electrical Modalities*, discusses the principles of electricity in Chapter 7, and applies these principles specifically to electrical stimulating currents and iontophoresis in Chapters 8 and 9. Part Four, *Mechanical Modalities*, includes chapters on sports massage (Chapter 10), intermittent compression (Chapter 11), and spinal traction (Chapter 12). Part Five, *Other Modalities*, looks at three seperate modalities that are less commonly used in an athletic training setting including biofeedback in Chapter 13, low-power lasers in Chapter 14, and ultraviolet therapy in Chapter 15. Each chapter includes discussions of (1) the physiologic basis for use, (2) clinical applications, and (3) specific techniques of application. Appendix B includes a comprehensive list of manufacturers and distributors of various types of therapeutic modalities and related equipment.

Based on Scientific Theory. This text discusses various concepts, principles, and theories that are supported by scientific research, factual evidence, and previous experience by the authors with injuries related to sport. The material presented in this text has been carefully researched by the contributing authors to provide the most up-to-date information on the theoretical basis for employing a particular modality in a specific injury situation. Additionally, the manuscript for this text has been carefully reviewed by both athletic trainers and physical therapists who are considered experts in their field to ensure that the material reflects factual and current concepts for modality use.

Timely and Practical. The first edition of this text filled a void that existed for quite some time in the athletic training education program curriculums. It was the first text ever published that focused on therapeutic modalities and their use by athletic trainers in a clinical setting. Since the first edition, several other texts on therapeutic modalities have been published. However, *Therapeutic*

Modalities for Sports Medicine and Athletic Training remains unique since it is still the only textbook that provides the student with a comprehensive resource covering all of the therapeutic modalities that could be used by an athletic trainer.

During the preparation of this fifth edition, as well as previous editions of this text, we have received much encouragement from athletic training educators and students regarding the usability of this text in the classroom setting. It should serve as a needed guide for the athletic trainer who is interested in knowing not only how to use a modality but also why that particular modality is most effective in a given situation.

The authors who have contributed to this text have a great deal of clinical experience with sports-related injury. Each of these individuals has also at one time or another been involved with the formal classroom education of the student athletic trainer. Thus, this text has been developed for the student of sports-injury rehabilitation who will be asked to apply the theoretical basis of modality use to the clinical setting.

Pertinent to the Athletic Trainer. Although it is certainly true that therapeutic modalities are important and necessary tools that should be used with physical problems of all varieties, this text specifically addresses how and why these modalities are best used in the treatment and rehabilitation of injuries related to sport. Several other texts are available that discuss the use of selected physical modalities with patient populations other than athletes. With the expanded content in this fifth edition, this is the most comprehensive text on therapeutic modalities available in any specific discipline.

Pedagogical Aids. This text includes the following aids to facilitate its use by students and instructors:

Objectives. These goals are listed at the beginning of each chapter to introduce students to the points that will be emphasized. The objectives have been rewritten to cover the entire spectrum of Bloom's Taxonomy and thus to challenge the student to go beyond knowing and comprehending the material, to be able to apply, analyze, synthesize, and evaluate the important concepts they have learned.

Figures and tables. Essential points of each chapter are illustrated with clear visual materials.

Glossary of key terms. A glossary of terms for quick reference is provided.

Analogies. A series of analogies is presented to help the reader more easily comprehend more difficult concepts.

Clinical decision-making exercises. New exercises have been added to the previous exercises in each chapter to help the athletic trainer with his or her decision-making abilities about how a specific modality may best be used clinically.

Summaries. The important points or concepts of each chapter are succinctly re-emphasized in the summary list.

Review questions. A series of questions has been developed for each chapter that help the student review the critical points to remember.

Self-quizzes. New with this edition is a series of objective questions in every chapter that can be used to prepare for a written examination and to assess student comprehension. Answers are located in Appendix D.

References. A list of up-to-date references is provided at the end of each chapter for the student who wishes to read further on the subject being discussed.

Suggested readings. A comprehensive list of journal articles and textbooks provides additional information related to the chapter material.

Appendices. A chart of motor points, a comprehensive list of manufacturers of therapeutic modality equipment, a table for unit conversions, and answers to the self-quizzes are provided.

ANCILLARIES

Laboratory Manual

With this fifth edition, a separate laboratory manual accompanies the text to facilitate and demonstrate the content presented. This manual includes practical laboratory exercises and case studies designed to enhance student understanding of therapeutic modality use. It illustrates the principles and theories of modality use through practical demonstrations and experiences. The lab manual is packaged at no charge with each new purchase of the fifth edition.

Image Presentation CD-ROM

The McGraw-Hill Image Presentation CD-ROM (IPCD) is an electronic library of visual resources. The CD-ROM includes (1) images from the text in PowerPoint, which allows the user to view, sort, search, use, and print catalog images, and (2) preset PowerPoint presentations, which allow the user to play chapter-specific slideshows. Images for the fifth edition will be available on the IPCD that accompanies *Arnheim's Principles of Athletic Training*, eleventh edition, also by William E. Prentice.

PowerPoint Presentation

A comprehensive and extensively illustrated PowerPoint presentation accompanies this text for use in classroom discussion. The PowerPoint presentation may also be converted to outlines and given to students as a handout. You can easily download the PowerPoint presentation from the McGraw-Hill website at *www.mhhe.com*. Adopters of the text can obtain the login and password to access this presentation by contacting your local McGraw-Hill sales representative.

eSims

eSims is an online assessment tool providing students not only with computerized simulation tests that imitate the actual Athletic Training Certification Exam but also with instant feedback. Check out eSims at www.mhhe.com/esims.

And Much More . . .

Check out the competency information found at www.mhhe.com/prentice11e. For more online study resources, visit the McGraw-Hill Health and Human Performance website at www.mhhe.com/hhp.

ACKNOWLEDGMENTS

Since the first edition, there have been many individuals who have collectively contributed to the evolution of this text. All have contributed in their own way, but a few deserve special thanks.

Michelle Turenne, my developmental editor at McGraw-Hill, has been responsible for coordinating the efforts between the publisher and myself. She has been very supportive and has taken care of many of the details in the completion of this text.

When assembling a group of contributors for a project such as this, it is essential to select individuals who are both knowledgeable and well-respected in their fields. It also helps if you can count them as friends, and I want to let them know that I hold each of them in the highest regard, both personally and professionally.

The following individuals have invested a great amount of time and effort in reviewing this manuscript. Their contributions are present throughout the text. I would like to thank each one of them for all their valuable insight.

Janet Balowski *Eastern Michigan University*
Suzanne Pero *University of Nevada–Las Vegas*
Jeffrey S. Monroe *Michigan State University*
Charles J. Redmond *Springfield College*
Patricia Aronson *Lynchburg College*

And finally, I would like to thank my wife Tena and my sons Brian and Zachary for being understanding, patient, and supportive while I pursue a career and a life that I truly enjoy.

William E. Prentice
Chapel Hill, North Carolina

Contributors

Gerald W. Bell, Ed.D., P.T., A.T.C.
Associate Professor
Departmet of Kinesiology
University of Illinois at Urbana–Champaign
Urbana, Illinois

J. Marc Davis, P.T., A.T.C.
Physical Therapist/Athletic Trainer
Division of Sports Medicine
Student Health Service
The University of North Carolina
Chapel Hill, North Carolina

Craig Denegar, Ph.D., P.T., A.T.C.
Associate Professor of Athletic Training
Department of Kinesiology
Penn State University
State College, Pennsylvania

David O. Draper, Ed.D., A.T.C.
Associate Professor
Department of Physical Education
Brigham Young University
Provo, Utah

Phillip B. Donley, M.S., P.T., A.T.C.
Director
Chester County Orthopaedic and Sports Physical
Therapy
West Chester, Pennsylvania

Daniel N. Hooker, Ph.D., P.T., Sc.S, A.T.C.
Coordinator of Athletic Training and Physical
Therapy
Division of Sports Medicine
Student Health Service
The University of North Carolina,
Chapel Hill, North Carolina

Clairbeth Lehn, P.T., A.T.C.
Physical Therapist/Athletic Trainer
Division of Sports Medicine
Student Health Service
The University of North Carolina
Chapel Hill, North Carolina

William E. Prentice, Ph.D., P.T., A.T.C.
Professor, Coordinator of Sports Medicine
Specialization
Department of Exercise and Sport Science
Clinical Professor, Division of Physical Therapy
Department of Medical Allied Health Professions
Associate Professor, Department of Orthopaedics
School of Medicine
The University of North Carolina
Chapel Hill, North Carolina

Ethan N. Saliba, Ph.D., P.T., A.T.C.
Head Athletic Trainer
Department of Athletics
Assistant Professor
Department of Kinesiology
University of Virginia
Charlottesville, Virginia

Susan H. Foreman Saliba, Ph.D., P.T., A.T.C.
Head Associate Athletic Trainer
McCue Sports Medicine Center
Sports Medicine Instructor
Department of Kinesiology
University of Virginia
Charlottesville, Virginia

Mastering the Competencies

The National Athletic Trainers' Association Athletic Training Educational Competencies originated from the need to have specific educational knowledge and skills common to all entry-level athletic trainers. These skills are deemed necessary by the NATA for all newly graduated athletic trainers and demonstrate to the public that the athletic trainer has been educated and has shown proficiency on specific standards prior to sitting for the National Athletic Trainers' Association Board of Certification (NATABOC) exam.

EVOLUTION OF THE COMPETENCIES

The original competencies were written in the form of behavioral objectives in 1983 by Gary Delforge of the Professional Education Committee of the National Athletic Trainers' Association. They were printed in the "Guidelines For Development and Implementation of NATA Approved Undergraduate Athletic Training Education Programs." This generation of behavioral objectives was first revised in 1988. In 1992, they were renamed the "Competencies in Athletic Training," were rewritten by the Professional Education Committee, and reviewed by the Joint Review Committee on Educational Programs in Athletic Training (JRC-AT). The 1992 revision divided the competencies into six areas pertaining to injuries and illnesses common to athletes. The areas were Prevention, Recognition and Evaluation, Management/Treatment and Disposition, Rehabilitation, Organization and Administration, and finally, Education and Counseling. Within each area were three domains: cognitive (knowledge), psychomotor (motor skills), and affective (attitudes and values), and each had specific behavioral objectives assigned to the domain. Students graduating from NATA approved educational programs were introduced to the competencies in classes and during clinical assignments.

In 1997, the Education Council formed the Competencies in Education Committee consisting of ten certified athletic trainers from all over the country representing all levels of education (high school through college) as well as the clinical setting. This Committee worked for a year to identify current skills and knowledge vital for the entry-level athletic trainer. Corresponding with the revision of the competencies was the new focus on competency-based education for the undergraduate preparation of the athletic trainer. The Committee identified 12 general areas of knowledge/skills that all athletic trainers should possess after completing their formal education and clinical experience. These content areas are Risk Management and Injury Prevention, Pathology of Injury and Illnesses, Assessment and Evaluation, Acute Care of Injury and Illness, Pharmacology, Therapeutic Modalities, Therapeutic Exercise, General Medical Conditions and Disabilities, Nutritional Aspects of Injury and Illnesses, Psychosocial Intervention and Referral, Health Care Administration, and Professional Development and Responsibility. The competencies were written according to content area, domain (cognitive, psychomotor, and affective), and a separate committee worked on clinical proficiencies for each content area.

Clinical proficiencies are linked to the content areas and consist of the common skills that all entry-level athletic trainers need to possess. The majority of the clinical proficiencies are psychomotor in nature, requiring demonstration of the ability to physically evaluate or treat an injury and create or use a particular item such as a protective device. The addition of clinical proficiencies to the Competencies document signifies the move from a purely quantitative education to an outcomes-based education.

Drafts of both the competency and clinical proficiency documents were sent for review to subject-area experts, as well as posted on the athletic training education web sites. By 1999, the competencies and clinical proficiencies, revised through several drafts and approved by NATA Board of Directors, were published as the "National Athletic Trainers' Association Athletic Training Educational Competencies." The difference in the 1999 edition is the inclusion of clinical proficiencies as well as newly identified content area that athletic trainers saw as critical for entry-level athletic trainers to possess when they enter the work force.

The new competency-based model of learning assures that no matter where a student did his or her athletic training education, whether at a big university or small college, he or she would have a common knowledge base and skill proficiency in specific areas. Since certified athletic trainers are currently working in high schools, clinics, industry, corporations, and with professional teams, competency-based education sets a baseline of proficiency that all athletic trainers must achieve.

TODAY'S COMPETENCY-BASED EDUCATION

Competency-based education now sets a baseline of proficiency that all athletic trainers must be able to achieve. Regarding curricula, the athletic training educational programs that have been accredited by the Commission on Accreditation of Allied Health Education Programs (CAAHEP), or seek this accreditation, have been charged with the task of finding a way to integrate the extensive list of educational competencies and clinical proficiencies into their curricula. For students seeking certification, all of the competencies must be learned, demonstrated, and the proficiencies mastered over time for any student taking the NATA Board of Certification Examination.

To access an index that correlates the educational competencies and clinical proficiencies related to the therapeutic modalities, visit the McGraw-Hill Online Learning Center at www.mhhe.com/prentice11e.

Katie Walsh, EdD, ATC-L
Director of Sports Medicine/Athletic Training
East Carolina University

PART ONE

Foundations of Therapeutic Modalities

CHAPTER 1

How Are Therapeutic Modalities Related to One Another? The Basic Science

William E. Prentice

Study Resources

Refer to the lab exercises in the accompanying Laboratory Manual, as well as eSims which simulates the athletic training certification exam at www.mhhe.com/esims. Also, check out the competency information found at www.mhhe.com/prentice11e. For more online study resources, visit our Health and Human Performance Website at www.mhhe.com/hhp/.

Following completion of this chapter, the student athletic trainer will be able to

- Define what radiant energy is and how it is produced.

- Analyze the relationship between wavelength and frequency.

- Apply the laws governing the effects of the electromagnetic radiations to the various therapeutic modalities.

- Argue how the athletic trainer can make use of electromagnetic radiations to affect the biologic tissues of the body.

- Compare the physiologic effects produced by each therapeutic modality.

- Differentiate between the electromagnetic and acoustic spectra.

- Categorize the indications and contraindications for using the various modalities that will be discussed throughout this text.

For the athletic trainer who chooses to incorporate a therapeutic modality into his or her clinical practice, some knowledge and understanding of the basic theories and principles of science that relate to the use of these physical agents is essential. The truly outstanding athletic training clinician has the ability to integrate a strong theoretical knowledge base with the ability to correctly apply this knowledge in a clinical setting.

Even among experienced clinicians there is often considerable confusion regarding the relationship of the various therapeutic modalities to the **electromagnetic** and **acoustic spectra**. Electrical stimulating currents, shortwave and microwave **diathermy**, the **infrared** modalities, **ultraviolet** therapy, and low-power lasers are all therapeutic agents that emit a type of energy with wavelengths and frequencies that can be classified as electromagnetic radiations. **Ultrasound** is a form of radiation whose wavelength and frequency of vibration are best classified in the acoustic spectrum rather than in the electromagnetic spectrum. Each of the modalities that makes use of these varying types of energy will be discussed in the following chapters.

RADIANT ENERGY

Radiation is a process by which energy in various forms travels through space. Most of us are familiar with the effects of radiation from the sun. Sunlight is a type of radiant energy, and we know that it not

Electromagnetic modalities

- Electrical stimulating currents
- Biofeedback
- Iontophoresis
- Shortwave diathermy
- Microwave diathermy
- Infrared modalities
- Ultraviolet therapy
- Low-power laser

Acoustic modalities

- Ultrasound

only makes objects visible but also produces heat. The sun emits radiant energy as a result of high-intensity chemical reactions. Radiant energy in the form of sunlight travels through space at about 300,000,000 meters per second and eventually reaches earth where its effects may be felt or seen. But the sun is not the only source capable of producing this radiant energy.

All matter produces energy that radiates in the form of heat. The sun produces radiation through chemical reactions. But when a sufficiently intense chemical or electrical force is applied to any object, radiant energy in various forms can be produced by movement of electrons. Many of the therapeutic modalities to be discussed in this text produce radiant energy (i.e., the infrared, diathermy, ultraviolet, lasers, and electrical stimulating modalities).[1,8]

The Electromagnetic Spectrum

If a ray of sunlight is passed through a prism, it will be broken down into various regions of colors (Figure 1-1). Each of these colors represents a different form of radiant energy. They appear because the various forms of radiant energy are **refracted**, or change direction, as a result of differences in wavelength and frequency of each color, thus resulting in distinct bands of color called a **spectrum**. These

electromagnetic spectrum   The range of frequencies and wavelengths associated with radiant energy.

acoustic spectrum   The range of frequencies and wavelengths of sound waves.

diathermy   The application of high-frequency electrical energy that is used to generate heat in body tissue as a result of the resistance of the tissue to the passage of energy.

infrared   The portion of the electromagnetic spectrum associated with thermal changes located adjacent to the red portion of the visible light spectrum.

ultraviolet   The portion of the electromagnetic spectrum associated with chemical changes located adjacent to the violet portion of the visible light spectrum.

ultrasound   A portion of the acoustic spectrum located above audible sound.

radiation   The process of emitting energy from some source in the form of waves. A method of heat transfer through which heat can be either gained or lost.

refraction   The change in direction of a sound wave or radiation wave when it passes from one medium or type of tissue to another.

spectrum   A charted band of wavelengths of electromagnetic energy forms.

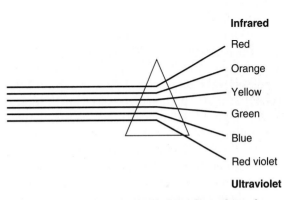

Infrared
Red
Orange
Yellow
Green
Blue
Red violet
Ultraviolet

Figure 1-1   When a beam of light is shone through a prism, the various electromagnetic radiations in visible light are refracted and appear as a distinct band of color called a spectrum.

color variations that we can detect with our eyes are referred to as visible light or luminous radiations. It becomes apparent when looking at this colorful display that there is a region of red at one end of the spectrum and a region of violet at the other end. When passed through a prism, the type of radiant energy refracted the least appears as the color red, while that refracted the most is violet.[1]

This beam of sunlight passing through the prism is also propagating forms of radiant energy that are not visible to our eyes. If a thermometer is placed close to the red end of the spectrum, heat will be detected. Likewise, a photographic plate placed close to the violet end of the spectrum will indicate chemical changes. The form of radiant energy that produces heat and is located in the spectrum beyond the visible red portion is referred to as the *infrared radiation region*. The form of radiant energy that produces chemical changes and is located beyond the violet end of the visible spectrum is called the *ultraviolet radiation region* (Figure 1-1).

Ultraviolet, infrared, and visible light rays are produced by heat. As the temperature increases in a particular substance, the vibration of molecules tends to increase the activity of the electrons. The movement of electrons produces electromagnetic waves. The higher the temperature, the greater the frequency of electromagnetic waves produced. These electromagnetic waves produced by heat are usually absorbed by many objects and have little penetration.[7]

Other forms of radiation beyond the infrared and ultraviolet portions of the spectrum may be produced when an electrical force is applied.[8] Beyond the infrared portion of the spectrum lie several large regions of radiations known as the diathermies—these include radio, television, and nerve- and muscle-stimulating currents. Beyond the ultraviolet end of the spectrum lie the high-frequency ionizing and penetration radiation regions (i.e., x-ray, alpha, beta, and gamma rays).

> • Visible light represents only a portion of the electromagnetic energy within the electromagnetic spectrum

ELECTROMAGNETIC RADIATIONS

All of these various classifications of radiations collectively constitute the electromagnetic spectrum (Table 1-1). All of the electromagnetic radiations lying within this spectrum have several theoretical characteristics in common:[2]

1. They may be produced when sufficiently intense electrical or chemical forces are applied to any material.
2. They all travel readily through space at an equal velocity.
3. Their direction of travel through space is always in a straight line and will alter this straight line travel only when they come in contact with some other surface.
4. They may be reflected, refracted, absorbed, or transmitted, depending on the specific medium that they strike.

The luminous, infrared, and ultraviolet rays in sunlight travel in waves through a vacuum or through space at a velocity of about 300 million meters per second and all reach the earth at about the same time. These rays are emitted from chemical reactions taking place on the sun, and each type of radiation processes its own individual physical characteristics. The basis of differentiation between the different regions of the electromagnetic spectrum is defined by analyzing the wavelengths and frequencies of the radiations within this spectrum.

The electromagnetic radiations produced by the different modalities all share the same physical characteristics as any other type of electromagnetic radiation.[3] However, when these radiations come in contact with various biologic tissues, the velocity and direction of travel will be altered within the various types of tissues.

■ **TABLE 1-1**   Electromagnetic Spectrum

REGION	CLINICALLY USED WAVELENGTH	CLINICALLY USED FREQUENCY*	ESTIMATED EFFECTIVE DEPTH OF PENETRATION	PHYSIOLOGIC EFFECTS
Electrical stimulating currents	3×10^8 Km to 75,000 Km	1–4000 Hz	Effects may occur anywhere between electrodes	Pain modulation, muscle contraction, relaxation, ion movement
Commercial radio and television frequencies‡				
Shortwave diathermy	22 m 11 m	13.56 MHz 27.12 MHz	3 cm	Deep tissue temperature increase, vasodilation, increased blood flow
Microwave diathermy	69 cm 33 cm 12 cm	433.9 MHz 915 MHz 2450 MHz	5 cm	Deep tissue temperature increase, vasodilation, increased blood flow
Infrared				Superficial temperature decrease
Cold packs (8° F)	111,000 Å	2.7×10^{12} Hz		
Cold whirlpool (63° F)	99,514 Å	3.01×10^{12} Hz		
Hot whirlpool (99° F)	93,097 Å	3.22×10^{12} Hz	1 cm	Vasoconstriction— decreased blood flow
Paraffin bath (117° F)	90,187 Å	3.32×10^{12} Hz		
Hydrocollar (170° F)	82,457 Å	3.63×10^{12} Hz		Analgesia
Luminous IR (1341° F)	28,860 Å	1.04×10^{13} Hz		Superficial temperature increase
Nonluminous IR (3140° F)	14,430 Å	2.08×10^{13} Hz		Vasodilation— increased blood flow
Red	Laser			
Visible light	GaAs 9100 Å HeNe 6328 Å	3.3×10^{13} Hz 4.74×10^{13} Hz	5 cm 10–15 mm	Pain modulation and wound healing
Violet				
Ultraviolet				Superficial chemical changes
UV-A	3200–4000 Å	9.38×10^{13}–7.5×10^{13} Hz		
UV-B	2900–3200 Å	1.03×10^{14}–9.38×10^{13} Hz	1 mm	Tanning effects
UV-C	2000–2900 Å	1.50×10^{14}–1.03×10^{14} Hz		Bactericidal
Ionizing radiation (x-ray, gamma rays, cosmic rays)‡				

*Calculated using $C = \lambda \times F$, C = velocity (3×10 m/sec), λ = wavelength, F = frequency.
‡Although these fall under the classification of electromagnetic energy, they have nothing to do with therapeutic modalities and thus warrant no further discussion in this text.

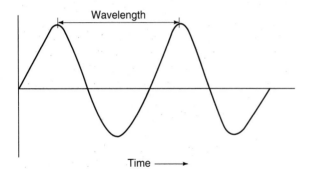

Figure 1-2 Wavelength and frequency.

WAVELENGTH AND FREQUENCY

Wavelength is defined as the distance between the peak of one wave and the peak of either the preceding or succeeding wave.[10] **Frequency** is defined as the number of wave oscillations or vibrations occurring in one second and is expressed in hertz (Hz) units (Figure 1-2).[10]

Each of the various types of radiation in the electromagnetic spectrum has a specific wavelength and frequency of vibration. Since it is theoretically accepted that all forms of electromagnetic radiation are produced simultaneously, travel at a constant velocity through space, and reach earth at the same time, it stands that longer wavelengths must have shorter frequencies and shorter wavelengths must have higher frequencies.

$$\text{velocity} = \text{wavelength} \times \text{frequency}$$
$$C = \lambda \times F$$

Thus, an inverse or reciprocal relationship exists between wavelength and frequency. Velocity is a constant 3×10^8 m/sec.[9] Therefore, if we know the wavelength, frequency can be calculated.

LAWS GOVERNING THE EFFECTS OF ELECTROMAGNETIC RADIATIONS

When electromagnetic radiations strike or come in contact with various objects, several things may happen. Some rays may be **reflected**, while others are **transmitted** through the tissues where they

■ Analogy *1-1*

The relationship between velocity, wavelength, and frequency is similar to that of a 7-foot tall basketball player and a 5-foot tall gymnast who are asked to run a 50-meter race and finish at the same time. Because his legs are longer, the basketball player will take longer strides (wavelength) but fewer steps (frequency) to get to the finish line. Conversely, the gymnast has a short stride length (wavelength) and therefore must take more steps (frequency) if she is to travel an equal distance in the same time as the basketball player. Thus, since velocity is a constant, there is an inverse relationship between wavelength and frequency.

wavelength The distance from one point in a propagating wave to the same point in the next wave.

frequency The number of cycles or pulses per second.

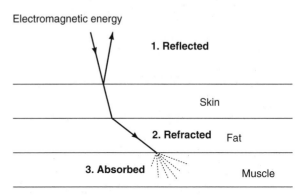

Figure 1-3 When electromagnetic radiations contact human tissues, they may be reflected, refracted, or absorbed. Energy that is transmitted through the tissues must be absorbed before any physiologic changes can take place.

may be **refracted**. Some rays that penetrate to deeper layers may be **absorbed** (Figure 1-3). Generally, those radiations that have the longest wavelengths tend to have the greatest depths of penetration, regardless of their frequency. It must be added, however, that a number of other factors, which will

- Longer wavelengths have greater depth of penetration

reflection The bending back of light or sound waves from a surface that they strike.

transmission The propagation of energy through a particular biologic tissue into deeper tissues.

absorption Energy that stimulates a particular tissue to perform its normal function.

Arndt-Schultz principle No reactions or changes can occur in the body if the amount of energy absorbed is not sufficient to stimulate the absorbing tissues.

Law of Grotthus-Draper Energy not absorbed by the tissues must be transmitted.

be discussed later, can also contribute to the depth of penetration. See Table 1-2 for a summary of laws governing electromagnetic radiations.

Arndt-Schultz Principle

The purpose of using therapeutic modalities is to stimulate a specific body tissue to perform its normal function. This stimulation will only occur if the tissue absorbs energy produced by the electrotherapeutic device. The **Arndt-Schultz principle** states that *no reactions or changes can occur in the body tissues if the amount of energy absorbed is insufficient to stimulate the absorbing tissues*. The goal of the athletic trainer should be to deliver sufficient energy in one form or another to stimulate the tissues to perform their normal function, while realizing that too much energy absorbed in a given period of time may seriously impair normal function and, if severe enough, may cause irreparable damage.[2]

An example would be using an electrical stimulating current to create a muscle contraction. To achieve a depolarization of a motor nerve, the intensity of the current must be increased until

■ **Analogy** *1-2*

The colors of a rainbow are created when sunlight (electromagnetic energy) is refracted through water droplets. The different colors appear because of varying wavelengths and frequencies, which are refracted differently.

■ **TABLE 1-2** Summary of Laws Governing Electromagnetic Radiations

Arndt-Schultz principle	No reactions or changes can occur in the body tissues if the amount of energy absorbed is insufficient to stimulate the absorbing tissues.
Law of Grotthus-Draper	If the therapeutic energy is not absorbed by the superficial tissues, it will penetrate to deeper tissues.
Cosine law	The smaller the angle between the propagating ray and the right angle, the less radiation reflected and the greater the absorption.
Inverse square law	The intensity of the radiation striking a particular surface is known to vary inversely with the square of the distance from the source.

enough energy is made available and is absorbed by that nerve to facilitate a depolarization.

Law of Grotthus-Draper

The inverse relationship that exists between energy absorption by a tissue and energy penetration to deeper layers is described by the **Law of Grotthus-Draper**.[6] When electromagnetic energy strikes the surface of the skin, several things can happen to it. A portion of the energy may be *reflected* (bounce off)

- The greater the amount of energy absorbed, the less penetration

from the surface producing no physiological response. That portion of the electromagnetic energy that is not reflected will penetrate into the tissues (i.e., skin layers), and some of it will be absorbed superficially. Again if the amount of energy absorbed is sufficient to stimulate that target tissue, some physiologic response will occur (i.e., vasodilation of a blood vessel).

The energy that is not absorbed superficially will continue to penetrate through the deeper layers of tissue (i.e., fat and muscle). At tissue interfaces (i.e., where skin meets fat or where fat meets muscle), the differences in density of the two tissues can cause that penetrating electromagnetic energy to be *refracted*, to alter its direction of transmission. If the target tissue is a motor nerve and your treatment goal is to provide enough energy to cause a depolarization of that motor nerve, then once again enough energy must be absorbed by that nerve to cause a depolarization.

An example showing application of the Law of Grotthus-Draper could be when using an ultrasound treatment to increase tissue temperature in the gluteus maximus muscle. Using ultrasound at a frequency of 3MHz (megahertz) would be more effective that at 1MHz since less than 3MHz would be absorbed superficially and thus more energy would penetrate to the deeper muscle tissue.

Cosine Law

Radiant energy is more easily transmitted to deeper tissues if the source of radiation is at a right angle to the area being radiated. Thus, the smaller the angle between the propagating ray and the right angle, the less radiation reflected and the greater the absorption. This principle, known as the **cosine law**, will be extremely important in the chapters dealing

cosine law Optimal radiation occurs when the source of radiation is at right angles to the center of the area being radiated.

■ Analogy *1-3*

When you go to the beach and are lying in the sun, you are more likely to get sunburned during the middle of the day when the sun's rays are striking your skin at closer to a right angle than later in the afternoon when sunlight is at more of an oblique angle.

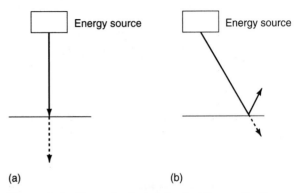

(a)   (b)

Figure 1-4 The cosine law states that the smaller the angle between the propagating ray and the right angle, the less radiation reflected and the greater absorbed. Thus the energy absorbed in *a* would be greater than in *b*.

with the diathermies, ultraviolet light, and infrared heating, since the effectiveness of these modalities is based to a large extent on how they are positioned with regard to the athlete (Figure 1-4).

An example showing the application of the cosine law could be when doing an ultrasound treatment, the surface of the applicator should be kept as flat on the skin surface as possible. This al-

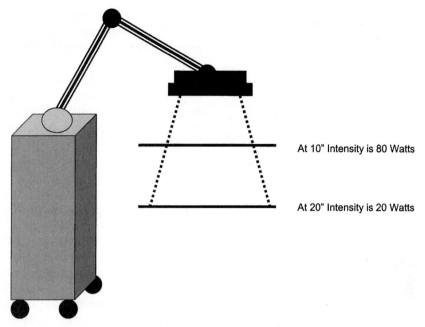

At 10" Intensity is 80 Watts

At 20" Intensity is 20 Watts

Figure 1-5   The inverse square law states that the intensity of the radiation striking a particular surface varies inversely with the square of the distance from the source.

lows the acoustic energy coming from the applicator to strike the surface as close to 90 degrees as possible, thus minimizing the amount of energy reflected.

Inverse Square Law

The intensity of the radiation striking a particular surface is known to vary inversely with the square of the distance from the source. For example, when using an infrared heating lamp to heat the low back region, the intensity of heat energy at the skin surface with the lamp positioned at a distance of 10 inches will be four times greater than if the lamp is placed at a 20-inch distance. This principle, known as the **inverse square law**, will obviously be of great consequence when setting up a specific modality to achieve a desired physiologic effect

inverse square law   The intensity of radiation striking a particular surface varies inversely with the square of the distance from the radiating source.

(Figure 1-5). Regardless of the path this transmitted energy takes, the physiologic effects will only be apparent when the energy is absorbed by a specific tissue.

All physical modalities emitting electromagnetic radiations are subject to the relationship between absorption and transmission of energy. The modalities that emit radiations with relatively longer wavelengths have the ability to transmit energy through the superficial tissue layers, thus penetrating to the deeper tissues where they are absorbed.

THE APPLICATION OF THE ELECTROMAGNETIC SPECTRUM TO THERAPEUTIC MODALITIES

The therapeutic modalities discussed in detail in later chapters (with the exception of ultrasound, massage, traction, and intermittent compression) all emit radiations with physical characteristics that may be classified as electromagnetic radiations.

Table 1-1 represents the electromagnetic spectrum and places all of the modalities in order based on wavelengths and corresponding frequencies. It is apparent, for example, that the electrical stimulating currents have the longest wavelength and the lowest frequency and, all other factors being equal, should therefore have the greatest depth of penetration. As we move down the chart, the wavelengths in each region become progressively shorter and the frequencies progressively higher. Shortwave and microwave diathermy, the various sources of infrared heating, and the ultraviolet regions have progressively less depth of penetration.

It should be noted that the regions labeled as radio and television frequencies, visible light, and high-frequency ionizing and penetrating radiations certainly fall under the classification of electromagnetic radiations. However, they do not have application as therapeutic modalities and, while extremely important to our everyday way of life, warrant no further consideration in the context of this discussion.

Infrared Modalities

Perhaps the greatest confusion over this relationship between electromagnetic radiations and therapeutic modalities is associated with the infrared region. We tend to think of the infrared modalities as being the luminous and nonluminous infrared bakers or lamps only, when in fact the largest number of modalities used by athletic trainers actually emit radiations with wavelengths and frequencies that clearly fall within this infrared region. Cold packs, hydrocollator packs, whirlpools, paraffin baths, and contrast baths are all infrared modalities.[5]

Earlier we explained that any object heated (or cooled) to a temperature different than the surrounding environment will dissipate heat through radiation to the other materials with which it comes in contact. The infrared modalities are used to produce a local and occasionally a generalized heating or cooling of the superficial tissues. It is generally accepted that the infrared modalities have a maximum depth of penetration of 1 cm or less. The infrared modalities can elicit either increases or decreases in circulation, depending on whether heat or cold is used. They are also known to have analgesic effects as a result of stimulation of sensory cutaneous nerve endings.

The infrared region of the spectrum is located adjacent to the red end of the visible light region. The wavelengths of the infrared modalities are obviously much shorter than are those of the electrical stimulating currents and the diathermies and are expressed in angstrom (Å) units; 1 Å is equal to 10^{-10} meters (m).

Both the infrared and ultraviolet wavelengths are temperature dependent. Those modalities with lower temperatures have longer wavelengths. This means that an ice pack will have a longer wavelength and thus a greater depth of penetration than will a hydrocollator pack. Temperatures used with the infrared modalities range from 0° C with ice to more than 3000° C with the infrared lamps. The wavelengths in this temperature range fall between 10,000 and 105,000 Å with corresponding frequencies ranging between 2×10^{12} and 4×10^{13} Hz.

An angstrom unit is an extremely small unit of measure, and thus the differences in depth of penetration are not great between any of the infrared modalities. The critical factor is the superficial increase or decrease in tissue temperature that elicits the same physiologic response regardless of wavelength. Infrared modalities will be discussed in Chapter 4.

Shortwave and Microwave Diathermy

The diathermies are considered to be high-frequency currents because they have more than a million cycles per second. When impulses of such a short duration come in contact with human tis-

■ **Clinical Decision-Making**   *Exercise 1-1*

There are several modalities that can be used to manage pain. Of the modalities discussed, which may be used to modulate pain and which should an athletic trainer recommend as the best to use immediately following injury?

sue, there is not sufficient time for ion movement to take place. Consequently, there is no stimulation of either motor or sensory nerves. The energy of this rapidly vibrating electrical current produces heat as it passes through tissue cells, resulting in a temperature increase. Shortwave diathermy may be either continuous or pulsed. Both continuous shortwave and microwave diathermy are used primarily for their thermal effects, while pulsed shortwave is used for its nonthermal effects.

The electrotherapeutic shortwave and microwave devices have preset frequencies and wavelengths that cannot be altered. Shortwave diathermy units are set at either (1) 13.56 MHz (1 MHz = 10 million Hz), with a corresponding wavelength of 22 m, or (2) 27.12 MHz, with a wavelength of 11 m.[2]

Microwave units have shorter wavelengths than do shortwave diathermy units and are set at wavelengths of 33 or 12 cm with respective frequencies of 915 or 2450 MHz. The depth of penetration with microwave is a bit deeper than with shortwave because the amount of energy when using microwave is concentrated in one spot rather than spread out over a large area.[2] This will be discussed in more detail in Chapter 6.

Electrical Stimulating Currents

The electrical stimulating currents that affect nerve and muscle tissue have the longest wavelengths and the lowest frequencies of any of the modalities. The wavelengths of electrical stimulating units are extremely long, ranging about 15,000 km. Clini-

cally used frequencies range from 1 to 4000 Hz. Most stimulators have the flexibility to alter the frequency output of the device to elicit a desired physiologic response. The nerve and muscle stimulating currents are capable of (1) pain modulation, either through stimulation of cutaneous sensory nerves at high frequencies (TENS) or through production of β-endorphin at lower frequencies (electroacutherapy); (2) producing muscle contraction and relaxation or tetany, depending on the type of current (alternating or direct) and frequency (Russian currents); (3) facilitating soft tissue and bone healing through the use of subsensory microcurrents (LIS); and (4) producing a net movement of ions through the use of continuous direct current and thus eliciting a chemical change in the tissues (iontophoresis see Chapter 9).[9]

The electrical stimulating currents and their various physiologic effects will be discussed in detail in Chapter 8.

Electromyographic Biofeedback.   Electromyographic biofeedback using surface EMG (electromyography) is a therapeutic procedure that uses electronic or electromechanical instruments to accurately measure, process, and feed back reinforcing information via auditory or visual signals. Clinically, it is used to help the athlete develop greater voluntary control in terms of either neuromuscular relaxation or muscle reeducation following injury. Biofeedback is discussed in Chapter 13.

Laser

Of the modalities discussed in this text, the low-power laser is certainly the newest used by the athletic trainer. The word *laser* is an acronym for **l**ight **a**mplification by **s**timulated **e**mission of **r**adiation. Laser is a form of electromagnetic radiation that is classified within both the infrared and visible light portions of the spectrum.

Lasers are either high power or low power. High-power lasers are used in surgery for purposes of incision, coagulation of vessels, and thermolysis, owing to their thermal effects. The low-power or cold laser produces little or no thermal effects but

The athletic trainer is treating an athlete with a chronic low back strain. At this point it has been decided that heating the area is the treatment of choice. Which of the modalities discussed briefly in this chapter may be used as heating modalities? Which of these modalities would you choose to provide the greatest depth of penetration?

seems to have some significant clinical effect on soft tissue and fracture healing as well as pain management through stimulation of acupuncture and trigger points.

Two types of low-power lasers are used by athletic trainers: the helium-neon laser (HeNe), and the gallium-arsenide laser (GaAs). The HeNe laser has a wavelength of 632.8 nanometers (nm) and a direct depth of penetration to 0.8 mm, although there may be some indirect effects up to 10 to 15 mm. The GaAs laser has a wavelength of 910 nm and can penetrate indirectly as much as 5 cm. The laser as a therapeutic tool will be discussed in Chapter 14.

Ultraviolet Therapy

The ultraviolet portion of the electromagnetic spectrum is adjacent to the violet end of the visible light region. As noted previously, the radiations in the ultraviolet region are undetectable by the human eye. However, if a photographic plate is placed at the ultraviolet end, chemical changes will be apparent. Although an extremely hot source (7000° to 9000° C) is required to produce ultraviolet wavelengths, the physiologic effects of ultraviolet are mainly chemical in nature and occur entirely in the cutaneous layers of skin. The maximum depth of penetration with ultraviolet is about 1 mm. The wavelengths with ultraviolet range between 2000 and 4000 Å. The ultraviolet region is subdivided

into three different areas: near ultraviolet or UV-A (3200 to 4000 Å), middle ultraviolet or UV-B (2900 to 3200 Å), and far ultraviolet or UV-C (2000 to 2900 Å). Clinically used frequencies with ultraviolet range between 7×10^{13} and 7×10^{14} Hz.[2,6,9] Although rarely used by the athletic trainer, the application of ultraviolet therapy is discussed in Chapter 15.

THE ACOUSTIC SPECTRUM AND ULTRASOUND

One additional therapeutic modality frequently used by athletic trainers is ultrasound. Ultrasound devices produce a type of energy that must be classified as acoustic rather than electromagnetic energy. Ultrasound is frequently classified along with shortwave and microwave diathermy as a deep-heating, "conversion" type modality, and it is certainly true that all of these are capable of producing a temperature increase in human tissue to a considerable depth. However, ultrasound is a mechanical vibration—a sound wave—produced and transformed from high-frequency electrical energy.[2] Ultrasound must be considered a type of acoustic vibration rather than a type of electromagnetic radiation.

Acoustic and electromagnetic radiations have very different physical characteristics. When acoustic vibrations are produced, they travel at a velocity that is significantly lower than electromagnetic radiations. Electromagnetic waves travel at approximately 300 million meters per second while sound waves travel at speeds from hundreds to several thousand meters per second.

The relationship between velocity, wavelength, and frequency is a bit different with acoustic energy than with electromagnetic energy even though the inverse relationship between wavelength and frequency still exists. The distinction lies in the fact that the velocity of travel is much greater for electromagnetic energy than for acoustic energy. Therefore, wavelengths are considerably shorter in acoustic vibrations than in electromagnetic radia-

■ **Clinical Decision-Making**   *Exercise 1-3*

With which of the modalities described briefly in this chapter are the cosine law and the inverse square law of greatest consideration?

■ **Clinical Decision-Making**   *Exercise 1-4*

Why would the athletic trainer choose to use ultraviolet therapy to treat a skin lesion?

indication   A sign or circumstance that determines the proper treatment.[10]

contraindication   Any symptom or circumstance that determines the inappropriateness of an otherwise proper treatment.

tions at any given frequency.[2] For example, ultrasound traveling in the atmosphere has a wavelength of approximately 0.3 mm, while electromagnetic radiations have wavelengths of 297 m at a similar frequency.

As noted earlier, electromagnetic radiations are capable of traveling through space or through a vacuum. As the density of the transmitting medium is increased, the velocity of travel significantly decreases as a result of refraction, reflection, or absorption by the molecules in the medium. Conversely, acoustic vibrations will not be transmitted at all through a vacuum, since they depend on conduction through molecular collisions. The more dense the transmitting medium, the greater the velocity of travel. In human tissue, ultrasound has a much greater velocity of transmission in bone tissue (3500 m per second), for example, than in fat tissue (1500 m per second).

Frequencies of ultrasound wave production are between 700,000 and 1,000,000 cycles per second. Frequencies up to around 20,000 Hz are detectable by the human ear. Thus, the ultrasound portion of the acoustic spectrum is inaudible. Ultrasound generators are generally set at a standard frequency of 1 to 3 MHz (1000 KHz). The depth of penetration with ultrasound is much greater than with any of the electromagnetic radiations. At a frequency of 1 MHz, 50% of the energy produced will penetrate to a depth of about 5 cm. The reason for this great depth of penetration is that ultrasound travels very well through homogeneous tissue (e.g., fat tissue), while electromagnetic radiations are almost entirely absorbed. Thus, when therapeutic

penetration to deeper tissues is desired, ultrasound is the modality of choice.[4,7]

Therapeutic ultrasound has traditionally been used to produce a tissue temperature increase through thermal physiologic effects. However, it is also capable of enhancing healing at the cellular level as a result of its nonthermal physiologic effects. The clinical usefulness of therapeutic ultrasound will be discussed in greater detail in Chapter 5.

INDICATIONS AND CONTRAINDICATIONS FOR USING DIFFERENT MODALITIES

Table 1-3 is a summary list of *indications* for use, *contraindications* and precautions in using the various modalities. This list should aid the athletic trainer in making decisions regarding the appropriate use of a therapeutic modality in a given clinical situation. Specific clinical uses and indications, as well as contraindications for different modalities, will be discussed in greater detail in the following chapters.

■ **TABLE 1-3** Indications and Contraindications for Therapeutic Modalities

THERAPEUTIC MODALITY	PHYSIOLOGIC RESOURCES (INDICATIONS FOR USE)	CONTRAINDICATIONS AND PRECAUTIONS
Electrical stimulating currents—high voltage	Pain modulation Muscle re-education Muscle pumping contractions Retard atrophy Muscle strengthening Increase range of motion Fracture healing Acute injury	Pacemakers Thrombophlebitis Superficial skin lesions
Electrical stimulating currents—low voltage	Wound healing Fracture healing Iontophoresis	Malignancy Skin hypersensitivities Allergies to certain drugs
Electrical stimulating currents—interferential	Pain modulation Muscle re-education Muscle pumping contractions Fracture healing Increase range of motion	Same as high-voltage
Electrical stimulating currents—Russian	Muscle strengthening	Pacemakers
Electrical stimulating currents—LIS (MENS)	Fracture healing Wound healing	Malignancy Infections
Shortwave and microwave diathermy	Increase deep circulation Increase metabolic activity Reduce muscle guarding/spasm Reduce inflammation Facilitate wound healing Analgesia Increase tissue temperatures over a large area	Metal implants Pacemakers Malignancy Wet dressings Anesthetized areas Pregnancy Acute injury and inflammation Eyes Areas of reduced blood flow Anesthetized areas
Cryotherapy—cold packs, ice massage	Acute injury Vasoconstriction—decreased blood flow Analgesia Reduce inflammation Reduce muscle guarding/spasm	Allergy to cold Circulatory impairments Wound healing Hypertension
Thermotherapy—hot whirlpool, paraffin, hydrocollator, infrared lamps	Vasodilation—increased blood flow Analgesia Reduce muscle guarding/spasm Reduce inflammation Increase metabolic activity Facilitate tissue healing	Acute and postacute trauma Poor circulation Circulatory impairments Malignancy
Low-power laser	Pain modulation (trigger points) Facilitate wound healing	Pregnancy Eyes

■ **TABLE 1-3**   Indications and Contraindications for Therapeutic Modalities—*continued*

THERAPEUTIC MODALITY	PHYSIOLOGIC RESOURCES (INDICATIONS FOR USE)	CONTRAINDICATIONS AND PRECAUTIONSS
Ultraviolet	Acne Aseptic wounds Folliculitis Pityriasis rosea Tinea Septic wounds Sinusitis Increase calcium metabolism	Psoriasis Eczema Herpes Diabetes Pellagra Lupus erythematosus Hyperthyroidism Renal and hepatic insufficiency Generalized dermatitis Advanced atherosclerosis
Ultrasound	Increase connective tissue extensibility Deep heat Increased circulation Treatment of most soft tissue injuries Reduce inflammation Reduce muscle spasm	Infection Acute and postacute injury Epiphyseal areas Pregnancy Thrombophlebitis Impaired sensation Eyes
Intermittent compression	Decrease acute bleeding Decrease edema	Circulatory impairment

Summary

1. Radiant energy may be produced when a sufficiently intense chemical or electrical force is applied to any object.
2. Electrical stimulating currents, shortwave and microwave diathermy, the infrared modalities, and ultraviolet therapy are all classified as portions of the electromagnetic spectrum according to corresponding wavelengths and frequencies associated with each region.
3. All electromagnetic radiations travel at the same velocity; thus, wavelength and frequency are inversely related.
4. Radiations may be reflected, refracted, absorbed, or transmitted in the various tissues.
5. Those radiations with the longer wavelengths tend to have the greatest depth of penetration.
6. The purpose of using any therapeutic modality is to stimulate a specific tissue to perform its normal function.
7. Ultrasound is part of the acoustic spectrum and is best propagated through dense tissue such as biologic tissue; thus, it is extremely effective in reaching deep tissues.

Review Questions

1. What is radiant energy and how is it produced?
2. What is the relationship between wavelength and frequency?
3. What are the characteristics of electromagnetic energy?
4. Which of the therapeutic modalities produce electromagnetic energy?

5. What is the purpose of using a therapeutic modality?
6. According to the Law of Grotthus-Draper, what happens to electromagnetic energy when it comes in contact with and/or penetrates human biologic tissue?

 ## Self-Test Questions

T/F
1. Wavelength is defined as the number of cycles per second.
2. To achieve deeper tissue penetration, the wavelength must be increased.
3. Continuous shortwave and microwave diathermy produce thermal effects.

Multiple Choice
4. Which of the following is NOT an electromagnetic modality?
   a. iontophoresis
   b. ultrasound
   c. low-power laser
   d. shortwave diathermy
5. Sound or radiation waves that change direction when passing from one type of tissue to another are said to _____ .
   a. transmit
   b. absorb
   c. reflect
   d. refract
6. The _____ states that if superficial tissue does not absorb energy, it must be transmitted deeper.
   a. Law of Grotthus-Draper
   b. cosine law
   c. inverse square law
   d. Arndt-Schultz principle

7. Explain the cosine and inverse square laws relative to tissue penetration of electromagnetic energy.
8. Which of the therapeutic modalities produces acoustic energy?
9. What are the differences between electromagnetic energy and acoustic energy?

7. According to the cosine law, to minimize reflection and maximize absorption, the energy source must be at a _____ angle to the surface.
   a. 45 degree
   b. 90 degree
   c. 180 degree
   d. 0 degree
8. Electrical stimulating currents may produce the following effects:
   a. muscle contraction
   b. net ion movement
   c. decrease in pain
   d. all of the above
9. Infrared modalities generally affect superficial tissue up to _____ cm deep.
   a. 5 cm
   b. 0.5 cm
   c. 1 cm
   d. 10 cm
10. Based on their different characteristics, which of the following travels at greater velocity through human tissue?
    a. acoustic vibrations
    b. electromagnetic radiation
    c. a and b travel at the same rate
    d. neither a nor b travel through human tissue

Solutions to Clinical Decision-Making Exercises

1-1 Superficial heat and cold, electrical stimulating currents, and low-power laser may all be effective for modulating pain. However, ice is likely the best choice immediately following injury because it will not only modulate pain but will also cause vasoconstriction and will thus help to control swelling.

1-2   The athletic trainer may choose to use infrared heating modalities, shortwave or microwave diathermy, or ultrasound—all of which have the ability to produce heat in the tissues. Ultrasound has a greater depth of penetration than any of the electromagnetic modalities since acoustic energy is more effectively transmitted through dense tissue than is electromagnetic energy.

1-3   When setting up an athlete for treatment using either microwave diathermy or ultraviolet therapy, it is critical that the athletic trainer consider the angle at which the electromagnetic energy is striking the body surface to ensure that most of the energy will be absorbed and not reflected. It is also essential to know the distance that these modalities should be placed from the surface to achieve the desired amount of energy in the target tissues.

1-4   Since the wavelength of ultraviolet energy is short, the depth of penetration is minimal, and thus the therapeutic effects are going to be primarily superficial. Also, the ultraviolet region of the electromagnetic spectrum is known to produce a chemical effect in biologic tissue that may be helpful in facilitating healing.

References

1. Goldman, L: *Introduction to modern phototherapy*, Springfield, Ill., 1978, Charles C Thomas.
2. Griffin, J, and Karselis, T: *Physical agents for physical athletic trainers*, Springfield, Ill., 1978, Charles C Thomas.
3. Hitchcock, RT, and Patterson RM: *Radiofrequency and ELF electromagnetic energies: A handbook for healthcare professionals*, New York, 1995, Van Nostrand Reinhold.
4. Lehmann, JF, and Guy, AW: *Ultrasound therapy*. Proc workshop on interaction of ultrasound and biological tissues. Washington, DC, HEW Pub. (FDA 73:8008), Sept., 1972.
5. Lehmann, J, editor: *Therapeutic heat and cold*, ed 2, New Haven, 1982, Elizabeth Licht.
6. Licht, S: *Therapeutic electricity and ultraviolet radiation*, New Haven, 1959, Elizabeth Licht.
7. Schriber, W: *A manual of electrotherapy*, Philadelphia, 1975, Lea & Febiger.
8. Sears, F, Zemansky, M, and Young, H: *University physics*, Reading, Mass., 1976, Addison-Wesley.
9. Stillwell, K: *Therapeutic electricity and ultraviolet radiation*, Baltimore, 1983, Williams & Wilkins.
10. Venes D, and Thomas, CL: *Taber's Cyclopedic Medical Dictionary*, Philadelphia, 2001, FA Davis.

Suggested Readings

Goodgold, J, and Eberstein, A: *Electrodiagnosis of neuromuscular diseases*, Baltimore, 1972, Williams & Wilkins.

Jehle, H: Charge fluctuation forces in biological systems, *Ann. NY Acad. Sci.* 158:240–255, 1969.

Koracs, R: *Light therapy*, Springfield, Ill., 1950, Charles C Thomas.

Licht, S, editor: *Electrodiagnosis and electromyography*, ed 3, New Haven, 1971, Elizabeth Licht.

Scott, P, and Cooksey, F: *Clayton's electrotherapy and actinotherapy*, London, 1962, Bailliere, Tindall and Cox..

CHAPTER 2

Using Therapeutic Modalities to Effect the Healing Process

William E. Prentice

Study Resources

Refer to the lab exercises in the accompanying Laboratory Manual, as well as eSims which simulates the athletic training certification exam at www.mhhe.com/esims. Also, check out the competency information found at www.mhhe.com/prentice11e. For more online study resources, visit our Health and Human Performance Website at www.mhhe.com/hhp/.

Following completion of this chapter, the student athletic trainer will be able to

- Define inflammation and its associated signs and symptoms.

- Clarify how therapeutic modalities should be used in rehabilitation of various conditions.

- Compare the physiological events associated with the different phases of the healing process.

- Formulate a plan for how specific modalities can be used effectively during each phase of healing and provide a rationale for their use.

- Identify those factors that can interfere with the healing process.

HOW SHOULD THE ATHLETIC TRAINER USE THERAPEUTIC MODALITIES IN REHABILITATION?

Therapeutic modalities, when used appropriately, can be extremely useful tools in the rehabilitation of the injured athlete. Like any other tool, their effectiveness is limited by the knowledge, skill, and experience of the clinician using them. For the athletic trainer, decisions regarding how and when a modality may best be incorporated should be based on a combination of theoretical knowledge and practical experience. As a clinician, you should not use therapeutic modalities at random, nor should you base their use on what has always been done before. Instead, you must always give consideration to what should work best in a specific injury situation.

There are many different approaches and ideas regarding the use of modalities in injury rehabilitation. Therefore, no "cookbook" exists for modality use. In a given clinical situation, you as an athletic trainer should make your own decision about which modality will be most effective.

In any program of rehabilitation, modalities should be used primarily as adjuncts to therapeutic exercise and certainly not at the exclusion of range-of-motion or strengthening exercises. Rehabilitation protocols and progressions must be based primarily on the physiological responses of the tissues to injury and on an understanding of how various tissues heal (Figure 2-1). Thus, the athletic trainer must understand the healing process to be effective in incorporating therapeutic modalities into the rehabilitative process.

In the athletic population, injuries most often involve the musculoskeletal system and in fewer instances the nervous system. In sports medicine, *primary injuries* are almost always described as being either chronic or acute in nature resulting from *macrotraumatic* or *microtraumatic* forces. Injuries classified as macrotraumatic occur as a result of acute trauma and produce immediate pain and disability. Macrotraumatic injuries include fractures, dislocations, subluxations, sprains, strains, and contusions. Microtraumatic injuries are most often called overuse injuries and result from repetitive overloading or incorrect mechanics associated with

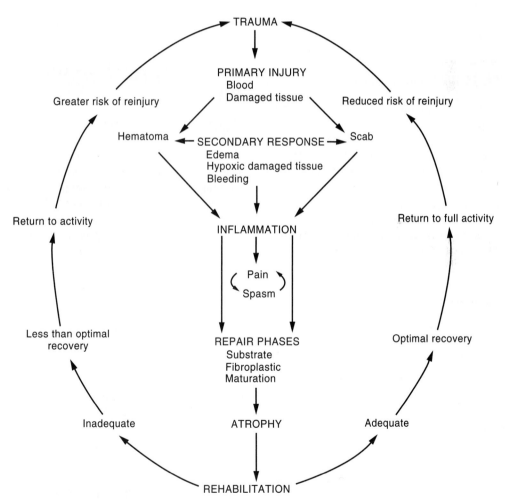

Figure 2-1   A cycle of sport-related injury.
(From Booher and Thibadeau, *Athletic Injury Assessment*, 1994)

The healing process is a continuum consisting of three phases

• Inflammatory-response phase
• Fibroblastic-repair phase
• Maturation-remodeling phase

continuous training or competition. Microtraumatic injuries include tendinitis, tenosynovitis, bursitis, and so on. A *secondary injury* is essentially the inflammatory or hypoxia response that occurs with the primary injury.

THE IMPORTANCE OF UNDERSTANDING THE HEALING PROCESS

The decisions made by the athletic trainer on how and when therapeutic modalities may best be used should be based on recognition of signs and symptoms as well as some awareness of the time frames associated with the different phases of the healing process.[1,14] The athletic trainer must have a sound understanding of that process in terms of the sequence of the phases of healing that take place.

The healing process consists of the inflammatory-response phase, the fibroblastic-repair phase,

Signs of inflammation

• Redness
• Swelling
• Tenderness to touch
• Increased temperature
• Loss of functions

and the maturation-remodeling phase. It must be stressed that although the phases of healing are presented as three separate entities, *the healing process is a continuum*. Phases of the healing process overlap one another and have no definitive beginning or end points[7] (Figure 2-2).

INFLAMMATORY-RESPONSE PHASE

When you hear the term inflammation, you automatically think of something negative. The fact is that inflammation is a very important part of the healing process. Without the physiological changes that take place during the inflammatory process, the later stages of healing cannot occur. Once a tissue is injured, the process of healing begins immediately.[2] The destruction of tissue produces direct injury to the cells of the various soft tissues. Cellular injury re-

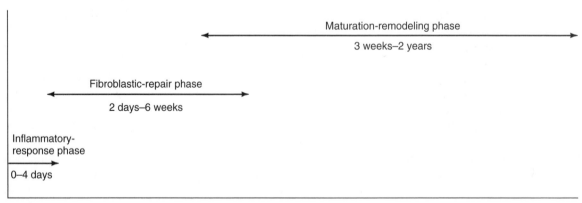

Figure 2-2   The three phases of the healing process fall along an overlapping time continuum.

sults in altered metabolism and the liberation of materials that initiate the inflammatory response.

Signs and Symptoms.   It is characterized symptomatically by redness, swelling, tenderness, increased temperature, and loss of function.[3,14]

Cellular Response.   Inflammation is a process during which **leukocytes** and other **phagocytic cells** and exudate are delivered to the injured tissue. This cellular reaction is generally protective, tending to localize or dispose of injury by-products (for example, blood or damaged cells) through phagocytosis, thus setting the stage for repair. Locally, vascular effects, disturbances of fluid exchange, and migration of leukocytes from the blood to the tissues occur.[12]

Vascular Reaction.   The vascular reaction involves vascular spasm, formation of a platelet plug, blood coagulation, and growth of fibrous tissue.[20] The immediate response to damage is a vasoconstriction of the vascular walls that lasts for approximately 5 to 10 minutes. This spasm presses the opposing endothelial linings together to produce a local anemia that is rapidly replaced by hyperemia of the area resulting from dilation. This increase in blood flow is transitory and gives way to slowing of the flow in the dilated vessels, which then progresses to stagnation and stasis.[16] The initial effusion of blood and plasma lasts for 24 to 36 hours.

The Chemical Mediators.   Three chemical mediators—histamine, leucotaxin, and necrosin—are important in limiting the amount of exudate, and thus swelling, following injury. *Histamine* released from the injured mast cells causes vasodilation and increased cell permeability, owing to swelling of endothelial cells and then separation between the cells. *Leucotaxin* is responsible for margination in which leukocytes line up along the cell walls. It also increases cell permeability locally, thus affecting passage of the fluid and white blood cells through cell walls via diapedesis to form exudate. Therefore, vasodilation and active hyperemia are important in exudate (plasma) formation and in supplying leukocytes to the injured area. *Necrosin* is responsible for phagocytic activity. The amount of swelling that occurs is directly related to the extent of vessel damage.

Chemical mediators

- Histamine
- Leucotaxin
- Necrosin

---

leukocytes   A white blood cell that is the primary effector cell against infection and tissue damage that functions to clean up damaged cells.

phagocytic cells   A cell that has the ability to destroy and ingest cellular debris.

The Function of Platelets.   Platelets do not normally adhere to the vascular wall. However, injury to a vessel disrupts the endothelium and exposes the collagen fibers. Platelets adhere to the collagen fibers to create a sticky matrix on the vascular wall, to which additional platelets and leukocytes adhere and eventually form a plug. These plugs obstruct local lymphatic fluid drainage and thus localize the injury response.

The Clotting Process.   The initial event that precipitates clot formation is the conversion of fibrinogen to fibrin. This transformation results from a cascading effect, beginning with the release of a protein molecule called thromboplastin, from the damaged cell. Thromboplastin causes prothrombin to be changed into thrombin, which in turn causes the conversion of fibrinogen into a very sticky fibrin clot that shuts off blood supply to the injured area. Clot formation begins around 12 hours following injury and is completed by 48 hours[8] (Figure 2-3).

As a result of a combination of these factors, the injured area becomes walled off during the inflammatory stage of healing. The leukocytes phagocytize most of the foreign debris toward the end of the inflammatory phase, setting the stage for the fibroblastic phase. This initial inflammatory response lasts for approximately 2 to 4 days following initial injury.

Chronic Inflammation.   A distinction must be made between the acute inflammatory response

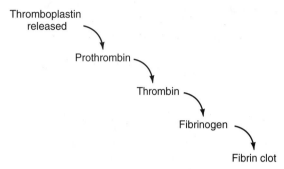

Figure 2-3 placement

Figure 2-3   The clotting process involves a series of physiologic events that require as long as 48 hours to complete.

as described previously and chronic inflammation. If an acute inflammation reaction fails to be resolved in 1 month, it is termed a subacute inflammation. If it lasts for months or even years, the condition is termed chronic. Chronic inflammation results from repeated acute microtraumas and overuse.[11] Prominent features that are distinct from acute inflammation are proliferation of connective tissue and tissue degeneration. The primary cells during chronic inflammation are *lymphocytes*, *plasma cells*, and *macrophages* (monocytes), in contrast to neutrophil leukocytes in acute inflammation.[13] It has been suggested that lymphocytes, although not normally phagocytic, may be used to stimulate fibroblasts to heal and to form scar tissue. The role of plasma cells is not clearly understood, however. Macrophages, present in both acute and chronic inflammation, are definitely phagocytic and actively engaged in repair and healing.[6,11,13]

Using Modalities in the Immediate First Aid Management of Injury

Table 2-1 summarizes the various modalilities that may be used in the difference phases of the healing process. Modality use in the initial treatment of injury should be directed toward limiting the amount of swelling and reducing pain that occurs acutely. The acute phase is marked by swelling, pain to touch or with pressure, and pain on both active and

In chronic inflammation, leukocytes are replaced with

- Macrophages
- Lymphocytes
- Plasma cells

passive motion. In general, the less initial swelling, the less the time required for rehabilitation. Traditionally, the modality of choice has been and still is *RICE* (rest, ice, compression, elevation).

Cryotherapy is known to produce vasoconstriction, at least superficially and perhaps indirectly in the deeper tissues, and thus limits the bleeding that always occurs with injury. Ice bags, cryocuffs, cold packs, and ice massage may all be used effectively. Cold baths should be avoided because the extremities must be placed in a gravity-dependent position. Cold whirlpools also place the extremities in the gravity-dependent position and produce a massaging action that is likely to retard clotting. The importance of applying ice immediately following injury for limiting acute swelling through vasoconstriction has probably been overemphasized. The initial use of ice is more important for decreasing the secondary hypoxic response associated with tissue injury (see Chapter 4). Analgesia, which occurs through stimulation of sensory cutaneous nerves that, via the gating mechanism, blocks or reduces pain.

Immediate compression has been demonstrated to be an effective technique for limiting swelling. An intermittent compression device may be used to provide even pressure around an injured extremity. The pressurized sleeve mechanically reduces the amount of space available for swelling to accumulate. Units that combine both compression and cold have been shown to be more effective in reducing swelling than using compression alone. Regardless of the specific techniques selected, cold and compression should always be combined with elevation to avoid any additional pooling of blood in the injured area due to the effects of gravity.

Electrical stimulating currents may also be used in the initial phase for pain reduction. Para-

■ **TABLE 2-1**   Athletic Training Decision-Making on the Use of Various Therapeutic Modalities in Treatment of Acute Injury

PHASE	APPROXIMATE TIME FRAME	CLINICAL PICTURE	POSSIBLE MODALITIES USED	RATIONALE FOR USE
Initial acute	Injury–day 3	Swelling, pain to touch, pain on motion	CRYO	↓ Swelling, ↓ pain
			ESC	↓ Pain
			IC	↓ Swelling
			LPL	↓ Pain
			ULTRA	Nonthermal effects to ↑ healing
			Rest	
Inflammatory response	Day 1–day 6	Swelling subsides, warm to touch, discoloration, pain to touch, pain on motion	CRYO	↓ Swelling, ↓ pain
			ESC	↓ Pain
			IC	↓ Swelling
			LPL	↓ Pain
			ULTRA	Nonthermal effects to ↑ healing.
			Range of motion	
Fibroblastic-repair*	Day 4–day 10	Pain to touch, pain on motion, swollen	THERMO	Mildly ↑ circulation
			ESC	↓ Pain—muscle pumping
			LPL	↓ Pain
			IC	Facilitate lymphatic flow
			ULTRA	Nonthermal effects to ↑ healing
			Range of motion	
			Strengthening	
Maturation-remodeling*	Day 7–recovery	Swollen, no more pain to touch, decreasing pain on motion	ULTRA	Deep heating to ↑ circulation
			ESC	↑ Range of motion, ↑ strength
			LPL	↓ Pain
			SWD	↓ Pain
			MWD	Deep heating to ↑ circulation
			Range of motion	Deep heating to ↑ circulation
			Strenghtening	
			Functional activities	

CRYO Cryotherapy; *ESC*, electrical stimulating currents; *IC*, intermittent compression; *LPL*, low-power laser; *MWD*, microwave diathermy; *SWD*, shortwave diathermy; *THERMO*, thermotherapy; *ULTRA*, ultrasound; ↓, decrease; ↑, increase.
* Anti-inflammatory medication prescribed by the team physician is recommended.

meters should be adjusted to maximally stimulate sensory cutaneous nerve fibers, again to take advantage of the gate control mechanism of pain modulation. Intensities that produce muscle contractions should be avoided because they may increase clotting time.

Ultrasound has been demonstrated to be effective in facilitating the healing process when used immediately following injury and certainly within the first 48 hours. Low spatial-averaged intensities below .2 W/cm^2 produce nonthermal physiologic effects that alter the permeability of cell membranes to sodium and calcium ions important in healing.

The low-power laser has also been shown to be effective in pain modulation through the stimulation of trigger points and may be used acutely.

The injured part should be rested and protected for at least the first 48 to 72 hours to allow the inflammatory phase of the healing process to do what it is supposed to.

Modality Use in the Inflammatory-Response Phase

The inflammatory-response phase begins immediately with injury and may last as long as day 6 following injury. With appropriate care, swelling begins to subside and eventually stops altogether. The injured area may feel warm to the touch, and some discoloration is usually apparent. The injury is still painful to the touch, and pain is elicited on movement of the injured part.

As in the initial injury management stage, modalities should be used to control pain and reduce swelling. Cryotherapy should still be used during the inflammatory stage. Ice bags, cold packs, or ice massages provide analgesic effects. The use of cold also reduces the likelihood of swelling, which may continue during this stage. Swelling does subside completely by the end of this phase.

It must be emphasized that heating an injury too soon is a bigger mistake than using ice on an injury for too long. Many athletic trainers elect to stay with cryotherapy for weeks following injury; in fact, some never switch to the superficial heating techniques. This procedure is simply a matter of personal preference that should be dictated by experience. Once swelling has stopped, the athletic trainer may elect to begin contrast baths with a longer cold-to-hot ratio.

An intermittent compression device may be used to decrease swelling by facilitating resorption of the by-products of inflammatory process

■ Analogy *2-1*

....

The physiologic events that occur during the inflammatory-response phase are similar to creating and rebuilding a fort. The injured area is essentially shut off from the outside environment, and soldiers (phagocytic cells) come inside the fort to clean up the debris before the reinforcement troops (fibroblastic cells) show up to rebuild the structures inside.

by the lymphatic system. Electrical stimulating currents and low-power laser can be used to help reduce pain.

After the initial stage, the athlete should begin to work on active and passive range of motion. Decisions regarding how rapidly to progress exercise should be determined by the response of the injury to that exercise. If exercise produces additional swelling and markedly exacerbates pain, then the level or intensity of the exercise is too great and should be reduced. Athletic trainers should be aggressive in their approach to rehabilitation, but the healing process will always limit the approach.

FIBROBLASTIC-REPAIR PHASE

During the fibroblastic phase of healing, proliferative and regenerative activity leading to scar formation and repair of the injured tissue follows the vascular and exudative phenomena of inflammation.[10] The period of scar formation referred to as **fibroplasia** begins within the first few hours following injury and may last for as long as 4 to 6 weeks.

Signs and Symptoms. During this period many of the signs and symptoms associated with the inflammatory response subside. The athlete may still indicate some tenderness to touch and will usually complain of pain when particular movements stress the injured structure. As scar formation progresses, complaints of tenderness or pain will gradually disappear.[17]

Revascularization. During this phase, growth of endothelial capillary buds into the

fibroplasia   The period of scar formation that occurs during the fibroblastic-repair phase.

wound is stimulated by a lack of oxygen. Thus, the wound is now capable of healing aerobically. Along with increased oxygen delivery comes an increase in blood flow, which delivers nutrients essential for tissue regeneration in the area.[4]

Formation of Scar.   The formation of a delicate connective tissue called granulation tissue occurs with the breakdown of the fibrin clot. Granulation tissue consists of fibroblasts, collagen, and capillaries. It appears as a reddish granular mass of connective tissue that fills in the gaps during the healing process.

As the capillaries continue to grow into the area, fibroblasts accumulate at the wound site, arranging themselves parallel to the capillaries. Fibroblastic cells begin to synthesize an extracellular matrix, which contains protein fibers of collagen and elastin, a ground substance that consists of nonfibrous proteins called proteoglycans, glycosaminoglycans, and fluid. On about day 6 or 7, fibroblasts also begin producing collagen fibers that are deposited in a random fashion throughout the forming scar. As the collagen continues to proliferate, the tensile strength of the wound rapidly increases in proportion to the rate of collagen synthesis. As the tensile strength increases, the number of fibroblasts diminishes to signal the beginning of the maturation phase.[5]

This normal sequence of events in the repair phase leads to the formation of minimal scar tissue. Occasionally, a persistent inflammatory response and continued release of inflammatory products can promote extended fibroplasia and excessive fibrogenesis that can lead to irreversible tissue damage.[21] Fibrosis can occur in synovial structures, as is the case with adhesive capsulitis in the shoulder; in extra-articular tissues, including tendons and ligaments; in bursa; or in muscle.

A mature scar will be devoid of physiologic function, it will have less tensile strength than the original tissue, and it is not as well vascularized.

■ **Granulation tissue consists of**

- Capillaries
- Collagen
- Fibroblasts

■ **The extracellular matrix contains**

- Collagen
- Elastin
- Ground substance

■ Analogy   *2-2*

The physiologic events that occur during the fibroblastic-repair phase are similar to taking spaghetti out of a pot of boiling water and laying it on a table at random. Initially the spaghetti is weak and tender. In a short time, the spaghetti begins to dry out and becomes more solid, a little dryer, and harder to disturb (as in the transition between the fibroblastic repair and maturation-remodeling phases).

Modality Use in the Fibroblastic-Repair Phase

Once the inflammatory response has subsided, the fibroblastic-repair phase begins. This stage may begin as early as 4 days after the injury and may last for several weeks. At this point, swelling has stopped completely. The injury is still tender to the touch but is not as painful as during the last stage. Pain is also less on active and passive motion.

Treatments may change during this stage from cold to heat, once again using increased swelling as a precautionary indicator. Thermotherapy techniques including hydrocollator packs, paraffin, or eventually warm whirlpool may be safely employed. The purpose of thermotherapy is to increase circulation to the injured area to promote healing.

■ **Clinical Decision-Making** *Exercise 2-1*

A woman soccer player sprains her ankle, and the team physician diagnoses it as a grade 1 sprain. The coach wants to know how long the athlete will be out. On what information should the athletic trainer base his or her response.

These modalities can also produce some degree of analgesia.

Intermittent compression can once again be used to facilitate removal of injury by-products from the area. Electrical stimulating currents can be used to assist this process by eliciting a muscle contraction and thus inducing a muscle pumping action. This aids in facilitating lymphatic flow. Electrical currents can once again be used for modulation of pain, as can stimulation of trigger points with the low-powered laser.

The athletic trainer must continue to stress the importance of range-of-motion and strengthening exercises and progress them appropriately during this phase.

MATURATION-REMODELING PHASE

The maturation-remodeling phase of healing is a long-term process. This phase features a realignment or remodeling of the collagen fibers that make up the scar tissue according to the tensile forces to which that scar is subjected. Ongoing breakdown and synthesis of collagen occur with a steady increase in the tensile strength of the scar matrix. With increased stress and strain, the collagen fibers will realign in a position of maximum efficiency parallel to the lines of tension.[19] The tissue gradually assumes normal appearance and function, although a scar is rarely as strong as the normal injured tissue. Usually by the end of approximately 3 weeks, a firm, strong, contracted, nonvascular scar exists. The maturation phase of healing may require several years to be totally complete.

Modality Use in the Maturation-Remodeling Phase

The maturation-remodeling phase is the longest of the four phases and may last for several years, depending on the severity of the injury. The ultimate goal during this maturation stage of the healing process is return to activity. The injury is no longer painful to the touch, although some progressively decreasing pain may still be felt on motion. The collagen fibers must be realigned according to tensile stresses and strains placed upon them. Virtually all modalities may be safely used during this stage; thus, decisions should be based on what seems to work most effectively in a given situation.

At this point some type of heating modality is beneficial to the healing process. The deep-heating modalities, ultrasound, or short-wave and microwave diathermy should be used to increase circulation to the deeper tissues. Ultrasound is particularly useful during this period since collagen absorbs a high percentage of the available acoustic energy. Increased blood flow delivers the essential nutrients to the injured area to promote healing, and increased lymphatic flow assists in breakdown and removal of waste products. The superficial heating modalities are certainly less effective at this point.

Electrical stimulating currents can be used for a number of purposes. As before, they may be used in pain modulation. They may also be used to stimulate muscle contractions for the purpose of increasing both range of motion and muscular strength.

Low-power laser can also assist in modulating pain. If pain is reduced, therapeutic exercises may be progressed more quickly.

The Role of Progressive Controlled Mobility in the Maturation Phase. **Wolff's Law** states that both bone and soft tissue will respond to the physical demands placed upon them causing them to remodel or realign along lines of tensile force.[1] Therefore, it is critical that injured structures be exposed to progressively increasing loads, particularly during the remodeling phase. Controlled mobilization has been shown to be superior to immobilization for scar formation, revasculariza-

■ **Clinical Decision-Making**   *Exercise 2-2*

A male lacrosse player is 8 days post strain of the quadriceps muscle of the thigh. The athletic trainer feels that it is time to change from cold therapy to some form of heat. What criteria should be used to determine if this athlete is ready to change to heat?

■ **Clinical Decision-Making**   *Exercise 2-3*

In the rehabilitative process for a sprain of the medial collateral ligament in the knee, at what point should the athletic trainer decide to add therapeutic exercises to modality use?

tion, muscle regeneration, and reorientation of muscle fibers and tensile properties in animal models.[2] However, immobilization of the injured tissue during the inflammatory-response phase will likely facilitate the process of healing by controlling inflammation, thus reducing athletic training symptoms. As healing progresses to the repair phase, controlled activity directed toward return-to-normal flexibility and strength should be combined with protective support or bracing. Generally, clinical signs and symptoms disappear at the end of this phase.

As the remodeling phase begins, aggressive active range-of-motion and strengthening exercises should be incorporated to facilitate tissue remodeling and realignment. To a great extent, pain will dictate rate of progression. With initial injury, pain is intense and tends to decrease and eventually subside altogether as healing progresses. Any exacerbation of either pain, swelling, or other athletic training symptoms during or following a particular exercise or activity indicates that the load is too great for the level of tissue repair or remodeling. The athletic trainer must be aware of the timelines required for the process of healing and realize that being overly aggressive can interfere with that process.

microtears   Minor damage to soft tissue most often associated with overuse.

macrotears   Significant damage to the soft tissues caused by acute trauma that results in clinical symptoms and functional alterations.

■ **Clinical Decision-Making**   *Exercise 2-4*

The athletic trainer decides to allow an athlete with a grade 1 ankle sprain to be full weight bearing immediately following injury. Is this the best decision based on your knowledge of the healing process?

OTHER CONSIDERATIONS IN TREATING INJURY

During the rehabilitation period following injury, athletes must alter their daily routines to allow the injury to heal sufficiently. Consideration must be given to maintaining levels of strength, flexibility, neuromuscular control, balance, and cardiorespiratory endurance. Modality use should be combined with the use of anti-inflammatory medications prescribed by the team physician, particularly during the initial acute and inflammatory-response phases of rehabilitation.

FACTORS THAT IMPEDE HEALING

See Table 2-2 for a list of factors that impede healing.

Extent of Injury.   The nature or amount of the inflammatory response is determined by the extent of the tissue injury. **Microtears** of soft tissue involve only minor damage and are most often associated with overuse. **Macrotears** involve significantly greater destruction of soft tissue and result in clinical symptoms and functional alterations. Macrotears are generally caused by acute trauma.

Edema.   The increased pressure caused by swelling retards the healing process, causes separation of tissues, inhibits neuromuscular control,

■ **TABLE 2-2** Factors That Impede Healing

Extent of injury
Edema
Hemorrhage
Poor vascular supply
Separation of tissue
Muscle spasm
Atrophy
Corticosteroids
Keloids and hypertrophic scars
Infection
Humidity, climate, and oxygen tension
Health, age, and nutrition

produces reflexive neurological changes, and impedes nutrition in the injured part. Edema is best controlled and managed during the initial first aid management period.[22]

Hemorrhage. Bleeding occurs with even the smallest amount of damage to the capillaries. Bleeding produces the same negative effects on healing as does the accumulation of edema, and its presence produces additional tissue damage and thus exacerbation of the injury.

Poor Vascular Supply. Injuries to tissues with a poor vascular supply heal poorly and at a slow rate. This is likely related to a failure in the delivery of phagocytic cells initially and also of fibroblasts necessary for formation of scar.

Separation of Tissue. Mechanical separation of tissue can significantly impact the course of healing. A wound that has smooth edges that are in good apposition will tend to heal by primary intention with minimal scaring. Conversely, a wound that has jagged separated edges must heal by second intention, with granulation tissue filling the defect and causing excessive scarring.[18]

Muscle Spasm. Muscle spasm causes traction on the torn tissue, separates the two ends, and prevents approximation. Both local and generalized ischemia may result from spasm.

Atrophy. Wasting away of muscle tissue begins immediately with injury. Strengthening and early mobilization of the injured structure retards atrophy.

■ Analogy *2-3*

The physiologic events that occur during the maturation-remodeling phase are similar to an artist sculpting a statue out of a mass of clay. As the artist's hands produce stresses and strains on the clay, it is reshaped and realigned until the artist is satisfied with the finished product (as would occur when the athletic trainer incorporates specific therapeutic exercises designed to realign collagen fibers along lines of tensile force).

Corticosteroids. Use of corticosteroids such as cortisone in the treatment of inflammation is controversial. Steroid use in the early stages of healing has been demonstrated to inhibit fibroplasia, capillary proliferation, collagen synthesis, and increases in tensile strength of the healing scar. Their use in the later stages of healing and with chronic inflammation is debatable.

Keloids and Hypertrophic Scars. Keloids occur when the rate of collagen production exceeds the rate of collagen breakdown during the maturation phase of healing. This process leads to hypertrophy of scar tissue, particularly around the periphery of the wound, that is out of proportion to normal scarring. The result is a raised, firm, thickened, red scar.

Infection. The presence of bacteria in the wound can delay healing, can cause excessive granulation tissue, and can frequently cause large deformed scars.

Humidity, Climate, and Oxygen Tension. Humidity significantly influences the process of epithelization. Occlusive dressings stimulate the epithelium to migrate twice as fast without crust or scab formation. The formation of a scab occurs with dehydration of the wound and traps wound drainage, which promotes infection. Keeping the wound moist provides an advantage for the necrotic debris to go to the surface and be shed.

Oxygen tension relates to the neovascularization of the wound, which translates into optimal saturation and maximal tensile strength development. Circulation to the wound can be affected by ischemia, venous stasis, hematomas, and vessel trauma.

Health, Age, and Nutrition.   The elastic qualities of the skin decrease with aging. Degenerative diseases, such as diabetes and arteriosclerosis, also become a concern of the older athlete and may affect wound healing. Nutrition is important for wound healing. In particular, vitamin C, vitamin K, vitamins A and E, zinc, and amino acids play critical roles in the healing process.

Summary

1. Clinical decisions on how and when therapeutic modalities may best be used should be based on recognition of signs and symptoms, as well as some awareness of the time frames associated with the various phases of the healing process.
2. Once an acute injury has occurred, the healing process consists of the inflammatory-response phase, the fibroblastic-repair phase, and the maturation-remodeling phase.
3. There are a number of pathologic factors that can impede the healing process.
4. Modality use in the initial treatment phase should be directed toward limiting the amount of swelling and reducing pain.
5. It is critical to use logic and common sense based on sound theoretical knowledge when selecting the appropriate modalities to use during the different phases of healing.
6. During the rehabilitation period after injury, athletes must alter their training and conditioning habits to allow the injury to heal sufficiently.

Review Questions

1. How should the athletic trainer incorporate therapeutic modalities into a rehabilitation program for various sports-related injuries?
2. What are the physiological events associated with the inflammatory-response phase of the healing process?
3. How can you differentiate between acute and chronic inflammation?
4. How is collagen laid down in the area of injury during the fibroblastic-repair phase of healing?
5. Explain Wolff's Law and the importance of controlled mobility during the maturation-remodeling phase of healing.
6. What are some of the factors that can have a negative impact on the healing process?
7. Why is the immediate care provided following acute injury so important to the healing process and the course of rehabilitation?
8. What specific modalities may be incorporated into treatment during the inflammatory-response phase?
9. What specific modalities may be incorporated into treatment during the fibroblastic-repair phase?
10. What are the specific indications and contraindications for using the various modalities?

 ## Self-Test Questions

T/F

1. Loss of function is a sign of the inflammatory process.
2. Leukocytes are present in both the acute and chronic inflammatory responses.
3. An injured individual's health, age, and nutrition are factors that influence healing.

Multiple Choice

4. The three phases of the healing process, in order, are as follows:
   a. Fibroblastic-repair, inflammatory-response, maturation-remodeling
   b. Inflammatory-response, fibroblastic-repair, maturation-remodeling

   c. Inflammatory-response, maturation-remodeling, fibroblastic-repair

5. Which of the following type of cell has phagocytic characteristics?
   a. red blood cells
   b. platelets
   c. leukocytes
   d. endothelials

6. The extracellular matrix, formed by fibroblastic cells, consists of
   a. collagen
   b. elastin
   c. ground substance
   d. all of the above

7. During the inflammatory-response phase of the healing process, modalities are used to
   a. control pain
   b. reduce swelling
   c. both a and b
   d. neither a nor b

8. _____ states that bone and soft tissue remodel and realign according to the physical demands placed upon them.
   a. Wolff's Law
   b. Ohm's Law
   c. Meissner's Law
   d. McGill's Law

9. Approximately how long does the maturation-remodeling phase of the healing process last?
   a. less than 1 week
   b. 1 week
   c. 1 to 2 weeks
   d. 3 weeks to 2 years

10. Which of the following is NOT a chemical mediator involved in the inflammatory-response phase?
   a. testosterone
   b. histamine
   c. necrosin
   d. leukotaxin

Solutions to Clinical Decision-Making Exercises

2-1 The athletic trainer's response should be based on knowledge of the healing process and an understanding of the time frames necessary in that process.

2-2 The athletic trainer should use cryotherapy and some type of compression device, along with elevation, to control swelling initially. Additionally, electrical stimulating currents may be used to help provide analgesia, and ultrasound can be used to facilitate healing.

2-3 At this point, the athlete is in transition between the fibroblastic-repair phase and the maturation-remodeling phase. Although there is still some pain on active motion, all of the clinical signs of inflammation (tenderness to touch, increased warmth, redness, and so on) have disappeared, and thus it should be safe to go with heat. If changing to heat causes the athlete to have greater difficulty completing strengthening and flexibility exercises, then the change has likely been made too quickly.

2-4 Knowing how important it is for the inflammatory-response phase to accomplish what it needs to physiologically without interference, it is likely best to recommend minimal weight bearing for the first 24 to 48 hours.

2-5 Therapeutic exercises should begin on day 1 following injury. The point is that modalities should be used to facilitate the athlete's effort to actively exercise the injured part and not in place of the active exercise.

References

1. Arnheim, D, Prentice, W: *Principles of athletic training*, ed 10, Boston, 2000, McGraw-Hill.
2. Bryant, M: Wound healing, *CIBA Athletic Training Symposia* 29(3):2–36, 1977.
3. Carrico, T, Mehrhof A, and Cohen I: Biology and wound healing, *Surg Clin North Am* 64(4):721–734, 1984.
4. Cheng, N: The effects of electrocurrents on A.T.P. generation, protein synthesis and membrane transport, *J Orth Related Research* 171:264–272, 1982.
5. Daly, T: The repair phase of wound healing—re-epithelialization and contraction. In Kloth, L, McCulloch, J, Feedar, J: *Wound healing: alternatives in management*, Philadelphia, 1990, F. A. Davis.
6. Fantone, J: Basic concepts in inflammation. In Leadbetter, W, Buckwalter, J, Gordon, S, editors: *Sports-induced inflammation*, Park Ridge, Illinois, 1990, American Academy of Orthopaedic Surgeons.
7. Fernandez, A, and Finlew, J: Wound healing: helping a natural process, *Postgrad Med* 74(4):311–318, 1983.
8. Fisher, D: Ultrastructural events following acute muscle trauma, *Med Sci Sport Exercise* 22:185, 1990.
9. Fleischli, JG, and Laughlin, TJ: Electrical stimulation in wound healing, *Journal of Foot Ankle Surgery* 36(6): 457–461, 474–476, 1997.
10. Hettinga D: Inflammatory response of synovial joint structures. In Gould J, and Davies, G, editors: *Orthopaedic and sports physical therapy*, St Louis, 1990, Mosby.
11. Houghton, PE: Effects of therapeutic modalities on wound healing: A conservative approach to the management of chronic wounds *Physical Therapy Reviews* 4(3):167–182, 1999.
12. Kloth, L, and Miller, K: The inflammatory response to wounding. In Kloth, L, McCulloch, J, and Feedar, J: *Wound healing: alternatives in management*, Philadelphia, 1990, F. A. Davis.
13. Leadbetter, W: Introduction to sports-induced soft-tissue inflammation. In Leadbetter, W, Buckwalter, J, and Gordon, S, editors: *Sports-induced inflammation*, Park Ridge, Illinois, 1990, American Academy of Orthopaedic Surgeons.
14. Leadbetter, W, Buckwalter, J, and Gordon, S, editors: *Sports-induced inflammation*, Park Ridge, Illinois, 1990, American Academy of Orthopaedic Surgeons.
15. Marchesi V: Inflammation and healing. In Kissane J, editor: *Anderson's pathology*, ed 8, St Louis, 1985, Mosby.
16. Reed, B, Zarro, V: Inflammation and repair in the use of thermal agents. In Michlovitz, S: *Thermal agents in rehabilitation*, Philadelphia, 1990, FA Davis.
17. Riley W: Wound healing, *Am Fam Physician* 24:5, 1981.
18. Robbins, S, Cotran, R, and Kumar, V: *Pathologic basis of disease*, ed 3, Philadelphia, 1984, WB Saunders.
19. Russell, B: Repair of injured skeletal muscle: a molecular approach, *Med Sci Sport Exercise* 24:189, 1992.
20. Rywlin, A: Hemopoietic system. In Kissane, JM, editor: *Anderson's pathology*, ed 8, St Louis, 1985, Mosby.
21. Wahl, S, and Renstrom, P: Fibrosis in soft-tissue injuries. In Leadbetter, W, Buckwalter, J, and Gordon, S, editors: *Sports-induced inflammation*, Park Ridge, Illinois, 1990, American Academy of Orthopaedic Surgeons.
22. Woo, SL-Y, and Buckwalter, J, editors: *Injury and repair of musculoskeletal soft tissues*, Park Ridge, Illinois, 1988, American Academy of Orthopaedic Surgeons.
23. Zachezewski, J: Flexibility for sports. In Sanders, B, editor: *Sports physical therapy*, Norwalk, Connecticut, 1990, Appleton and Lange.

CHAPTER 3

Managing Pain with Therapeutic Modalities

Craig R. Denegar and Phillip B. Donley

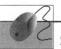

Study Resources

Refer to the lab exercises in the accompanying Laboratory Manual, as well as eSims which simulates the athletic training certification exam at www.mhhe.com/esims. Also, check out the competency information found at www.mhhe.com/prentice11e. For more online study resources, visit our Health and Human Performance Website at www.mhhe.com/hhp/.

Following completion of this chapter, the student athletic trainer will be able to

- Compare the various types of pain and appraise their positive and negative effects.

- Choose a technique for assessing pain.

- Analyze the characteristics of sensory receptors.

- Examine how the nervous system relays information about painful stimuli.

- Distinguish between the different neurophysiologic mechanisms for pain control for the therapeutic modalities used by athletic trainers.

- Predict how pain perception can be modified by cognitive factors.

UNDERSTANDING PAIN

The International Association for the Study of Pain defines pain as "an unpleasant sensory and emotional experience associated with actual or potential tissue damage, or described in terms of such damage."[22] Pain is a subjective sensation with more than one dimension and an abundance of descriptors of its qualities and characteristics. In spite of its universality, pain is composed of a variety of human discomforts, rather than being a single entity.[21] The perception of pain can be subjectively modified by past experiences and expectations. Much of what we do to treat athletes' pain is to change their perceptions of pain.[4]

Pain does have a purpose. It warns us that there is something wrong and can provoke a withdrawal response to avoid further injury. It also results in muscle spasm and guards or protects the injured part. Pain, however, can persist after it is no longer useful. It can become a means of enhancing disability and inhibiting efforts to rehabilitate the athlete. Prolonged spasm, which leads to circulatory deficiency, muscle atrophy, disuse habits, and conscious or unconscious guarding, may lead to a severe loss of function.[17] Chronic pain may become a disease state in itself. Often lacking an identifiable cause, chronic pain can totally disable an athlete.

Research in recent years has led to a better understanding of pain and pain relief. This research also has raised new questions, while leaving many unanswered. We now have better explanations for the analgesic properties of the physical agents we use, as well as a better understanding of the psychology of pain. Newer physical agents, such as LASER, and recent improvements to older agents such as diathermy and transcutaneous electrical nerve simulators, offer new approaches to the treatment of musculoskeletal injury and pain. The evolution of the treatment of pain is, however, incomplete. Not even the mechanisms for the analgesic response to the simplest therapeutic modalities, heat and cold, have been fully described.[31]

The control of pain is an essential aspect of caring for the injured athlete. The athletic trainer has several therapeutic agents with analgesic properties from which to choose. The selection of a therapeutic agent should be based on a sound understanding of its physical properties and physiologic effects. This chapter will not provide a complete explanation of neurophysiology, pain, and pain relief. Several physiology textbooks provide extensive discussions of human neurophysiology and neurobiology to supplement this chapter. Instead, this chapter presents an overview of some theories of pain control, intended to provide a stimulus for the therapist to develop his or her own rationale for using modalities in the plan of care for patients he or she treats. Ideally, it will also facilitate growth in the body of evidence from which improved responses to the therapeutic agents used in the treatment of pain can be derived.

Many of the modalities discussed in later chapters have analgesic properties. Often, they are employed to reduce pain and permit the athlete to perform therapeutic exercises. Some understanding of what pain is, how it affects us, and how it is perceived is essential for the athletic trainer who uses these modalities.

TYPES OF PAIN

Traditionally, pain has been categorized as either *acute* or *chronic*. Acute pain is experienced when tissue damage is impending and after injury has occurred. Pain lasting for more than 6 months is gen-

---

referred pain (referred myofascial pain)   When nociceptive impulses reach the dorsal grey matter, they converge, and their summation can depolarize internuncial neurons over several spinal segments, causing the individual to feel pain in distal areas innervated by these segments.

trigger point   Localized deep tenderness in a palpable firm band of muscle. When stretched, a palpating finger can snap the band like a taut string, which produces local pain, a local twitch of that portion of the muscle, and a jump by the athlete. Sustained pressure on a trigger point reproduces the pattern of referred pain for that site.

sclerotome   A segment of bone innervated by a spinal segment.

---

erally classified as chronic.[6] More recently, the term *persistent pain* has been used to differentiate chronic pain that defies intervention from conditions where continuing (persistent) pain is a symptom of a treatable condition.[13,26] There is more research devoted to chronic pain and its treatment, but acute and persistent confront the therapist most often.

Referred pain, which also may be either acute or chronic, is pain that is perceived to be in an area that seems to have little relation to the existing pathology. For example, injury to the spleen often results in pain in the left shoulder. This pattern, known as Kehr's sign, is useful for identifying this serious injury and arranging prompt emergency care. Referred pain can outlast the causative events because of altered reflex patterns, continuing mechanical stress on muscles, learned habits of guarding, or the development of hypersensitive areas, called **trigger points**.

Irritation of nerves and nerve roots can cause *radiating pain*. Pressure on the lumbar nerve roots associated with a herniated disc or a contusion of the sciatic nerve can result in pain radiating down the lower extremity to the foot.

Deep somatic pain is a type that seems to be **sclerotomic** (associated with a sclerotome, a segment of bone innervated by a spinal segment). There is often a discrepancy between the site of the disorder and the site of the pain.

The athlete's perception of pain can differ markedly from person to person as can the terminology used to describe the type of pain the athlete is experiencing. The athletic trainer commonly asks the athlete to describe what his or her pain feels like during an injury evaluation. Term's like "sharp," "dull," "aching," "throbbing," "burning," "piercing," "localized," and "generalized" are often used by the athlete. It is sometimes difficult for the athletic trainer to infer what exactly is causing a particular type of pain. For example, "burning" pain is often associated with some injury to a nerve, but certainly there are other injuries that may produce what the athlete is perceiving as "burning" pain. Thus verbal descriptions of the type of pain should be applied with caution.

PAIN ASSESSMENT

Pain is a complex phenomenon that is difficult to evaluate and quantify because it is subjective and is influenced by attitudes and beliefs of the athletic trainer and the athlete. Quantification is hindered by the fact that pain is a very difficult concept to put into words.[1]

Obtaining an accurate and standardized assessment of pain is problematic. Several tools have been developed. These pain profiles identify the type of pain, quantify the intensity of pain, evaluate the effect of the pain experience on the athlete's level of function, and/or assess the psychosocial impact of pain.

The pain profiles are useful because they compel the athlete to verbalize the pain and thereby provide an outlet for the athlete and also provide the athletic trainer with a better understanding of the pain experience. They assess the psychosocial response to pain and injury. The pain profile can assist with the evaluation process by improving communication and directing the athletic trainer toward appropriate diagnostic tests. These assessments also assist the athletic trainer in identifying which therapeutic agents may be effective and

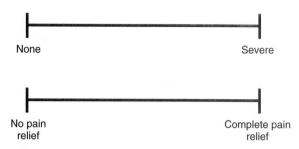

Figure 3-1 Visual analogue scales.

when they should be applied. Finally, these profiles provide a standard measure to monitor treatment progress.[13]

Pain Assessment Scales

The following profiles are used in the evaluation of acute and chronic pain associated with illnesses and injuries.

Visual Analogue Scales. *Visual analogue scales* are quick and simple tests to be completed by the athlete (Figure 3-1). These scales consist of a line, usually 10 cm in length, the extremes of which are taken to represent the limits of the pain experience. One end is defined as "No Pain" and the other as "Severe Pain." The athlete is asked to mark the line at a point corresponding to the severity of the pain. The distance between "No Pain" and the mark represents pain severity. A similar scale can be used to assess treatment effectiveness by placing "No Pain Relief" at one end of the scale and "Complete Pain Relief" at the other. These scales can be completed daily or more often as pre- and post-treatment assessments.[15]

Pain Charts. *Pain charts* can be used to establish spatial properties of pain. These two-dimensional graphic portrayals are completed by the athlete to assess the location of pain and a number of subjective components. Simple line drawings of the body in several postural positions are presented to the athlete (Figure 3-2). On these drawings, the athlete draws or colors in areas that correspond to his or her pain experience. Different

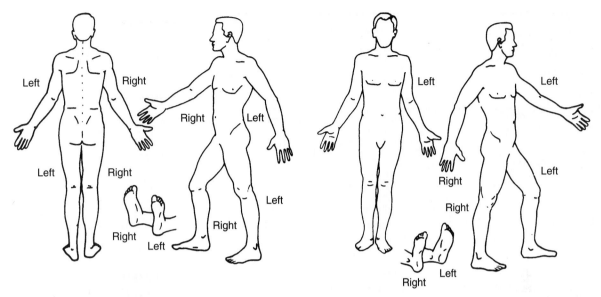

Figure 3-2   The pain chart. Use the following instructions: "Please use all of the figures to show me exactly where all your pains are, and where they radiate to. Shade or draw with *blue marker*. Only the athlete is to fill out this sheet. Please be as precise and detailed as possible. Use *yellow marker* for numbness and tingling. Use *red marker* for burning or hot areas, and *green marker* for cramping. Please remember: blue = pain, yellow = numbness and tingling, red = burning or hot areas, green = cramping."
Used with permission from Melzack, R: *Pain measurement and assessment*, New York, 1983, Raven Press.

colors are used for different sensations—for example, blue for aching pain, yellow for numbness or tingling, red for burning pain, and green for cramping pain. Descriptions can be added to the form to enhance the communication value. The form could be completed daily.[18]

McGill Pain Questionnaire.   The *McGill Pain Questionnaire* (MPQ) is a tool with 78 words that describe pain (Figure 3-3). These words are grouped into 20 sets that are divided into 4 categories representing dimensions of the pain experience. While completion of the MPQ may take only 20 minutes, it is often frustrating for athletes who do not speak English well. The MPQ is commonly administered to athletes with low back pain. When administered every 2 to 4 weeks, it demonstrated changes in status very clearly.[21]

Activity Pattern Indicators Pain Profile.
The *Activity Pattern Indicators Pain Profile* measures athlete activity. It is a 64-question, self-report tool that may be used to assess functional impairment associated with pain. The instrument measures the frequency of certain behaviors such as housework, recreation, and social activities.[13]

Numeric Pain Scale.   The most common acute pain profile used in sports medicine clinics today is a *numeric pain scale*. The athlete is asked to rate his or her pain on a scale from 1 to 10, with 10 representing the worst pain he or she has experienced or could imagine. The question is asked before and after treatment. When treatments provide pain relief, athletes are asked about the extent and duration of the relief. In addition, athletes may be asked to estimate the portion of the day that they experience pain and about specific activities that increase or decrease their pain. When pain affects sleep, athletes may be asked to estimate the amount of sleep they got in the previous 24 hours. In addition, the amount of medication required for pain can be noted. This information helps the athletic

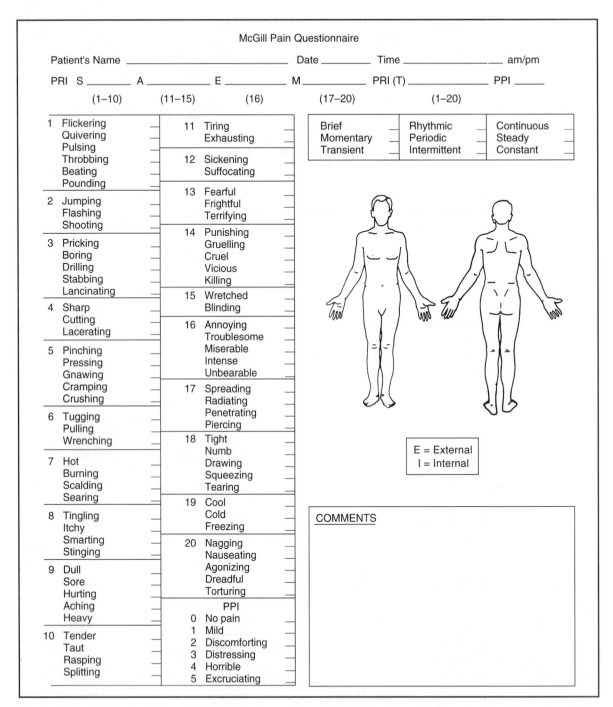

McGill Pain Questionnaire

Patient's Name _____ Date _____ Time _____ am/pm

PRI S _____ A _____ E _____ M_____ PRI (T) _____ PPI _____

   (1–10)   (11–15)   (16)   (17–20)   (1–20)

1 Flickering —
   Quivering —
   Pulsing —
   Throbbing —
   Beating —
   Pounding —
	11 Tiring —
	    Exhausting —

2 Jumping —
   Flashing —
   Shooting —
	12 Sickening —
	    Suffocating —

	13 Fearful —
	    Frightful —
	    Terrifying —

3 Pricking —
   Boring —
   Drilling —
   Stabbing —
   Lancinating —
	14 Punishing —
	    Gruelling —
	    Cruel —
	    Vicious —
	    Killing —

4 Sharp —
   Cutting —
   Lacerating —
	15 Wretched —
	    Blinding —

5 Pinching —
   Pressing —
   Gnawing —
   Cramping —
   Crushing —
	16 Annoying —
	    Troublesome —
	    Miserable —
	    Intense —
	    Unbearable —

6 Tugging —
   Pulling —
   Wrenching —
	17 Spreading —
	    Radiating —
	    Penetrating —
	    Piercing —

7 Hot —
   Burning —
   Scalding —
   Searing —
	18 Tight —
	    Numb —
	    Drawing —
	    Squeezing —
	    Tearing —

8 Tingling —
   Itchy —
   Smarting —
   Stinging —
	19 Cool —
	    Cold —
	    Freezing —

9 Dull —
   Sore —
   Hurting —
   Aching —
   Heavy —
	20 Nagging —
	    Nauseating —
	    Agonizing —
	    Dreadful —
	    Torturing —

10 Tender —
    Taut —
    Rasping —
    Splitting —
	PPI
	0 No pain —
	1 Mild —
	2 Discomforting —
	3 Distressing —
	4 Horrible —
	5 Excruciating —

Brief —	Rhythmic —	Continuous —
Momentary —	Periodic —	Steady —
Transient —	Intermittent —	Constant —

E = External
I = Internal

COMMENTS

Figure 3-3 McGill Pain Questionnaire. the descriptors fall into four major groups: Sensory, 1 to 10; affective, 11 to 15; evaluative, 16; and miscellaneous, 17 to 20. the rank value for each descriptor is based on its position in the word set. The sum of the rank values is the pain rating index (PRI). The present pain intensity (PPI) is based ona scale of 0 to 5.
Used with permission from Melzack, R: *Pain measurement and assessment*, New York, 1983, Raven Press.

Pain assessment techniques

- Visual analogue scales
- Pain charts
- McGill Pain Questionnaire
- Activity Pattern Indicators Pain Profile
- Numeric pain scales

periosteum   A highly vascularized and innervated membrane lining the surface of bone.

joint capsule   Ligamentous structure that surrounds and encapsulates a joint.

avulsion fracture   A fracture in which a small piece of bone is torn away by an attached tendon or ligament.

trainer assess changes in pain, select appropriate treatments, and communicate more clearly with the athlete about the course of recovery from injury or surgery.

All of these scales help athletes communicate the severity and duration of their pain and appreciate changes that occur. Often in a long recovery, athletes lose sight of how much progress has been made in terms of the pain experience and return to functional activities. A review of these pain scales often can serve to reassure the athlete; foster a brighter, more positive outlook; and reinforce the commitment to the plan of treatment.

Documentation.   The efficacy of many of the treatments used by athletic trainers has not been fully substantiated. These scales are one source of data that can help athletic trainers identify the most effective approaches to managing common injuries. These assessment tools can also be useful when reviewing an athlete's progress with physicians, and third-party payers. Thus, pain assessments should be routinely included as documentation in the athlete's note.

TISSUE SENSITIVITY

The structures most sensitive to damaging (noxious) stimuli are, first, the **periosteum** and **joint capsule;** second, subchondral bone, tendons, and ligament; third, muscle and cortical bone; and finally, the synovium and articular cartilage. A variety of "silent" fractures produce little or no pain. Different anatomic tissues exhibit varying degrees of sensitivity to pain. **Avulsion fractures** tend to be quite painful because they tear away the periosteum. Musculoskeletal pain is usually spread over a

large area unless it is close to the surface. For example, a hamstring strain usually results in pain over the posterior thigh, whereas an acromioclavicular sprain usually localizes over the joint.

GOALS IN MANAGING PAIN

Regardless of the cause of pain, its reduction is an essential part of treatment. Pain signals the athlete to seek assistance and is often useful in establishing a diagnosis. Once the injury or illness is diagnosed, pain serves little purpose. Medical or surgical treatment or immobilization is necessary to treat some conditions, but physical therapy and an early return to activity are appropriate following many injuries. The athletic trainer's objectives are to encourage the body to heal through exercise designed to progressively increase functional capacity and to return the athlete to work, recreational, and other activities as swiftly and safely as possible. Pain will inhibit therapeutic exercise. The challenge for the athletic trainer is to control acute pain and protect the athlete from further injury while encouraging progressive exercise in a supervised environment.

PAIN PERCEPTION

Sensory Receptors

A nerve ending is the termination of a nerve fiber in a peripheral structure. It may be a sensory ending (receptor) or a motor ending (effector). Sensory endings can be capsulated (e.g., free nerve endings, Merkel's corpuscles) or encapsulated (e.g., end bulbs of Krause Meissner's corpuscles).

■ **TABLE 3-1** Some Characteristics of Selected Sensory Receptors

TYPE OF SENSORY RECEPTORS	Stimulus		Receptor	
	GENERAL TERM	**SPECIFIC NATURE**	**TERM**	**LOCATION**
Mechanoreceptors	Pressure	Movement of hair in a hair follicle	Afferent nerve fiber	Base of hair follicles
		Light pressure	Meissner's corpuscle	Skin
		Deep pressure	Pacinian corpuscle	Skin
		Touch	Merkel's touch corpuscle	Skin
Nociceptors	Pain	Distension (stretch)	Free nerve endings	Wall of gastrointestinal tract, pharynx, skin
Proprioceptors	Tension	Distension	Corpuscles of Ruffini	Skin and capsules in joints and ligaments
		Length changes	Muscle spindles	Skeletal muscle
		Tension changes	Golgi tendon organs	Between muscles and tendons
Thermoreceptors	Temperature change	Cold	Krause's end bulbs	Skin
		Heat	Corpuscles of Ruffini	Skin and capsules in joints and ligaments

From Previte JJ: *Human Physiology*, New York, 1983, McGraw-Hill.

There are several types of sensory receptors in the body, and the athletic trainer should be aware of their existence as well as of the types of stimuli that activate them (Table 3-1). Activation of some of these sense organs with therapeutic agents will decrease the athlete's perception of pain.

Six different types of receptor nerve endings are commonly described:

1. Meissner's corpuscles are activated by light touch.
2. Pacinian corpuscles respond to deep pressure.
3. Merkel's corpuscles respond to deep pressure, but more slowly than pacinian corpuscles, and also are activated by hair follicle deflection.
4. Ruffini corpuscles in the skin are sensitive to touch, tension, and possibly heat; those in the joint capsules and ligaments are sensitive to change in position.
5. Krause's end bulbs are thermoreceptors that react to a decrease in temperature and touch.[28]
6. Pain receptors, called **nociceptors** or **free nerve endings**, are sensitive to extreme mechanical, thermal, or chemical energy.[4] They respond to noxious stimuli—in other words, to impending or actual tissue damage (for example, cuts, burns, sprains, and so on). The term *nociceptive* is from the Latin *nocere*, to damage, and is used to imply pain information. These organs respond to superficial forms of heat and cold, analgesic balms, and massage.

Proprioceptors found in muscles, joint capsules, ligaments, and tendons provide information regarding joint position and muscle tone. The muscle spindles react to changes in length and tension when the muscle is stretched or contracted. The Golgi tendon organs also react to changes in length

■ **Clinical Decision-Making**   *Exercise 3-1*

The athletic trainer is interested in an injured athlete's subjective perception of pain following a TENS treatment designed to reduce pain. Describe the steps you would take to evaluate pain and suggest which pain scale you might choose to use.

nociceptor   Pain information or signals of pain stimuli.

accommodation   Adaption by the sensory receptors to various stimuli over an extended period of time.

and tension within the muscle. See Table 3-1 for a more complete listing.

Some sensory receptors respond to phasic activity and produce an impulse when the stimulus is increasing or decreasing, but not during a sustained stimulus. They adapt to a constant stimulus. Meissner's corpuscles and Pacinian corpuscles are examples of such receptors.

Tonic receptors produce impulses as long as the stimulus is present. Examples of tonic receptors are muscle spindles, free nerve endings, and Krause's end bulbs. The initial impulse is at a higher frequency than later impulses that occur during sustained stimulation.

Accommodation is the decline in generator potential and the reduction of frequency that occurs with a prolonged stimulus or with frequently repeated stimuli. If some physical agents are used too often or for too long, the receptors may adapt to or accommodate the stimulus and reduce their impulses. The **accommodation** phenomenon can be observed with the use of superficial hot and cold agents, such as ice packs and hydrocollator packs.

As a stimulus becomes stronger, the number or receptors excited increases, and the frequency of the impulses increases. This provides more electrical activity at the spinal cord level, which may facilitate the effects of some physical agents.

afferent   Conduction of a nerve impulse toward an organ.

efferent   Conduction of a nerve impulse away from an organ.

NEURAL TRANSMISSION

Afferent nerve fibers transmit impulses from the sensory receptors toward the brain while **efferent** fibers, such as motor neurons, transmit impulses from the brain toward the periphery.[31] First order or primary afferents transmit the impulses from the sensory receptor to the dorsal horn of the spinal cord (Figure 3-4). There are four different types of first order neurons (Table 3-2). A-alpha and A-beta are large diameter afferents that have a *high* (fast) conduction velocity, and A-delta and C fibers are small diameter fibers with *low* (slow) conduction velocity.

Second order afferent fibers carry sensory messages from the dorsal horn to the brain. Second order afferent fibers are categorized as wide dynamic range or nociceptive specific. The wide dynamic range second order afferents receive input from A-beta, A-delta, and C fibers. These second order afferents serve relatively large, overlapping receptor fields. The nociceptive specific second order afferents respond exclusively to noxious stimulation. They receive input only from A-delta and C fibers. These afferents serve smaller receptor fields that do not overlap. All of these neurons synapse with third order neurons, which carry information to various brain centers where the input is integrated, interpreted, and acted upon.

Facilitators and Inhibitors of Synaptic Transmission

For information to pass between neurons, a transmitter substance must be released from one neuron terminal (presynaptic membrane), enter the synaptic cleft, and attach to a receptor site on the next

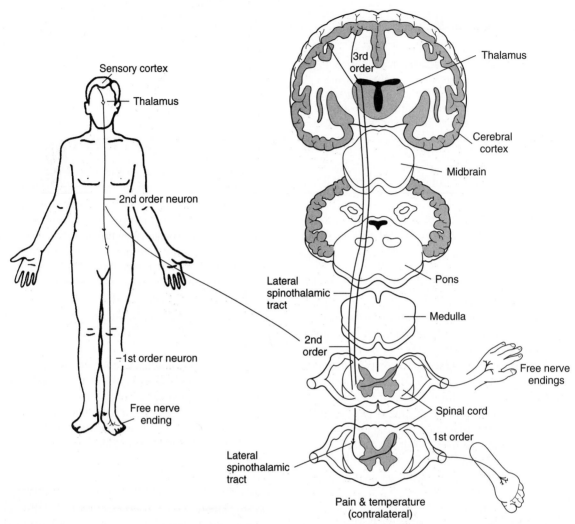

Figure 3-4 The lateral spinothalamic tract carries impulses of pain and temperature from the sensory receptors to the cortex.

neuron (postsynaptic membrane). In the past, all the activity within the synapse was attributed to **neurotransmitters**, such as acetylcholine. The neurotransmitters, when released in sufficient quantities, are known to cause depolarization of the postsynaptic neuron. In the absence of the neurotransmitter, no depolarization occurs.

It is now apparent that several compounds that are not true neurotransmitters can facilitate or inhibit synaptic activity. These compounds are classified as biogenic amine transmitters or neuroactive peptides. Serotonin and norepinephrine are examples of biogenic amine transmitters. About two dozen neuroactive peptides have been identified, including **substance P, glutamate enkephalins,** and **β-endorphin.**[3]

Serotonin and enkephalins are active in descending (efferent) pathways that block the pain

■ **TABLE 3-2**   Classification of Afferent Neurons

SIZE	TYPE	GROUP	SUBGROUP	DIAMETER (MICROMETERS)	CONDUCTION VELOCITY	RECEPTOR	STIMULUS
Large	A α	I	1a	12–20 (22)	70–120	Proprioceptive mechanoreceptor	Muscle velocity and length change, muscle shortening of rapid speed
	A α	I	1b				
	A β	II	Muscle	6–12	36–72	Proprioceptive mechanoreceptor	Muscle length information from touch and pacinian corpuscles
	A β	II	Skin			Cutaneous receptors	Touch, vibration, hair receptors
	A δ	III	Muscle	1–5 (6)	6(12)–36(80)	75% mechano-receptors and thermoreceptors	Temperature change
Small	A δ	III	Skin			25% nociceptors, mechanoreceptors and thermorecep-tors (hot and cold)	Noxious mechanical and temperature (> 45° C, < 10° C)
	C	IV	Muscle	0.3–1.0	0.4–1.0	50% mechano-receptors and thermoreceptors	Touch and Temperature
	C	IV	Skin			50% nociceptors, 20% mechano-receptors, and 30% thermoreceptors (hot and cold)	Noxious mechanical and temperature (> 45° C, < 10° C)

neurotransmitter   Substance that passes information between neurons. It is released from one neuron terminal (presynaptic membrane), enters the synaptic cleft, and attaches (binds) to a receptor on the next neuron (postsynaptic membrane). Substance P, enkephalins, serotonin, methionine, acetylcholine, and leucine enkephalin are neurotransmitters.

substance P   A peptide believed to be the neurotransmitter of small-diameter primary afferent. It is released from both ends of the neuron.

glutamate enkephalin   Neurotransmitter proteins that block the passage of noxious stimuli from first order to second order afferents. They inhibit the release of substance P and are produced by enkephalinergic neurons.

β-endorphin   A neurohormone derived from proopiomelanocortin (POMC). It is similar in structure and properties to morphine.

serotonin   A neurotransmitter found in neurons descending in the dorsolateral tract. The dorsolateral tract is thought to play a significant role in pain control. Serotonin is found in the vesicles in nerve endings that bind when released to postsynaptic membranes. Its action is terminated by re-uptake into presynaptic membranes. It is probably involved in both endogenous pain control and opiate analgesia. Increased levels of serotonin in the central nervous system are generally associated with increased analgesia.

....

endogenous opioids Opiate-like neuroactive peptide substances made by the body.

interneurons Neurons contained entirely in the central nervous system. They have no projections outside the spinal cord. Their function is to serve as relay stations within the central nervous system.

substantia gelatinosa (SG) Lamina II of the dorsal horn of the grey matter. Melzack and Wall[20] proposed that the SG is responsible for closing the gate to painful stimuli.

norepinephrine A neurotransmitter.

dynorphin An endogenous opioid derived from the prohormone prodynorphin.

....

message.[7] Enkephalin is an **endogenous** (made by the body) **opioid** that inhibits the depolarization of second order nociceptive nerve fibers. It is released from **interneurons**, enkephalin neurons with short axons. The enkephalins are stored in nerve-ending vesicles found in the **substantia gelatinosa (SG)** and in several areas of the brain. When released, enkephalin may bind to presynaptic or postsynaptic membranes.[3]

Norepinephrine is a biogenic amine transmitter that is released by the depolarization of some neurons and that binds to the postsynaptic membranes. Norepinephrine is found in several areas of the nervous system, including a tract that descends from the pons, which inhibits synaptic transmission between first order and second order nociceptive fibers, thus decreasing pain sensation.[16]

Other endogenous opioids may be active analgesic agents. These neuroactive peptides are released into the central nervous system and have an action similar to that of morphine, an opiate analgesic. There are specific opiate receptors located at strategic sites, called binding sites, to receive these compounds. β-endorphin, a 31-amino acid peptide, and **dynorphin** have potent analgesic effects. These are released within the central nervous system by mechanisms that are not fully understood at this time.

Nociception

A nociceptive neuron is one that transmits pain signals. Its cell body is in the dorsal root ganglion near the spinal cord. Approximately 25% of the myelinated A-delta and 50% of the unmyelinated C fibers contact nociceptors and are considered nociceptive, afferent neurons (see Table 3-2). Pain is initiated by a chemical stimulus. Injury to a cell due to trauma triggers the formation and release of *prostaglandin* and *bradykinin* that sensitize the nociceptors in and around the area of injury by lowering the depolarization threshold. This is referred to as *primary hyperalgesia*, in which the nerve's threshold to noxious stimuli is lowered, thus enhancing the pain response. Over a period of several hours, *secondary hyperalgesia* occurs as chemicals spread throughout the surrounding tissues, increasing the size of the painful area and creating hypersensitivity. Once a nociceptor is stimulated, it releases a neuropeptide (substance P) that initiates the electrical impulses along the afferent fiber toward the spinal cord. Substance P also serves as a transmitter substance between the first order afferent fiber and a second order afferent fiber (see Figure 3-4) at the dorsal horn of the spinal column.

The A-delta and C fibers that transmit sensations of pain and temperature have different diameters (A-delta are larger) and different conduction velocities (A-delta are faster). The C fibers also are connected to more of the nociceptive specific second order afferents. These differences result in two qualitatively different types of pain, termed fast and slow.[3] Fast pain is brief, well-localized, and well-matched to the stimulus—for example, the initial pain of an unexpected pinprick. Slow pain is an aching, throbbing, or burning sensation that is poorly localized and less specifically related to the stimulus. There is a delay in the perception of slow pain following injury, but the pain will continue long after the noxious stimulus is removed. Fast pain is transmitted over the larger, faster-conducting A-delta afferent neurons and originates from receptors located in the skin. Slow pain is transmitted by the C afferent neurons and originates from both superficial tissue (skin) and deeper tissue (ligaments and muscle).[3]

The various types of afferent fibers follow different courses as they ascend toward the brain. Some A-delta and most C afferent neurons enter the spinal cord through the dorsolateral tract of Lissauer and synapse in marginal zone (lamina 1) or the substantia gelatinosa (lamina 2) with a second order neuron.[16] Most nociceptive second order neurons ascend to higher centers along one of three tracts: (1) lateral spinothalamic tract, (2) spinoreticular tract, (3) and spinoencephalic tract, with the remainder ascending along the spinocervical tract or as projections to the cuneate and gracile nuclei of the medulla.[16] Approximately 90% of the wide dynamic range second order afferents terminate in the thalamus.[16] Third order neurons project to the sensory cortex and numerous other centers in the central nervous system. These projections allow us to perceive pain. They also permit the intergration of past experiences and emotions, which form our response to the pain experience. These connections are also believed to be parts of complex circuits that the athletic trainer may stimulate to pain management. Most analgesic physical agents are believed to slow or block the impulses ascending along the A-delta and C afferent neuron pathways through direct input into the dorsal horn or through descending mechanisms. These pathways are discussed in more detail in the following section.

NEUROPHYSIOLOGICAL EXPLANATIONS OF PAIN CONTROL

The neurophysiologic mechanisms of pain control through stimulation of cutaneous receptors have not been fully explained.[32] Much of what is known—and current theory—is the result of work involving electroacupuncture and transcutaneous electrical nerve stimulation. However, this information often provides an explanation for the analgesic response to other modalities, such as massage, analgesic balms, and moist heat.

The concepts of the analgesic response to cutaneous receptor stimulation presented here were first proposed by Melzack and Wall[20] and Castel.[7] These models essentially present three analgesic mechanisms:

1. Stimulation from ascending A-beta afferents results in the blocking of impulses (pain messages) carried along A-delta and C afferent fibers.
2. Stimulation of descending pathways in the dorsolateral tract of the spinal cord by A-delta and C fiber afferent input results in a blocking of the impulses carried along the A-delta and C afferent fibers.
3. The stimulation of A-delta and C afferent fibers causes the release of endogenous opioids (β-endorphin), resulting in a prolonged activation of descending analgesic pathways.

These theories or models are not necessarily mutually exclusive. Recent evidence suggests that pain relief may result from combinations of dorsal horn and central nervous system activity.[2,10]

A decrease in input along nociceptive afferents also results in pain relief. Cooling afferent fibers decreases the rate at which they conduct impulses. Thus, a 20-minute application of cold is effective in relieving pain because of the decrease in activity, rather than an increase in activity, along afferent pathways. In athletic training, the use of ice or cryotherapy to modulate pain is perhaps the most commonly used technique involving gate control.

Blocking the Pain Impulses with Ascending A-beta Input

Pain modulation due to sensory stimulation and the resultant increase in the impulses in the large diameter (A-beta) afferent fibers was proposed by the *gate control theory of pain*[20] (Figure 3-5). Impulses ascending on these fibers stimulate the substantia gelatinosa as they enter the dorsal horn of the spinal cord. Stimulation of the substantia gelatinosa inhibits synaptic transmission in the large and small (A-delta and C) fiber afferent pathways. The

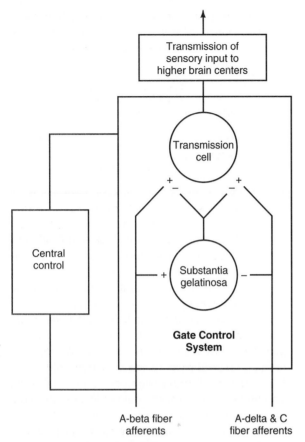

Figure 3-5 The gate control system. Increases A-beta input and stimulates the substantia gelatinosa, which inhibits the flow of afferent input to sensory centers.

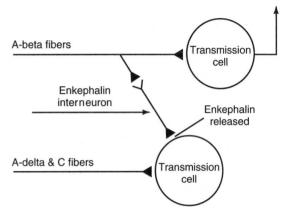

Figure 3-6 Presynaptic inhibition of dorsal horn synapse transmission due to A-beta fiber stimulation at enkephalin interneurons.

"pain message" carried along the smaller diameter fibers is not transmitted to the second order neurons and never reaches sensory centers. The balance between the input from the small- and large-diameter afferents determines how much of the pain message is blocked or gated.

The concept of sensory stimulation for pain relief, as proposed by the gate control theory, has empirical support. Rubbing a contusion, applying moist heat, or massaging sore muscles decreases the perception of pain. The analgesic response to these treatments is attributed to the increased stimulation of large-diameter afferent fibers.

The gate control theory also proposes that A-delta and C fiber impulses inhibit the substantia gelatinosa, facilitating the perception of pain. The sensation of pain does not diminish rapidly because free nerve endings do not accommodate and the afferent impulses from them "open the gate" to further pain message transmission.

The discovery and isolation of endogenous opioids in the 1970s led to new theories of pain relief. Castel[8] introduced an endogenous opioid analogue to the gate control theory (Figure 3-6).[8] This theory proposes that increased neural activity in A-alpha and A-beta primary afferent pathways trigger a release of enkephalin from enkephalin interneurons found in the dorsal horn. These neuroactive amines inhibit synaptic transmission in the A-delta and C fiber afferent pathways. The end result, as in the gate control theory, is that the pain message is blocked before it reaches sensory levels.

Descending Pain Control Mechanisms

The gate control theory[20] proposed a second analgesic mechanism that involves descending efferent fibers. The central control, originating in higher centers of the central nervous system, could affect the dorsal horn gating process. Impulses from the thalamus and brain stem **(central biasing)** are

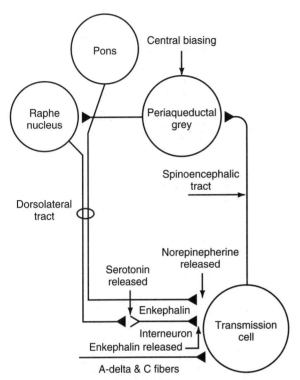

Figure 3-7 Stimulation of the periaqueductal grey region of the midbrain and the raphe nucleus in the pons and medulla by ascending neural input, especially from A-delta and C fiber afferents, and possibly central biasing, activates the descending mechanism.

central biasing A theory of pain modulation where higher centers, such as the cerebral cortex, influence the perception of and response to pain.

periaqueductal grey A midbrain structure that plays an important role in descending tracts that inhibit synaptic transmission of noxious input in the dorsal horn.

raphe nucleus Part of the brain that is known to inhibit pain impulses being transmitted through the ascending system.

enkephalinergic interneurons Neurons with short axons that release enkephalin. They are widespread in the central nervous system and are found in the substantia gelatinosa, nucleus raphae magnus, and periaqueductual grey matter.

carried into the dorsal horn on efferent fibers in the dorsal or dorsal lateral paths (or tracts). Impulses from the higher centers act to close the gate and block transmission of the pain message at the dorsal horn synapse. Through this system, it was theorized, previous experiences, emotional influences, sensory perception, and other factors could influence the transmission of the pain message and the perception of pain.

Castel[7] offers an endogenous opioid model of descending influence over dorsal horn synapse activity (Figure 3-7). Stimulation of the **periaqueductal grey** region of the midbrain and the **raphe nucleus** in the pons and medulla by ascending neural input, especially from A-delta and C fiber afferents and possibly central biasing, activates the descending mechanism. The periaqueductal grey stimulates the raphe nucleus. The raphe nucleus in turn sends impulses along serontonergic efferent fibers in the dorsal lateral tract, which synapse with **enkephalin interneurons**. The interneurons release enkephalin into the dorsal horn, inhibiting the synaptic transmission of impulses to the second order afferent neurons.

More recently, a second descending, norandrenergic pathway projecting from the pons to the dorsal horn has been identified.[16] The significance of these parallel pathways is not fully understood. It is also not known if these norandrenergic fibers directly inhibit dorsal horn synapses or stimulate the enkephalin interneurons.

This model provides a physiologic explanation for the analgesic response to brief, intense stimulation. The analgesia following accupressure and the use of some transcutaneous electrical nerve simulators (TENS), such as point simulators, is attributed to this descending pain control mechanism.

β-Endorphin and Dynorphin

There is evidence that stimulation of the small-diameter afferents (A-delta and C) can stimulate the release of other endogenous opioids.[8,10,19,23,25,27,29]

■ Analogy   *3-1*

Blocking pain along ascending and descending pathways is like closing a gate to certain types of sensory information and opening a gate to allow the passage of other types of sensory input. The athletic trainer can use different modalities set at specific treatment parameters to open or close that gate according to specific desired treatment responses.

β-endorphin (BEP) and dynorphin are neuroactive peptides with potent analgesic affects. The term **endorphin** refers to an opiate-like substance produced by the body. The mechanisms regulating the release of BEP and dynorphin have not been fully elucidated. However, it is apparent that these large endogenous substances play a role in the analgesic response to some forms of stimuli used in the treatment of athletes in pain.

One of the sources of BEP is the anterior pituitary. Here it shares the prohormone propiomelanocortin (POMC) with **adrenocorticotropin (ACTH)**. Prolonged (20 to 40 minutes) small-diameter afferent fiber stimulation has been thought to trigger the release of BEP from the anterior pituitary gland. Electro-acupuncture, and possibly TENS with long phase durations and low pulse rates (1 to 5 pulses/second), will cause small-diameter afferent fiber depolarization necessary for BEP release.[29] The anterior pituitary gland may not, however, be a source of BEP in low pulse rate, long pulse width, TENS-induced analgesia.[11] These results and the recognition that BEP does not readily cross the blood-brain barrier[3] suggest that if BEP or other endogenous opioids are active analgesic agents within the central nervous system, they are released from areas within the brain.

The neurons in the hypothalamus that send projections to the PAG and noradrenergic nuclei in the brain stem contain BEP. It is possible that BEP released from these neurons by stimulation of the hypothalamus is responsible for the analgesic response to the treatments[6] (Figure 3-8).

Dynorphin, a more recently isolated endogenous opioid, is found in the PAG, rostroventral medulla, and the dorsal horn.[16] It has been demon-

■ **Clinical Decision-Making**   *Exercise 3-2*

A female gymnast is complaining of pain in the low back from a muscle strain. The athletic trainer plans to incorporate a modality that will affect the ascending pathways, in effect "closing the gate" to ascending pain fibers. What modalities can be used to take advantage of the gate control theory of pain modulation?

endorphins   Endogenous opioids whose actions have analgesic properties (i.e., β-endorphin).

ACTH   Adrenocorticotropic hormone. This hormone stimulates the release of glucocorticoids (cortisol) from the adrenal glands.

strated that dynorphin is released during electroacupuncture.[14] Dynorphin may be responsible for suppressing the response to noxious mechanical stimulation.[16]

Summary of Pain Control Mechanisms

The body's pain control mechanisms are probably not mutually exclusive. Rather, analgesia is the result of overlapping processes. It is also important to realize that the theories presented are only models. They are useful in conceptualizing the perception of pain and pain relief. These models will help the athletic trainer understand the effects of therapeutic modalities and form a sound rationale for modality application. As more research is conducted and as the mysteries of pain and neurophysiology are solved, new models will emerge. The athletic trainer should adapt these models to fit new developments.

Cognitive Influences

Pain perception and the response to a painful experience may be influenced by a variety of cognitive processes, including anxiety, attention, depression, past pain experiences, and cultural influences.

■ **Clinical Decision-Making**   *Exercise 3-3*

In addition to managing pain through the use of therapeutic modalities, the athletic trainer should make every effort to encourage central biasing the cognitive processes. What techniques can be taught to the athlete to take advantage of the cognitive aspects of pain modulation?

■ **Clinical Decision-Making**   *Exercise 3-4*

An athlete asks the athletic trainer to explain why electric stimulation of a trigger point can help reduce pain in her shoulder. What is the explanation?

Mechanisms of pain control

- Blocking ascending pathways
- Blocking descending pathways
- Release of β-endorphin

These individual aspects of pain expression are mediated by higher centers in the cortex in ways that are not clearly understood. They may influence both the sensory discriminative and motivational affective dimensions of pain.

Many mental processes modulate the perception of pain through descending systems. Behavior modification, the excitement of the moment, happiness, positive feelings, **focusing** (directed attention toward specific stimuli), hypnosis, and suggestion may modulate pain perception. Past experiences, cultural background, personality, motivation to play, aggression, anger, and fear are all factors that could facilitate or inhibit pain perception. Strong central inhibition may mask severe injury for a period of time. At such times, evaluation of the injury is quite difficult.

Athletes with chronic pain may become very depressed and experience a loss of fitness. They tend to be less active and may have altered ap-

focusing   Narrowing attention to the appropriate stimuli in the environment.

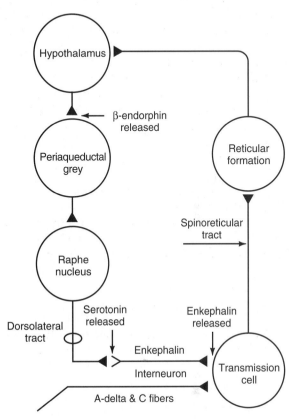

Figure 3-8   The neurons in the hypothalamus that send projections to the periaqueductal grey and noradrenergic nuclei in the brain stem contain β-endorphin. It is possible that β-endorphin released from these neurons by stimulation of the hypothalamus is responsible for the analgesic response to the treatments.

petites and sleep habits. They have a decreased will to work and exercise and often develop a reduced sex drive. They may turn to self-abusive patterns of behavior. Tricyclic drugs are often used to inhibit serotonin depletion for the athlete with chronic pain.

Just as pain may be inhibited by central modulation, it may also arise from central origins. Phobias, fear, depression, anger, grief, and hostility are all capable of producing pain in the absence of local pathologic processes. In addition, pain memory, which is associated with old injuries, may result in pain perception and pain response that are out of proportion to a new, often minor, injury. Substance abuse can also alter and confound the perception of pain. Substance abuse may cause the chronic pain athlete to become more depressed or may lead to depression and psychosomatic pain.

PAIN MANAGEMENT

How should the athletic trainer approach pain? First, the source of the pain must be identified. Unidentified pain may hide a serious disorder, and treatment of such pain may delay the appropriate treatment of the disorder. Once a diagnosis has been made, many physical agents can provide pain relief. The athletic trainer should match the therapeutic agent to each athlete's situation. Casts and braces may prevent the application of ice or moist heat. However, TENS electrodes often can be positioned under a cast or brace for pain relief. Following acute injuries, ice may be the therapeutic agent of choice because of the effect of cold on the inflammatory process. There is not one "best" therapeutic agent for pain control. The athletic trainer must select the therapeutic agent that is most appropriate for each athlete, based on the knowledge of the modalities and professional judgment. In no situation should the athletic trainer apply a therapeutic agent without first developing a clear rationale for the treatment.

In general, physical agents can be used to
1. Stimulate large-diameter afferent fibers. This can be done with TENS, massage, and analgesic balms.
2. Decrease pain fiber transmission velocity with cold or ultrasound.
3. Stimulate small-diameter afferent fibers and descending pain control mechanisms with accupressure, deep massage, or TENS over acupuncture points or trigger points.

4. Stimulate a release of BEP or other endogenous opioids through prolonged small-diameter fiber stimulation with TENS.[28]

Other useful pain control strategies include the following:
1. Encourage central biasing through cognitive processes, such as motivation, tension diversion, focusing, relaxation techniques, positive thinking, thought stopping, and self-control.
2. Minimize the tissue damage through the application of proper first aid and immobilization.
3. Maintain a line of communication with the athlete. Let the athlete know what to expect following an injury. Pain, swelling, dysfunction, and atrophy will occur following injury. The athlete's anxiety over these events will increase his or her perception of pain. Often, an athlete who has been told what to expect by someone he or she trusts will be less anxious and suffer less pain.
4. Recognize that all pain, even psychosomatic pain, is very real to the athlete.
5. Encourage supervised exercise to encourage blood flow, promote nutrition, increase metabolic activity, and reduce stiffness and guarding if the activity will not cause further harm to the athlete.

The physician may choose to prescribe oral or injectable medications in the treatment of the athlete. The most commonly used medications are classified as analgesics, anti-inflammatory agents, or both. The athletic trainer should become familiar with these drugs and note if the athlete is taking any medications. It is also important to work with the referring physician to assure that the athlete takes the medications appropriately.

The athletic trainer's approach to the athlete has a great impact on the success of the treatment. The athlete will not be convinced of the efficacy and importance of the treatment unless the athletic trainer appears confident about it. The athletic trainer must make the athlete a participant rather than a passive spectator in the treatment and rehabilitation process.

The goal of most treatment programs is to encourage early pain-free exercise. The physical agents used to control pain do little to promote tissue healing. They should be used to relieve acute pain following injury or surgery or to control pain and other symptoms, such as swelling, to promote progressive exercise. The athletic trainer should not lose sight of the effects of the physical agents or the importance of progressive exercise in restoring the athlete's functional ability.

Reducing the perception of pain is as much an art as a science. Selection of the proper physical agent, proper application, and marketing are all important and will continue to be so even as we increase our understanding of the neurophysiology of pain. There is still the need for a good empirical rationale for the use of a physical agent. The athletic trainer is encouraged to keep abreast of the neurophysiology of pain and the physiology of tissue healing to maintain a current scientific basis for selecting modalities and managing the pain experienced by his or her athletes.

Summary

1. Pain is a response to a noxious stimulus that is subjectively modified by past experiences and expectations.
2. Pain is classified as either acute or chronic and can exhibit many different patterns.
3. Early reduction of pain in a treatment program will facilitate therapeutic exercise.
4. Stimulation of sensory receptors via the therapeutic modalities can modify the athlete's perception of pain.
5. Four mechanisms of pain control may explain the analgesic affects of physical agents:
   a. Decreased transmission of input along nociceptive pathways.
   b. Dorsal horn modulation due to the input from large-diameter afferents through a gate control system, the release of enkephalins, or both.
   c. Descending efferent fiber activation due to the effects of small-fiber afferent input on higher centers including the thalamus, raphe nucleus, and periaqueductal grey region.
   d. The central release of endogenous opioids including β-endorphin through prolonged small diameter afferent stimulation.
6. Pain perception may be influenced by a variety of cognitive processes mediated by the higher brain centers.
7. The selection of a therapeutic modality for controlling pain should be based on current knowledge of neurophysiology and the psychology of pain.
8. The application of physical agents for the control of pain should not occur until the diagnosis of the injury has been established.
9. The selection of a therapeutic modality for managing pain should be based on establishing the primary cause of pain.

Review Questions

1. What is a basic definition of pain?
2. What are the different types of pain?
3. What are the different assessment scales available to help the athletic trainer determine the extent of pain perception?
4. What are the characteristics of the various sensory receptors?
5. How does the nervous system relay information about painful stimuli?
6. Describe how the gate control mechanism of pain modulation may be used to modulate pain.
7. How do the descending pain control mechanisms function to modulate pain?

8. What are the opiate-like substances and how do they act to modulate pain?
9. How can pain perception be modified by cognitive factors?

10. How can the athletic trainer help modulate pain during a rehabilitation program?

 ## Self-Test Questions

T/F

1. Both sclerotomic and radiating pain may cause pain away from the site of the disorder.
2. Afferent nerve fibers conduct impulses from the brain to peripheral sites.
3. Both biogenic amines, such as serotonin, and neuroactive peptides, such as β-endorphin, affect synaptic activity.

Multiple Choice

4. Which of the following is NOT a method of pain assessment?
   a. McGill pain questionnaire
   b. Snellen test
   c. visual analogue scales
   d. numeric pain scale
5. Pain receptors in the body are called _____ .
   a. Meissner's corpuscles
   b. Krause's end bulbs
   c. Pacinian corpuscles
   d. nociceptors
6. Which of the following plays a role in transmitting sensations of pain?
   a. substance P
   b. enkephalin
   c. dynorphin
   d. serotonin

7. Which of the following is/are characteristic(s) of A-delta fibers?
   a. large-diameter fibers
   b. fast conduction velocities
   c. transmit brief, localized pain
   d. all of the above
8. Stimulation of the substantia gelatinosa occurs in the _____ theory of pain.
   a. central biasing
   b. descending
   c. gate control
   d. enkephalin release
9. β-endorphin, an endogenous opioid, is released from the _____ .
   a. hypothalamus
   b. anterior pituitary gland
   c. raphe nucleus
   d. a and b
10. Which of the following cognitive processes may affect pain perception?
   a. depression
   b. past pain experiences
   c. both a and b
   d. neither a nor b

Solutions to Clinical Decision-Making Exercises

3-1 After conducting a detailed evaluation, there are a number of available options including visual analogue scales, pain charts, the McGill Pain Questionnaire, the Activity Pattern Indicators Pain Profile, and numeric pain scales. Numeric pain scales, in which the athlete is asked to rate his or her pain on a scale from 1 to 10, are perhaps the most widely used in the athletic training setting.

3-2 The modality selected should provide a significant amount of cutaneous input that would be transmitted to the spinal cord along A-beta fibers. The modalities of choice may include various types of heat or cold, electrical stimulating currents, counterirritants (analgesic balms), or massage.

3-3 The athletic trainer may choose to use relaxation techniques, tension diversion, focusing, positive thinking, thought stopping, and self-control techniques. Certainly the cognitive perception of pain and the ability to control that perception is an aspect of rehabilitation

that should be taken very seriously by the athletic trainer.

3-4 The athletic trainer should explain that stimulating the trigger point with an electrical stimulating current will trigger the release of a chemical (β-endorphin) in the brain that will act to modulate pain in the shoulder.

References

1. Addison, R: Chronic pain syndrome, *Am. J. Med.* 77:54, 1985.

2. Anderson, S, Ericson, T, and Holmgren, E: Electroacupuncture affects pain threshold measured with electrical stimulation of teeth, *Brain* 63:393–396, 1973.

3. Berne, R, and Levy, M: *Physiology*, St. Louis, 1988, Mosby.

4. Bishop, B: Pain: its physiology and rationale for management, *Phys Ther* 60:13–37, 1980.

5. Bonica, J: *The management of pain.* Philadelphia, 1990, Lea & Febiger.

6. Bowsher, D: Central pain mechanisms. In Wells, P, Frampton, V, and Bowsher, D, editors: *Pain management in physical therapy.* Norwalk, Conn. 1988, Appleton & Lange.

7. Castel, J: *Pain management: acupuncture and transcutaneous electrical nerve stimulation techniques,* Lake Bluff, Ill., 1979, Pain Control Services.

8. Chapman, C, and Benedetti, C: Analgesia following electrical stimulation: partial reversal by a narcotic antagonist, *Life Sci.* 26:44–48, 1979.

9. Cheng, R, and Pomeranz, B: Electroacupuncture analgesia could be mediated by at least two pain relieving mechanisms: endorphin and non-endorphin systems, *Life Sci.* 25:1957–1962, 1979.

10. Clement-Jones, V, McLaughlin, L, and Tomlin, S: Increased beta-endorphin but not met-enkephalin levels in human cerebrospinal fluid after electroacupuncture for recurrent pain, *Lancet* 2:946–948, 1980.

11. Denegar, G, Perrin, D, and Rogol, A: Influence of transcutaneous electrical nerve stimulation on pain, range of motion and serum cortisol concentration in females with induced delayed onset muscle soreness, *JOSPT* 11:101–103, 1989.

12. Dickerman, J: The use of pain profiles in sports medicine practice, *Family Practice Recertification* 14(3): 35–44, 1992.

13. Gatchel, R: Million behavioral health inventory: its utility in predicting physical functioning athletes with low back pain, *Arch Phys Med Rehab* 67:878, 1986.

14. Ho, W, and Wen, H: Opioid-like activity in the cerebrospinal fluid of pain athletes treated by electroacupuncture, *Neuropharmacology* 28: 961–966, 1989.

15. Huskisson, E: Visual Analogue scales. Pain measurement and assessment. In Melzack, R, editor: *Pain measurement and assessment,* New York, 1983, Raven Press.

16. Jessell, T, and Kelly, D: Pain and Analgesia. In Kandel, E, Schwartz, J, and Jessell T, editors: *Principles of neural science.* Norwalk, Conn., 1991, Appleton & Lange.

17. Kuland, DN: The injured athletes' pain, *Curr Concepts Pain* 1:3–10, 1983.

18. Margoles, M: The pain chart: spatial properties of pain. Pain measurement and assessment. In Melzack, R., editor: *Pain measurement and assessment,* New York, 1983, Raven Press.

19. Mayer, D, Price, D, and Rafii, A: Antagonism of acupuncture analgesia in man by the narcotic antagonist naloxone, *Brain Res.* 121:368–372, 1977.

20. Melzack, R, and Wall, P: Pain mechanisms: a new theory, *Science* 150:971–979, 1965.

21. Melzack, R: Concepts of pain measurement. In Melzack, R., editor: *Pain measurement and assessment,* New York, 1983, Raven Press.

22. Merskey, H, Albe Fessard, D, and Bonica, J: Pain terms: a list with definitions and notes on usage, *Pain* 6:249–252, 1979.

23. Pomeranz, B, and Paley, D: Brain opiates at work in acupuncture, *New Scientist* 73:12–13, 1975.

24. Pomeranz, B, and Chiu, D: Naloxone blockade of acupuncture analgesia: enkephalin implicated, *Life Sci.* 19:1757–1762, 1976.

25. Pomeranz, B, and Paley, D: Electro-acupuncture hypoalgesia is mediated by afferent impulses: an electrophysiological study in mice, *Exp. Neurol.* 66:398–402, 1979.

26. Previte, J: *Human physiology,* New York, 1983, McGraw-Hill, Inc.

27. Salar, G, Job, I, and Mingringo, S: Effects of transcutaneous electrotherapy on CSF beta-endorphin content in athletes without pain problems, *Pain* 10:169–172, 1981.

28. Sjolund, B, and Eriksson, M: Electroacupuncture and endogenous morphines, *Lancet* 2:1085, 1976.

29. Sjoland, B, and Eriksson, M: Increased cerebrospinal fluid levels of endorphins after electro-acupuncture, *Acta Physiol. Scand.* 100:382–384, 1977.

30. Wen, H, Ho, W, and Ling, N: The influence of electroacupuncture on naloxone: induces morphine with-

drawal: elevation of immunoassayable beta-endorphin activity in the brain but not in the blood, *Am. J. Clin. Med.* 7:237–240, 1979.

31. Willis, W, and Grossman, R: *Medical Neurobiology*, ed 3, St. Louis, 1981, Mosby.

32. Wolf, S: Neurophysiologic mechanisms in pain modulation: relevance to TENS. In Manheimer, J, and Lampe, G, editors: *Sports medicine applications of TENS*, Philadelphia, 1984, FA Davis Co.

PART TWO

Thermal Modalities

CHAPTER 4

Infrared Modalities (Therapeutic Heat and Cold)

Gerald W. Bell and William E. Prentice

Study Resources

Refer to the lab exercises in the accompanying Laboratory Manual, as well as eSims which simulates the athletic training certification exam at www.mhhe.com/esims. Also, check out the competency information found at www.mhhe.com/prentice11e. For more online study resources, visit our Health and Human Performance Website at www.mhhe.com/hhp/.

Following completion of this chapter, the student athletic trainer will be able to

- Explain how the infrared modalities are classified in the electromagnetic spectrum.

- Differentiate between the physiologic effects of therapeutic heat and cold.

- Describe the contemporary modalities of the infrared spectrum in cryotherapy and thermotherapy.

- Categorize the indications and contraindications for each infrared modality discussed.

- Indicate how these various infrared modalities may be applied.

- Explain how the athletic trainer can use the infrared modalities to reduce pain.

Of the therapeutic modalities discussed in this text, perhaps none are more commonly used by athletic trainers than infrared modalities. As indicated in Chapter 1, the infrared region of the electromagnetic spectrum falls between the microwave diathermy and the visible light portions of the spectrum in terms of wavelength and frequency. There seems to be a great deal of misunderstanding regarding which of the modalities used in a sports medicine setting are actually classified as infrared modalities. Traditionally, the term infrared heating conjures up visions of infrared lamps and bakers. However, it must be re-emphasized that most of the heat and cold modalities, such as hydrocollator packs, paraffin baths, hot and cold whirlpools, and ice packs, as well as infrared lamps, produce forms of radiant energy that have wavelengths and frequencies that fall into the infrared region (see Table 1-4). This chapter will include a discussion of all the modalities that fall into the infrared portion of the electromagnetic spectrum.

MECHANISMS OF HEAT TRANSFER

Easy application and convenience of use of hot and cold modalities provide the athletic trainer with the necessary tools for primary care of sports injuries. Heat is defined as the internal vibration of the molecules within a body. The transmission of heat oc-

■ **TABLE 4-1**   Mechanisms of Heat Transfer of the Various Modalities

CONDUCTION	CONVECTION	RADIATION	CONVERSION
Ice massage	Hot whirlpool	Infrared lamps	Ultrasound
Cold packs	Cold whirlpool	LASER	Diathermy
Hydrocollator packs	Fluidotherapy	Ultraviolet light**	
Cold spray			
Ice immersion			
Contrast baths*			
Cryo-Cuff			
Cryokinetics			
Paraffin bath			

*Contrast Baths could also involve convection if hot or cold whirlpools are being used.
**Ultraviolet therapy does not involve a tissue temperature change, but the energy from the ultraviolet source radiates to the skin surface

Mechanisms of heat transfer

- Conduction
- Convection
- Radiation
- Conversion

curs by three mechanisms: **conduction, convection**, and **radiation**. A fourth mechanism of heat transfer, **conversion**, is discussed in Chapter 15.

Conduction occurs when the body is in direct contact with the heat or cold source. Convection occurs when particles (air or water) move across the body, thus creating a temperature variation. Radiation is the transfer of heat from a warmer source to a cooler source through a conducting medium, such as air (e.g., infrared lamps). The body may either gain or lose heat through any of these processes of heat transfer. The **infrared** modalities discussed in this chapter use these methods of heat transfer to effect a tissue temperature increase or decrease.

A fourth method of heat transfer, **conversion**, in which heat is generated from another energy form such as sound, electricity or chemical agents is more applicable to ultrasound (Chapter 5) and diathermy (Chapter 6). Table 4-1 Summarizes the mechanisms of heat transfer for the various modalities.

conduction   Heat loss or gain through direct contact.

convection   Heat loss or gain through the movement of water molecules across the skin.

radiation   The process of emitting energy from some source, in the form of waves. A method of heat transfer through which heat can either be gained or lost.

infrared   That portion of the electromagnetic spectrum associated with thermal changes; located adjacent to the red portion of the visible light spectrum.

conversion   Changing from one energy form into another.

thermotherapy   The use of heat in the treatment of pathology or disease.

USING THE INFRARED MODALITIES APPROPRIATELY

The athletic trainer should not use an infrared modality randomly without reviewing its benefits. Placing the athlete in the whirlpool or a slush bucket of ice simply because these two modalities are available is not an acceptable treatment technique.

Heating techniques used for therapeutic purposes are referred to as **thermotherapy**.

cryotherapy The use of cold in the treatment of pathology or diseases.

hydrotherapy Cryotherapy and thermotherapy techniques that use water as the medium for heat transfer.

analgesia Loss of sensitivity to pain.

Thermotherapy is used when a rise in tissue temperature is the goal of treatment. The use of cold, or **cryotherapy**, is most effective in the acute stages of the healing process immediately following injury, when a loss of tissue temperature is the goal of therapy. Cold applications can be continued into the reconditioning stage of injury management. Thermotherapy and cryotherapy are included in this section on the basis of their classification in the electromagnetic spectrum. The term **hydrotherapy** can be applied to any cryotherapy or thermotherapy technique that uses water as the medium for tissue temperature exchange.

The electromagnetic spectrum has a relatively large region of radiations designated as infrared. The infrared wavelength provides the radiant energy that is used therapeutically (see Table 1-2). Penetration of the energy is dependent on the source but is generally considered to be a superficial form of treatment.

While this chapter is concerned primarily with application of the infrared modalities and their physiologic effects, several of the other modalities discussed in this text (e.g., the diathermies and ultrasound) cause similar physiologic responses. Specifically, the effects of heat and cold therapy discussed in this chapter may be applied to any modality that alters tissue temperature.

Heating and cooling agents can be used successfully to treat injuries and trauma.[26] The athletic trainer must know the injury mechanism and specific pathology as well as the physiologic effects of the heating and cooling agents to establish a consistent treatment schedule.

CLINICAL APPLICATIONS FOR THE INFRARED MODALITIES

The physiologic effects that occur from using heat and cold are rarely the result of direct absorption of infrared energy. There is general agreement that no form of infrared energy can have a depth of penetration greater than 1 cm.[1] Thus, the effects of the infrared modalities are primarily superficial and directly affect the cutaneous blood vessels and the cutaneous nerve receptors.[66]

Absorption of infrared energy cutaneously increases and decreases circulation subcutaneously in both the muscle and fat layers. If the energy is absorbed cutaneously over a long enough period of time to raise the temperature of the circulating blood, the hypothalamus will reflexively increase blood flow to the underlying tissue. Likewise, absorption of cold cutaneously can decrease blood flow via a similar mechanism in the area of treatment.[1]

Thus, if the primary treatment goal is a tissue temperature increase with a corresponding increase in blood flow to the deeper tissues, it is perhaps wiser to choose a modality, such as diathermy or ultrasound, that produces energy that can penetrate the cutaneous tissues and be directly absorbed by the deep tissues. If the primary treatment goal is to reduce tissue temperature and decrease blood flow to an injured area, the superficial application of ice or cold is the only modality capable of producing such a response.

Perhaps the most effective use of the infrared modalities should be to provide **analgesia** or to reduce the sensation of pain associated with injury. The infrared modalities stimulate primarily the cutaneous nerve receptors. Through one of the mechanisms of pain modulation discussed in Chapter 3, most likely the gate control theory, hyperstimulation of these nerve receptors by heating or cooling reduces pain. Within the sports medicine philosophy of an aggressive program of rehabilitation, the reduction of pain as a means of facilitating therapeutic exercise is a common practice. As emphasized in the preface to this text, therapeutic modalities are perhaps best used as an adjunct to therapeutic exercise.

- Infrared modalities should be used primarily to provide analgesia and reduce pain

Certainly, this should be a prime consideration when selecting an infrared modality for use in any treatment program.

Continued investigation and research into the use of heat and cold is warranted to provide useful guidance for the athletic trainer. Heat and cold applications, when used properly and efficiently, will provide the athletic trainer with the tools to enhance recovery and provide the athlete with optimal health care management. Thermotherapy and cryotherapy are only two of the tools available to assist in the well-being and reconditioning of the injured athlete.

Effects of Tissue Temperature Change on Circulation

Local application of heat or cold is indicated for thermal physiologic effects. The main physiologic effect is on superficial circulation because of the response of the temperature receptors in the skin and the sympathetic nervous system.

Circulation through the skin serves two major functions: (1) nutrition of the skin tissues and (2) conduction of heat from internal structures of the body to the skin so that heat can be removed from the body.[36] The circulatory apparatus is composed of two major vessel types: (1) arteries, capillaries, and veins, and (2) vascular structures for heating the skin. Two types of vascular structures are the subcutaneous venous plexus, which holds large quantities of blood that heat the surface of the skin, and the arteriovenous anastomosis, which provides vascular communication between arteries and venous plexuses.[24] The walls of the plexuses have strong muscular coats innervated by sympathetic vasoconstrictor nerve fibers that secrete norepinephrine. When constricted, blood flow is reduced in the venous plexus to almost nothing. When maximally dilated, there is an extremely rapid flow of blood into the plexuses. The arteriovenous anastomoses are found principally in the volar or palmar surfaces of the hands and feet, the lips, the nose, and the ears.

When cold is applied directly to the skin, the skin vessels progressively constrict to a temperature of about 10° C (50° F), at which point they reach their maximum constriction. This constriction results primarily from increased sensitivity of the vessels to nerve stimulation, but it probably also results at least partly from a reflex that passes to the spinal cord and then back to the vessels. At temperatures below 10° C (50° F), the vessels begin to dilate. This dilation is caused by a direct local effect of the cold on the vessels themselves, producing paralysis of the contractile mechanism of the vessel wall or blockage of the nerve impulses coming to the vessels. At temperatures approaching 0° C (32° F), the skin vessels frequently reach maximum vasodilation.

Skin plexuses are supplied with sympathetic vasoconstrictor innervation. In times of circulatory stress, such as exercise, hemorrhage, or anxiety, sympathetic stimulation of these skin plexuses forces large quantities of blood into internal vessels. Thus, the subcutaneous veins of the skin act as an important blood reservoir, often providing blood to serve other circulatory functions when needed.[36]

Three types of sensory receptors are found in the subepithelial tissue: cold, warm, and pain. The pain receptors are free nerve endings. Temperature and pain are transmitted to the brain via the lateral spinothalamic tract (see Chapter 3). The nerve fibers respond differently at different temperatures. Both cold and warm receptors discharge minimally at 33° C (91.4° F). Cold receptors discharge between 10° C and 41° C (50° F and 105.8° F), with a maximum discharge in the 37.5° C to 40° C (99.5° F to 104° F) range. Above 45° C (113° F), cold receptors begin to discharge again and pain receptors are stimulated. Nerve fibers transmitting sensations of pain respond to the temperature extremes. Both warm and cold receptors adapt

■ Analogy *4-1*

....

Using heat or cold can be like an on/off switching mechanism for blood flow. Heat is the on switch that may be used to increase circulation, while cold is the off switch that minimizes circulation.

rapidly to temperature change; the more rapid the temperature change, the more rapid the receptor adaptation. The number of warm and cold receptors in any given small surface area is thought to be few. Therefore, small temperature changes are difficult to perceive in localized areas. Larger surface areas stimulate summation of thermal signals. These larger patterns of excitation activate the vasomotor centers and the hypothalamic center.[60,63] Stimulation of the anterior hypothalamus causes cutaneous vasodilation, while stimulation of the posterior hypothalamus causes cutaneous vasoconstriction.[36,87]

The cutaneous blood flow depends on the discharge of the sympathetic nervous system. These sympathetic impulses are transmitted simultaneously to the blood vessels for cutaneous vasoconstriction and to the adrenal medulla. Both norepinephrine and epinephrine are secreted into the blood vessels and induce vessel constriction.[36] Most of the sympathetic constriction influences are mediated chemically through these neural transmitters. General exposure to cold elicits cutaneous vasoconstriction, shivering, piloerection, and an increase in epinephrine secretion, so vascular contraction occurs. Simultaneously, metabolism and heat production are increased to maintain the body temperature.[36]

Increased blood flow supplies additional oxygen to the area, thus explaining the analgesic and relaxation effects on muscle spasm. An increased proprioceptive reflex mechanism may explain these effects. Receptor end organs located in the muscle spindle are inhibited by heat temporarily, while sudden cooling tends to excite the receptor end organ.[60,63]

Effects of Tissue Temperature Change on Muscle Spasm

Numerous studies deal with the effects of heat and cold in the treatment of many musculoskeletal conditions. While it is true that the use of heat as a therapeutic modality has long been accepted and documented in the literature, it is apparent that most recent research has been directed toward the use of cold. There seems to be general agreement that the physiologic mechanisms underlying the effectiveness of heat and cold treatments in reducing muscle spasm lie at the level of the muscle spindle, Golgi tendon organs, and the gamma system.[84]

Heat is believed to have a relaxing effect on skeletal muscle tone.[30] Local application of heat relaxes muscles throughout the skeletal system by simultaneously lessening the stimulus threshold of muscle spindles and by decreasing the gamma efferent firing rate. This suggests that the muscle spindles are more easily excited. Consequently, the muscles may be electromyographically silent while at rest during the application of heat, but the slightest amount of voluntary or passive movement may cause the efferents to fire, thus increasing muscular resistance to stretch. If this is indeed the case, then it seems logical that decreasing the afferent impulses by raising the threshold of the muscle spindles might be effective in facilitating muscle relaxation as long as there is no movement.

The rate of firing of both primary and secondary endings is directly proportional to temperature. Local applications of cold decrease local neural activity. Annulospiral, flower-spray (small fibers located in the muscle spindle that detect changes in muscle position), and Golgi tendon organ endings all fire more slowly when cooled. Cooling actually decreases the rate of afferent activity even more, with an increase in the amount of tension on the muscle. Thus, cold appears to raise the threshold stimulus of muscle spindles, and heat tends to lower it.[28] While firing of the primary spindle afferents increases abruptly with the application of cold, a subsequent decrease in spindle afferent activity occurs and persists as the temperature is lowered.[64]

- Cold may be better for reducing muscle spasm

Simultaneous use of heat and cold in the treatment of muscle spasm has also been studied.[24] Local cooling with ice, while maintaining body temperature to prevent shivering, results in a significant reduction of muscle spasm, greater than that which occurs with the use of heat or cold independently. This effect was attributed to maintenance of body temperature, which decreases efferent activity while local cooling decreases afferent activity. If the core temperature of the body was not maintained, the reflex shivering would result in increased muscle tone, thus inhibiting relaxation.

There is a substantial reduction in the frequency of action potential (stimulus intensity necessary for firing muscle fibers) firing of the motor unit when the muscle temperature is reduced. Muscle spindle activity is most significantly reduced when the muscle is cooled while normal body temperature is maintained.[72]

Miglietta[72] presented a slightly different perspective on the effect of cold in reducing muscle spasm. He performed an electromyographic analysis of the effects of cold on the reduction of clonus (increased muscle tone) or spasticity in a group of 15 athletes. After immersion of the spastic extremity in a cold whirlpool for 15 minutes, it was observed that electromyographic activity dropped significantly and in some cases disappeared altogether. The cold was thought to induce an afferent bombardment of cold impulses, which modify the cortical excitatory state and block the stream of painful impulses from the muscle. Thus, relaxation of skeletal muscle is assumed to occur with the disappearance of pain.[98] It is not certain whether it is the excitability of the motor neurons or the hyperactivity of the gamma system, which is changed either at the muscle spindle level or at the spinal cord level, that is responsible for the reduction of spasticity. However, it is certain that cold is effective in reducing spasticity by reducing or modifying the highly sensitive stretch-reflex mechanism in muscle.

Another factor that may be important to the reduction of spasticity is reduction in the nerve conduction velocity as a result of the application of cold.[19] These changes may result from a slowing of motor and sensory nerve conduction velocity and a decrease of the afferent discharges from cutaneous receptors.

Several studies investigated the use of cold followed by some type of exercise in the treatment of various injuries to the musculotendinous unit.[33,52] Each of these studies indicated that the use of cold and exercise was extremely effective in the treatment of acute pathologies of the musculoskeletal system that produced restrictions of muscle action. However, if stretching was indicated, it has been stressed that stretching is more important for increasing flexibility than using either heat or cold.[27,94] Following treatment with heat "stretching window" has been identified (see Chapter 5) in which the stretching of a muscle is optimal. The most effective time to stretch is immediately following treatment.

Effects of Temperature Change on Performance

Several recent studies have examined the effects of altering tissue temperature on physical performance capabilities. Changes in the ability to produce torque during isokinetic testing following the application of heat and cold have been demonstrated, although there appears to be some disagreement relative to the degree of change in concentric and eccentric torque capabilities.[45] One study observed that the strength of an eccentric contraction was improved with the application of ice,[18] while another indicated the ice helped to facilitate concentric but not eccentric strength.[88] This may be due to an increase in the ability to recruit additional motorneurons during and after cooling.[56] It also appears that higher torque values can be produced following the application of cold packs and then of hot packs.[14] The use of cryotherapy doesn't seem to effect peak torque but may increase endurance.[97] Cold appears to have some effect on muscular power. It has been shown that performance in vertical jumping is decreased following the application of cold.[31,34] Cold water immersion does not seem to effect range of motion.[15]

It seems that heating or cooling of an extremity has minimal or no effects on proprioception, joint position sense, and balance.[10,58,61,82,88,89,95,96,104] Thus, it follows that tissue temperature changes have no effect on agility or the ability to change direction.[29,49,90]

CRYOTHERAPY

Physiologic Effects of Tissue Cooling

The physiologic effects of cold are for the most part opposite those of heat, the primary effect being a local decrease in temperature. Cold has its greatest benefit in acute athletic injury.[6,35,44,47,69] There is general agreement that the use of cold is the initial treatment for most conditions in the musculoskeletal system. *The primary reason for using cold in acute injury is to lower the temperature in the injured area, thus reducing the metabolic rate with a corresponding decrease in production of metabolites and metabolic heat.*[41] This helps the injured tissue survive the hypoxia and limits further tissue injury that may occur.[45,47] Cold when applied along with compression has been demonstrated to be more effective than using ice alone for reducing metabolism in injured tissue.[69,70] It is also used immediately after injury to decrease pain and promote local vasoconstriction, thus controlling hemorrhage and edema.[67,81] Cold is also used in the acute phase of inflammatory conditions, such as bursitis, tenosynovitis, and tendinitis, in which heat may cause additional pain and swelling.[63]

Cold is also used to reduce pain and the reflex muscle spasm and spastic conditions that accompany it.[69] Its analgesic effect is probably one of its greatest benefits.[25,64,84] One explanation of the analgesic effect is that cold decreases the velocity of nerve conduction, although it does not entirely eliminate it.[15,48,49] It is also possible that cold bombards central pain receptor areas with so many cold impulses that pain impulses are lost through the gate control theory of pain modulation. With ice treatments, the athlete usually reports an uncomfortable sensation of cold followed by stinging or burning, then an aching sensation, and finally complete numbness.[48]

Cold also has been demonstrated to be effective in the treatment of **myofascial pain**.[99] This type of pain is referred from active myofascial trigger points with various symptoms, including pain on active movement and decreased range of motion. Trigger points may result from muscle strain or tension, which sensitizes nerves in a localized area. A trigger point may be palpated as a small nodule or as a strip of tense muscle tissue.[100]

It appears that cold is more effective in treating acute muscle pain as opposed to delayed onset muscle soreness (DOMS), which occurs following exercise.[13] Ultrasound has been shown to be more effective than ice for treating DOMS.[71]

Cold depresses the excitability of free nerve endings and peripheral nerve fibers, and this increases the pain threshold.[54] This is of great value in short-term treatment. Cold applications can also enhance voluntary control in spastic conditions, and in acute traumatic conditions they may decrease painful spasms that result from local muscle irritability.[3]

Reduction in muscle guarding relative to acute trauma has been observed by all active athletic trainers. Literature reviewed indicates various reasons behind reduced muscle guarding with the common thought of decreased muscle spindle activity.[53]

The initial reaction to cold is local vasoconstriction of all smooth muscle by the central nervous system to conserve heat.[81] Localized vasoconstriction is responsible for the decrease in the tendency toward formation and accumulation of edema,[93] probably as a result of a decrease in local hydrostatic pressure. There is also a decrease in the amount of **nutrients** and phagocytes delivered to the area, thus reducing phagocytic activity.[93]

myofascial pain A type of referred pain associated with trigger points.

nutrients Essential or nonessential food substance.

hunting response A reflex vasodilation that occurs in response to cold approximately 15 minutes into the treatment. This has been demonstrated to be only an increase in temperature and not necessarily a change in blood flow.

It has been hypothesized that when local temperature is lowered considerably for a period of about 30 minutes, intermittent periods of cold-induced vasodilation (CIVD) occur, lasting 4 to 6 minutes. Then vasoconstriction recurs for a 15- to 30-minute cycle, followed again by vasodilation. This phenomenon was originally referred to as the **hunting response**, and it hypothesized that this was necessary to prevent local tissue injury caused by cold.[12,16,50,62,74,81] The hunting response has been accepted for a number of years as fact; in reality, however, these investigations have talked about measured temperature changes rather than circulatory changes. Thus, the hunting response is more likely a measurement artifact than an actual change in blood flow in response to cold.[2,48] Even if some cold-induced vasodilation does occur, the effects are negligible.[45]

If a large area is cooled, the hypothalamus (the temperature-regulating center in the brain) will reflexly induce shivering, which raises the core temperature as a result of increased production of heat. Cooling of a large area might also cause arterial vasoconstriction in other remote parts of the body, resulting in an increased blood pressure.[93] Because of the low thermal conductivity of underlying subcutaneous fat tissue, applications of cold for short periods of time will probably be ineffective in cooling deeper tissues.[81] It has also been shown that using cold for too long may be detrimental to the healing process.[35]

The length of treatment time needed to cool tissue effectively depends on differences in subcutaneous tissue thickness. Athletes with thick subcutaneous tissue should be treated with cold applications for longer than 5 minutes to produce a significant drop in intramuscular temperature. Grant[33] treated acute and chronic conditions of the musculoskeletal system and found that thin people require shorter icing periods and that response was more successful. McMaster[67] supported these findings. Recommended treatment times range from direct contact of 5 to 45 minutes to obtain adequate cooling. While a treatment as short as 5 minutes may allow for analgesia to occur, it is generally accepted that vasoconstriction takes a minimum of 12 minutes.

It is generally believed that cold treatments are more effective in reaching deep tissue than most forms of heat. Cold applied to the skin is capable of significantly lowering the temperature of tissue at a considerable depth. The extent of this lowered tissue temperature is dependent on the type of cold applied to the skin, the duration of its application, the thickness of the subcutaneous fat, and the region of the body on which it is applied. Figure 4-1 shows the temperature changes in various tissues associated with an ice pack treatment.

The application of cold decreases cell permeability, decreases cellular metabolism, and decreases accumulation of edema and should be continued in 5- to 45-minute applications for at least 72 hours

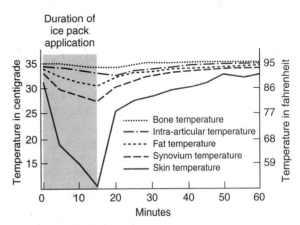

Figure 4-1 Temperature changes in various tissues during ice application.
(From Bocobo, et al. The effect of ice on intra-articular temperature in the knee of a dog. *AMJ Phys. Rehab.* 70:181, 1991)

■ **TABLE 4-2**   Physiologic Effects of Heat and Cold

EFFECTS OF COLD

Decreased local temperature, in some cases
   to a considerable depth
Decreased cell metabolism
Vasoconstriction of arterioles and capillaries (at first)
Decreased blood flow (at first)
Decreased nerve conduction velocity
Decreased delivery of leukocytes and phagocytes
Decreased lymphatic and venous drainage
Decreased muscle excitability
Decreased muscle spindle depolarization
Decreased formation and accumulation of edema
Extreme anesthetic effects

EFFECTS OF HEAT

Increased local temperature superficially
Increased local metabolism
Vasodilation of arterioles and capillaries
Increased blood flow to part heated
Increased leukocytes and phagocytosis
Increased capillary permeability
Increased lymphatic and venous drainage
Increased metabolic wastes
Increased axon reflex activity
Increased elasticity of muscles, ligaments, and capsule
   fibers
Analgesia
Increased formation of edema
Decreased muscle tone
Decreased muscle spasm

after initial trauma.[45] Care should be taken to avoid aggressive cold treatment to prevent disruption of the healing sequence.

The physiologic effects of cold are summarized in Table 4-2 above.

CRYOTHERAPY TECHNIQUES

Cryotherapy is the use of cold in the treatment of acute trauma and subacute injury and for the decrease of discomfort after reconditioning and rehabilitation.[46] Tools of cryotherapy include ice packs, cold whirlpool, ice whirlpool, ice massage, commercial chemical cold spray, and contrast baths. Application of cryotherapy produces a 3- to 4-stage sensation. First there is an uncomfortable sensation of cold followed by a stinging, then a burning or aching feeling, and finally numbness. Each stage is related to the nerve endings as they temporarily cease to function as a result of both decreased blood flow and decreased nerve conduction velocity. The time required for this sequence varies, but several authors indicate that it occurs within 5 to 15 minutes. Thus, a minimum of 15 minutes is necessary to achieve extreme analgesic effects.[2,4,7,33,38,48,74–76,81]

Application of ice is safe, simple, and inexpensive. Cryotherapy is contraindicated in athletes with cold allergies (hives, joint pain, nausea), Raynaud's phenomenon (arterial spasm), and some rheumatoid conditions.[2,26,33,36,42]

Depth of penetration depends on the amount of cold and the length of the treatment time because the body is well-equipped to maintain skin and subcutaneous tissue viability through the capillary bed by reflex vasodilation of up to 4 times normal blood flow. The body has the ability to decrease blood flow to the body segment that is supposedly losing too much body heat by shunting the blood flow. Depth of penetration is also related to intensity and duration of cold application and the circulatory response to the body segment exposed. If the person has normal circulatory responses, frostbite should not be a concern. Even so, caution should be exercised when applying intense cold directly to the skin. If deeper penetration is desired, ice therapy is most effective using ice towels, ice packs, ice massage, and ice whirlpools. Athletes should be advised of the four stages of sensation associated with cryotherapy and the discomfort they will experience. The athletic trainer should explain this sequence and advise the

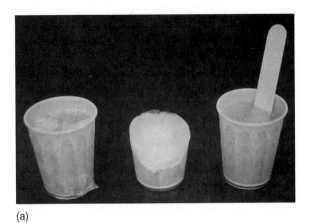
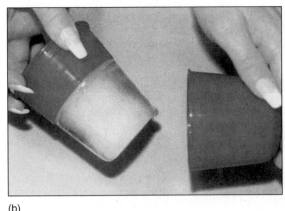

(a)   (b)

Figure 4-2   (a) Water may be frozen in a paper cup, Styrofoam cup, or on a tongue depressor for the purpose of ice massage. (b) Cyrocup is a commercially produced product for ice massage. (Courtesy Cryocup)

athlete of the expected outcome, which may include a rapid decrease in pain.[2,19,33,40]

Frostbite.   Frostbite is defined as freezing of a body part and occurs when tissue temperatures fall below 0° C (32° F). Symptoms of frostbite initially include tingling and redness from hyperemia, which indicate blood is still circulating to the superficial tissues, followed by pallor, (a lack of color in the skin) and numbness, which indicate that vasoconsriction has occurred and blood is no longer circulating to the superficial tissues.

When using a cryotherapy technique, the chances of frostbite are minimal if the recommended procedures are followed. However, if treatment time exceeds recommendations or if the temperature of the modality is below what is recommended, the chances of frostbite will be increased. Certainly if there is circulatory insufficiency, the chances of frostbite are also increased. Using commercial chemical cold packs or Fluoromethane spray can also lower tissue temperature substantially, and caution should be applied when using these techniques.

If frostbite is suspected the body part should be immediately removed from the cold source and immersed in water at 38° to 40° C (100° to 104° F). It is also advisable to refer the athlete to a physician.

Ice Massage

Ice massage can be applied by the athletic trainer or the athlete if the athlete can reach the area of application to administer self-treatment. It is best for the first three treatments to be administered by the athletic trainer to give the athlete the full benefit of the treatment. When positioning the athlete's body segment to be treated, it should be relaxed and the athlete should be made comfortable. If possible the body part to be treated should be elevated. Appropriate seating and positioning should be taken into consideration with the application of ice. Administration must be thorough to get maximal treatment. Ice massage is perhaps best indicated in conditions in which some type of stretching activity is to be used. It appears that ice message cools muscle more rapidly than an ice bag.[106]

EQUIPMENT NEEDED (FIGURES 4-2 AND 4-3)

A. Styrofoam cups. A regular 6- to 8-ounce styrofoam cup should be filled with water and placed in the freezer. After it is frozen, all the styrofoam on the sides should be removed down to 1 inch from the bottom. A frozen cup of ice with a tongue depressor

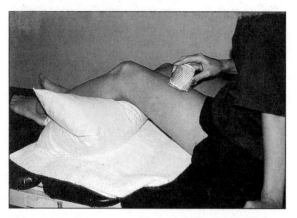

Figure 4-3 Ice massage may be applied using either circular or longitudinal strokes.

erythema Redness of the skin.

vasodilation Dilation of the blood vessels.

thermopane An insulating layer of water next to the skin.

inserted is preferred because it has a handle with which to hold the block of ice.

B. Popsicle ice cups. Cups are filled with water, and a wooden tongue blade is placed in each cup. The cups are then placed in the freezer. After the water is frozen, the paper cup is torn off. A block of ice on a stick is now ready to be used for massage.

C. Paper cups. Same technique as the styrofoam cups, except toweling may be needed to insulate the athletic trainer's hand holding the paper cup.

D. Towels. These are used for positioning and absorbing the melting water in the area of the ice massage application.

TREATMENT

A. Athlete position. Sidelying, prone, supine, hooklying, or sitting, depending on the area to be treated.

B. Self-treatment. Used when athletes can comfortably reach the area to be treated by themselves.

C. Circular motion. Application of ice massage in a circular pattern with each succeeding stroke covering half the previous stroke.

D. Longitudinal strokes. Application of ice massage in a longitudinal motion with

each stroke overlapping half the previous stroke.

E. Peripheral coverage. Ice should be applied for 15 to 20 minutes; consistent patterning of circular and longitudinal strokes includes the sequence described in the clinical uses section.

PHYSIOLOGIC RESPONSES

A. Cold progression proceeds through the four stages: cold, stinging, burning, and numbness.

B. Reddening of the skin **(erythema)** occurs as a result of blanching or lack of blood in the capillary bed. A common example occurs when one works outside in the cold without gloves or appropriate footwear and returns inside to find the toes beet red. The body is attempting to pool blood in the area to prevent further temperature loss.

C. Ice applications of 5 to 15 minutes and greater than 10° C (50° F) will not stimulate the hunting response and do not stimulate the reflex **vasodilation** that creates the body's own physically induced heat or increased blood flow.

CONSIDERATIONS

A. The time necessary for the surface area to be numbed will depend on the body area to be massaged. Approximate time will depend on how fast the ice melts and what **thermopane** develops between the skin and ice massage.

B. Athlete comfort should be considered at all times.

C. If adequate circulation is present, frostbite should not be a concern. However, if the athlete has diabetes, the extremities, especially the toes, may require reduced temperature and adjustment of the intensity and duration of the cold.

Application.   After the type of cold applicator for ice massage is selected, the athlete should be positioned comfortably and clothing should be removed from the area to be treated. The area should be set up before positioning the athlete. Remove the top two thirds of paper from the ice-filled paper or styrofoam cup, leaving 1 inch on the bottom of the cup as a handle for the athletic trainer or athlete to use as a handgrip. The athletic trainer should smooth the rough edges of the ice cup by gently rubbing along the edges. Ice should be applied to the athlete's exposed skin in circular or longitudinal strokes, with each stroke overlapping the previous stroke. The application should be continued until the athlete goes through the cold progression sequence of cold, stinging, burning or aching, and numbness. Once the skin is numb to fine touch, ice application can be terminated. The cold progression is the response of the sensory nerve fibers in the skin. The difference between cold and burning is primarily between the dropping out (sensory deficit) of the cold and warm nerve endings. Standard treatments allow the athlete to place cold applications every other 20 minutes, thus facilitating the hunting response. Some thermobarrier is developed during the ice massage in the layer of water directly on the skin, but this allows the ice cup to move smoothly over the skin. The time from application to numbing of the body segment depends on the size of the segment, but progression to numbing should be around 7 to 10 minutes.

Commercial (Cold) Hydrocollator Packs

Cold hydrocollator packs (Figure 4-4) are indicated in any acute injury to a musculoskeletal structure.

EQUIPMENT NEEDED
A.   Hydrocollator cold pack. This must be cooled to 8° F (15° C). It needs plastic liners or protective toweling for placement on a

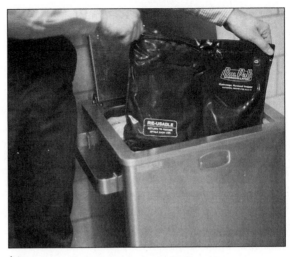

(a)

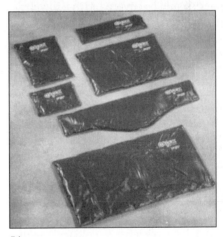

(b)

Figure 4-4   Commercial cold pack. (a) Stored in a refrigeration unit. (b) Come in a variety of sizes. (Courtesy ColPaC)

body segment. Petroleum distillate gel is the substance contained in the plastic pouch design.
B.   Moist cold towels. Towels may be immersed in ice water and molded to the skin surface, or they can be packed in ice and allowed to remain in place. The commercial cold pack should be placed on top of a moist towel.

C. Plastic bag. The hydrocollator should be placed in the bag. Air should be removed from the bag. The plastic bag may then be molded around the body segment.

D. Dry towel. To prevent the cold hydrocollator from losing heat rapidly, the towel is used as a covering to insulate the cold pack.

TREATMENT

A. Athlete position. Sidelying, prone, supine, hooklying, or sitting, depending on the area to be treated.

B. The athlete must remain still during the treatment to maintain appropriate positioning of the cold pack.

C. Cold pack must be molded onto the skin.

D. The pack should be covered with a towel to limit loss of cold.

E. A timer should be set, or time should otherwise be noted.

F. Treatment time should be 20 minutes.

PHYSIOLOGIC RESPONSES

A. Cold progression proceeds through the four stages.

B. Erythema occurs.

CONSIDERATIONS

A. Body area should be covered to prevent unnecessary exposure.

B. The physiologic response to cold treatment is immediate.

C. Athlete comfort should be considered at all times.

D. There is no thermopane so caution should be applied to prevent frostbite.

E. The athlete should not lie on top of the cold pack.

Application.   The athlete should be positioned with treatment area exposed and towel draped to protect clothing. The commercial cold pack should be placed against wet toweling to enhance transfer of cold to the body segment. If the injury is acute or subacute, the body segment should be elevated to reduce gravity-dependent swelling.[103]

Pack the cold pack around the joint in a manner designed to remove all air and ensure placement directly against wet toweling. Cold progression will be the same as with ice massage but not as quick because of the toweling between the skin and cold pack.[101] General treatment time required for numbing is about 20 minutes. The importance of a comfortable, properly positioned athlete is evident. Checking the sensory area after application is important. With proper treatment technique frostbite should not be a concern if circulation is intact. If swelling is a concern, a wet compression (elastic) wrap could be applied under the cold pack. A sequence of 20 minutes on and 20 minutes off should be repeated for 2 hours; the same sequence can be used in home treatment. Elevation is a key adjunct therapy during the sleeping hours.

Ice Packs

Like cold hydrocollator packs, ice packs (Figure 4-5) are indicated in acute stages of injury as well as for prevention of additional swelling after exercise of the injured part. It appears that ice packs may lower intramuscular temperatures more than commercial gel packs.[68]

EQUIPMENT NEEDED

A. Small plastic bags. Vegetable or bread bags may be used.

B. Ice flaker machine. Flaked or crushed ice is easier to mold than cubed ice.

C. Moist towels. These are used to facilitate cold transmission and should be placed directly on the skin.

D. Elastic bandaging. Bandaging holds the plastic ice pack in place and applies compression. The body segment may be elevated.

TREATMENT

A. Athlete position. Position depends on the part to be treated.

B. The athlete must remain still during treatment.

C. Pack must be placed on skin.

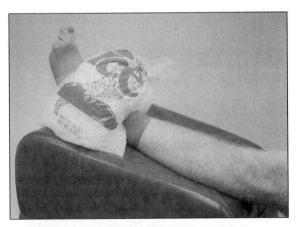

Figure 4-5   Ice pack molded to fit the injured part.

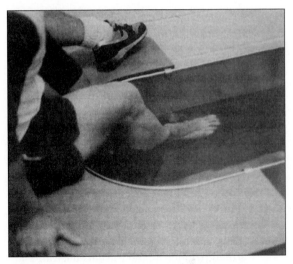

Figure 4-6   The cold whirlpool should have the ice melted before it is turned on.

D. Pack should be secured in place with toweling or elastic bandage.
E. Pack should be covered with towel to limit cold loss.
F. A timer should be set, or time should otherwise be noted.
G. Treatment time should be 20 minutes.

PHYSIOLOGIC RESPONSES
A. Cold progression proceeds through the four stages.
B. Erythema occurs.

CONSIDERATIONS
A. Body area should be covered to prevent unnecessary exposure.
B. The physiologic response to cold is immediate.
C. Athlete comfort should be considered at all times.
D. Frostbite should not be a concern unless circulation is inadequate.
E. The athlete should not lie on top of the ice pack.

Application.   Application of ice packs is similar to the use of commercial cold hydrocollator packs; the equipment to be set up in the treatment area consists of flaked or cubed ice in a plastic bag large enough for the area to be treated. The plastic bag can be applied directly to the skin and held in place by a moist or dry elastic wrap. Athlete comfort is of the utmost importance during this application to facilitate athlete relaxation. The athletic trainer may want to add salt to the ice to facilitate melting of the ice to create a colder slush mixture. Melting ice gives off more energy because of its less stable state, and it is therefore colder. A towel should be placed over the ice pack to decrease the warming effect of the environmental air, thus facilitating the cold application. The normal physiologic response will be cold/stinging/burning/numbness, at which time the set up can be terminated. Because of the pliability of the flaked ice pack, it can be molded to the body segment treated. If cubed ice is used instead of flaked ice, it can still be molded, but it will not readily hold its position and will need to be secured via elastic wrap or toweling.

Cold Whirlpool

The cold whirlpool (Figure 4-6) is indicated in acute and subacute conditions in which exercise of the injured part during a cold treatment is desired.

■ **Clinical Decision-Making** *Exercise 4-1*

....

The athletic trainer is treating an acute inversion ankle sprain and has placed an elastic wrap around the ankle for compression. Crushed ice bags have been applied to both sides of the ankle and it has been elevated. How long should the ice bags be left in place?

EQUIPMENT NEEDED

A. Whirlpool. The appropriate size whirlpool must be filled with cold water or ice to lower the temperature to 50° F to 60° F. The athletic trainer should use flaked ice and make sure the ice melts completely, since pieces of ice could become projectiles if a body segment is in the pool.

B. Ice machine. Flaked ice acts faster than cubed to lower the water temperature.

C. Toweling. Sufficient toweling is needed for padding the body segment on the whirlpool and for drying off after treatment.

D. Appropriate set up in area. A chair, whirlpool, and a bench in the whirlpool must be arranged before treatment.

TREATMENT

A. Temperature should be set at 50° F to 60° F.

B. Body segment must be immersed.

C. For total body immersion the water temperature should be set at 65° F to 80° F.

D. Treatment time should be 5 to 15 minutes.

PHYSIOLOGIC RESPONSES

A. Cold progression proceeds through the four stages.

B. Erythema occurs.

CONSIDERATIONS

A. Caution: Although the immediate application of cold will help to control edema if applied immediately following injury,[16] the gravity-dependent positions should be avoided with acute and subacute injuries.[16,21,23,102] Cold wet compression or elastic wrap should be put in place before treatment.

B. The body area treated should be completely immersed.

C. A cold whirlpool allows exercises to be done during treatment.

D. Athlete comfort should be considered at all times.

E. Frostbite should not be a concern unless circulation is inadequate.

F. A toe cap made of neoprene can be used to make the athlete more comfortable in the cold whirlpool.[73]

Application and Safety. The unit should be turned on after it has been established that the ground fault interrupter (GFI) is functioning. The athlete should be positioned in the whirlpool area, and appropriate padding should be provided for the athlete's comfort. The athlete should be cautioned to use care when standing or walking on slippery floors, and particularly when getting into and out of the whirlpool. The timer should be set for the amount of time desired, depending on the size of the body part to be treated. Treatment should continue until the body segment becomes numb (approximately 15 minutes). Numbness is the cutaneous (skin or superficial) response. Frostbite should not be a concern unless the individual has a history of circulatory deficiencies or has diabetes. Treatment time will be between 7 and 15 minutes to allow the complete circulatory response. Caution is indicated in the gravity-dependent position because of the likelihood of additional swelling if the body segment is already swollen.[16] This is the most intense application of cold of the cryotherapy techniques listed. Therefore, the first two or three treatments should be administered with the athletic trainer remaining in the area. One of several reasons for the intensity of cold is that the body cannot develop a thermopane (insulating layer of water) on the skin because of the convection effect of the whirlpool. Cold whirlpools have been shown to be more effective than ice packs for maintaining prolonged significant temperature reduction for at least 30 minutes post-treatment.[79] Additional benefits include the massaging and vibrating effect of the water flow. Removal of the part being treated from the whirlpool will necessitate a review of the skin surface and an assessment of edema in the extremities. If total body immersion is used, care should be taken for the intensity and duration of the whirlpool and for protection of the genitals from direct water flow. Applications can be repeated following rewarming of the body segment after sensation has returned. If the cold application is administered before practice, it should be done before the application of preventive strapping. Enough time should also be allowed for sensation to return before taping. Studies have indicated that the reflex vasodilation lasts up to 2 hours. An athlete could practice, then return to the training room and receive additional treatment without additional edema created by **congestion** as a result of vascular and capillary insufficiency occurring during the healing process. Increased heart rate and blood pressure are associated with cold application. Conditioned athletes should not have a problem with dizziness after cold applications, but care should be taken when transferring the athlete from the whirlpool area.

Whirlpool Maintenance.   Safety considerations for using both a cold and hot whirlpool have been discussed previously. It is equally important to mention the importance of maintaining the cleanliness of the whirlpools, particularly in an athletic training clinical setting.

It is not uncommon for several individuals to use a whirlpool, particularly a cold whirlpool, simultaneously. This practice is certainly not recommended and in fact is contrary to standards of most health regulatory agencies in many states.

It is recommended that the whirlpool be drained and cleaned after each treatment to minimize the potential risks of spreading fungal, viral, or bacterial infections, especially in those individuals who have open lesions. Whirlpools should be cleaned by filling the basin above the level of the turbine, adding a commercial antibiotic solution,

---

congestion   Presence of an abnormal amount of blood in the vessels resulting from an increase in blood flow or obstructed venous return.

---

disinfecting agent, or chlorine bleach and then running the turbine for at least 1 minute. The turbine and drain filter should be scrubbed and the tub thoroughly rinsed. The outside surface of the whirlpool should be cleaned daily.

To keep bacterial and fungal growth in check, whirlpool cultures should be taken monthly.

Cold Spray

Cold sprays, such as Fluoromethane (liquid ethyl chloride spray is no longer used), do not provide adequate deep penetration, but they do provide adjunctive therapy for acupressure techniques to reduce muscle spasm. Physiologically this is accomplished by stimulating the A fibers involved in the gate control theory. The primary action of a cold spray is reduction of the pain spasm sequence secondary to direct trauma. It will, however, not reduce hemorrhage because it works on the superficial nerve endings to reduce the spasm via the stimulation of A fibers to reduce the so-called painful arc. Cold spray is an extremely effective technique in the treatment of myofascial trigger points. Precautions concerning the use of cold spray include protecting the athlete's face from the fumes and spraying the skin at an acute angle rather than at a perpendicular angle.[99] Cold spray is indicated when stretching of an injured part is desired along with cold treatment.

EQUIPMENT NEEDED
A.   Fluoromethane.
B.   Toweling.
C.   Padding.

TREATMENT
A.   The area to be treated should be sprayed and then stretched.
B.   Spasm should be reduced.

C.   Treatment should be distal to proximal.
D.   A quick jetstream spray or stroking motion should be used.
E.   Cooling should be superficial; no frosting should occur.
F.   Cold sprays may be used in conjunction with acupressure.
G.   Treatment time should be set according to body segment.

PHYSIOLOGIC RESPONSES

A.   Muscle spasm is reduced.
B.   Golgi tendon organ response is facilitated.
C.   Muscle spindle response is inhibited.
D.   Musculoskeletal structures may be stimulated.

CONSIDERATIONS

A.   Both the acute and the subacute response should be positive.
B.   The room should be well ventilated to avoid the accumulation of fumes.
C.   Athlete comfort should be considered at all times.

Application.   The application of Fluoromethane (Figure 4-7) is typical of the application of other cold sprays. The following application procedures apply specifically to Fluoromethane, but they provide an outline of the procedures, indications, and precautions applicable to all cold sprays. The athletic trainer should follow the manufacturer's instructions in the use of any cold spray.

Fluoromethane is a topical vapocoolant that acts as a counterirritant to block pain impulses of muscles in spasm. When used in conjunction with the "spray-and-stretch" technique, Fluoromethane can break the pain cycle, allowing the muscle to be stretched to its normal length (pain-free state). The application of the "spray-and-stretch" technique is a therapeutic technique that involves three stages: evaluation, spraying, and stretching. The therapeutic value of "spray and stretch" becomes most effective when the athletic trainer has mastered all stages and applies them in the proper sequence.

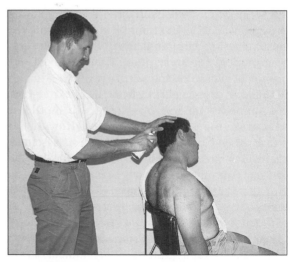

Figure 4-7   Spray-and-stretch technique using Fluoromethane.

Evaluation.   During the evaluation phase the cause of pain is determined as local spasm of an irritated trigger point. The method of applying "spray and stretch" to a muscle spasm differs slightly from application to a trigger point. The trigger point is a deep hypersensitive localized spot in a muscle that causes a referred pain pattern. With trigger points, the source of pain is seldom the site of the pain. A trigger point may be detected by a snapping palpation over the muscle, causing the muscle in which the irritated trigger point is situated to "jump." In the case of muscle spasm, the source and site of pain are identical. A trigger point may also be treated effectively using ultrasound and electrical stimulation.[59]

Spraying.   To apply Fluoromethane, (a) Athletes should assume a comfortable position; (b) take precautions to cover the patient's eyes, nose, and mouth if spraying near face; (c) hold spray can or spray bottle (upside down) 12 to 18 inches away from the treatment surface, allowing the jetstream of vapocoolant to meet the skin at an acute angle; (d) apply the spray in one direction only—not back and forth—at a rate of 4 inches (10 cm) per second. Three or four sweeps of the spray in one direction are sufficient to treat the trigger point or to overcome painful muscle spasms. It is possible but not very likely that the intense cold (−15° C) of the Fluoromethane can freeze the skin. Certainly the chances of this occurring are not nearly as likely as when using ethyl chloride. In the case of a trigger point, spray should be applied from the trigger point to the area of referred pain. If there is no trigger point, the spray should be applied from the affected muscle to its insertion. The spray should be applied in an even sweep, using two to four parallel sweeps, but not overlapping. Sweeps of spray should be enough to cover the skin over the affected muscle or trigger point.

Stretching.   A static stretch should begin as you start spraying from the origin to the insertion (simple muscle spasm pain) or from the trigger point to the referred pain when the trigger point is present holding the position of stretch for 30 to 60 seconds. Spray and stretch until the muscle reaches its maximal or normal resting length. You will usually feel a gradual increase in range of motion. The spraying and stretching may require two to four spray applications to achieve the therapeutic results in any treatment session. An athlete may have multiple treatment sessions in any one day.

The "spray-and-stretch" technique outlined here must be considered a therapeutic system. The practitioner should spend some time each day practicing until the technique is mastered.

Composition.   Fluoromethane is a combination of two chlorofluorocarbons: 15% dichlorodifluoromethane and 85% trichloromonofluoromethane. The combination is not flammable and at room temperature is only volatile enough to expel the contents from the inverted container. Fluoromethane is supplied in amber Dispenseal bottles that emit a jetstream from a calibrated nozzle.

Indications.   Fluoromethane is a vapocoolant intended for topical application in the management of myofascial pain, restricted motion, and muscle spasm. Clinical conditions that may respond to "spray and stretch" include low back pain (caused by muscle spasm), acute stiff neck, torticollis, acute

---

■ **Clinical Decision-Making**   *Exercise 4-2*

....

A gymnast is diagnosed with a myofascial trigger point in her middle trapezius. What infrared therapeutic modality would likely be a good choice for treating this condition?

....

anesthesia   Loss of sensation.

contrast bath   Hot (106° F) and cold (50° F) treatments in a combined sequence to stimulate superficial capillary vasodilation or vasoconstriction.

....

bursitis of shoulder, muscle spasm associated with osteoarthritis, ankle sprain, tight hamstring, masseter muscle spasm, certain types of headache, and referred pain from trigger points.

Precautions.   Federal law prohibits dispensing without a prescription. Although Fluoromethane is safe for topical application to the skin, care should be taken to minimize inhalation of vapors, especially when it is being applied to the head or neck. Fluoromethane is not intended for production of local **anesthesia** and should not be applied to the point of frost formation. Freezing can occasionally alter pigmentation.*

Contrast Baths

Contrast baths are used to treat subacute swelling by using alternating hot and cold immersions. It has been suggested that this treatment induces alternating vasoconstriction/vasodilation and thus a "pumping" action that is useful for removal of edema. However, research has not shown that this "pumping" actually occurs.[45]

*Modified with permission of the Gebauer Chemical Company, Cleveland, Ohio, 44104, (800) 321-9348; Ohio, (216) 271-5252.

■ **Clinical Decision-Making** *Exercise 4-3*

An athlete is about 1 week post quadriceps contusion. To this point the athlete has had only cryotherapy and some mild stretching exercises. At what point should the athletic trainer choose to switch to heat?

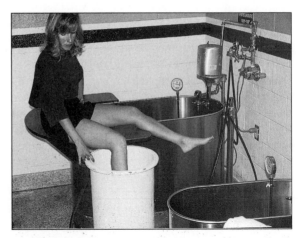

Figure 4-8 Contrast bath using a warm whirlpool and ice immersion cylinder.

However, both contrast herbs and cold whirlpool have been shown to be more effective than hot whirlpool in alleviating delayed onset muscle soreness.[51]

A Contrast therapy technique using hot and cold packs has been shown to have little or no effect on deep muscle temperatures.[78]

EQUIPMENT NEEDED (FIGURE 4-8)
A. Two containers. One container is used to hold cold water (50° F to 60° F), and the other is used to hold warm water (98° F to 110° F). Whirlpools may be used for one or both containers.
B. Ice machine.
C. Towels.
D. Chair.

TREATMENT
A. Hot and cold immersions are alternated.
B. Treatment time should be at least 20 minutes. Treatments should consist of five 1-minute cold immersions and five 3-minute warm immersions, although the exact ratio of cold to hot treatment is highly variable.

PHYSIOLOGIC RESPONSES
A. Vasoconstriction and vasodilation occur.
B. There is a reduction of necrotic cells at the cellular level.
C. Edema is decreased.

CONSIDERATIONS
A. The temperatures of the baths must be maintained.
B. A large area is required for treatment.
C. Athlete comfort must be considered at all times.

Application. After the area is set up, a whirlpool can be used for either hot or cold application, with the opposite method of treatment contained in a bucket or sterile container. The temperatures of these immersion baths must be maintained (cold at 50° F to 60° F, hot at 98° F to 110° F) by adding ice or warm water. It is generally easier to use a large whirlpool for the warm water application and a bucket for the cold water application.

There has been considerable controversy regarding the use of contrast baths to control swelling. The theory that contrast baths induce a type of pumping action by alternating vasoconstriction with vasodilation has no credibility. Contrast baths probably cause only a superficial capillary response, resulting from inability of the larger deep blood vessels to constrict and dilate in response to superficial heating.[77,92]

Thus, it is recommended that during the initial stages of contrast bath treatment the ratio of hot to cold treatment begins with a relatively brief period in the hot bath, gradually increasing the length of time in the hot bath during subsequent treatments. Recommendations as to specific lengths of time are extremely variable. However, it would appear that a 3:1 ratio (3 minutes in hot, 1 minute in cold) or 4:1 ratio for 19 to 20 minutes is fairly well accepted. Whether the treatment is ended with cold or hot depends to some extent on the degree of tissue temperature increase desired. Other athletic trainers prefer to use the same ratios of 3:1 or 4:1, beginning with cold. The technique may certainly be modified to meet specific needs. Since the extremity is in the gravity-dependent position, once the injured part is removed from the contrast bath, skin sensation and the amount of edema accumulation should be assessed to make sure that the treatment has not actually increased the amount of edema.[5]

Ice Immersion

Ice buckets allow ease of application for the athletic trainer. Again, a wet area should be selected (where spilled water is not a concern), with the patient positioned for comfort. The immersion, like the contrast bath, should be maintained until desired results are reached. If cryokinetics are part of the treatment, then the container should be large enough to allow for the movement of the body segment. Although ice immersion has been shown to be effective in controlling post-traumatic edema,[22] ice immersion is similar to cold whirlpool in that the body segment may be subject to gravity-dependent position. Cold pain may be somewhat worse during ice immersion than during cold pack application.[51]

Cryo-Cuff

The Cryo-Cuff is a device that uses both cold and compression simultaneously (Figure 4-9). The Cryo-Cuff is used both acutely following injury and post surgically.[20] Originally developed by Aircast, it is made of a nylon sleeve that connects via a tube to a one gallon cooler/jug. Cold water flows into the sleeve from the cooler. As the cooler is raised the pressure in the cuff is increased. During the treatment the water warms and can be rechilled by lowering the cooler to drain the cuff, mixing the warmer water with the colder water and then

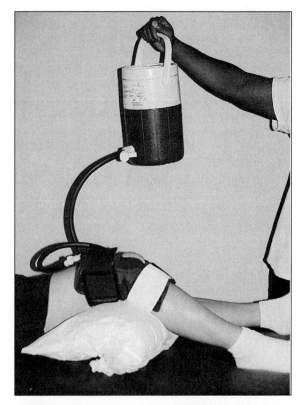

Figure 4-9   Cyro-Cuff combines cold and pressure.

....

cryokinetics   The use of cold and exercise in the treatment of pathology or diseases.

....

again raising the jug to increase pressure in the cuff. The only drawback to this simple yet effective piece of equipment is that you must continually rechill the water in the cuff. However, the Cyro-Cuff is portable, easy to use, and inexpensive.[45]

Cryokinetics

Cryokinetics is a technique that combines cryotherapy or the application of cold with exercise.[45,47] The goal of cryokinetics is to numb the injured part to the point of analgesia and then work toward achieving normal range of motion through progressive active exercise.

The technique begins by numbing the body part via ice immersion, cold packs, or ice massage. Most athletes will report a feeling of numbness within 12 to 20 minutes. If numbness is not perceived within 20 minutes, the therapist should proceed with exercise regardless. The numbness usually will last for 3 to 5 minutes, at which point ice should be reapplied for an additional 3 to 5 minutes until numbness returns. This sequence should be repeated five times.

Exercises are performed during the periods of numbness. The exercises selected should be pain free and progressive in intensity, concentrating on both flexibility and strength.[83] Changes in the intensity of the activity should be limited by both the nature of the healing process and by individual athlete differences in perception of pain. However, progression always should be encouraged within the framework of those limiting factors, the ultimate goal being a return to full athletic activities.[45]

THERMOTHERAPY

Physiologic Effects of Tissue Heating

Local superficial heating (infrared heat) is recommended in subacute conditions for reducing pain and inflammation through analgesic effects. Superficial heating produces lower tissue temperatures at the site of the pathology (injury) relative to the higher temperatures in the superficial tissues, resulting in analgesia. During the later stages of injury healing, a deeper heating effect is usually desirable; it can be achieved by using the diathermies or ultrasound. Heat dilates blood vessels, causing the patent capillaries to open up and increase circulation. The skin is supplied with sympathetic **vasoconstricton** fibers that secrete norepinephrine at their endings (especially evident in feet, hands, lips, nose, and ears). At normal body temperature, the sympathetic vasoconstrictor nerves keep vascular anastomoses almost totally closed, but when the superficial tissue is heated, the number of sympathetic impulses is greatly reduced so that the anastomoses dilate and allow large quantities of blood to flow into the venous plexuses. This increases blood flow about twofold, which can promote heat loss from the body.[36]

vasoconstriction Narrowing of the blood vessels.

hyperemia Presence of an increased amount of blood in part of the body.

metabolites Waste products of metabolism or catabolism.

inflammation A redness of the skin caused by capillary dilation.

The **hyperemia** created by heat has a beneficial effect on injury. This is based on increases of blood flow and pooling of blood during the metabolic processes. Recent hematomas (blood clots) should never be treated with heat until resolution of bleeding is completed. Some clinicians have advocated never using heat during any therapeutic modality application because of the chance of creating an increase in blood flow that may exacerbate swelling.[42,45,47,50]

The rate of metabolism of tissues depends partly on temperature. The metabolic rate has increased approximately 13% for each 1° C (1.8° F) increase in temperature.[42] A similar decrease in metabolism has been demonstrated when temperatures are lowered.

A primary effect of local heating is an increase in the local metabolic rate with a resulting increase in the production of **metabolites** and additional heat. These two factors lead to an increased intravascular hydrostatic pressure, causing arteriolar vasodilation and increased capillary blood flow.[93] However, with increased hydrostatic pressure, there is a tendency toward formation of edema, which may increase the time required for rehabilitation of a particular injury. Increased capillary blood flow is important with many types of injury in which there is mild or moderate **inflammation**, since it causes an increase in the supply of oxygen, antibodies, leukocytes, and other necessary nutrients and enzymes, along with an increased clearing of metabolites. With higher heat intensities, vasodilation and

consensual heat vasodilation Vasodilation and increased blood flow will spread to remote areas, causing increased metabolism in the unheated area.

edema Excessive fluid in cells.

increased blood flow will spread to remote areas, causing increased metabolism in the unheated area. This is known as **consensual heat vasodilation** and may be useful in many conditions where local heating is contraindicated.[30]

The application of heat can produce an analgesic effect, resulting in a reduction in the intensity of pain. The analgesic effect is the most frequent indication for the use.[93] Although the mechanisms underlying this phenomenon are not completely understood, it is in some way related to the gate control theory of pain modulation.

Heat is applied in musculoskeletal and neuromuscular disorders, such as sprains, strains, articular (joint-related) problems, and muscle spasms, which all describe various types of muscle pain.[30] Heat generally is considered to produce a relaxation effect and a reduction in guarding in skeletal muscle. It also increases the elasticity and decreases the viscosity of connective tissue, which is an important consideration in postacute joint injuries or after long periods of immobilization. Many athletic trainers empirically believe that in these types of disorders, heat has little effect on the condition itself but serves merely to facilitate further treatment by producing relaxation.[30] This is accomplished by relieving pain; lessening hypertonicity of muscles; producing sedation, which decreases spasticity, tenderness, and spasm; and decreasing tightness in muscles and related structures. The physiologic effects of heat are summarized in Table 4-2.

Heat is still used as a universal treatment for pain and discomfort. Much of the benefit is derived from the treatment simply feeling good. However, in the early stages after injury, heat causes increased capillary blood pressure and increased cellular permeability; this results in additional swelling or edema accu-

■ **Clinical Decision-Making** *Exercise 4-4*

On day 2 following an ankle sprain, the athletic trainer decides to put the athlete in a cold whirlpool to have her do exercises. At this point in a rehabilitation program is this really the best course of action?

mulation.[2,11,33,48,105] *No athlete with moderate or severe edema should be treated with any heat modality until the reasons for the edema are determined.* It is in the best interest of the athletic trainer to use cryotherapy techniques to reduce the **edema** before applying heat. Superficial heat applications seem to feel more comfortable for complaints of the neck, back, low back, and pelvic areas and may be most appropriate for the athlete who exhibits some allergic response to cold applications. However, the tissues in these areas are absolutely no different from those in the extremities. Thus, the same physiologic responses to the use of heat or cold will be elicited in all areas of the body.

Primary goals of thermotherapy include increased blood flow and increased muscle temperature to stimulate analgesia, increased nutrition to the damaged cells, reduction of edema, and removal of metabolites and other products of the inflammatory process.

THERMOTHERAPY TECHNIQUES

Warm Whirlpool

EQUIPMENT NEEDED
A.   Whirlpool. The whirlpool must be the correct size for the body segment to be treated.
B.   Towels. These are to be used for padding and drying off.
C.   Chair.
D.   Padding. This is to be placed on the side of the whirlpool.

TREATMENT

A. The athlete should be positioned comfortably, allowing the injured part to be immersed in the whirlpool.

B. Direct flow should be 6 to 8 inches from the body segment.

C. Temperature should be 98° F to 110° F (37° C to 45° C) for treatment of the arm and hand. For treatment of the leg, the temperature should be 98° F to 104° F (37° C to 40° C), and for full body treatment, the temperature should be 98° F to 102° F (37° C to 39° C).

D. Time of application should be 15 to 20 minutes.

CONSIDERATIONS

A. Athlete positioning should allow for exercise of the injured part.

B. The size of the body segment to be treated will determine whether an upper extremity, lower extremity, or full body whirlpool should be used.

   Application (Figure 4-10). The temperature range of a warm whirlpool is 100° F to 110° F (39° C to 45° C). It is similar in set up to a cold whirlpool. The athlete must be positioned in the whirlpool, with appropriate padding provided for the athlete's comfort. The unit should be turned on after it has been ascertained that the GFI is functioning. The timer should be set for the amount of time desired, depending on the size of the body part to be treated (10 to 30 minutes). Treatment time should be long enough to stimulate vasodilation and reduce muscle spasm (approximately 20 minutes).[85] Again, caution is indicated in the gravity-dependent position in subacute injuries. If some pitting edema exists (i.e., finger pressure on the skin leaves an indentation), cold or contrast baths are better indicated. In addition to increased circulation and reduction of spasm, benefits of the warm whirlpool include the massaging and vibrating effects of the water movement. On removal of the body segment from the whirlpool, it is necessary to review the skin surface and limb girth to see if the

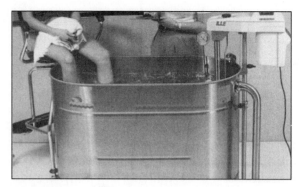

Figure 4-10 Warm whirlpool.
(Courtesy Ferno-Ille)

■ **Clinical Decision-Making**   *Exercise 4-5*

....

The athletic trainer is treating an athlete with a grade 2 MCL sprain. After the first week there is still considerable swelling on the medial side of the knee just below the joint line. He decides to use a contrast bath to take advantage of the "pumping action" of vasoconstriction/vasodilation. Is this technique likely to be effective?

---

warm whirlpool increased swelling; this step is indicated even if the athlete is past the subacute stage. After allowing the body segment to cool down, the athlete can have appropriate preventive strapping or padding placed on the body segment. If the athlete receives the treatment before exercising, it is recommended that he or she gently do range-of-motion exercises to reduce congestion and increase proprioception (sense of position) in all joints. If the athlete is complaining of muscle soreness, it would be more appropriate to recommend swimming pool exercises. The whirlpool provides a sedative effect. It is recommended that the athlete shower or clean the body surface before using a whirlpool. Random access to the whirlpool is not warranted.

   The warm whirlpool is an excellent postsurgical modality to increase systemic blood flow and mobilization of the affected body part. The appropriate-

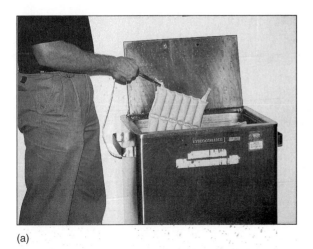

(a)

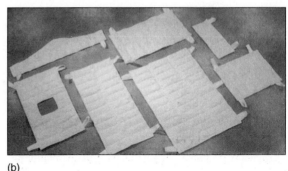

(b)

Figure 4-11   (a) Hydrocollator packs stored in tank. (b) Come in a variety of sizes. (Courtesy Chattanooga Corp)

ness of whirlpool therapy needs to be addressed by the athletic trainer because it is the most commonly abused physical therapy modality. An example of this abuse is the practice of placing an individual in the whirlpool without taking the time to assess the specific physiologic responses desired. However, it is an excellent adjunctive modality when used appropriately in the clinical setting. Again, whirlpools should be cleaned frequently to prevent the bacterial growth. When an athlete with any open or infected lesion uses the whirlpool, it must be drained and cleaned immediately. Cleaning should be done using both a disinfecting and antibacterial agent. Particular attention should be paid to cleaning the turbine by placing the intake valves in a bucket containing the disinfecting solution and turning the power on. Bacterial cultures should be monitored periodically from the tank, drain, and jets.

Commercial (Warm) Hydrocollator Packs

EQUIPMENT NEEDED

A.   Unit heat packs. These are canvas pouches of petroleum distillate (Figure 4-11). A thermostat maintains the high temperature

■   **Clinical Decision-Making**   *Exercise 4-6*

A volleyball player has an acute strain of the erector spinae muscles in the low back. The athletic trainer feels that using ice on the low back will cause the athlete to be uncomfortable and perhaps induce muscle guarding in the injured muscle. Thus, the athletic trainer chooses to use a hot hydrocollator pack instead of an ice pack. Is this the appropriate clinical decision?

(170° F) and helps prevent burns. Unit heat packs come in three sizes: (1) regular size is 12 × 12 inches for most body segments; (2) double size is 24 × 24 inches, for the back, low back, and buttocks; and (3) cervical is 6 × 8 inches for the cervical spine. Packs are removed by tongs or scissor handles.

B.   Towels. Regular bath towels and commercial double pad towels are required. Commercial double pad toweling has a pouch for pack placement and 1-inch thick toweling to be placed in cross fashion, tags on the edge of packs folded in, toweling

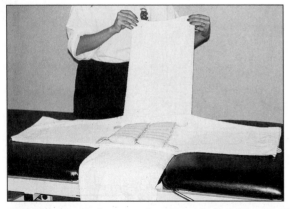 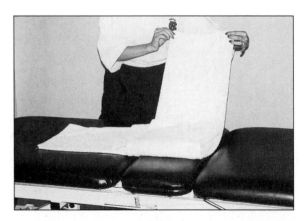

Figure 4-12 Techniques of wrapping hydrocollator packs.

overlapped on one side and four layers on the opposite side. Six layers equal 1 inch of toweling. Additional toweling may be needed depending on total body surface covered.

TREATMENT
A. Position six layers of toweling as described in (Figure 4-12).
B. Sufficient toweling should be provided to protect the athlete from burns.
C. Athlete position should be comfortable.
D. Treatment time should be 15 to 20 minutes.

PHYSIOLOGIC RESPONSES
A. Circulation is increased.
B. Muscle temperature is increased.
C. Tissue temperature is increased.
D. Spasms are relaxed.

CONSIDERATIONS
A. The size of the body segment to be treated should determine how many packs are needed.
B. Athlete comfort is always a consideration.
C. Time of application should be 15 to 20 minutes.
D. The athlete should not lie on top of the hot pack.

Application. Appropriate toweling and positioning of the athlete is necessary for a comfortable treatment. The moist heat pack tends to stimulate the circulatory response. Dry heat, as discussed in the infrared section, has a tendency to force blood away from the cutaneous capillary bed, thus increasing the possibility of a burn with the skin's inability to dissipate heat. The athlete must not be allowed to lie on the packs because of an increased risk of burn. If the athlete cannot tolerate the weight of the moist heat pack, alternate methods, such as placing the athlete sidelying with the majority of the weight of the hot pack on the side of the pack and the pack held in place by additional towels or sheets wrapped around the athlete, can be used. The most common indications are for muscular spasm, back pain, or as a preliminary treatment to other modalities.

Paraffin Bath

A **paraffin bath** is a simple and efficient, though somewhat messy, technique for applying a fairly high degree of localized heat. Paraffin treatments provide six times the amount of heat available in water because the mineral oil in the paraffin lowers the melting point of the paraffin. The combination of paraffin and mineral oil has a low specific heat, which enhances the athlete's ability to tolerate heat

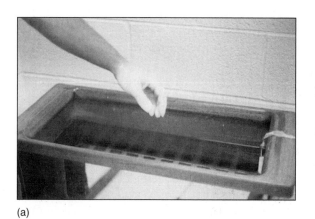
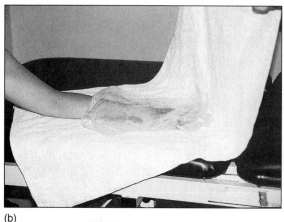

(a)   (b)

Figure 4-13   (a) Hand being dipped in paraffin bath. (b) After being dipped in paraffin, the hand should be wrapped in plastic bags and toweling.
(Courtesy Parabath)

paraffin bath   A combined paraffin and mineral oil immersion technique in which the paraffin substance is heated to 126° F for conductive heat gains: commonly used on the hands and feet for distal temperature gains in blood flow and temperature.

from paraffin better than from water of the same temperature.

The risk of a burn with paraffin is substantial. The athletic trainer should weigh heavily the considerations between a paraffin bath and warm whirlpool bath in the athletic setting. The majority of paraffin baths are used for chronic arthritis athletes, hands and feet. If the athlete has a chronic hand or foot problem, the use of paraffin instead of water usually gives longer lasting pain relief.[8,48]

EQUIPMENT NEEDED
A.   Paraffin bath (Figure 4-13a).
B.   Plastic bags and paper towels.
C.   Towels.

TREATMENT
A.   Dipping. The extremity should be dipped into the paraffin for a couple of seconds,

then removed to allow the paraffin to harden slightly for a few seconds. This procedure is repeated until 6 layers have accumulated on the part to be treated.
B.   Wrapping. The paraffin-coated extremity should be wrapped in a plastic bag with several layers of toweling around it to act as insulation (Figure 4-13b). Treatment time should be 20 to 30 minutes.

PHYSIOLOGIC RESPONSES
A.   There is an increase in tissue temperature.
B.   Pain relief occurs.
C.   Thermal hyperthermia occurs.

CONSIDERATIONS
A.   Some units are equipped with thermostats that may elevate the temperature to 212° F, thus killing any bacteria that may grow in the paraffin. Otherwise, the temperature should be set at 126° F.
B.   If the paraffin becomes soiled, it should be dumped and replaced at no longer than 6-month intervals.
   Application.   The purchase of a paraffin bath for the clinic requires that the bath have a built-in

thermostat. Before treatment, the athlete's body segment should be cleaned thoroughly with soap, water, and finally alcohol to remove any soap residue. This will prevent bacterial build-up in the bottom of the paraffin bath, which is an excellent medium for culture growth.

The mixture ratio of paraffin to mineral oil is 1 gallon of mineral oil to 2 pounds of paraffin. The mineral oil reduces the ambient temperature of the paraffin, which is 126° F (at which temperature a burn could occur). It is important to build six layers of paraffin, with the first layer highest on the body segment and each successive layer lower than the previous one. This is important because when dipping the extremity in the paraffin, if the second layer of paraffin is allowed to get between the skin and the first layer of paraffin, the heat will not dissipate and the athlete could be burned. Because heat is retained in the body and is also radiated from the paraffin, there is an increase in capillary dilation and blood supply in the treated segment. The athletic trainer should place the athlete in a comfortable position and enclose the paraffin in paper towels, plastic bags, and toweling to maintain the heat. Treatment is applied for approximately 20 to 30 minutes. Removal of the paraffin calls for extra care not to contaminate the used portion so that it does not contaminate the entire bath when it is returned.

Removal of paraffin involves removing towels, plastic bag, and paper towels, then using a tongue depressor to split the paraffin to allow easy removal. If the paraffin has not touched the floor, remove the paraffin cast over the open paraffin bath. It will dissolve on returning to the remaining liquid paraffin. Clean the body segment with soap and water or, if a postsurgical athlete is being treated, give a massage, since the mineral oil will make the skin moist and supple. When cleaning the skin, the athletic trainer must examine the surface for burns or **mottling** (a blotchy reddening of the skin). The thermostat will raise the temperature of the paraffin to 212° F, destroy any bacteria, and maintain a sterile contact medium.

---

mottling   A reddening of the skin in a blotchy pattern.

A less safe but likely more effective technique for increasing tissue temperature is to immerse the body part in the paraffin bath. The treatment begins by repeatedly dipping the body part in the paraffin until at least six layers have accumulated and then placing the body part in the paraffin for the remainder of the treatment time. The athlete should be instructed not to move the body part so there is no cracking and not to touch the bottom or the sides of the paraffin unit.

Paraffin baths require a large amount of supervision to prevent contamination, but they do provide a special type of treatment that is well adapted to the athlete with injuries of the hands and feet.

Infrared Lamps

When talking about infrared modalities, the athletic trainer most typically thinks of the infrared lamp. The biggest advantages of an infrared lamp and an increasing superficial tissue temperature, is that the unit does not touch the athlete. However, radiant heat is seldom used because it is limited in depth of skin penetration to less than 1 mm. Dry heat from an infrared lamp tends to elevate superficial skin temperatures more than moist heat; however, moist heat probably has a greater depth of penetration.

Superficial skin burns occasionally occur because of intense infrared radiation and the reflectors becoming extremely hot (4000° F). It is recommended that a warm moist towel be placed over the body segment to be treated to enhance the heating effects. Dry towels should cover the remainder of the body not being treated. This will allow a greater blood/tissue exchange by trapping the heat buildup in the moist towel and reducing the stagnant air over the body segment. Caution should be used, and the skin should be checked every few minutes for mottling.

Infrared generators may be divided into two categories: luminous and nonluminous. Nonluminous generators consist of a spiral coil of resistant metal wire wound around a cone-shaped piece of nonconducting material. The resistance of the wire to the electric flow produces heat and a dull red glow. A properly shaped reflector then radiates the heat to the body. All incandescent bodies and tungsten and carbon filament lamps are in the category of luminous generators. No nonluminous lamps are currently being manufactured since infrared at a wavelength of 12,000 A will penetrate slightly more deeply than either longer or shorter waves, due to a certain unique characteristic of human skin. Tungsten filament and special quartz red sources produce significant amounts of infrared heat at 12,000 A. Flare as a result of reflection off the skin can be a real problem.

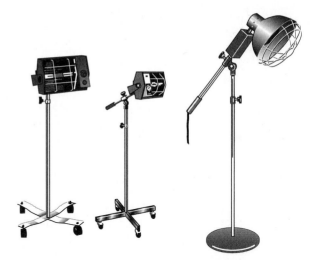

Figure 4-14   Various infrared heating lamps. (Courtesy of G. E. Millan Inc. Yonkers, NY)

EQUIPMENT NEEDED
A. Infrared lamp.
B. Dry toweling. This is to be used for draping the parts of the body not being treated.
C. Moist toweling. Moist towels are used to cover the area to be treated.
D. A GFI should be used with an infrared lamp.

TREATMENT
A. The athlete should be positioned 20 inches from the source.
B. Protective toweling should be put in place.
C. Treatment time should be 15 to 20 minutes.
D. Skin should be checked every few minutes for mottling.
E. Areas that are not to be treated must be protected.

PHYSIOLOGIC RESPONSES
A. A superficial rise in tissue temperature occurs.
B. There is some decrease in pain.
C. Moisture and sweat appear on the skin surface.

CONSIDERATIONS
A. To avoid a generalized temperature rise, only the portion that is injured should be treated.
B. The infrared lamp should be used primarily when an athlete cannot tolerate pressure from another type of modality (e.g., hydrocollator packs).
C. Caution must be exercised to avoid burns.

Application (Figure 4-14).   The athlete should be placed in a comfortable position. Moist heat should be used to stimulate blood flow. It is recommended to prevent blood from being forced away from the area as with dry heat. A moist, warm towel should be applied to the area to be treated. A squirt bottle is needed to keep the towel moist. All areas not to be treated should be draped. The distance from the area to be treated to the lamp should be adjusted according to treatment time: the standard formula is 20 inches distance = 20 minutes treatment time. After treatment, the skin surface should be checked. This type of treatment tends to force the blood away from the capillary bed and should be used only in superficial skin complaints related to dry heat requirements.

fluidotherapy A modality of dry heat using a finely divided solid suspended in a stream with the properties of liquid.

Fluidotherapy

Fluidotherapy is a unique, multifunctional physical medicine modality. The fluidotherapy unit is a dry heat modality that uses a suspended air stream, which has the properties of a liquid. Its therapeutic effectiveness in rehabilitation and healing is based on its ability to simultaneously apply heat, massage, sensory stimulation for desensitization, levitation, and pressure oscillations. Unlike water, the dry, natural medium does not irritate the skin or produce thermal shocks. This allows for much higher treatment temperatures than with aqueous or paraffin heat transfer. The pressure oscillations may actually minimize edema, even at very high treatment temperatures. Outstanding clinical success has been reported in treatment of pain, range of motion, wounds, acute injuries, swelling, and blood flow insufficiency. Fluidotherapy treatment of the hand at 115° F (46.2° C) results in a sixfold increase in blood flow and a fourfold increase in metabolic rates in a normal adult. These properties will increase blood flow, sedate, decrease blood pressure, and promote healing by accelerating biochemical reactions.[8]

Counterirritation, through mechanoreceptor and thermoreceptor stimulation, reduces pain sensitivity, thus permitting high temperatures without painful heat sensations. Pronounced hyperthermia accelerates the chemical metabolic processes and stimulates the normal healing process. The high temperatures enhance tissue elasticity and reduce tissue viscosity, which improves musculoskeletal mobility. Vascular responses are stimulated by long-lasting hyperthermia and pressure fluctuations, resulting in increased blood flow to the injured area.

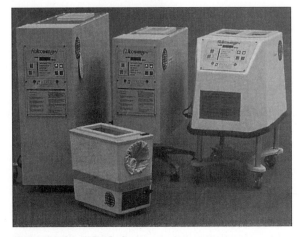

Figure 4-15 Fluidotherapy treatment units. (Photo courtesy of Fluidotherapy Corporation, 6113 Aletha Lane, Houston, TX 77081.)

EQUIPMENT NEEDED
A. Fluidotherapy model 104 (Figure 4-15).
B. Toweling.

TREATMENT
A. The athlete must be positioned for comfort.
B. The athlete should place the body segment to be treated (hand or foot) in the fluidotherapy unit.
C. Protective toweling must be placed at the unit interface and body segment.
D. Treatment time should be 15 to 20 minutes.

PHYSIOLOGIC RESPONSES
A. Tissue temperature increases.
B. Pain relief occurs.
C. Thermal hyperthermia occurs.

CONSIDERATIONS
A. Fluidotherapy unit must be kept clean.
B. All knobs must be returned to zero after treatment.

Application. The athlete should be positioned comfortably. The treated body segment should be submerged in the medium before the unit

■ **TABLE 4-3** Summary of Indications and Contraindications for Cryotherapy

INDICATIONS	CONTRAINDICATIONS
During acute or subacute inflammation	Impaired circulation
Acute pain	Peripheral vascular disease
Chronic pain	Hypersensitivity to cold
Acute swelling (controlling hemorrhage and edema)	Skin anesthesia
	Open wounds or skin conditions (cold whirlpools and contrast baths)
Myofascial trigger points	
Muscle guarding	Infection
Muscle spasm	
Acute muscle strain	
Acute ligament sprain	
Acute contusion	
Bursitis	
Tenosynovitis	
Tendinitis	
Delayed onset muscle soreness	

■ **TABLE 4-4** Summary of Indications and Contraindications for Thermotherapy

INDICATIONS	CONTRAINDICATIONS
Subacute and chronic inflammatory conditions	Acute musculoskeletal conditions
Subacute or chronic pain	Impaired circulation
Subacute edema removal	Peripheral vascular disease
Decreased ROM	Skin anesthesia
Resolution of swelling	Open wounds or skin conditions (cold whirlpools and contrast baths)
Myofascial trigger points	
Muscle guarding	
Muscle spasm	
Subacute muscle strain	
Subacute ligament sprain	
Subacute contusion	
Infection	

is turned on. There is no thermal shock when heat is applied. Treatments are approximately 20 minutes. Recommended temperature varies by body part and athlete tolerance, with a range of 110° F to 125° F (43° C to 53° C). Maximum temperature rise in the treated part occurs after 15 minutes of treatment. Unless contraindicated, active and passive exercise is encouraged during treatment.

In case of open lesions or infections, a protective dressing is recommended to prevent soiling or contaminating the cloth entry ports. Athletes with splints, bandages, tape, orthopedic pins, plastic joint replacement, and artificial tendons may be treated with fluidotherapy. The medium is clean and will not soil clothing. It is not necessary to disrobe to get the full benefit of heat and massage; however, direct contact between skin and the medium is desirable to maximize heat transfer.

In treating the hands, muscles, ankles, and conditions that manifest themselves relatively near the surface of the skin, appreciably higher body temperatures can be achieved using superficial heating modalities.[8] Further, the superficial modalities treat a larger area of the body than ultrasound or microwave diathermies; thus, the total amount of heat absorbed will be much higher. Fluidotherapy, hydrotherapy, and paraffin cause about the same amount of temperature increase.[26]

COUNTERIRRITANTS

Although counterirritants are not an infrared modality, they are often associated with ice and heat because of their common sensations. Counterirritants are topically applied ointments that chemically stimulate sensory receptors in the skin. There are four major active ingredients found in counterirritants. Menthol and methyl salicylate, which are found in peppermint and wintergreen oils respectively, are the two most common and are often combined. Camphor is another irritant that is usually combined with these first two, producing a chemical irritant. Perhaps the most promising irritant is capsaicin, which is derived from hot peppers.

Capsaicin, the most researched, has been shown to be effective in reducing chronic pain.[37] Skin counterirritants are used by allied health professionals, along with an increasing active population, to relieve some pain from the strains and sprains of their jobs and recreational activities.

The mechanism of pain relief from the counterirritants is not exactly known. It is very probable that there could be multiple methods of pain control at work. Some speculate that the rubbing application stimulates the large myelinated mechanoreceptors and works by the gate control theory. Because the irritants produce a noxious stimulus and a cool/warming sensation, the application is also thought to stimulate both noxious and thermal receptors. By applying a noxious stimulus and superficial thermal response, the thin A-delta and C afferent fibers are stimulated and inhibit pain similar to acupuncture. There is no evidence of tissue temperature response or a significant increase in blood flow from the application of a counterirritant. Capsaicin is thought to have a preferential action on C fibers by stimulating the release and depletion of substance P stores in the nociceptors, which is responsible for transmitting the pain signal. There is strong evidence that capsaicin affects synapses in the spinothalmic tract.[9] Counterirritants have been shown in clinical trials to decrease pain and increase range of motion[39] when compared to warm placebo ointment. Some others speculate that they may act in a similar way to the spray-and-stretch technique.

Methods of application include massaging, vigorous rubbing, and combine padding. The most common method used is massaging a generous amount on the affected area until no ointment is visible. Counterirritants can be applied with vigorous rubbing or friction massage for the benefit of soft tissue treatment. The combine padding method involves applying a generous amount of counterirritant, between 1/4 to 1/2 inch, on the pad and applying it to the affected area with a wrap. Manufac-

tured counterirritant packs with self-adhesive are now available.

Counterirritants should not be confused with other similar products containing trolamine salicylate, which has not been shown to be effective. They do not produce a chemical irritation and should be used with skeptical optimism. It is proposed that they work in a similar way to nonsteroidal anti-inflammatory medication by limiting prostaglandin production. It is also recommended to be cautious with people who are sensitive to anti-inflammatory medication.

CONCLUSIONS

Infrared sources transmit thermal energy to or from the athlete. In most cases, they are simple, efficient, and inexpensive. Athletic trainers who choose to compare modalities and use the most appropriate technique for their athletes will be providing quality care for that athlete. A haphazard approach to the use of infrared modalities will only reflect a disregard for the health care of the athlete.

Questioning, thinking athletic trainers will determine which procedure is best and most appropriate clinically. They will take responsibility for seeing that the most appropriate therapeutic modality is applied to enhance the athlete's reconditioning and rehabilitation. Regardless of which infrared modality athletic trainers choose, they should be aware of (1) the physiologic implications relative to circulation, (2) the ease of application, and (3) the short- and long-term benefits of treatment.

Additional areas of concern relate to (1) benefits of the infrared modality application, whether cryotherapy or thermotherapy, (2) economy of modality application, and (3) repeatability of applications. Common sense in the application of these modalities will provide optimum injury management and modality usage for tissue healing of athletic trauma.

Summary

1. Any modalities that radiate energy with wavelengths and frequencies that fall into the infrared region of the electromagnetic spectrum are referred to as infrared modalities.
2. When infrared modalities are applied to connective tissue or muscle and soft tissue, they will cause either a tissue temperature decrease or tissue temperature increase.
3. The infrared energies have a depth of penetration of less than 1 cm, thus the physiologic effects are primarily superficial and directly affect the cutaneous blood vessels and nerve receptors.
4. The primary physiologic effects of cold are vasoconstriction of capillaries with decreased blood flow, decreased metabolic activity, and analgesia with reduction of muscle spasm.

5. Examples of cryotherapy techniques are ice massage, commercial cold packs, ice packs, cold whirlpool, cold spray, contrast bath, ice immersion, Cryo-Cuff, and cryokinetics.
6. The primary physiologic effect of heat is vasodilation of capillaries with increased blood flow, increased metabolic activity, and relaxation of muscle spasm.
7. Examples of thermotherapy are whirlpools, moist heat packs, infrared lamps, heating pads, and fluidotherapy.
8. Counterirritants are not an infrared modality. They are topically applied ointments that stimulate sensory receptors in the skin. Their effects are similar to heat and cold modulating pain.

Review Questions

1. What is the definition of an infrared modality and how are these modalities classified within the electromagnetic spectrum?
2. What are the two basic therapeutic clinical uses for the infrared modalities?
3. What is the depth of penetration into the tissues of the infrared modalities?
4. What are the effects of changing temperatures on circulation?
5. How does changing tissue temperature affect muscle spasm?

6. What are the physiological effects of both therapeutic heat and cold?
7. What are the differences between the terms cryotherapy, thermotherapy, and hydrotherapy?
8. What are the various cryotherapy techniques that can be used by the athletic trainer?
9. What are the various thermotherapy techniques that can be used by the athletic trainer?

Self-Test Questions

T/F
1. Applying heat or cold to an extremity will affect balance, proprioception, and performance.
2. Cold whirlpools should be set at temperatures of 50 to 60 degrees Fahrenheit.
3. Cryokinetics is a therapeutic technique that combines cryotherapy and exercise.

Multiple Choice
4. This mechanism of heat transfer is through direct contact.
   a. radiation
   b. convection
   c. conduction
   d. conversion

5. _____ should be used on acute injuries to _____ temperature and thus slow metabolic rate.
   a. cold, decrease
   b. cold, increase
   c. heat, decrease
   d. heat, increase
6. The three to four stages of sensation following cold application, in order, are the following:
   a. sting, cold, burn/ache, numb
   b. cold, sting, numb, burn/ache
   c. burn/ache, cold, sting, numb
   d. cold, sting, burn/ache, numb
7. An insulating layer of water next to the skin is called which of the following?.
   a. erythema
   b. thermopane
   c. anesthesia
   d. inflammation

8. Which of the following is NOT an effect of thermotherapy?
   a. increased circulation
   b. spasms are relaxed
   c. decreased cell metabolism
   d. increased soft-tissue elasticity
9. Which of the following is a contraindication for cryotherapy?
   a. acute pain
   b. skin anesthesia
   c. muscle spasm
   d. acute ligament sprain
10. In what condition would thermotherapy be indicated?
    a. decreased range of motion
    b. skin anesthesia
    c. acute musculoskeletal injury
    d. acute pain

Solutions to Clinical Decision-Making Exercises

4-1 Because the elastic wrap has been placed underneath the ice bags there is an insulating layer through which the cold must penetrate. The passage of cold can be facilitated if the elastic wrap is wet. It is likely that the ice can be left in place for up to an hour as long as the athlete does not have any type of sensitivity reaction to the cold.

4-2 A spray-and-stretch technique has been recommended as an effective technique for dealing with myofascial trigger points. Using Fluoromethane spray, the athletic trainer should make strokes parallel with the direction of fibers and then stretch the middle trapezius immediately following the application of the cold spray.

4-3 At day 7, the likelihood of any additional swelling is minimal. As long as the athlete is not complaining of tenderness to touch it is probably safe to switch to some form of heat, but it would be recommended that either ultrasound or shortwave diathermy be used since the depth of penetration of both is greater than any infrared modality.

4-4 It is likely that the combined effects of placing the ankle in a dependent position, the massaging action of the whirlpool jets, and the active exercise may cause some additional swelling, especially only 2 days post injury. It would be more advisable to simply use an ice bag with elevation followed by whatever active exercises are appropriate.

4-5 It is clear that a contrast bath produces little or no "pumping action" and thus would not be effective in treating swelling. A better alternative would be to use cryokinetics, which involves cold followed by active muscle contractions and relaxation to help eliminate swelling.

4-6 The athletic trainer should have chosen to use an ice pack. Remember this is an acute injury. Muscle strains in the low back are no different than any other muscle, and just because the athlete might be a little uncomfortable is not a good reason to make an incorrect decision about which modality is the most appropriate.

References

1. Abramson, D, Tuck, S, and Lee, S: Vascular basis for pain due to cold, *Arch Phys Med Rehab* 47:300–305, 1966.

2. Baker, R, and Bell, G: The effect of therapeutic modalities on blood flow in the human calf, *JOSPT* 13:23, 1991.

3. Basset, S, and Lake, B: Use of cold applications in management of spasticity, *Phys Ther* 38(5):333–334, 1958.

4. Behnke, R: Cold therapy, *Ath Train* 9(4):178–179, 1974.

5. Bibi, KW, Dolan, MG, and Harrington, K: Effects of hot, cold, contrast therapy whirlpools on non-traumatized ankle volumes, *Journal of Athletic Training* 34(2):S-17, 1999.

6. Bierman, W, and Friendiander, M: The penetrative effect of cold, *Arch Phys Med Rehab* 21:585–592, 1940.

7. Braswell, S. Frazzini, M, and Knuth, A: Optimal duration of ice massage for skin anesthesia, *Phys Ther* 74(5):S156, 1994.

8. Chambers, R: Clinical uses of cryotherapy, *Phys Ther* 49(3):145–149, 1969.

9. Chung, JM, Lee, KH, Hori, Y, and Willis, WD: Effects of capsaicin applied to a peripheral nerve on the responses of primate spinothalamic tract cells, *Brain Res* 329(1–2):27–38, 1985.

10. Clarke, D: Effect of immersion in hot and cold water upon recovery of muscular strength following fatiguing isometric exercise, *Arch Phys Med Rehab* 44:565–568, 1963.

11. Clarke, D, and Stelmach, G: Muscle fatigue and recovery curve parameters at various temperatures, *Res Quart* 37(4):468–479, 1966.

12. Clarke, R, Hellon, R, and Lind, A: Vascular reactions of the human forearm to cold, *Clin Sci* 17:165–179, 1958.

13. Clark, R, Lephardt, S, and Baker, C: Cryotherapy and compression treatment protocols in the prevention of delayed onset muscle soreness, *J Ath Train* 31(2):S33, 1996.

14. Clemente, F, Frampton, R, and Temoshenka, A: The effects of hot and cold packs on peak isometric torque generated by the back extensor musculature, *Phys Ther* 74(5):S70, 1994.

15. Comeau, MJ, and Potteiger, JA: The effects of cold water immersion on parameters of skeletal muscle damage and delayed onset muscle soreness, *Journal of Athletic Training* 35(2):S-46, 2000.

16. Cote, D, Prentice, W, and Hooker, D: A comparison of three treatment procedures for minimizing ankle edema, *Phys Ther* 68(7):1072–1076, 1988.

17. Curl, WW, Smith, BP, Marr, A, Rosencrance, E, Holden, M, and Smith TL: The effect of contusion and cryotherapy on skeletal muscle microcirculation, *Journal of Sports Medicine & Physical Fitness* 37(4):279–286, 1997.

18. Cutlaw, K, Arnold, B, and Perrin, D: Effect of cold treatment on concentric and eccentric force velocity relationship of the quads, *J Ath Train* 30(2):S31, 1995.

19. DeJong, R, Hershey, W, and Wagman, I: Nerve conduction velocity during hypothermia in man, *Anes* 27:805–810, 1966.

20. Dervin, GF, Taylor, DE, and Keene, GC: Effects of cold and compression dressings on early postoperative outcomes for the athroscopic ACL reconstruction patient, *Journal of Orthopedic and Sports Physical Therapy* 27(6):403–411, 1998.

21. Dolan, MG, Mendel, FM, and Teprovich, JM: Effects of dependent positioning and cold water immersions on nontraumatized ankle volumes, *Journal of Athletic Training* 34(2): S-17, 1999.

22. Dolan, MG, Thornton, RM, and Fish, DR: Effects of cold water immersion on edema formation after blunt injury to the hind limbs of rats, *Journal of Athletic Training* 32(3): 233–237, 1997.

23. Dolan, M, Thornton, R, and Mendel, F: Cold water immersion effects on edema formation following impact injury to hind limbs of rats, *J Ath Train* 31(2):S48, 1996.

24. Dontigny R, and Sheldon K: Simultaneous use of heat and cold in treatment of muscle spasm, *Arch Phys Med Rehab* 43:235–237, 1962.

25. Downer, A: *Physical therapy procedures*, ed 3, Springfield, I11. 1978. Charles C Thomas.

26. Downey, J: Physiological effects of heat and cold, *J Am Phys Ther Assoc* 44(8):713–717, 1964.

27. Dufresne, T, Jarzabaski, K, and Simmons, D: Comparison of superficial and deep heating agents followed by a passive stretch on increasing the flexibility of the hamstring muscle group, *Phys Ther* 74(5):S70, 1994.

28. Eldred, E, Lindsley, D, and Buchwald, J: The effect of cooling on mammalian muscle spindles, *Exp Neurol* 2:144–157, 1960.

29. Evans, T, Ingersoll, C, and Knight, K: Agility following the application of cold therapy, *J Ath Train* 30(3):231–234, 1995.

30. Fischer, E, and Soloman, S: Physiologic responses to heat and cold. In Licht S, editor: *Therapeutic heat*, New Haven, Conn, 1965, Elizabeth Licht.

31. Gallant, S, Knight, K, and Ingersoll, C: Cryotherapy effects on leg press and vertical jump force production, *J Ath Train* 31(2):S18, 1996.

32. Golestani, S, Pyle, M, and Threlkeld, AJ: Joint position sense in the knee following 30 min of cryotherapy, *Journal of Athletic Training* 34(2):S-68, 1999.

33. Grant, A: Massage with ice (cryokinetics) in the treatment of painful conditions of the musculoskeletal system, *Arch Phys Med Rehab* 45:233–238, 1964.

34. Grecier, M, Kendrick, Z, and Kimura, I: Immediate and delayed effects of cryotherapy on functional power and agility, *J Ath Train* 31 supp:S-32, 1996.

35. Griffin, J, and Karselis, T: *Physical agents for physical athletic trainers*, ed 2, Springfield, I ll. 1988, Charles C Thomas.

36. Guyton, A: *Medical physiology*, ed 6, Philadelphia, 1991, WB Saunders.

37. Hautkappe, M, Roizen, M, Toledano, A, Roth, S, Jefferies, J, and Andreas, M: Review of the effectiveness of capsaicin for painful cutaneous disorders and neural dysfunction, *Clinical Journal of Pain* 14(2):97–106, 1998.

38. Hayden, C: Cryokinetics in an early treatment program, *J Am Phys Ther Assoc* 44:11, 1964.

39. Haynes, S C, and Perrin, D H: Effects of a counterirritant on pain and restricted range of motion associated with delayed onset muscle soreness, *Journal of Sport Rehabilitation* (1):13–18, 1992.

40. Hedenberg, L: Functional improvement of the spastic hemiplegic arm after cooling, *Scand J Rehab Med* 2:154–158, 1970.

41. Ho, S, Illgen, R, and Meyer, R: Comparison of various icing times in decreasing bone metabolism and blood in the knee, *Am J Sports Med* 23(1):74–76, 1995.

42. Hocutt, J, Jaffe, R, and Rylander, C: Cryotherapy in ankle sprains, *Am J Sports Med* 10(3):316–319, 1992.

43. Kimura, IF, Gulick, DT, and Thompson, GT: The effect of cryotherapy on eccentric plantar flexion peak torque and endurance, *Journal of Athletic Training* 32(2):124–126, 1997.

44. Knight, K: Effects of hypothermia on inflammation and swelling, *Ath Train* 11:7–10, 1976.

45. Knight, K: *Cryotherapy in sports injury management*, Champaign, 1995, Human Kinetics.

46. Knight, K: Ice for immediate care of injuries, *Phys Sports Med* 10(2):137, 1982.

47. Knight, K: *Cryotherapy: theory, technique and physiology*, Chattanooga, 1985, Chattanooga Corporation.

48. Knight, K, Aquino, J, and Johannes S: A re-examination of Lewis' cold induced vasodilation in the finger and the ankle, *Ath Train* 15:248–250, 1980.

49. Knight, K, Ingersoll, C, and Trowbridge, C: The effects of cooling the ankle, the triceps surae or both on functional agility, *J Ath Train* 29(2):165, 1994.

50. Knight, K, and Londeree, B: Comparison of blood flow in the ankle of uninjured subjects during therapeutic applications of heat, cold, and exercise, *Med Sci Sports Exerc* 12(1):76–80, 1980.

51. Knight, KL, Rubley, MD, and Ingersoll, CD: Pain perception is greater during ankle ice immersion than during ice pack application, *Journal of Athletic Training* 35(2):S-45, 2000.

52. Knott, M, and Barufaldi, D: Treatment of whiplash injuries, *Phys Ther* 41:8, 1961.

53. Knutsson, E: Topical cryotherapy in spasticity, *Scand J Rehab Med* 2:159–163, 1970.

54. Knutsson, E, and Mattson, E: Effects of local cooling on monosynaptic reflexes in man, *Scand J Rehab Med* 1:126–132, 1969.

55. Kolb, P, and Denegar, C: Traumatic edema and the lymphatic system, *Ath Train* 18:339–341, 1983.

56. Krause, BA, Hopkins, JT, Ingersoll, CD: The relationship of ankle temperature during cooling and rewarming to the human soleus H reflex, *Journal of Sport Rehabilitation*, 9(3):253–262, 2000.

57. Kuligowski, LA, Lephart, SM, and Frank, P: Effect of whirlpool therapy on the signs and symptoms of delayed-onset muscle soreness, *Journal of Athletic Training* 33(3):222–228, 1998.

58. LaRiviere, J, and Osternig, L: The effect of ice immersion on joint position sense, *J Sport Rehab* 3(1):58–67, 1994.

59. Lee, JC, Lin, DT, and Hong, C: The effectiveness of simultaneous thermotherapy with ultrasound and electrotherapy with combined AC and DC current on the immediate pain relief of myofascial trigger points, *Journal of Musculoskeletal Pain* 5(1):81–90, 1997.

60. Lehman, J: *Therapeutic heat and cold*, ed 3, Baltimore, 1982, Williams & Wilkins.

61. Leonard, K, Horodyski, MB, and Kaminski, T: Changes in dynamic postural stability following cryotherapy to the ankle and knee, *Journal of Athletic Training* 34(2):S-68, 99.

62. Lewis, T: Observations upon the reactions of the vessels of the human skin to cold, *Heart* 15:177–208, 1930.

63. Licht, S: *Therapeutic heat and cold*, New Haven, Conn., 1965, Elizabeth Licht.

64. Lippold, O, Nicholls, J, and Redfearn, J: A study of the afferent discharge produced by cooling a mammalian muscle spindle, *J Physiol* 153:218–231, 1960.

65. Lowdon, B, and Moore, R: Determinants and nature of intramuscular temperature changes during cold therapy, *Am J Phys Med* 54(5):223–233, 1975.

66. Mancuso, D, and Knight, K: Effects of prior skin surface temperature response of the ankle during and after a 30-minute ice pack application, *J Ath Train* 27:242–249, 1992.

67. McMaster, W: A literary review on ice therapy in injuries, *Am J Sports Med* 5(3):124–126, 1977.

68. Merrick, MA, Jutte, LS, and Smith, ME: Intramuscular temperatures during cryotherapy with three different cold modalities, *Journal of Athletic Training* 35(2):S-45, 2000.

69. Merrick, M, Knight, K, and Ingersoll, C: The effects of ice and compression wraps on intramuscular temperatures at various depths, *J Ath Train* 28(3):236–245, 1993.

70. Merrick, M, Knight, K, and Ingersoll, C: The effects of ice and elastic wraps on intratissue temperatures at various depths, *J Ath Train* 28(2):156, 1993.

71. Mickey, C, Bernier, J, and Perrin, D: Ice and ice with nonthermal ultrasound effects on delayed onset muscle soreness, *J Ath Train* 31(2):S19, 1996.

72. Miglietta, O: Electromyographic characteristics of clonus and influence of cold, *Arch Phys Med Rehab* 45:508, 1964.

73. Misasi, S, Morin, G, and Kemler, D: The effect of a toe cap and bias on perceived pain during cold water immersion, *J Ath Train* 30(1):149–156, 1995.

74. Moore, R: *Uses of cold therapy in the rehabilitation of athletes: recent advances*, Proceedings 19th American Medical Association National Conference on the medical aspects of sports, San Francisco, June 1977.

75. Moore, R, Nicolette, R, and Behnke, R: The therapeutic use of cold (cryotherapy) in the care of athletic injuries, *Ath Train* 2:613, 1967.

76. Murphy, A: The physiological effects of cold application, *Phys Ther* 40(2):112–115, 1960.

77. Myrer, J, Draper, D, and Durrant, E: The effect of contrast therapy on intramuscular temperature in the human lower leg, *J Ath Train* 29(4):318–322, 1994.

78. Myrer, JW, Measom, G, Durrant, E, and Fellingham, GW: Cold- and hot-pack contrast therapy: subcutaneous and intramuscular temperature change, *Journal of Athletic Training* 32(3):238–241, 1997.

79. Myrer, JW, Meason, G, and Fellingham, GW: Temperature changes in the human leg during and after two methods of cryotherapy, *Journal of Athletic Training* 33(1):25–29, 1998.

80. Myrer, KA, Myrer, JW, and Measom, GJ: Overlying adipose significantly affects intramuscular temperature change during crushed ice pack therapy, *Journal of Athletic Training* 34(2):S-69, 1999.

81. Olson, J, and Stravino, V: A review of cryotherapy, *Phys Ther* 62(8):840–853, 1972.

82. Paduano, R, and Crothers, J: The effects of whirlpool treatments and age on a one-leg balance test, *Phys Ther* 74(5): S70, 1994.

83. Pincivero, D, Gieck, J, and Saliba, E: Rehabilitation of a lateral ankle sprain with cryokinetic and functional progressive exercise, *J Sport Rehab* 2(3):200–207, 1993.

84. Prentice, W: An electromyographic analysis of the effectiveness of heat or cold and stretching for inducing relaxation in injured muscle *JOSPT* 3(3):133–146, 1982.

85. Ragan, BG, Marvar, PJ, and Dolan, MG: Effects of magnesium sulfate and warm baths on nontraumatized ankle volumes, *Journal of Athletic Training* 35(2):S-43, 2000.

86. Rivers, D, Kimura, I, and Sitler, M: The influence of cryotherapy and Aircast bracing on total body balance and proprioception, *J Ath Train* 30(2):S15, 1995.

87. Rocks, A: Intrinsic shoulder pain syndrome, *Phys Ther* 59(2):153–159, 1979.

88. Ruiz, D, Myrer, J, and Durrant, E: Cryotherapy and sequential exercise bouts following cryotherapy on concentric and eccentric strength in the quadriceps, *J Ath Train* 28(4):320–323, 1993.

89. Schnatz, A, Kimura, I, and Sitler, M: Influence of cryotherapy, thermotherapy, and neoprene ankle sleeve on total body balance and proprioception, *J Ath Train* 31(2):S32, 1996.

90. Schuler, D, Ingersoll, C, and Knight, K: Local cold application to foot and ankle, lower leg of both effects on a cutting drill, *J Ath Train* 31(2):S35, 1996.

91. Smith, K, Draper, D, and Schulthies, S: The effect of silicate gel hot packs on human muscle temperature, *J Ath Train* 30(2):S33, 1995.

92. Smith, K, and Newton, R: The immediate effect of contrast baths on edema, temperature and pain in post surgical hand injuries, *Phys Ther* 74(5):S157, 1994.

93. Stillwell, K: Therapeutic heat and cold. In Krusen, F, Kootke, F, and Ellwood, P, editors: *Handbook of physical medicine and rehabilitation*, Philadelphia, 1971, WB Saunders.

94. Taylor, B, Waring, C, and Brasher, T: The effects of therapeutic application of heat or cold followed by static stretch on hamstring muscle length, *JOSPT* 21(5):283–286, 1995.

95. Thieme, H, Ingersoll, C, and Knight, K: The effect of cooling on proprioception of the knee, *J Ath Train* 28(2):158, 1993.

96. Thieme, H, Ingersoll, C, and Knight, K: Cooling does not affect knee proprioception, *J Ath Train* 31(1):8–11, 1996.

97. Thompson, G, Kimura, I, and Sitler, M: Effect of cryotherapy on eccentric and peak torque and endurance, *J Ath Train* 29(2):180, 1994.

98. Travell, J: Rapid relief of acute "stiff neck" by ethyl chloride spray, *Am Med Wom Assoc* 4(3):89–95, 1949.

99. Travell, J: Ethyl chloride spray for painful muscle spasm, *Arch Phys Med Rehabil* 32:291–298, 1952.

100. Travell, J, and Simons, D: *Myofascial pain and dysfunction: the trigger point manual*, Baltimore, 1983, Williams & Wilkins.

101. Tsang, KKW, Buxton, BP, Guion, WK, Joyner, AB, and Browder KD: The effects of cryotherapy applied through various barriers, *Journal of Sport Rehabilitation* 6(4):343–354, 1997.

102. Tsang, KH, Hertel, J, and Denegar, C: The effects of gravity-dependent positioning following elevation on the volume of the uninjured ankle, *Journal of Athletic Training* 35(2) S-50, 2000.

103. Weston, M, Taber, C, and Casagranda, L: Changes in local blood volume during cold gel pack application to traumatized ankles, *JOSPT* 19(4):197–199, 1994.

104. Whittaker, T, Lander, J, and Brubaker, D: The effect of cryotherapy on selected balance parameters, *J Ath Train* 29(2):180, 1994.

105. Zankel, H: Effect of physical agents on motor conduction velocity of the ulnar nerve, *Arch Phys Med Rehab* 47(12):787–792, 1966.

106. Zemke, JE, Andersen, JC, and Guion, K: Intramuscular temperature responses in the human leg to two forms of cryotherapy: ice massage and icebag, *Journal of Orthopedic and Sports Physical Therapy* 27(4):301–307, 1998.

Suggested Readings

Abraham, E: Whirlpool therapy for treatment of soft tissue wounds complicated by extremity fractures, *J Trauma* 4:222, 1974.

Abraham, W: Heat vs. cold therapy for the treatment of muscle injuries, *Ath Train* 9(4):177, 1974.

Abramson, D, Bell, B, and Tuck, S: Changes in blood flow, oxygen uptake and tissue temperatures produced by therapeutic physical agents: effect of indirect or reflex vasodilation, *Am J Phys Med* 40:5–13, 1961.

Abramson, D, Mitchell, R, and Tuck, S: Changes in blood flow, oxygen uptake and tissue temperatures produced by a topical application of wet heat, *Arch Phys Med Rehab* 42:305, 1961.

Abramson, D, Tuck, S, and Zayas, A: The effect of altering limb position on blood flow, oxygen uptake and skin temperature, *J App Physiol* 17:191, 1962.

Abramson, D, Tuck, S, and Chu, L: Effect of paraffin bath and hot fomentation on local tissue temperature, *Arch Phys Med Rehab* 45:87, 1964.

Abramson, D, Tuck, S, and Chu, L: Indirect vasodilation in thermotherapy, *Arch Phys Med Rehab* 46:412, 1965.

Abramson, D: Physiologic basis for the use of physical agents in peripheral vascular disorders, *Arch Phys Med Rehab* 46:216, 1965.

Abramson, D, Chu, L, and Tuck, S: Effect of tissue temperatures and blood flow on motor nerve conduction velocity, *JAMA* 198:1082, 1966.

Abramson, D, Tuck, S, and Lee, S: Comparison of wet and dry heat in raising temperature of tissues, *Arch Phys Med Rehab* 48:654, 1967.

Airhihenbuwa, C, St. Pierre R, and Winchell D: Cold vs. heat therapy: a physician's recommendations for first aid treatment of strain, *Emergency* 19(1):40–43, 1987.

Arnheim, D, and Prentice, W: *Principles of athletic training*, ed 9, New York, 1997, McGraw-Hill.

Ascenzi, J: *The need for decontamination and disinfection of hydrotherapy equipment*, vol 1, Surgikos Inc, 1980, Asepsis Monograph.

Austin, K: Diseases of immediate type hypersensitivity. In Isselbacher, K, Adams, R, and Braumwald, E, editors: *Harrison's principles of internal medicine*, ed 9, New York, 1980, McGraw-Hill.

Barnes, L: Cryotherapy: putting injury on ice, *Phys Sportsmed* 7(6):130–136, 1979.

Barr, E, Gibbs, C, and Knight, K: Effect of different types of cold applications on surface and intramuscular temperatures, *J Ath Train* 32(2):S-33, 1997.

Basur, R, Shephard, E, and Mouzos, G: A cooling method in the treatment of ankle sprains, *Practitioner* 216:708, 1976.

Beasley, R, and Kester, N: Principles of medical-surgical rehabilitation of the hand, *Med Clin North Am* 53:645, 1969.

Belitsky, R, Odam, S, and Humbley-Kozey, C: Evaluation of the effectiveness of wet ice, dry ice, and cryogen packs in reducing skin temperature, *Phys Ther* 67:1080, 1987.

Benoit, T, Martin, D, and Perrin, D: Effect of clinical application of heat and cold on knee joint laxity, *J Ath Train* 31(3):242–244, 1996.

Benson, T, and Copp, E: The effects of therapeutic forms of heat and ice on the pain threshold of the normal shoulder, *Rheumatol Rehab* 13:101, 1974.

Berne, R, and Levy, M: *Cardiovascular physiology*, ed 4, St Louis, 1981, Mosby.

Bickle, R: Swimming pool management, *Physiotherapy* 57:475, 1971.

Bierman, W: Therapeutic use of cold, *JAMA* 157:1189–1192, 1955.

Bocobo, C: The effect of ice on intra-articular temperature in the knee of the dog, *Am J Phys Med Rehab* 70:181, 1991.

Boes, M: Reduction of spasticity by cold, *J Am Phys Ther Assoc* 42(1):29–32, 1962.

Boland, A: Rehabilitation of the injured athlete. In Strauss, R, editor: *Physiology*, Philadelphia, 1979, WB Saunders.

Borrell, R, Henley, E, and Purvis, H: Fluidotherapy: evaluation of a new heat modality, *Arch Phys Med Rehab* 58:69, 1977.

Borrell, R, Parker, R, and Henley, E: Comparison of in vivo temperatures produced by hydrotherapy, paraffin wax treatment, and fluidotherapy, *Phys Ther* 60(10):1273–1276, 1980.

Boyer, T, Fraser, R, and Doyle, A: The haemodynamic effects of cold immersion, *Clin Sci* 19:539, 1980.

Boyle, R, Balisteri, F, and Osborne, F: The value of the Hubbard tank as a diuretic agent, *Arch Phys Med Rehab* 45:505, 1964.

Burke, D, Holt, L, and Rasmussen, R: Effects of hot or cold water immersion and modified PNF flexibility exercise on hamstring length, *Journal of Athletic Training* 36(1):16–19, 2001.

Chastain, P: The effect of deep heat on isometric strength, *Phys Ther* 58:543, 1978.

Clarke, K, editor: *Fundamentals of athletic training: physical therapy procedures*, Chicago, 1971, AMA Press.

Claus-Walker J: Physiological responses to cold stress in healthy subjects and in subjects with cervical cord injuries, *Arch Phys Med Rehab* 55:485, 1974.

Clendenin, M, and Szumski, A: Influence of cutaneous ice application on single motor units in humans, *Phys Ther* 51(2):166–175, 1971.

Cobb, C, DeVries, H, and Urban, R: Electrical activity in muscle pain, *Am J Phys Med* 54:80, 1975.

Cobbold, A, and Lewis, O: Blood flow to the knee joint of the dog: effect of heating, cooling and adrenaline, *J Physiol* 132:379, 1956.

Cohen, A, Martin, G, and Waldin, K: The effect of whirlpool bath with and without agitation on the circulation in normal and diseased extremities, *Arch Phys Med Rehab* 30:212, 1949.

Conolly, W, Paltos, N, and Tooth, R: Cold therapy: an improved method, *Med J Aust* 2:424, 1972.

Cook, D, and Georgouras K: Complications of cutaneous cryotherapy, *Med J Australia* 161(3):210–213, 1994.

Cordray, Y, and Krusen, E: Use of hydrocollator packs in the treatment of neck and shoulder pains, *Arch Phys Med Rehab* 39:105, 1959.

Coulombe, B, Swakik, C, and Raylman, R: Quantification of musculoskeletal blood flow changes in response to cryotherapy using positron emmission tomography, *Journal of Athletic Training* 36(2 supp): S-49, 2001.

Covington, D, and Bassett, F: When cryotherapy injures, *Phys Sportsmed* 21(3):78–79, 1993.

Crockford, G, and Hellon, R: Vascular responses of human skin to infrared radiation, *J Physiol* 149:424, 1959.

Crockford, G, Hellon, R, and Parkhouse, J: Thermal vasomotor response in human skin mediated by local mechanism, *J Physiol* 161:10, 1962.

Cross, K, Wilson, R, and Perrin, D: Functional performance following ice immersion to the lower extremity, *J Ath Train* 31(2):113–118, 1996.

Culp, R, and Taras, J: The effect of ice application versus controlled cold therapy on skin temperature when used with postoperative bulky hand and wrist dressings: a preliminary study, *J Hand Ther* 8(4):249–251, 1995.

Currier, D, and Kramer, J: Sensory nerve conduction: heating effects of ultrasound and infrared, *Physiother Can* 34:241, 1982.

Danielson, R, Jaeger, J, and Rippletoe, J: Differences in skin surface temperature and pressure during the application of various cold and compression devices, *J Ath Train* 32(2):S-34, 1997.

Dawson, W, Kottke, F, and Kubicek, W: Evaluation of cardiac output, cardiac work, and metabolic rate during hydrotherapy exercise in normal subjects, *Arch Phys Med Rehab* 46:605, 1965.

Day, M: Hypersensitive response to ice massage: report of a case, *Phys Ther* 54:592, 1974.

DeLateur, B, and Lehmann, J: Cryotherapy. In Lehmann, J, editor: *Therapeutic heat and cold*, ed 3, Baltimore, 1982, Williams & Wilkins.

DeVries, H: Quantitative electromyographic investigation of the spasms theory of muscle pain, *Am J Phys Med* 45:119, 1966.

Draper, D, Schulthies, S, and Sorvisto, P: Temperature changes in deep muscles of humans during ice and ultrasound therapies: an in vivo study, *JOSPT* 21(3):153–157, 1995.

Drez, D: *Therapeutic modalities for sports injuries*, Chicago, 1989, Yearbook.

Drez, D, Faust, DC, and Evans, J: Cryotherapy and nerve palsy, *Am J Sports Med* 9:256, 1981.

Edwards, H, Harris, R, and Hultman, E: Effect of temperature on muscle energy metabolism and endurance during successive isometric contractions, sustained to fatigue, of the quadriceps muscle in man, *J Physiol* 220:335, 1972.

Epstein, M: Water immersion: modern researchers discover the secrets of an old folk remedy, *Sciences* 205:12, 1979.

Eyring, E, and Murray, W: The effect of joint position on the pressure of intraarticular effusion, *J Bone Joint Surg* 46[A](6):1235, 1964.

Farry, P, and Prentice, N: Ice treatment of injured ligaments: an experimental model, *NZ Med J* 9:12, 1950.

Folkow, B, Fox, R, and Krog, J: Studies on the reactions of the cutaneous vessels to cold exposure, *Acta Physiol Scand* 58:342, 1963.

Fountain, F, Gersten, J, and Senger, O: Decrease in muscle spasm produced by ultrasound, hot packs and IR, *Arch Phys Med Rehab* 41:293, 1960.

Fox, R: Local cooling in man, *Brit Med Bull* 17(1):14–18, 1961.

Fox, R, and Wyatt, H: Cold induced vasodilation in various areas of the body surface in man, *J Physiol* 162:259, 1962.

Gammon, G, and Starr, I: Studies on the relief of pain by counterirritation, *J Clin Invest* 20:13, 1941.

Gerig, B: The effects of cryotherapy upon ankle proprioception (abstract), *Ath Train* 25:119, 1990.

Gieck, J: Precautions for hydrotherapeutic devices, *Clin Manage* 3:44, 1953.

Golland, A: Basic hydrotherapy, *Physiotherapy* 67:258, 1951.

Green, G, Zachazewski, J, and Jordan, S: A case conference: peroneal nerve palsy induced by cryotherapy, *Phys Sportsmed* 17:63, 1989.

Greenberg, R: The effects of hot packs and exercise on local blood flow, *Phys Ther* 52:273, 1972.

Halkovich, I, Personius, W, and Clamann, H: Effect of fluoromethane spray on passive hip flexion, *Phys Ther* 61:185, 1981.

Halvorson, G: Therapeutic heat and cold for athletic injuries, *Phys Sportsmed* 18:87, 1990.

Harb, G: The effect of paraffin bath submersion on digital blood flow in athletes with Raynaud's syndrome, *Phys Ther* 73(6):S9, 1993.

Harrison, R: Tolerance of pool therapy by ankylosing spondylitis athletes with low vital capacity, *Physiotherapy* 67:296, 1981.

Hatzel, B, Weidner, T, and Gehlsen, G: Mechanical power and velocity following cryotherapy and ankle taping, *Journal of Athletic Training* 36(2 supp): S-89, 2001.

Hayes, K: Heat and cold in the management of rheumatoid arthritis, *Arthritis Care Research* 6(3):156–166, 1993.

Head, M, and Helms, P: Paraffin and sustained stretching in the treatment of burn contractures, *Burns* 4:136, 1977.

Healy, W, Seidman, J, and Pfeifer, B: Cold compressive dressing after total knee arthroplasty, *Clin Ortho Related Research* (299):143–146, 1994.

Hellerbrand, T, Holutz, S, and Eubarik, I: Measurement of whirlpool temperature, pressure and turbulence, *Arch Phys Med Rehab* 32:17, 1950.

Hendier, E, Crosbie, R, and Hardy, J: Measurement of heating of the skin during exposure to infrared radiation *J Appl Physiol* 12:177, 1958.

Henrickson, A, Fredricksson, K, and Persson, I: The effect of heat and stretching on the range of hip motion, *JOSPT* 6:110, 1984.

Higgins, D, Kaminski, T, and Lacey, D: The effects of contrast therapy on the intermuscular temperature of the human gastrocnemius muscle, *J Ath Train* 32(2):S-5, 1997.

Ho, S, Coel, M, and Kagawa, R: The effects of ice on blood flow and bone metabolism in knees, *Am J Sports Med* 22(4):537–540, 1994.

Hocutt, J, Jaffe, R, and Rylander, R: Cryotherapy in ankle sprains, *Am J Sports Med* 10:316, 1982.

Holcomb, W, Mangus, B, and Tandy, R: The effect of icing with the Pro-Stim Edema Management System on cutaneous cooling, *J Ath Train* 31(2):126–129, 1996.

Holmes, G: Hydrotherapy as a means of rehabilitation, *Brit J Phys Med* 5:93, 1942.

Hopkins, J, Ingersoll, C, and Edwards, J: The effects of cryotherapy and TENS on arthrogenic muscle inhibition of the quadriceps, *Journal of Athletic Training* 36(2 supp): S-49, 2001.

Horton, B, Brown, G, and Roth, G: Hypersensitiveness to cold with local and systemic manifestations of a histamine-like character: its amenability to treatment, *JAMA* 107:1263, 1936.

Horvath, S, and Hollander, J: Intra-articular temperature as a measure of joint reaction, *J Clin Invest* 28:469, 1949.

Hunter, J, and Mackin, E: Edema and bandaging. In Hunter, J, editor: *Rehabilitation of the hand*, ed 1, St Louis, 1978, Mosby.

Ingersoll, C, and Mangus, B: Sensations of cold reexamined: a study using the McGill pain questionnaire, *Ath Train* 26:240, 1991.

Ingersoll, C, Mangus, B, and Wolf, S: Cold-induced pain: habituation to cold immersion (abstract), *Ath Train* 25:126, 1990.

Jamison, C, Merrick, M, and Ingersoll, C: The effects of post cryotherapy exercise on surface and capsular temperature, *Journal of Athletic Training* 36(2 supp): S-9 1, 2001.

Jessup, G: Muscle soreness: temporary distress of injury? *Ath Train* 15(4):260, 1950.

Jezdirisky, J, Marek, J, and Ochonsky, P: Effects of local cold and heat therapy on traumatic oedema of the rat hind paw. 1. Effects of cooling on the course of traumatic oedema, *Acta Universitatis Palackianae Olomucensis Facultatis Medicae* 66:155, 1973.

Johnson, D: Effect of cold submersion on intramuscular temperature of the gastrocnemius muscle, *Phys Ther* 59:1238, 1979.

Johnson, J, and Leider, F: Influence of cold bath on maximum handgrip strength, *Percept Mot Skills* 44:323, 1977.

Kaempffe, F: Skin surface temperature after cryotherapy to a casted extremity, *JOSPT* 10(11):448–450, 1989.

Kaul, M, and Herring, S: Superficial heat and cold: how to maximize the benefits, *Phys Sportsmed* 22(12):65–72, 74, 1994.

Kessler, R, and Hertling, D: *Management of common musculoskeletal disorders*, Philadelphia, 1953, Harper & Row.

Knight, K, Okuda, I, and Ingersoll, C: The effects of cold application on nerve conduction velocity and muscle force, *J Ath Train* 32(2):S-5, 1997.

Knight, K: Ankle rehabilitation with cryotherapy, *Phys Sportsmed* 7(11):133, 1979.

Knight, K, Rubley, M, and Brucker, J: Knee surface temperature changes on uninjured subjects during and following application of three post operative cryotherapy devices, *Journal of Athletic Training* 36(2 supp): S-90, 2001.

Kowal, M: Review of physiological effects of cryotherapy, *JOSPT* 6(2):66–73, 1953.

Kramer, J, and Mendryk, S: Cold in the initial treatment of injuries sustained in physical activity programs, *Can Assoc Health Phys Ed Rec J* 45(4):27–29, 38–40, 1979.

Krause, B, Ingersoll, C, and Edwards, J: Ankle joint and triceps surae muscle cooling produces similar changes in the soleus H:M ratio, *Journal of Athletic Training* 36(2 supp): S-50, 2001.

Krusen, E: Effects of hot packs on peripheral circulation, *Arch Phys Med Rehab* 31:145, 1950.

Landen, B: Heat or cold for the relief of low back pain? *Phys Ther* 47:1126, 1967.

Lane, L: Localized hypothermia for the relief of pain in musculoskeletal injuries, *Phys Ther* 51:182, 1971.

Lee, J, Warren, M, and Mason, S: Effects of ice on nerve conduction velocity, *Physiotherapy* 64:2, 1978.

Lehmann, J: Effect of therapeutic temperatures on tendon extensibility, *Arch Phys Med Rehab* 51:481, 1970.

Lehmann, J, Brurmer, G, and Stow, R: Pain threshold measurements after therapeutic application of ultrasound, microwaves and infrared, *Arch Phys Med Rehab* 39:560, 1958.

Lehmann, J, Silverman, J, and Baum, B: Temperature distributions in the human thigh produced by infrared, hot pack and microwave applications, *Arch Phys Med Rehab* 47:291, 1966.

Levine, M, Kabat, H, and Knott, M: Relaxation of spasticity by physiological techniques, *Arch Phys Med Rehab* 35:214, 1954.

Levy, A, and Marmar, E: The role of cold compression dressings in the postoperative treatment of total knee arthroplasty, *Clin Ortho Related Res* (297):174–178, 1993.

Lundgren, C, Muren, A, and Zederfeldt, B: Effect of cold vasoconstriction on wound healing in the rabbit, *Acta Cbir Scand* 118:1, 1959.

Magness, J, Garrett, T, and Erickson, D: Swelling of the upper extremity during whirlpool baths, *Arch Phys Med Rehab* 51:297, 1970.

Major, T, Schwingharner, J, and Winston, S: Cutaneous and skeletal muscle vascular responses to hypothermia, *Am J Physiol* 240 (Heart Circ. Physiol. 9):H868, 1981.

Marek, I, Jezdinsky, J, and Ochonsky, P: Effects of local cold and heat therapy on traumatic oedema of the rat hind paw. II. Effects of various kinds of compresses on the course of traumatic oedema. *Acta Universitatis Palackianae Olomucensis Facultatis Medicae* 66:203, 1973.

Matsen, F, Questad, K, and Matsen, A: The effect of local cooling on post fracture swelling, *Clin Orthop* 109:201, 1975.

McDowell, J, McFarland, E, and Nalli, B: Use of cryotherapy for orthropaedic athletes, *Orthopaedic Nursing* 13(5):21–30, 1994.

McGowen, H: Effects of cold application on maximal isometric contraction, *Phys Ther* 47:185, 1967.

McGray, R, and Patton, N: Pain relief at trigger points: a comparison of moist heat and shortwave diathermy, *JOSPT* 5:175, 1984.

McMaster, W: Cryotherapy, *Phys Sports Med* 10(11):112–119, 1982.

McMaster, W, and Liddie, S: Cryotherapy influence on posttraumatic limb edema, *Clin Orthop* 150:283–287, 1980.

McMaster, W, Liddie, S, and Waugh T: Laboratory evaluation of various cold therapy modalities, *Am J Sports Med* 6(5): 291–294, 1978.

Mense, S: Effects of temperature on the discharges of muscle spindles and tendon organs, *Pflugers Arch* 374:159, 1978.

Mermel, J: The therapeutic use of cold, *J Am Osteopathic Assoc* 74:1146–1157, 1975.

Michalski, W, Sequin, J: The effects of muscle cooling and stretch on muscle spindle secondary endings in the cat, *J Physiol* 253:341–356, 1975.

Michlovitz, S: *Thermal agents in rehabilitation*, Philadelphia, 1995, FA Davis.

Miglietta, O: Action of cold on spasticity, *Am J Phys Med* 52(4):198–205, 1973.

Myrer, J, Measom, G, and Fellingham, G: A comparison of subcutaneous and intramuscular temperature change between ice pack and cold whirlpool cryotherapy, *J Ath Train* 32(2):S-5, 1997.

Myrer, W, Myrer, K, and Measom, G: Muscle temperature is affected by overlying adipose when cryotherapy is administered, *Journal of Athletic Training* 36(1): 32–36, 2001.

Newton, M, and Lchnikuhi, D: Muscle spindle response to body heating and localized muscle cooling: implications for relief of spasticity, *J Am Phys Ther Assoc* 45(2):91, 105, 1965.

Noonan, T: Best, T, and Seaber, A: Thermal effects on skeletal muscle tensile behavior, *Am J Sports Med* 21(4):517–522, 1993.

Nylin, J: The use of water in therapeutics, *Arch Phys Med Rehab* 13:261, 1932.

Oliver, R, Johnson, D, and Wheelhouse, W: Isometric muscle contraction response during recovery from reduced intramuscular temperature, *Arch Phys Med Rehab* 60:126–129, 1979.

Otte, J, Merrick, M, and Ingersoll, C: Subcutaneous adipose tissue thickness changes cooling time during cryotherapy, *Journal of Athletic Training* 36(2 supp): S-91, 2001.

Palmer, J, and Knight, K: Ankle and thigh skin surface temperature changes with repeated ice pack application, *J Ath Train* 31(4):319–323, 1996.

Panus, P, Carroll, J, and Gilbert, R: Gender dependent responses in humans to dry and wet cryotherapy, *Phys Ther* 74(5): S156, 1994.

Perkins, J, Mao-Chih, L, and Nicholas, C: Cooling and contraction of smooth muscle, *Am J Physiol* 163:14, 1950.

Petajan, J, and Watts, N: Effects of cooling on the triceps surae reflex, *Am J Phys Med* 42:240–251, 1962.

Pope, C: Physiologic action and therapeutic value of general and local whirlpool baths, *Arch Phys Med Rehab* 10:498, 1929.

Preston, D, Irrgang, J, and Bullock, A: Effect of cold and compression on swelling following ACL reconstruction, *J Ath Train* 28(2):166, 1993.

Price, R: Influence of muscle cooling on the vasoelastic response of the human ankle to sinusoidal displacement, *Arch Phys Med Rehabil* 71(10):745–748, 1990.

Price, R, Lehmann, J, and Boswell, S: Influence of cryotherapy on spasticity at the human ankle, *Arch Phys Med Rehab* 74(3):300–304, 1993.

Randall, B, Imig, C, and Hines, H: Effects of some physical therapies on blood flow, *Arch Phys Med Rehabil* 33:73, 1952.

Randt, G: Hot tub folliculitis, *Phys Sports Med* 11:75, 1983.

Ritzmann, S, and Levin, W: Cryopathies: a review, *Arch Intern Med* 107:186, 1961.

Roberts, P: Hydrotherapy: its history, theory and practice, *Occup Health* 235:5, 1981.

Rogers, J, Knight, K, and Draper, D: Increased pressure of application during ice massage results in an increase in calf skin numbering, *Journal of Athletic Training* 36(2 supp): S-90, 2001.

Rubley, M, West, T, and Newell, K: The effects of cryotherapy on fine motor control in the finger, *J Ath Train* 32(2):S-6, 1997.

Schaubel, H: Local use of ice after orthopedic procedures, *Am J Surg* 72:711, 1946.

Schultz, K: *The effect of active exercise during whirlpool on the hand*, Unpublished thesis. San Jose, Calif, 1982, San Jose State University.

Serwa, J, Rancourt, L, and Merrick, M: Effect of varying application pressures on skin surface and intramuscular temperatures during cryotherapy, *Journal of Athletic Training* 36 (2 supp): S-90, 2001.

Shelley, W, and Caro W: Cold erythema: a new hypersensitivity syndrome, *JAMA* 180:639, 1962.

Simonetti, A, Miller, R, and Gristina, J: Efficacy of povidone-iodine in the disinfection of whirlpool baths and hubbard tanks, *Phys Ther* 52:450, 1972.

Steve, L, Goodhart, P, and Alexander, J: Hydrotherapy burn treatment: use of chloramine-T against resistant microorganisms, *Arch Phys Med Rehab* 60:301, 1979.

Stewart, B, and Basmajian, J: Exercises in water. In Basmajian, J, editor: *Therapeutic exercise*, ed 3, Baltimore, 1978, Williams & Wilkins.

Strandness, D: Vascular diseases of the extremities. In Isselbacher, K, Adams, R, and Braunwald, E, editors: *Harrison's principles of internal medicine*, ed 9, New York, 1980, McGraw-Hill.

Streator, S, Ingersoll, C, and Knight, K: The effects of sensory information on the perception of cold-induced pain, *J Ath Train* 29(2):166, 1994.

Taber, C, Contryman, K, and Fahrenbach, J: Measurement of reactive vasodilation during cold gel pack application to nontraumatized ankles, *Phys Ther* 72:294, 1992.

Thieme, H, Ingersoll, C, and Knight, K: Cooling does not affect knee proprioception, *J Ath Train* 31(1):8–11, 1996.

Travell, J, and Simons, D: *Myofascial pain and dysfunction: the trigger point manual*, Baltimore, 1983, Williams & Wilkins.

Tremblay, E, Estephan, L, and Legendre, M: Influence of local cooling on proprioceptive acuity in the quadriceps muscle, *Journal of Athletic Training* 36(2):119–123, 2001.

Tsang, K, Buxton, B, and Guion, K: Effects of cryotherapy applied through various barriers on skin temperature, heart rate, and blood pressure, *J Ath Train* 32(2):S-6, 1997.

Urbscheit, N, Johnston, R, and Bishop, B: Effects of cooling on the ankle jerk and H-response in hemiplegic athletes, *Phys Ther* 51:983, 1971.

Wakim, K, Porter, A, and Krusen, K: Influence of physical agents and of certain drugs on intra-articular temperature, *Arch Phys Med Rehab* 32:714, 1951.

Walsh, M: *Relationship of hand edema to upper extremity position and water temperature during whirlpool treatments in normals*, Unpublished thesis. Philadelphia, 1983, Temple University.

Warren, G: The use of heat and cold in the treatment of common musculoskeletal disorders. In Kessler, R, and Hertling, D: *Management of common musculoskeletal disorders*, Philadelphia, 1983, Harper & Row.

Warren, G, Lehmann, J, and Koblanski, N: Heat and stretch procedures: an evaluation using rat tail tendon, *Arch Phys Med Rehab* 57:122, 1976.

Watkins, A: *A manual of electrotherapy*, ed 3, Philadelphia, 1972, Lea & Febiger.

Waylonis, G: The physiological effect of ice massage, *Arch Phys Med Rehab* 48:37–42, 1967.

Weinberger, A, and Lev, A: Temperature elevation of connective tissue by physical modalities, *Crit Rev Phys Rehab Med* 3:121, 1991.

Wertz, A, Myrer, J, and Measom, G: Intramuscular and subcutaneous temperature changes in the human leg due to contrast therapy, *J Ath Train* 32(2):S-33, 1997.

Wessman, M, and Kottke, F: The effect of indirect heating on peripheral blood flow, pulse rate, blood pressure and temperature, *Arch Phys Med Rehab* 48:567, 1967.

Whitelaw, G, DeMuth, K, and Demos, H: The use of the Cryo/Cuff versus ice and elastic wrap in the postoperative care of knee arthroscopy athletes, *Am J. Knee Surgery* 8(1):28–30, 1995.

Whitney, S: Physical agents: heat and cold modalities. In Scully, R, and Barnes, M, editors: *Physical therapy*, Philadelphia, 1987, JB Lippencott.

Whyte, H, and Reader, S: Effectiveness of different forms of heating, *Ann Rheum Dis* 10:449, 1951.

Wickstrom, R, and Polk, C: Effect of whirlpool on the strength endurance of the quadriceps muscle in trained male adolescents, *Am J Phys Med* 40:91, 1961.

Wilkerson, G: Treatment of inversion ankle sprain through synchronous application of focal compression and cold, *Ath Train* 26:220, 1991.

Wolf, S, Basmajian, J: Intramuscular temperature changes deep to localized cutaneous cold stimulation, *Phys Ther* 53(12):1284–1288, 1973.

Wolf, S, and Ledbetter, W: Effect of skin cooling on spontaneous EMG activity in triceps surae of the decerebrate cat, *Brain Res* 91:151–155, 1975.

Wright, V, and Johns, R: Physical factors concerned with the stiffness of normal and diseased joints, *Bull Johns Hopkins Hosp* 106:215, 1960.

Wyper, D, and McNiven, D: Effects of some physiotherapeutic agents on skeletal muscle blood flow, *Physiotherapy* 62:83, 1976.

Yackzan, L, Adams, C, and Francis, K: The effects of ice massage in delayed muscle soreness, *Am J Sports Med* 12(2):159–165, 1984.

Zankel, H: Effect of physical agents on motor conduction velocity of the ulnar nerve, *Arch Phys Med Rehab* 47:787, 1966.

Zeiter, V: Clinical application of the paraffin bath, *Arch Phys Ther* 20:469, 1939.

Zislis, J: Hydrotherapy. In Krusen, F, editor: *Handbook of physical medicine and rehabilitation*, ed 2, Philadelphia, 1971, WB Saunders.

CHAPTER 5

Therapeutic Ultrasound

David O. Draper and William E. Prentice

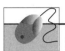

Study Resources

Refer to the lab exercises in the accompanying Laboratory
Manual, as well as eSims which simulates the athletic
training certification exam at www.mhhe.com/esims.
Also, check out the competency information found at
www.mhhe.com/prentice11e. For more online study
resources, visit our Health and Human Performance
Website at www.mhhe.com/hhp/.

**Following completion of this chapter the
student athletic trainer will be able to**

- Analyze the transmission of acoustical energy
  in biologic tissues relative to waveforms,
  frequency, velocity, and attenuation.

- Break down the basic physics involved in the
  production of a beam of therapeutic ultrasound.

- Compare the thermal and nonthermal
  physiological effects of therapeutic ultrasound.

- Evaluate specific techniques of application of
  therapeutic ultrasound and how they may be
  modified to achieve treatment goals.

- Choose the most appropriate and clinically
  effective uses for therapeutic ultrasound.

- Explain the technique and clinical application
  of phonophoresis.

- Identify the contraindications and precautions
  that should be observed with therapeutic
  ultrasound.

- Ultrasound is one of the most widely
  used modalities in sports medicine

I n the medical community, ultrasound is a modality that is used for a number of different purposes
including diagnosis, destruction of tissue, and as a
therapeutic agent. Diagnostic ultrasound has been
used for more than 30 years for the purpose of imaging internal structures. Most typically, diagnostic ultrasound is used to image the fetus during pregnancy.
Ultrasound has also been used to produce extreme tissue hyperthermia, which has been demonstrated to
have tumoricidal effects in cancer patients.

In sports medicine, ultrasound is one of the most
widely used therapeutic modalities,[26] in addition to
superficial heat and cold and electrical stimulating
currents. It has been used for therapeutic purposes as
a valuable tool in the rehabilitation of many different
injuries, primarily for the purpose of stimulating the
repair of soft tissue injuries and for relief of pain.[37]

As discussed in Chapter 1, ultrasound is a form
of acoustic rather than electromagnetic energy. Ultrasound is defined as inaudible, acoustic vibrations
of high frequency that may produce either thermal
or nonthermal physiologic effects.[51] The use of ultrasound as a therapeutic agent may be extremely
effective if the athletic trainer has an adequate understanding of its effects on biologic tissues and of
the physical mechanisms by which these effects are
produced.[37]

ULTRASOUND AS A THERMAL MODALITY

In Chapter 4, we discussed heat as a treatment modality. Warm whirlpools, paraffin baths and hot packs, to name a few, all produce therapeutic heat. However, the depth of penetration of these modalities is superficial and, at best, only 1 to 2 cm.[87] Ultrasound, along with diathermy, has traditionally been classified as a "deep heating modality" and has been used primarily for the purpose of elevating tissue temperatures.

Suppose an athlete is lacking dorsiflexion. It is determined, through evaluation, that a tight soleus is the problem, and as a athletic trainer your desire is to use thermotherapy followed by stretching. Will superficial heat adequately prepare this muscle to be stretched? Since the soleus lies deep under the gastrocnemius muscle, it is beyond the reach of superficial heat.

One of the advantages of using ultrasound over other thermal modalities is that it can provide deep heating.[87] The heating effects of silicate gel hot packs and warm whirlpools have been compared with ultrasound. At an intramuscular depth of 3 cms, a 10-minute hot pack treatment yielded an increase of .8° C[111] whereas at this same depth, 1 MHz ultrasound has raised muscle temperature nearly 4° C in 10 minutes.[91] At 1 cm below the fat surface, a 4-minute warm whirlpool (40.6° C) raised the temperature 1.1° C,[93] however, at this same depth, 3 MHz ultrasound raised the temperature 4° C in 4 minutes.[31,33,93]

TRANSMISSION OF ACOUSTICAL ENERGY IN BIOLOGICAL TISSUES

Unlike electromagnetic energy, which travels most effectively through a vacuum, acoustical energy relies on molecular collision for transmission. When set into vibration, molecules in a conducting medium will cause vibration and minimal displacement of other surrounding molecules so that eventually this "wave" of vibration has propagated through the entire medium. Sound

- Ultrasound and diathermy = deep heating modalities

■ Analogy *5-1*

Acoustic energy emitted from a single source travels in waves in all directions much like a rock that is thrown into a pond. The waves travel outward and away from the spot where the rock entered the water. As they move outward, they become smaller and smaller until they eventually disappear.

- Ultrasound = acoustic energy

longitudinal wave   The primary waveform in which ultrasound energy travels in soft tissue with the molecular displacement along the direction in which the wave travels.

transverse wave   Occurring only in bone, the molecules are displaced in a direction perpendicular to the direction in which the ultrasound wave is moving.

waves travel in a manner similar to waves created by a stone thrown into a pool of water. Ultrasound is a mechanical wave in which energy is transmitted by the vibrations of the molecules of the biological medium through which the wave is traveling.[117]

Transverse versus Longitudinal Waves

There are two types of waves that can travel through a solid medium: **longitudinal** and **transverse waves**. In a longitudinal wave, the molecular displacement is along the direction in which the wave travels. Within this longitudinal wave pathway are regions of high molecular density referred

··

compressions   Regions of high molecular density within the longitudinal wave.

rarefactions   Regions of lower molecular density within a longitudinal wave.

··

to as **compressions** (the molecules are squeezed together), and regions of lower molecular density are called **rarefactions** (the molecules spread out) (Figure 5-1). In a transverse wave, the molecules are displaced in a direction perpendicular to the di-

rection in which the wave is moving. While longitudinal waves travel both in solids and liquids, transverse waves can travel only in solids. Since soft tissues are more like liquids, ultrasound travels primarily as a longitudinal wave; however, when it contacts bone, a transverse wave results.[117]

Frequency of Wave Transmission

The *frequency* of audible sound ranges between 16 kHz and 20 kHz (kilohertz = 1000 cycles per second). Ultrasound has a frequency above 20 kHz.

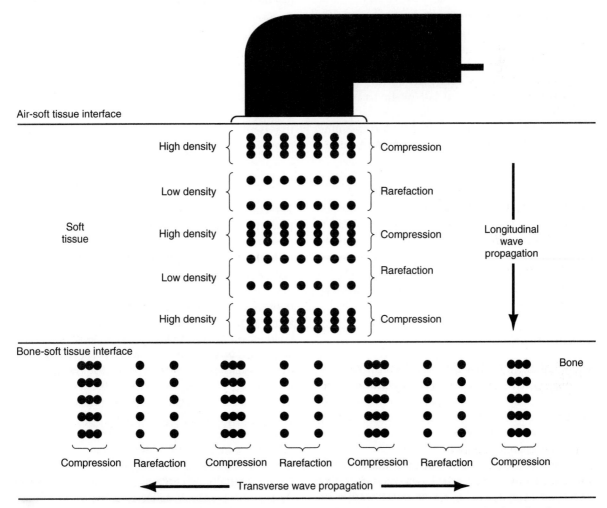

Figure 5-1   Ultrasound travels through soft tissue as a longitudinal wave alternating regions of high molecular density (compressions) and areas of low molecular density (rarefactions). Transverse waves are found primarily in bone.

■ Analogy   5-2

Longitudinal and transverse waves move through tissue in a series of compressions and rarefactions in much the same manner as the squeezing together and spreading apart of a child's toy slinky.

> • Penetration and absorption are inversely related

The frequency range for therapeutic ultrasound is between 0.75 and 3 MHz (megahertz = 1,000,000 cycles per second). The higher the frequency of the sound waves emitted from a sound source, the less the sound will diverge and thus a more focused beam of sound is produced. In biologic tissues, the lower the frequency of the sound waves the greater the depth of penetration. Higher frequency sound waves are absorbed in the more superficial tissues.

Velocity

The *velocity* at which this vibration or sound wave is propagated through the conducting medium is directly related to the density. Denser and more rigid materials will have a higher velocity of transmission. At a frequency of 1 MHz, sound travels through soft tissue at 1540 m/sec and through compact bone at 4000 m/sec.[128]

Attenuation

As the ultrasound wave is transmitted through the various tissues, there will be **attenuation**, or a decrease in energy intensity. This decrease is due to either *absorption* of energy by the tissues or *dispersion* and *scattering* of the sound wave, which results from reflection or refraction.[117]

Ultrasound penetrates through tissue high in water content and is absorbed in dense tissues high in protein where it will have its greatest heating potential.[57] The capability of acoustic energy to pene-

attenuation   A decrease in energy intensity as the ultrasound wave is transmitted through various tissues due to scattering and dispersion.

acoustic impedance   Determines the amount of ultrasound energy reflected at tissue interfaces.

trate or be transmitted to deeper tissues is determined by the frequency of the ultrasound as well as the characteristics of the tissues through which ultrasound is traveling. Penetration and absorption are inversely related. Absorption increases as the frequency increases, thus less energy is transmitted to the deeper tissues.[73] Tissues that are high in water content have a low rate of absorption, while tissues high in protein have a high absorption rate.[38] Fat has a relatively low absorption rate, and muscle absorbs considerably more. Peripheral nerve absorbs at a rate twice that of muscle. Bone that is relatively superficial absorbs more ultrasonic energy than any of the other tissues (Table 5-1).

When a sound wave encounters a boundary or an interface between different tissues, some of the energy will scatter due to reflection or refraction. The amount of energy reflected, and conversely the amount of energy which will be transmitted to deeper tissues, is determined by the relative magnitude of the **acoustic impedances** of the two materials on either side of the interface. Acoustic impedance may be determined by multiplying the density of the material by the speed at which sound travels inside it. If the acoustic impedance of the two materials forming the interface is the same, all of the sound will be transmitted and none will be reflected. The larger the difference between the two acoustic impedances the more energy is reflected and the less that can enter a second medium[123] (see Table 5-2).

Sound passing from the transducer to air will be almost completely reflected. Ultrasound is transmitted through fat. It is both reflected and refracted at the muscular interface. At the soft tissue-bone interface virtually all of the sound is reflected. As the ultrasound energy is reflected at tissue interfaces with different acoustical impedances, the intensity

■ **TABLE 5-1**   Relationship between Penetration and Absorption (1 MHz)

MEDIA	ABSORPTION	PENETRATION
Water	1	1200
Blood plasma	23	52
Whole blood	60	20
Fat	390	4
Skeletal muscle	663	2
Peripheral nerve	1193	1

From Griffin, JE: *J Am Phys Ther* 46(1):18–26, 1966. Reprinted with permission of the American Physical Therapy Association.

■ **TABLE 5-2**   The Percentage of the Incident Energy Reflected at Tissue Interfaces[121]

INTERFACE	PERCENT REFLECTION
Soft tissue/air	99.9
Water/soft tissue	0.2
Soft tissue/fat	1.0
Soft tissue/bone	15–40

of the energy is increased as the reflected energy meets new energy being transmitted, creating what is referred to as a **standing wave** or a "hot spot." This increased level of energy has the potential to produce tissue damage. Moving the sound transducer or using pulsed wave ultrasound can help to minimize the development of **hot spots**.[38]

BASIC PHYSICS OF THERAPEUTIC ULTRASOUND

Components of a Therapeutic Ultrasound Generator

An ultrasound generator consists of a high frequency electrical generator connected through an oscillator circuit and a transformer via a coaxial cable to a transducer housed in a type of insulated

standing wave   As the ultrasound energy is reflected at tissue interfaces with different acoustical impedances, the intensity of the energy is increased as the reflected energy meets new energy being transmitted forming waves of high energy, that can potentially damage surrounding tissues.

hot spots   Areas at tissue interfaces that may become overheated.

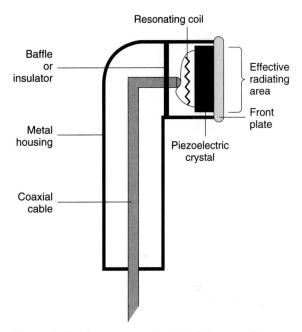

Figure 5-2   The anatomy of a typical ultrasound transducer.

applicator (Figure 5-2). The oscillator circuit produces a sound beam at a specific frequency that is adjusted by the manufacturer to the frequency requirements of the transducer. The control panel of an ultrasound unit usually has a timer that can be preset, a power meter, an intensity control, a duty cycle control switch, a selector for continuous or pulsed modes, possibly output power in response to tissue loading, and automatic shut-off in case of overheating of the transducer. Recently dual soundheads and dual frequency choices have become standard equipment on ultrasound units

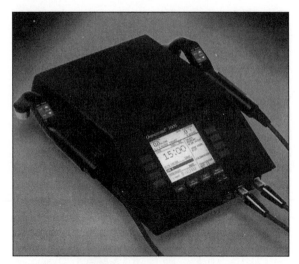

Figure 5-3 State-of-the-art ultrasound unit with dual soundheads, dual frequencies, intensity and frequency controls located on transducers and preprogrammed temperature increase settings.
(Manufactured by Physio Technology Inc., Topeka, Kans.)

(Figure 5-3). Table 5-3 provides a list of the most desirable features in an ultrasound generator.

Transducer

The transducer, also referred to as an applicator or a sound head, must be matched to particular units and is generally not interchangeable.[23] The transducer consists of some piezoelectric crystal, such as quartz, or synthetic ceramic crystals made of lead zirconate or titanate, barium titanate, or nickel-cobalt ferrite, approximately 2 to 3 mm in thickness. It is the crystal within the transducer which converts electrical energy to acoustic energy through mechanical deformation of the piezoelectric crystal.

Piezoelectric Effect. When an alternating electrical current generated at the same frequency as the crystal resonance is passed through the piezoelectric crystal, the crystal will expand and contract creating what is referred to as the **piezoelectric effect**. There are two forms of this piezoelectric effect (Figure 5-4). A *direct* piezoelectric effect is the generation of an electrical voltage across the crystal when it is compressed or expanded. An *indirect* or *reverse* piezoelectric effect is created when

■ **TABLE 5-3** The State-of-the-Art "Ultimate" Ultrasound Machine Would Contain the Following:

1. Low BNR (< 4:1)
2. High ERA (nearly matches the size of the soundhead)
3. Multiple frequencies (1 and 3 MHz)
4. Multiple sized soundheads
5. Sensing device that shuts off the unit when overheating
6. Good insulation that can be used underwater
7. Output jack for combination therapy
8. Several pulsed duty cycles
9. High-quality synthetic crystal
10. Transducer handle that maintains the operator's wrist in a natural, relaxed position
11. Durable transducer face that will protect the crystal if dropped
12. Computer controlled timer that makes adjustments in treatment duration as the intensity is adjusted (much like iontophoresis where the treatment time adjusts according to the dose applied)

an alternating current moves through the crystal, producing compression or expansion. It is this change in voltage polarity that causes the crystal to expand and contract and thus vibrate at the frequency of the electrical oscillation. Thus, the reverse piezoelectric effect is used to generate ultrasound at a desired frequency.

Effective Radiating Area (ERA). That portion of the surface of the transducer that actually produces the sound wave is referred to as the **effective radiating area** (ERA). ERA is dependent on the surface area of the crystal and ideally nearly matches the diameter of the transducer faceplate[37] (Figure 5-5). The ERA is determined by scanning the transducer at a distance of 5 mm from the radiating surface and recording all areas in excess of 5% of the maximum power output found at any location on the surface of the transducer. The acoustic energy is contained with a focused cylindrical beam that is roughly the same diameter as the soundhead.[123]

Since the effective radiating area is always smaller than the transducer surface, the size of the

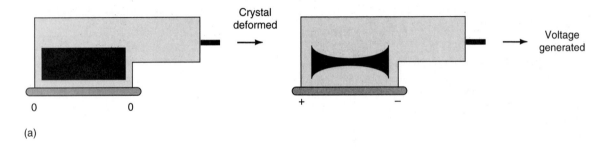

(a)

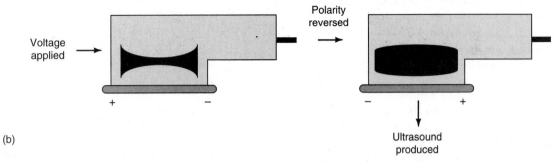

(b)

Figure 5-4   Piezoelectric effect. (a) In a direct piezoelectric effect, a mechanical deformation of the crystal generates a voltage. (b) In the reverse piezoelectric effect, as the alternating current reverses polarity, the crystal expands and contracts, producing ultrasound energy.

piezoelectric effect   When an alternating electrical current generated at the same frequency as the crystal resonance is passed through the piezoelectric crystal, the crystal will expand and contract or vibrate at the frequency of the electrical oscillation, thus generating ultrasound at a desired frequency.

effective radiating area   The total area of the surface of the transducer that actually produces the sound wave.

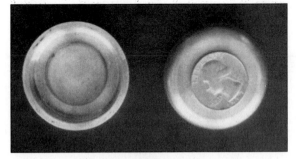

Figure 5-5   (left) Photo of a quarter-sized crystal mounted to the inside of the transducer faceplate. (right) A quarter is placed on the transducer face to illustrate that this crystal is smaller than the faceplate. Ideally, they should be closer to the same size.

- Treatment area = 2 to 3 ERA

transducer is not indicative of the actual radiating surface. A very common mistake is to assume that because you have a large transducer surface, the entire surface radiates ultrasound output. This is generally not true, particularly with larger 10 cm² transducers. There is really no point in having a large transducer with a small radiating surface, as it only mechanically limits the coupling in smaller areas (see Figure 5-5). The transducer ERA should match the total size of the soundhead as closely as possible for ease of application to various body surfaces to maintain the most effective coupling.

The appropriate size of the area to be treated using ultrasound is 2 to 3 times the size of the effective radiating area (ERA) of the crystal.[14,107] To support this premise, peak temperature in human muscle was measured during 10 minutes of 1 MHz ultrasound delivered at 1.5W/cm² (Figure 5-6). The treatment size for 10 subjects was 2 ERA, and for the other 10 it was 6 ERA. The 2 ERA group's temperature increased 3.6° C (moderate to vigorous heating), whereas the subject's temperature in the 6 ERA group only increased 1.1° C (mild heating). A similar study showed that 3 MHz ultrasound at an intensity of 1 W/cm² significantly increased patellar tendon temperature at both 2 times and 4 times ERA. However, the 2 ERA size provided higher and longer heating than the 4 ERA size.[15] Thus, ultrasound is most effectively used for treating small areas.[29] Hot packs, whirlpools, and shortwave diathermy have an advantage over ultrasound in that they can be used to heat much larger areas.

Frequency of Therapeutic Ultrasound

Therapeutic ultrasound produced by a piezoelectric transducer has a frequency range between 0.75 and 3.0 MHz. Frequency is the number of wave cycles completed each second. The majority of the

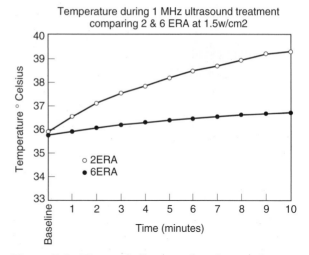

Figure 5-6 This graph illustrates that ultrasound is ineffective in heating areas much larger than twice the size of the transducer face. Mean temperature increase for 2 ERA was 3.4° C, and only 1.1° C for an area 6 times the effective radiating area (ERA).
(From: Chudliegh, D, Schulthies, SS, Draper, DO, and Myrer, JW: Muscle temperature rise with 1 MHz ultrasound in treatment sizes of 2 and 6 times the effective radiating area of the transducer. Master's Thesis, Brigham Young University, July, 1997)

■ **Clinical Decision-Making** *Exercise 5-1*

An athlete is complaining of pain at the lateral epicondyle of the elbow, which has been diagnosed as tennis elbow. The athletic trainer is trying to decide whether to use 1 MHz or 3 MHz ultrasound. Which would likely be most effective?

older ultrasound generators are set at a frequency of 1 MHz (meaning the crystal is deforming 1 million times per second), while some of the newer models also contain the 3 MHz frequency (the crystal is deforming 3 million times per second). Certainly, a generator which can be set between 1 and 3 MHz affords the athletic trainer the greatest treatment flexibility.

A common misconception is that intensity determines the depth of ultrasonic penetration, thus

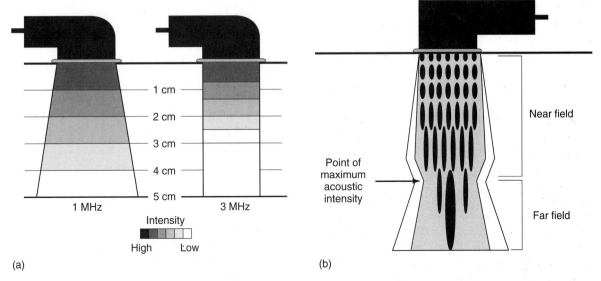

Figure 5-7   (a) The ultrasound energy attenuates as it travels through soft tissue. At 1 MHz, the energy can penetrate to the deeper tissues although the beam diverges slightly. At 3 MHz, the effects are primarily in the superficial tissues and the beam is less divergent. (b) In the near field the distribution of energy is nonuniform. In the far field energy distribution is more uniform but the beam is more divergent.

high intensities (1.5 or 2 W/cm²) are used for deep heating, and low intensities (1 W/cm²) are used for superficial heating. However, depth of tissue penetration is determined by ultrasound frequency and not by intensity.[49] Ultrasound energy generated at 1 MHz is transmitted through the more superficial tissues and absorbed primarily in the deeper tissues at depths of 2 to 5 cm[31] (Figure 5-7). A 1 MHz frequency is most useful in patients with high percent body fat cutaneously, and whenever desired effects are in the deeper structures, such as in the soleus or piriformis muscles.[51] At 3 MHz the energy is absorbed in the more superficial tissues, with a depth of penetration between 1 and 2 cm, making it ideal for treating superficial conditions such as plantar fasciitis, patellar tendinitis, and epicondylitis.[128]

As previously mentioned, attenuation is the decrease in the energy of ultrasound as the distance it travels through tissue increases. The rate of absorption, and therefore attenuation, increases as the frequency of the ultrasound increases.[67] The 3 MHz frequency is not only absorbed more superficially, it is also absorbed 3 times faster than 1 MHz ultra-

> **Ultrasound frequencies**
> ⋯⋯⋯⋯⋯⋯⋯⋯⋯⋯⋯⋯⋯⋯⋯⋯⋯⋯⋯⋯⋯⋯⋯
> - 3 MHz = superficial heat
> - IMHz = deep heat

sound. This faster rate of absorption results in faster peak heating in tissues. It has been demonstrated that 3 MHz ultrasound heats human muscle 3 times faster than 1 MHz ultrasound.[31]

The Ultrasound Beam

If the wavelength of the sound is larger than the source that produced it, then the sound will spread in all directions.[123] Such is the case with audible sound, thus explaining why it is possible for a person behind you to hear your voice almost as well as a person in front of you. In the case of therapeutic ultrasound, the sound is less divergent, thus concentrating energy in a limited area (1 MHz at a velocity 1540 m/sec in soft tissue and a wavelength of

1.5 mm, emitted from a transducer that is larger than the wavelength at approximately 25 mm in diameter).

The larger the diameter of the sound head, the more focused or **collimated** the **beam**. Smaller sound heads produce a more divergent beam. Also, the beam from ultrasound generated at a frequency of 1 MHz is more divergent than ultrasound generated at 3 MHz (Figure 5-7a).

Within this cylindrical beam the distribution of sound energy is highly nonuniform, particularly in an area close to the transducer, which is referred to as the *near field* or near zone (Figure 5-7b). The near field is a zone of spatially fluctuating ultrasound strength. The fluctuation occurs due to differences in pressure created by the waves emitted from the transducer. As the beam moves away from the transducer, the waves eventually become indistinguishable, arriving at a certain point simultaneously, creating a point of highest acoustic intensity.[123] The point of maximum acoustic intensity can be determined by calculating the distance (*L*) from the surface of the transducer:

$$L = D^2/4W$$

where *D* is the diameter of the transducer and *W* is the wavelength.[73] From this point, the beam moves into the *far field* or far zone, where the distribution of energy is much more uniform but the beam becomes more divergent.

Beam Nonuniformity Ratio (BNR). Ultrasound beams are not homogeneous along their longitudinal axis; some points are of higher intensity than others away from the transducer surface. The amount of variability of intensity within the ultrasound beam is indicated by the **beam nonuniformity ratio (BNR)**. This ratio is determined by using an underwater microphone (acoustic hydrophone) to measure the maximal point intensity of the transducer to the average intensity across the transducer surface. For example, a BNR of 2:1 means when the average output intensity is 1 W/cm^2, the peak or maximal point intensity of the beam is 2 W/cm^2. Optimally the BNR would be 1:1; however, since this is not possible,

collimated beam A focused, less divergent beam of ultrasound energy produced by a large diameter transducer.

beam nonuniformity ratio (BNR) Indicates the amount of variability of intensity within the ultrasound beam and is determined by the maximal point intensity of the transducer to the average intensity across the transducer surface.

- Ideal BNR = 1:1

the BNR should fall between 2 and 6. Some ultrasound units have BNRs as high as 8:1. Peak intensities of 8 W/cm^2 have been shown to damage tissue; therefore, the athlete runs a risk of tissue damage if intensities greater than 1 W/cm^2 are used on a machine with a 8:1 BNR. The lower the BNR the more uniform the output and therefore the lower the chance of developing "hot spots" of concentrated energy. The Food and Drug Administration requires all ultrasound units to list the BNR and the athletic trainer should be aware of the BNR for that particular unit.[46]

The high peak intensities associated with high BNRs are responsible for much of the discomfort or periosteal pain often associated with ultrasound treatment.[61] Therefore, the higher the BNR, the more important it is to move the transducer faster during treatment to avoid hot spots and areas of tissue damage or cavitation. Figure 5-8 shows the high beam homogeneity of a low BNR transducer and the typical beam profile of a high BNR transducer at 3 MHz output frequency.

Some researchers give little credence to BNR as a factor in good ultrasound equipment and say that it has little effect in treatment quality. Their

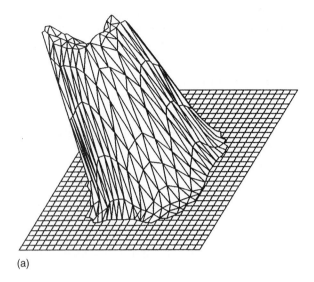

(a)

- Ultrasound may be continuous or pulsed

pulsed ultrasound   The intensity is periodically interrupted with no ultrasound energy being produced during the off period. When using pulsed ultrasound, the average intensity of the output over time is reduced.

continuous wave ultrasound   The sound intensity remains constant throughout the treatment, and the ultrasound energy is being produced 100% of the time.

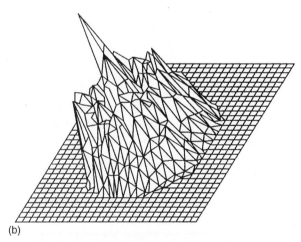

(b)

Figure 5-8   (a) Graphic representation of a low BNR of 2:1. (b) Graphic representation of a high BNR of 6:1.

rationale is that good treatment technique is much more important than the BNR.[52] However, most would agree that a continuous thermal ultrasound treatment is effective only if it is tolerated by the athlete, and if it produces uniform heating through the tissues. Some have speculated that a beam flowing from a poor quality ultrasound crystal might be a reason athletes experience pain and might cause uneven heating of tissue. Athlete compliance should be better when thermal ultrasound is delivered via an ultrasound device with a low beam nonuniformity ratio. This will encourage athletes to return for needed ultrasound treatments and allow the athletic trainer to increase the intensity to the point where the athlete feels local heat. When a heat modality is applied to tissue, it only makes sense that the athlete should feel heat. If warmth is not felt, either the athletic trainer is moving the soundhead too fast or the intensity is too low.

Pulsed versus Continuous Wave Ultrasound

Virtually all therapeutic ultrasound generators can emit either continuous or **pulsed ultrasound** waves. If **continuous wave ultrasound** is used, the sound intensity remains constant throughout the treatment, and the ultrasound energy is being produced 100 percent of the time (Figure 5-9).

With pulsed ultrasound, the intensity is periodically interrupted with no ultrasound energy being

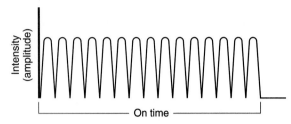

Figure 5-9 In continuous ultrasound, energy is constantly being generated.

produced during the off period (Figure 5-10). When using pulsed ultrasound, the average intensity of the output over time is reduced. The percentage of time that ultrasound is being generated (pulse duration) over one pulse period is referred to as the **duty cycle**.

$$\text{duty cycle} = \frac{\text{duration of pulse (on time)}}{\text{pulse period (on time} + \text{off time)}} \times 100$$

Thus, if the pulse duration is 1 msec and the total pulse period is 5 msec, the duty cycle would be 20%. Therefore, the total amount of energy being delivered to the tissues would be only 20% of the energy delivered if a continuous wave was being used. The majority of ultrasound generators have duty cycles that are preset at either 20% or 50%; however, some provide several optional duty cycles. Occasionally the duty cycle is also referred to as the mark:space ratio.

Continuous ultrasound is most commonly used when thermal effects are desired. The use of pulsed ultrasound results in a reduced average heating of the tissues. Pulsed ultrasound or continuous ultrasound at a low intensity will produce nonthermal or mechanical effects that may be associated with soft tissue healing.

Amplitude, Power, and Intensity

Amplitude is a term used to describe the magnitude of the vibration in a wave. It is the maximum distance from equilibrium that any particle reaches. Amplitude is used to describe either the movement of particles in the medium through

duty cycle The percentage of time that ultrasound is being generated (pulse duration) over one pulse period, which is also referred to as the mark:space ratio.

amplitude Describes the magnitude of the vibration in a wave. It is the maximum distance from equilibrium that any particle reaches.

power The total amount of ultrasound energy in the beam; is expressed in watts.

intensity A measure of the rate at which energy is being delivered per unit area.

which it travels in units of distance (centimeters or meters), or the variation in pressure found along the path of the wave in units of pressure (Newtons/meter^2).[23]

Power is the total amount of ultrasound energy in the beam and is expressed in watts. **Intensity** is a measure of the rate at which energy is being delivered per unit area. Since power and intensity are unevenly distributed in the beam, several varying types of intensities must be defined.

Spatial-averaged intensity is the intensity of the ultrasound beam averaged over the area of the transducer. It may be calculated by dividing the power output in watts by the total effective radiating area of the sound head in cm^2 and is indicated in watts per square centimeter (W/cm^2). If ultrasound is being produced at a power of 6 watts, and the effective radiating area of the transducer is 4 cm^2 the spatial-averaged intensity would be 1.5 W/cm^2. On many ultrasound units, both the power in watts and the spatial-average intensity in W/cm^2 may be displayed. If the power output is constant, increasing the size of the transducer will decrease the spatial-averaged intensity.

Spatial peak intensity is the highest value occurring within the beam over time. With therapeutic ultrasound, maximum intensities can range between 0.25 and 3.0 W/cm^2.

Temporal peak intensity, sometimes also referred to as *pulse average intensity*, is the maximum inten-

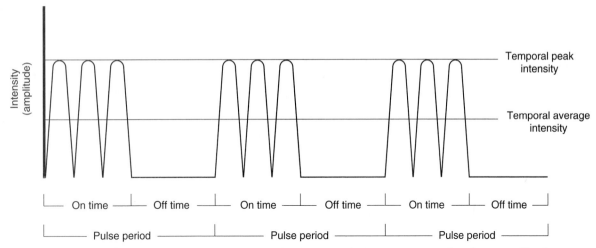

Figure 5-10   In pulsed ultrasound, energy is generated only during the on time. Duty cycle is determined by the ration of on time to pulse period.

sity during the on period with pulsed ultrasound, indicated in W/cm² (Figure 5-10).

Temporal-averaged intensity is important only with pulsed ultrasound and is calculated by averaging the power during both the on and off periods. For a pulsed sound beam with a duty cycle of 20% with a temporal peak intensity of 2.0 W/cm², temporal-averaged intensity would be 0.4 W/cm². It should be pointed out that on some machines, the intensity setting indicates the temporal peak intensity or on time, while on others it shows the temporal-averaged intensity or the mean of the on-off intensity[89] (Figure 5-10).

Spatial-averaged temporal peak intensity (SATP) is the maximum intensity occurring in time of the spatially-averaged intensity. The SATP intensity is simply the spatial-average during a single pulse.

There are no definitive rules that govern selection of specific ultrasound intensities during treatment, yet using too much may likely damage tissues and exacerbate the condition.[123] One recommendation is that the lowest intensity of ultrasound energy at the highest frequency that will transmit the energy to a specific tissue should be used to achieve a desired therapeutic effect.[89] Some guidance for selecting intensities has come from published reports

from those who have obtained successful yet subjective clinical outcomes. Table 5-4 provides a summary of various studies from the literature that have made recommendations regarding intensities, frequencies, and treatment mode.[89]

It is important to remember that everyone's tolerance to heat is different, and thus ultrasound intensity should always be adjusted to athlete tolerance.[61] At the beginning of the treatment, turn the intensity to the point where the athlete feels deep warmth, and then back the intensity down slightly until gentle heating is felt.[27,28] During the treatment, ask the athlete for feedback, and make the necessary intensity adjustments. This idea only applies to continuous mode ultrasound since pulsed ultrasound generally does not produce heat. Regardless, the treatment should never produce reports of pain. If the athlete reports that the transducer feels hot at the skin surface, it is likely that the coupling medium is inadequate, and possible that the piezoelectric crystal has been damaged and the transducer is overheating.

Ultrasound treatments should be temperature dependent, not time dependent. Thermal ultrasound is used to bring about certain desired effects, and tissues respond according to the amount of

■ **TABLE 5-4** Summary of Research Relating to Ultrasound

APPLICATION	AUTHORS	FREQUENCY	INTENSITY (SATP)	MODE	REGIMEN	OUTCOME
SOFT TISSUE LESIONS						
Acute injuries			*	P	*	
Sports injuries	Patrick (1978)	*			5 times a week	Significant improvement
Minor fractures			0.5–2.0	P		
Recent occupational soft tissue injuries	Middlemast and Chatterjee (1978)	1.5				Success with acute only
Subacute			2.0–4.0	*	up to 5 min daily × 3 then alternate days	
Acute subacromial bursitis	Bearzy (1953)	1.0	0.8–3.0	*	5–10 min × 12	Improvement
Bursitis shoulder	Newman et al. (1958)	1.0	1.2–1.3	CW	6 min 3 times a week × 4	No significant difference
Painful shoulder	Downing and Weinstein (1986)	1.0	0.5	CW	3–5 min × 10	Improvement
Subacromial bursitis	Munting (1978)	1.5	2.0	*	3 times a week × 3	0.89 MHz more successful
Chronic arthritis	Griffin et al. (1970)	0.89/1.0	1.0–2.5	CW	5 min × 8–10	Decreased pain
Plantar fasciitis	Clarke and Stenner (1976)	0.75/1.5	1.05–2.5	CW	5 min × 8–10	Size unchanged; pain decreased
Rheumatoid nodules		3.0				
Phonophoresis						
Arthritis	Griffin et al. (1967)	1.0	1.5 max	CW	1 time a week × 9 max	Successful
Epicondylitis/bursitis	Kleinkort and Wood (1975)	1.0	2.0 max	CW	6–9 min	Improvement
Wounds						
Episiotomies	Fieldhouse (1979)	*	0.5–0.8	*	5 min 3 times a week × 6	Improvement
Episiotomies and surgical wounds	Ferguson (1981)	1.0	0.5	P1:5	3 min daily × 2–4	Improvement
Episiotomies	McLaren (1984)	*	0.5	*	5 min	Improvement
Scars						
Contracture after hip fixation	Lehmann et al. (1961)	*	1.0–2.5	*	5 min daily up to 3 weeks	Significant improvement
Hand scars	Bierman (1954)	1.0	1.0–2.0	CW	6–8 min, alternate days	Improvement
Dupuytren's contracture	Markham et al. (1980)	1.0/3.0	0.25–0.75	*	4–10 min 1 time a week	Improvement
PAIN						
Low back pain	Patrick (1966)	*	1.0–1.5	P	5 min daily × 10 max	Improvement
Nerve root pain	Nwuga (1983)	*	1.0–2.0	*	10 min 3 times a week × 4	Significant improvement
Prolapsed intervertebral disc						

heat they receive.[77,78] **Any significant adjustment in the intensity must be countered with an adjustment in the treatment time.** It is possible that ultrasound treatments of the future will be like iontophoresis, where the treatment time is dependent upon the dosage delivered. For this reason, it is likely that the new generation of ultrasound generators will have the capability of automatically decreasing treatment time as the intensity is increased, and increasing treatment time as the intensity is decreased (see Figure 5-3).

PHYSIOLOGICAL EFFECTS OF ULTRASOUND

Therapeutic ultrasound when applied to biologic tissue may induce clinically significant responses in cells, tissues, and organs through both thermal effects and nonthermal biophysical effects.[10,37–39,49,67,97,117,123,128] Ultrasound will affect both normal and damaged biologic tissues. It has been suggested that damaged tissue may be more responsive to ultrasound than normal tissue.[41] When ultrasound is applied for its thermal effects, nonthermal biophysical effects that may damage normal tissues will also occur.[67] If appropriate treatment parameters are selected, however, nonthermal effects can occur with minimal thermal effects.

Thermal Effects

The ultrasound wave attenuates as it travels through the tissue. Attenuation is caused primarily by the conversion of ultrasound energy into heat through absorption and to some extent by scattering and beam deflection. Traditionally, ultrasound has been used primarily to produce a tissue temperature increase.[7,48,80,83,110,121] The clinical effects of using ultrasound to heat tissues are similar to other forms of heat that may be applied, including the following:[77]

1. An increase in the extensibility of collagen fibers found in tendons and joint capsules

2. Decrease in joint stiffness
3. Reduction of muscle spasm
4. Modulation of pain
5. Increased blood flow
6. Mild inflammatory response, which may help in the resolution of chronic inflammation

It has been suggested that for the majority of these effects to occur, the tissues must be raised to a level of 40 to 45° C for a minimum of 5 minutes.[38] Others are of the opinion that absolute temperatures aren't the key, but rather how much the temperature rises above baseline.[77–79] They report that tissue temperature increases of 1° C increase metabolism and healing, increases of 2° to 3° C decrease pain and muscle spasm, and increases of 4° C or greater increase extensibility of collagen and decrease joint stiffness.[13,14,77] It has been shown that temperatures above 45° C may be potentially damaging to tissues, yet athletes usually experience pain prior to these extreme temperatures.[31]

Ultrasound at 1 MHz with an intensity of 1 W/cm^2 has been reported to raise soft tissue temperature by as much as 0.86° C per minute in tissues with a poor vascular supply.[123] It has been shown that 3 MHz ultrasound at 1 W/cm^2 raise human patellar tendon temperatures 2° C per minute.[15] In muscle, which is quite vascular, 1 MHz and 3 MHz ultrasound at 1 W/cm^2 increase the temperature 0.2° C and 0.6° C per minute, respectively.[31]

The primary advantage of ultrasound over other nonacoustic heating modalities is that tissues high in collagen, such tendons, muscles, ligaments, joint capsules, joint menisci, intermuscular interfaces, nerve roots, periosteum, cortical bone and other deep tissues may be selectively heated to the therapeutic range without causing a significant tissue temperature increase in skin or fat.[80,118] Ultrasound will penetrate skin and fat with little attenuation.[36]

The thermal effects of ultrasound are related to frequency. As indicated earlier, an inverse relationship exists between depth of penetration and frequency. Most of the energy in a sound wave at

3 MHz will be absorbed in the superficial tissues. At 1 MHz there will be less attenuation and the energy will penetrate to the deeper tissues selectively heating them.

Heating will occur with both continuous and pulsed ultrasound depending on the intensity of the total current being delivered to the patient. Significant thermal effects will be induced whenever the upper end of the available intensity range is used. Regardless of whether ultrasound is pulsed or continuous, if the spatial-averaged, temporal-averaged intensity is in the 0.1 to 0.2 W/cm² range, the intensity is too low to produce a tissue temperature increase, and only nonthermal effects will occur.[38]

Unlike the other heating modalities discussed in this text, whenever ultrasound is used to produce thermal changes, nonthermal changes also simultaneously occur.[39] An understanding of these nonthermal changes, therefore, is essential.

Nonthermal Effects

The nonthermal effects of therapeutic ultrasound include **cavitation** and **acoustic microstreaming** (Figure 5-11). Cavitation is the formation of gasfilled bubbles that expand and compress due to ultrasonically induced pressure changes in tissue fluids.[38,117] Cavitation may be classified as being either *stable* or *unstable*. In stable cavitation, the bubbles expand and contract in response to regularly repeated pressure changes over many acoustic cycles. In unstable or transient cavitation, there are violent large excursions in bubble volume before implosion and collapse occurs after only a few cycles. Therapeutic benefits are derived only from stable cavitation while the collapse of bubbles is thought to create increased pressure and high temperatures, which may cause local tissue damage. Unstable cavitation should clearly be avoided. It is likely that high-intensity, low-frequency ultrasound may produce unstable cavitation, particularly if standing waves develop at tissue interfaces.[38]

Cavitation results in an increased flow in the fluid around these vibrating bubbles. Microstream-

cavitation The formation of gas-filled bubbles that expand and compress due to ultrasonically induced pressure changes in tissue fluids.

acoustic microstreaming The unidirectional movement of fluids along the boundaries of cell membranes resulting from the mechanical pressure wave in an ultrasonic field.

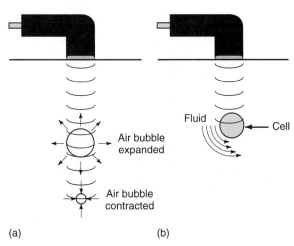

(a)   (b)

Figure 5-11 Nonthermal effects of ultrasound. (a) Cavitation is the formation of gas-filled bubbles which expand and compress due to ultrasonically induced pressure changes in tissue fluids. (b) Microstreaming is the unidirectional movement of fluids along the boundaries of cell membranes resulting from the mechanical pressure wave in an ultrasonic field.

ing is the unidirectional movement of fluids along the boundaries of cell membranes resulting from the mechanical pressure wave in an ultrasonic field.[38,117] Microstreaming produces high viscous stresses that can alter cell membrane structure and function due to changes in cell membrane permeability to sodium and calcium ions important in the healing process. As long as the cell membrane is not damaged, microstreaming can be of therapeutic value in accelerating the healing process.[38]

■ **Clinical Decision-Making**   *Exercise 5-2*

> An athletic trainer is treating an ankle sprain on day 2 post injury. To facilitate the healing process, she is using ultrasound for its nonthermal effects. What treatment parameters are required to ensure there will be no thermal effects during the treatment?

phonophoresis   A technique in which ultrasound is used to drive a topical application of a selected medication into the tissues.

It has been well documented that the nonthermal effects of therapeutic ultrasound in the treatment of injured tissues may be as important if not more important than the thermal effects. Therapeutically, significant nonthermal effects have been identified in soft tissue repair via stimulation of fibroblast activity, which produces an increase in protein synthesis,[41] tissue regeneration,[41] increased blood flow in chronically ischemic tissues,[62] bone healing and repair of nonunion fractures,[101] and **phonophoresis**.

The nonthermal effects of cavitation and microstreaming can be maximized while minimizing the thermal effects by using a spatial-averaged, temporal-averaged intensity of 0.1 to 0.2 W/cm^2 with continuous ultrasound. This range may also be achieved using a low temporal-averaged intensity by pulsing a higher temporal peak intensity of 1.0 W/cm^2 at a duty cycle of 20% to give a temporal average intensity of 0.2 W/cm^2.

TECHNIQUES OF APPLICATION

The principles and theories of therapeutic ultrasound are well understood and documented. However, specific practical recommendations as to how ultrasound may best be applied to an athlete therapeutically are quite controversial and are based primarily on the experience of the clinicians who have used it. Although there are numerous laboratory and clinically based reports in the literature, treatment procedures and parameters are highly variable, and many contradictory results and conclusions have been presented in the literature.[89]

Frequency of Treatment

It is generally accepted that acute conditions require more frequent treatments over a shorter period of time, while more chronic conditions require fewer treatments over a longer period of time.[89] Ultrasound treatments should begin as soon as possible following injury, ideally within hours but definitely within 48 hours to maximize effects on the healing process.[50,96,98] Acute conditions may be treated using low-intensity or pulsed ultrasound once or even twice daily for 6 to 8 days until acute symptoms such as pain and swelling subside. In chronic conditions, when acute symptoms have subsided, treatment may be done on alternating days.[115] Ultrasound treatment should continue as long as there is improvement. Assuming the appropriate treatment parameters are chosen and the ultrasound generator is functioning properly, if no improvement is noted following three or four treatments, ultrasound should be discontinued, or different parameters (i.e., duty cycle, frequency) should be employed.

The question is often asked, "How many ultrasound treatments can be given?" It must be pointed out that most of the research regarding treatment longevity has been performed on animals, and it takes quite a leap of logic to assume that the same negative effects would occur in humans. If the correct parameters are followed using a high-quality, recently calibrated ultrasound machine, treatments could occur daily for several weeks. In the past, it has been recommended that ultrasound be limited to 14 treatments in the majority of conditions, although this has not been documented scientifically. More than 14 treatments can reduce both red and white blood cell counts. After these 14 treatments, some authors advise avoiding ultrasound use for two weeks.[51]

Duration of Treatment

In the past, modality textbooks have been quite vague with respect to treatment time, and generally the suggested duration has been too short.[61,113] Typically, recommended treatment times have ranged between 5 and 10 minutes in length; however, these times may be insufficient. The length of the treatment is dependent on several factors: the size of the area to be treated, the intensity in W/cm^2, the frequency, and the desired temperature increase. As stated previously, specific temperature increases are required to achieve beneficial effects in tissue. The athletic trainer must determine what the desired effects of the treatment are before a treatment duration is set (Figure 5-12).

An accepted recommendation is that ultrasound be administered in an area 2 times the ERA (roughly twice the size of the soundhead). If thermal effects are desired in an area larger than this, obviously the treatment time needs to be increased.

The higher the intensity applied in W/cm^2, the shorter the treatment time, and vice versa. It just doesn't make clinical sense to treat one athlete at 1 W/cm^2 and another at 2 W/cm^2 at identical treatment durations when both athletes require vigorous heating. Based upon this scenario, athlete 2 will produce tissue temperature increases of twice that of athlete 1.

Ultrasound frequency (MHz) not only determines the depth of penetration, it also determines the rate of heating. The energy produced with 3 MHz ultrasound is absorbed three times faster than that produced from 1 MHz ultrasound, the result of which is faster heating. Ultrasound at 3 MHz consistently heats tissues three times faster than 1 MHz, thus reducing the required treatment duration by one third.[29,31]

The desired temperature increase is also a factor in determining the duration of an ultrasound treatment. Table 5-5[31] displays the rate of muscle

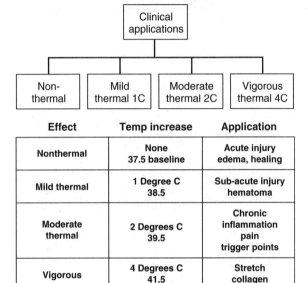

Basic therapeutic ultrasound applications

Effect	Temp increase	Application
Nonthermal	None 37.5 baseline	Acute injury edema, healing
Mild thermal	1 Degree C 38.5	Sub-acute injury hematoma
Moderate thermal	2 Degrees C 39.5	Chronic inflammation pain trigger points
Vigorous	4 Degrees C 41.5	Stretch collagen

Figure 5-12   It is important to have a treatment goal, and to adjust the ultrasound treatment time accordingly. (Courtesy of Castel, JC: *Sound advice*, PTI, Inc., 1995. Used by permission.)

■ **TABLE 5-5**   Ultrasound Rate of Heating per Minute (Human Muscle)[31]

INTENSITY (W/cm^2)	1 MHz	3 MHz
.5	.04° C	.3° C
1.0	.2° C	.6° C
1.5	.3° C	.9° C
2.0	.4° C	1.4° C

temperature increase per minute, per W/cm^2, at various intensities and frequencies. Based upon this information, the athletic trainer can determine the appropriate duration of an ultrasound treatment. For example, an athlete has limited range of motion due to scar tissue buildup from a chronic hamstring strain at the musculotendinous junction. An

■ **Clinical Decision-Making**   *Exercise 5-3*

An athlete is being treated with ultrasound for muscle guarding in the upper trapezius. The athletic trainer wishes to achieve a mild heating effect by increasing the temperature by 3° C. If 1 MHz ultrasound at an intensity of 1.5 W/cm^2 is being used, how long must the treatment be to achieve this temperature increase?

appropriate goal would be to vigorously heat the muscle (an increase of 4° C) and immediately perform passive hamstring stretching. If 1 MHz ultrasound were used at an intensity of 2 W/cm^2, the 4° C increase would take about 10 minutes. If at 2 minutes into the treatment, however, the athlete complains that the treatment is too hot, most of us would respond by decreasing the intensity, but we may forget to increase the treatment time. In this case, if we decreased the intensity to 1.5 W/cm^2, we would need to add 2 minutes to the treatment time to ensure a 4° C increase in muscle temperature. It is important to note that this chart requires a treatment size of 2 to 3 ERA, and these temperatures were reported in muscle. It has also been suggested that tendon heats over three times faster than muscle.[15]

Coupling Methods

The greatest amount of reflection of ultrasonic energy occurs at the air-tissue interface. To ensure that maximal energy will be transmitted to the athlete, the face of the transducer should be parallel with the surface of the skin so that the ultrasound will strike the surface at a 90° angle. If the angle between the transducer face and the skin is greater than 15°, a large percentage of the energy will be reflected and the treatment effects will be minimal.[115] Applying the ultrasound via the use of some coupling agent can further reduce reflection at the air-tissue interface. The purpose of the **coupling**

coupling medium   A substance used to decrease the acoustical impedance at the air-skin interface and thus facilitate the passage of ultrasound energy.

medium is to exclude air from the region between the athlete and the transducer so that ultrasound can get to the area to be treated.[123] The acoustical impedance of the coupling medium should match the impedance of the transducer and should be slightly higher than the skin. Also, the medium should have a low coefficient of absorption to minimize attenuation in the coupling medium. It is important that the medium remains free of air bubbles during treatment. The coupling agent should be viscous enough to act as a lubricant as the transducer is moved over the surface of the skin.[89]

The coupling medium should be applied to the skin surface, and the ultrasound transducer should be in contact with the coupling medium before the power is turned on. If the transducer is not in contact with the skin via the coupling medium, or if for some reason the transducer is lifted away from the treatment area, the piezoelectric crystal may be damaged, and the transducer can overheat.

A number of studies have looked at the efficacy of different coupling media in transmitting ultrasound.[3,35,38,107] Water, light oils, gel packs,[71,88] topical analgesics[94] (Biofreeze, Natures Chemist), and various brands of ultrasonic gel have been recommended as coupling agents. The recommendations of these studies have proven to be somewhat contradictory. Essentially, it appears that all of these agents have very similar acoustic properties and are effective as coupling agents.[24]

Water is an effective coupling medium, but its low viscosity reduces its suitability in surface application. Light oils, such as mineral oil and glycerol, have relatively higher absorption coefficients and are somewhat difficult to clean up following treatment. Water-soluble gels seem to have the most desirable properties necessary for a good coupling medium.[24,35] Perhaps the only disadvantage is that

• Water-soluble gels = best coupling medium

the salts in the gel may damage the metal face of the transducer with improper cleaning. Out of convenience, some athletic trainers have used massage lotion instead of ultrasound gel; however, experience has revealed that massage lotion is not an adequate ultrasound-conducting medium.

Table 5-6 indicates a technique that can be used to check the relative transmission capability of a medium.

Exposure Techniques

Direct Contact. Direct application of ultrasound involves actual contact between the applicator and the skin, with a thin film of couplant between. A layer of gel should be applied to the treatment area in sufficient amounts to maintain good contact and lubrication between the transducer and the skin, but not so much that air pockets may form from movement of the transducer. A thin film of gel should be applied directly to the transducer face before transmission begins[89] (Figure 5-13). A direct technique of exposure may be used as long as the surface being treated is larger than the diameter of the transducer. If a smaller surface area is to be treated, a smaller transducer should be used so that direct application can still be performed.

Heating of the ultrasound gel prior to treatment has been recommended to improve the thermal effects of ultrasound in deeper tissues; however, this is not the case. Since ultrasound heats only through conversion of mechanical vibration to heat and not through conduction, heating of the gel will have no effect in the deeper tissues.[51] The only rationale for heating cold ultrasound gel is strictly for athlete comfort and compliance.

Recently several manufacturers of analgesic creams have been promoting their use as ultra-

■ **TABLE 5-6** Technique That Can Be Used to Check the Relative Transmission Capability of a Medium

1. Encircle the transducer with tape while leaving about 2 cm of tape exposed (making a tape tube).
2. Fill the tape tube with 1 cm thickness of ultrasound gel medium.
3. Fill the tube to the top with water.
4. Adjust the intensity and watch the water bubble.
5. Repeat the procedure, yet substitute the gel with the medium you are testing.
6. If the water has little or no bubbles, your desired medium is not a good couplant after all.

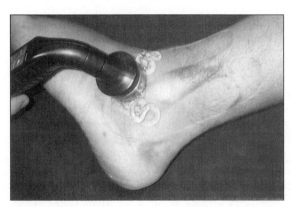

Figure 5-13 Ultrasound may be applied directly through some gel-like coupling medium.

sound couplants.[94] Patients are treated with ultrasound via a conducting medium of gel mixed with their product. One company recommended a mixture of two parts gel to one part analgesic cream (this has recently been changed to 80% gel/20% cream), while another recommended a 50/50 ratio of ultrasound gel and its analgesic cream. Small mixtures of analgesic creams with 80% or 90% gel may produce significant heating, but as yet have not been tested. Some of these products have been shown to actually impede the transmission of ultrasound. Many of these over-the-counter medications presently used are only minimally effective as ultra-

■ **Clinical Decision-Making**   *Exercise 5-4*

The athletic trainer is using ultrasound to treat an inversion ankle sprain. Unfortunately, the ultrasound generator only has a 10 cm^2 transducer, and the athletic trainer is worried about maintaining good direct contact over the treatment area. What alternative couple techniques could potentially be used?

Flex-All versus Biofreeze

Depth	50/50 flex-all; gel	50/50 biofreeze; gel	100% gel
3cm	2.8°C	1.8°C	3.4°C
5cm	1.8°C	1.3°C	2.5°C

Muscle temperature increase from continuous 1 MHz ultrasound at 1.5 W/cm^2 for 10 minutes.

Figure 5-14   Two popular analgesic creams were mixed with ultrasound gel and used as coupling media. Only the treatments that used 100% ultrasound gel as the couplant yielded temperatures consistent with vigorous heating. We conclude that these creams, although they might decrease pain perception, actually impede ultrasound transmission. Note: These manufacturers are now recommending mixtures of 80% ultrasound gel with 20% of their product.

sound couplants.[2] If an athlete wants the added benefits of heat and analgesia, first massage the balm into the area, then apply 100% ultrasound gel followed by ultrasound. Until further research is performed in this area, it is suggested that the practice of using analgesic creams mixed with ultrasound gel be discontinued when vigorous heating is desired. Figure 5-14 displays the results of research involving two such products and their effect on muscle temperature increase via ultrasound.

Immersion.   Although direct application with gel has been shown to be the most effective application technique, there are some instances where water immersion is warranted. The immersion technique is recommended if the area to be treated is smaller than the diameter of the available transducer or if the treatment area is irregular with boney prominences (Figure 5-15). A plastic, ceramic, or rubber basin should be used, since a metal basin or whirlpool will reflect some of the ultrasound, increasing the intensity near the basin walls. Tap water seems to be just as effective as degassed water as a coupling medium for the immersion technique[50] and less likely to produce surface heating than mineral oil or glycerin.[107] The transducer should be moved parallel to the surface being treated at a distance of 0.5 to 1 cm. If air bubbles accumulate on the transducer or over[128] the treatment area, they may be wiped away quickly during the treatment. To ensure adequate heating, the intensity should be increased, possibly as much as 50%.[35]

Bladder Technique.   If for some reason the treatment area cannot be immersed in water, a

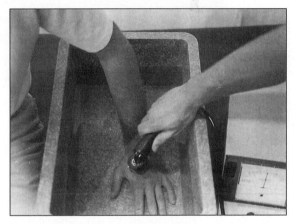

Figure 5-15   The immersion technique is recommended when using ultrasound over irregular surfaces.

bladder technique can be used in which a balloon, surgical glove, or even a condom has been filled with water, and the ultrasound energy is transmitted from the transducer to the treatment surface through this bladder (Figure 5-16). Both sides of the bladder should be coated with gel to assure better contact. Recently, commercial gel packs have gained popularity and several studies have demonstrated their efficacy as a coupling medium.[71,88] Treatments using a bladder filled with either gel or

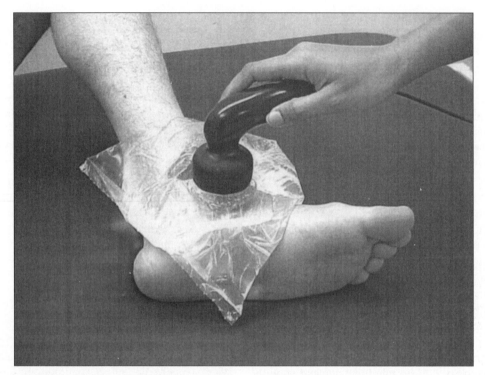

Figure 5-16 The bladder technique may also be used over irregular surfaces.

silicone have been recommended as effective at higher ultrasound intensities.[3]

Moving the Transducer

In the past, treatment techniques that involve both moving the transducer and holding the transducer stationary have been recommended. The stationary technique was most often used when the treatment area was small or when pulsed ultrasound was used at a low temporal-averaged intensity. However, because of the nonuniformity of the ultrasound beam, the energy distribution in the tissue is uneven, thus creating potential tissue damaging hot spots.[128] If the ultrasound beam is stationary, the spatial-peak intensity determines the point of maximal temperature increase. With the moving technique, the spatial-averaged intensity gives the most reasonable measure of the average rate of heating within the treatment area.[117] This station-

ary technique has been demonstrated to produce disruption of blood flow, platelet aggregation, and damage to the venous system; therefore, the stationary technique is no longer recommended.[127]

Moving the transducer during treatment leads to a more even distribution of energy within the treatment area, especially if the unit has a low BNR.[13] This can reduce the damaging effects of standing waves, particularly those that are most likely to occur at bone-tissue interfaces. Overlapping circular motions or a longitudinal stroking pattern can be used. The transducer should be moved slowly at approximately 4 cm per second,[72,87] covering a treatment area that is 2 to 3 times larger than the ERA of the transducer.[87] Movement speed of the transducer is BNR dependent, and the higher the BNR, the more important it is to move the transducer faster during treatment to avoid periosteal irritation and transient cavitation.[61,113] However, moving the transducer too rapidly decreases the total amount of energy absorbed per unit area. Rapid movement of the soundhead causes the athletic trainer to slip into treating a larger area, thus the desired temperatures may not be attained.

Equipment with a low BNR usually allows for a slower stroking movement of the ultrasound transducer. Slow strokes are more controlled, and can easily be contained to a small area (2 ERA). Slow movement of the applicator results in evenly distributed soundwaves throughout the area, whereas a fast moving transducer will not allow for adequate absorption of the soundwaves, and sufficient heating will not occur. If the athlete complains of pain, decrease the output intensity, while making the appropriate adjustments in treatment duration. The transducer should be kept in maximum contact with the skin via some coupling agent.

During the administration of ultrasound, it is possible that the amount of pressure at the transducer may effect the physiological response to and the outcome of the treatment.[70] It has been demonstrated that applying an excessive amount of pressure could decrease the acoustic transmissivity, damage the crystal in the transducer, or make the athlete uncomfortable. It is recommended that the athletic trainer apply firm consistent pressure during treatment.[70]

Recording Ultrasound Treatments

It is recommended that the athletic trainer report or record the specific parameters used in an ultrasound treatment when completing treatment records or progress notes so that the treatment may be reproduced or altered. The parameters that should be recorded include frequency, spatial-averaged temporal peak intensity, whether the beam is pulsed or continuous, the duty factor (if pulsed), effective radiating surface area of the transducer, duration of the treatment, and the number of treatments per week.[89]

A typical treatment might be recorded as 3 MHz, at 1.0 W/cm^2, pulsed at 20% (0.2) duty factor, 5 cm transducer head, 5 mins, 4 times per week.

CLINICAL APPLICATIONS OF THERAPEUTIC ULTRASOUND

Ultrasound is generally recognized clinically as one of the most effective and widely used modalities in the treatment of many soft tissue and boney lesions that occur with participation in sport activities. Considering the extensive use of ultrasound in treating sport-related injuries, until the past decade, there has been relatively little documented evidence from the medical community concerning the efficacy of this modality (however, research in this area is increasing). Many of the decisions as to how ultrasound should be used are empirically based on personal opinion and experience. This section summarizes the various clinical applications of therapeutic ultrasound used in a clinical setting.

Soft Tissue Healing and Repair

Soft tissue repair may be accelerated by both thermal and nonthermal ultrasound.[37,47] Repair of soft tissues involves three phases of healing, inflammation, proliferation, and remodeling. Ultrasound does not seem to have any anti-inflammatory effects; rather it is thought to accelerate the inflammatory phase of healing.

It has been shown that a single treatment with ultrasound can stimulate the release of histamine from mast cells.[60] The mechanism for this may be attributed primarily to nonthermal effects involving cavitation and streaming, which increase the transport of calcium ions across the cell membrane, thus stimulating release of histamine by the mast cells.[38] Histamine attracts polymorphonuclear leukocytes that "clean up" debris from the injured area, along with monocytes, whose primary function is to release chemotactic agents and growth factors that stimulate fibroblasts and endothelial cells to form a collagen-rich, well-vascularized tissue used for the development of new connective tissue that is essential for rapid repair. Thus, ultrasound can be effective in facilitating the process of inflammation, and therefore healing, if applied after bleeding has stopped but still within the first few

- Ultrasound accelerates the inflammatory process

hours after injury during the early stages of inflammation.[38] It has been suggested that this response occurs using pulsed ultrasound at 0.5 W/cm^2 with a duty cycle of 20% for 5 minutes or continuous ultrasound at 0.1 W/cm$^{2.39}$

These treatments have been described as being "pro-inflammatory" and are of value in accelerating repair in short-term or acute inflammation.[112] However, in chronic inflammatory conditions, the pro-inflammatory effects are of questionable value.[60] If an inflammatory stimulus, such as overuse, remains, the response to therapeutic ultrasound is of questionable value.[6]

Pitting edema is a condition that sometimes provides a challenge for athletic trainers. Pitting edema may be treated with continuous 3 MHz ultrasound at intensities of 1 to 1.5 W/cm^2. The heat seems to liquify the gel-like cellular debris. The limb is then elevated, massaged, or EMS is used to pump the fluid and promote lymphatic drainage.

During the proliferative phase of healing, a connective tissue matrix is produced into which new blood vessels will grow. Fibroblasts are mainly responsible for producing this connective tissue. Fibroblasts exposed to therapeutic ultrasound are stimulated to produce more collagen, which gives connective tissue most of its strength.[54] Again, cavitation and streaming alter cell membrane permeability to calcium ions which facilitate increases in collagen synthesis and in tensile strength. The intensity levels of therapeutic ultrasound that produce these changes during the proliferative phase are too low to be entirely thermal. It has been demonstrated that heating with continuous ultrasound may be more effective than stretching, alone for increasing the extensibility of dense connective tissue.[106]

Ultrasound does not appear to be effective in enhancing postexercise muscle strength recovery or in diminishing delayed onset muscle soreness.[18,102]

Although treatment with pulsed ultrasound can promote the satellite cell proliferation phase of the myoregeneration, it does not seem to have significant effects on the overall morphological manifestations of muscle regeneration.[105]

Scar Tissue and Joint Contracture

During remodeling, collagen fibers are realigned along lines of tensile stresses and strains forming scar tissue. This process may continue for months or even years. In scar tissue, collagen never attains the same pattern and remains weaker and less elastic than normal tissue prior to injury. Scar tissue in tendons, ligaments, and capsules surrounding joints can produce joint contractures that limit range of motion. Increased tissue temperatures increase the elasticity and decrease the viscosity of collagen fibers. Since the deeper tissues surrounding joints which most often restrict range are rich in collagen, ultrasound is the treatment modality of choice.[75,128]

A number of studies have investigated the effects of ultrasound treatment on scar tissue and joint contracture. Ultrasound has been demonstrated to increase mobility in mature scar.[5] A greater residual increase in tissue length with less potential damage is produced through preheating with ultrasound prior to stretching,[76] or by putting the joint on stretch while insonating.[33,109] Tissue extensibility increases when continuous ultrasound is applied at higher intensities causing vigorous heating of tissues.[53] Thigh, periarticular structures, and scar tissues become significantly more extensible following treatment with ultrasound involving thermal effects at intensities of 1.2 to 2.0 W/cm^2.[76] Scar tissue can be softened if treated with ultrasound at an early stage.[98] Dupuytren's contracture shows a beneficial effect on long standing contracted bands of scar and a decrease in pain when treated early on with ultrasound.[85]

The majority of the these earlier studies attributed the effectiveness of ultrasound to thermal effects and used continuous moderate intensities between 0.5 and 2.0 W/cm^2.

Stretching of Connective Tissue

Collagenous tissue, when stressed, is fairly rigid, yet when heated it becomes much more yielding.[53,76] However, the combination of heat and stretching produces a residual lengthening of connective tissue, which increases according to the force applied.

A common practice in sports medicine is to apply ultrasound, and then send the athlete out to exercise, warm up, or stretch.[86] However, quite often this process of heating followed by stretching is interrupted by team meetings, changing into uniforms, and even travel. What happens to the tissue that has just been heated with ultrasound during the 10, 20, or 60 minutes until the athlete actually begins to warm up? It may be assumed that the muscle temperature increase from the ultrasound treatment will last up to an hour; however, this idea is false.

The time period of vigorous heating when tissues will undergo the greatest extensibility and elongation is referred to as the **"stretching window."**[33,109] It should be added that the existence of this "stretching window" is theoretical and it has not been conclusively demonstrated to exist.[8] If tissue is heated vigorously it becomes more pliable and less resistant to stretch, yet as the tissue cools, it with-

....

stretching window   The time period of vigorous heating when tissues will undergo their greatest extensibility and elongation.

....

stands stretching and can actually be damaged if too great of a force is applied.

It appears that ultrasound combined with stretching increases the range of motion more than stretching alone immediately following treatment. However, there is no significant difference between the two techniques over the long term.[30]

The rate of tissue cooling following continuous ultrasound at both 1 MHz and 3 MHz frequencies has been determined[33,109] (Figure 5-17). Thermistor probes were inserted 1.2 cm below the skin's surface, and ultrasound was applied. The treatment raised the tissue temperature 5.3° C for the 3 MHz frequency. The average time it took for the temperature to drop each degree as expressed in minutes and seconds was the following: 1° C = 1:20; 2° C = 3:22; 3° C = 5:50; 4° C = 9:13; 5° C = 14:55. In this case, the temperature remained in the vigorous

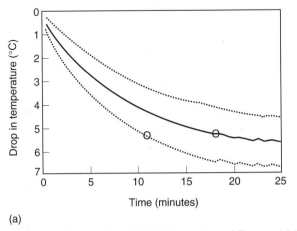

(a)

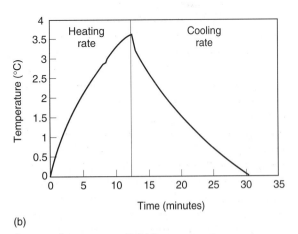

(b)

Figure 5-17   (a) Rate of temperature decay following 3 MHz ultrasound treatments. Solid line = mean temperature decay. Hatched line = 1 standard deviation above and below the mean. Oval = time to pre-ultrasound baseline. (b) Rate of temperature increase during 1 MHz ultrasound applied at 1.5W/cm², followed by the rate of temperature decay at termination of insonation. The thermistor was 4 cms deep in the triceps surae muscle.[34,108]

■ **Clinical Decision-Making** *Exercise 5-5*

How may the athletic trainer best use ultrasound to treat patellar tendinitis?

heating phase for only 3.3 minutes following an ultrasound treatment.

The same methods were used to determine the stretching window at 1 MHz. The temperature was recorded 4 centimeters deep in the muscle. It took two minutes for the temperature to drop 1° C, and a total of 5.5 minutes to drop 2° C. The deeper muscle cools at a slower rate than superficial muscle since the added tissue serves as a barrier to escaping heat. Regardless, tissue heated by ultrasound loses its heat at a fairly rapid rate; therefore, stretching, friction massage, or joint mobilization should be performed immediately post ultrasound. To increase the duration of the stretching window, it is recommended that stretching be done during and immediately after ultrasound application.

Chronic Inflammation

There are few clinical or experimental studies that discuss the effects of therapeutic ultrasound on the chronic inflammations (i.e., tendinitis, bursitis, epicondylitis). Treatment of bicipital tendinitis with ultrasound decreased pain and tenderness and increased range of motion.[43] While earlier studies have shown ultrasound to be effective in treating pain and increasing range of motion in subacromial bursitis, a more recent study shows no improvement in the general condition of the shoulder when using continuous ultrasound at 1.0 to 2.0 W/cm²[5]. Ultrasound applied at an intensity of 1.0 to 2.0 W/cm² at a 20% duty cycle significantly enhanced recovery in patients with epicondylitis.[6] In these chronic inflammatory conditions, ultrasound seems to be effective in increasing blood flow for healing and for pain reduction through heating.[128]

Bone Healing

Since bone is a type of connective tissue, damaged bone progresses through the same stages of healing as other soft tissues, the major difference being the deposition of bone salts.[126] Several researchers have observed acceleration of fracture repair following treatment with ultrasound.[101,114,122] It has been shown that the application of ultrasound within the first 2 weeks post fibular fracture during the inflammatory and proliferative stages increases the rate of healing. Treatment parameters were 0.5 W/cm² at a duty cycle of 20% for 5 minutes, 4 times per week.[40] Ultrasound was effectively used to stimulate bone repair following osteotomy and fixation of the tibia in rabbits.[11]

Treatment given during the first 2 weeks after injury is sufficient to accelerate boney union. However, ultrasound given to an unstable fracture during the phase of cartilage formation may cause proliferation of cartilage and consequent delayed boney union.[37] It appears that nonthermal mechanisms are most responsible for the accelerated bone healing.[89]

Several researchers have looked at the use of ultrasound over growing epiphyses.[21,57,120] While results have been somewhat inconsistent, some form of damage was observed in each study including premature closure of the epiphysis, epiphyseal displacement, widening of the epiphyseal, fractures, condyle erosion, and shortening of the bones. The degree of destruction appears to be unpredictable; therefore, it is not recommended that ultrasound be applied to growing bone.[51]

Absorption of Calcium Deposits. No documented evidence exists that ultrasound treatment can cause reabsorption of calcium deposits. However, it has been suggested that ultrasound may help to reduce inflammation surrounding a calcium deposit, thus reducing pain and improving function.[128]

Myositis ossificans is calcification within the muscle following acute or repeated trauma. Applying heat or massaging the area may exacerbate this condition. Thus, ultrasound is contraindicated in

■ Analogy   *5-3*

....

Stretching muscle following vigorous heating is like taking a plastic spoon and dipping it in hot water. It becomes soft and by pulling on the ends, we are able to stretch it. As the plastic cools, however, it hardens and is no longer able to be stretched. Likewise, if we vigorously heat tissue it becomes more pliable and less resistant to stretch, yet as the tissue cools, it withstands stretching and can actually be damaged if too great of a force is applied.

acute hematomas, and it is a large leap of logic to assume it capable of reducing the size of the mature calcification.

Ultrasound in Assessing Stress Fractures. The use of ultrasound as a reliable technique for identifying stress fractures has been recommended.[81] Using a continuous beam at 1 MHz with a small transducer and a water-based coupling medium, the athletic trainer moves the transducer slowly over the injured area while gradually increasing the intensity from 0 to 2.0 W/cm^2 until the athlete indicates that he or she feels uncomfortable (periosteal irritation) at which point the ultrasound is turned off. If the athlete reports a feeling of pressure, bruising, or aching, then a stress fracture may be present.

Another technique is to first apply 1 MHz continuous ultrasound in the stationary mode to the contralateral limb. The intensity is slowly increased until the individual reports pain. This is then repeated on the affected area. Typically with a stress fracture, pain will be reported at a lower intensity than on the opposite site. Either a radiograph or a bone scan is then necessary to confirm this diagnosis.

Pain Reduction

Many of the studies discussed previously have noted that reduction in pain occurs with ultrasound treatment even though the treatment was given for other purposes. Several mechanisms have

been proposed that might explain this pain reduction. Ultrasound is thought to elevate the threshold for activation of free nerve endings through thermal effects.[124] Heat produced by ultrasound in large-diameter myelinated nerve fibers may reduce pain through the gating mechanism.[19,89] Ultrasound may also increase nerve conduction velocity in normal nerves creating a counterirritant effect through thermal mechanisms.[68] There is no consensus of opinion in the literature as to the exact mechanism of pain reduction.

Pain reduction following application of ultrasound has been reported in patients with lateral epicondylitis,[5] shoulder pain,[92] plantar fasciitis,[17] surgical wounds,[47] bursitis,[55] prolapsed intervertebral disks,[95] ankle sprains,[84] reflex sympathetic dystrophy,[103] and in various other soft tissue injuries.[90]

Plantar Warts

Plantar warts are occasionally seen on the weight-bearing areas of the feet due to either a virus or to trauma. These lesions contain thrombosed capillaries in a whitish-colored soft core covered by hyperkeratotic epithelial tissue. Among other more conventional techniques, several studies have recommended ultrasound as being an effective painless method for eliminating plantar warts.[66,104,119] Intensities average 0.6 W/cm^2 for 7 to 15 minutes.[22]

Placebo Effects

While the physiologic effects of ultrasound have been discussed in detail, it should also be mentioned that ultrasound can have significant therapeutic psychologic effects.[38] A number of studies have demonstrated a placebo effect in patients receiving sham ultrasound.[44,60,82]

PHONOPHORESIS

Phonophoresis is a technique in which ultrasound is used to enhance delivery of a selected medication into the tissues.[9] Perhaps the greatest advantage of phonophoresis is that medication can be delivered via a safe, painless, noninvasive technique, as is the case with iontophoresis (to be discussed in Chapter 9), which uses electrical energy to deliver a medication. It is thought that active transport occurs as a result of both thermal and nonthermal mechanisms, which together increase permeability of the stratum corneum, although using thermal parameters seems to be most beneficial.[116] This allows a medication to diffuse across it because of differences in concentration from the outside to the inside during sonation. Although the medication tends to follow the path of the beam, it must be stressed that once the medication penetrates the stratum corneum, the vascular circulation will cause diffusion from the highly concentrated delivery site, spreading it throughout the body.[9]

Unlike iontophoresis, phonophoresis drives whole molecules into the tissues as opposed to ions.[1] Consequently, phonophoresis is not as likely to damage or burn skin. Also the potential depth of penetration with phonophoresis is substantially greater than with iontophoresis.

Medications commonly applied through phonophoresis most often are either anti-inflammatories such as hydrocortisone, cortisol, salicylates, or dexamethasone, or anagelsics such as lidocaine. When applying phonophoresis, it is important to select the appropriate drug for the pathology. Since phonophoresis may increase drug penetration, it may also increase the clinical benefits as well as the risks of topical drug application.[12] The athletic trainer should remember that most of the medications used in phonophoresis must be prescribed by a physicain.

The most widespread use of the phonophoresis technique in sports medicine has been to deliver hydrocortisone, which has anti-inflammatory effects. Typically, either 1% or 10% hydrocortisone cream is used in treatments along with thermal ultrasound.[45] The 10% hydrocortisone preparation appears to be superior to the 1% preparation.[69] Several studies have looked at the efficacy of this technique.[64] Using phonophoresis with hydrocortisone was shown to be superior to ultrasound alone in alleviating pain and reducing inflammation in patients with arthritic disorders.[56] It has been used in treating patients with various inflammatory dis-

orders including bursitis, tendinitis, and neuritis.[69] It has also been used to treat tempromandibular joint dysfunction.[65,125] Griffin[56] and Kleinkhort[69] have demonstrated the effective penetration of corticosteroids into tissue with ultrasound. However, Benson[4] and colleagues have shown that many phonophoresis treatments are ineffective.

It appears that many athletic trainers are now using dexamethasone sodium phosphate (Decadron) as an alternative to hydrocortisone.[20] Dexamethasone is best used with thermal ultrasound for 2 to 3 days.[116]

Salicylates are compounds that evoke a number of pharmacologic effects including analgesia and decreased inflammation due to a reduction in prostaglandins. There are few reports that suggest that phonophoresis using saliclyates enhances analgesic or anti-inflammatory effects. However, it has been reported that salicylate phonophoresis may be used to decrease delayed onset muscle soreness without promoting cellular changes that mimic an inflammatory response.[16]

Lidocaine is a commonly used local anesthetic drug. The use of phonophoresis with lidocaine was found to be effective in treating a series of trigger points.[91]

The efficacy of various coupling media has been discussed previously. The addition of an active ingredient into the coupling medium is common practice. However, topical pharmacologic products are usually not formulated to optimize their efficiency as ultrasound coupling media.[4] For example, 1% or 10% hydrocortisone usually comes in a thick white cream base, which has been demonstrated to be a poor conductor of ultrasound. Clinicians have tried mixing this preparation with ultrasound gel (which is known to be a good transmitter) without improvement in transmission capabilities. The use of topical preparations with poor transmission capabilities may negate the effectiveness of ultrasound therapy. Unfortunately, there are few suitable products available and there is clearly a need for appropriate active ingredients in gel form. Table 5-7 provides a list of transmission capabilities of various commercially available phonophoresis media.[12]

■ **TABLE 5-7**   Ultrasound Transmission by Phonophoresis Media

PRODUCT	TRANSMISSION RELATIVE TO WATER (%)
MEDIA THAT TRANSMIT ULTRASOUND WELL	
Lidex® gel, fluocinonide 0.05%[a]	97
Thera-Gesic® cream, methyl salicylate 15%[b]	97
Mineral oil[c]	97
US gel[d]	96
US lotion[e]	90
Betamethasone 0.05% in US gel[d]	88
MEDIA THAT TRANSMIT ULTRASOUND POORLY	
Diprolene® ointment, betamethasone 0.05%[g]	36
Hydrocortisone (HC) powder 1%[b] in US gel[d]	29
HC powder 10%[b] in US gel[d]	7
Cortril® ointment, HC 1%[i]	0
Eucerein® cream[j]	0
HC cream 1%[k]	0
HC cream 10%[k]	0
HC cream 10%[k] mixed with equal weight US gel[d]	0
Myoflex® cream, trolamine salicylate 10%[j]	0
Triamcinolone acetonide cream 0.1%[k]	0
Velva HC cream 10%[b]	0
Velva HC cream 10%[b] with equal weight US gel[d]	0
White petrolatum[m]	0
OTHER	
Chempad-L®[n]	68
Polyethylene wrap[o]	98

[a]Syntex Laboratories Inc. 3401 Hillview Ave, PO Box 10850, Palo Alto, CA 94303.
[b]Missions Pharmacal Co, 1325 E Durango, San Antonio, TX 78210.
[c]Pennex Corp, Eastern Ave at Pennex Dr, Verona, PA 15147.
[d]Ultraphonic®, Pharmaceutical Innovations Inc, 897 Frelinghuysen Dr, Newark, NJ 07114.
[e]Polysonic, Parker Laboratories Inc, 307 Washington St, Orange NJ 07050.
[g]Pharmfair Inc, 110 Kennedy Dr, Hauppauge, NY 11788.
[h]Schering Corp, Galloping Hill Rd, Kenilworth, NJ 07033.
[i]Purepace Pharmaceutical Co, 200 Elmora Ave, Elizabeth, NJ 07207.
[j]Pfizer Labs Division, Pfizer Inc, 253 E. 42nd St, New York, NY 10017.
[k]Beiersdorf Inc, PO Box 5529, Norwalk, CT 06856-5529.
[l]E Fougera & Co, 60 Baylis Rd, Melville, NY 11747.
[l]Rorer Consumer Pharmaceuticals, Div of Rhône-Poulenc Rorer Pharmaceuticals Inc, 500 Virginia Dr, Fort Washington, PA 19034.
[m]Universal Cooperatives Inc, 7801 Metro Pkwy, Minneapolis, MN 55420.
[n]Henley International, 104 Industrial Blvd, Sugar Land, TX 77478.
[o]Saran Wrap®, Dow Brands Inc, 9550 Zionsville Rd, Indianapolis, IN 46268.
From Cameron, M, and Monroe, L: Relative transmission of ultrasound by media customarily used for phonophoresis, *Phys Ther* 72(2): 142–148, 1992. Reprinted with permission from the American Physical Therapy Association.

Since research has shown some of these medications to impede the sound,[2] one suggestion is to apply the medication and gel separately. This is accomplished by rubbing the medication directly onto the surface of the treatment area, then applying gel couplant followed by sonation. With the direct technique, transmission gel should be applied. With immersion, the treatment area with the preparation already applied is simply treated underwater.

■ **Clinical Decision-Making**   *Exercise 5-6*

....

An athletic trainer is treating an athlete with a myofascial trigger point. She has been using thermal ultrasound for about 1 week with less than desirable results. How might she alter the treatment to possibly achieve better results?

Both pulsed and continuous ultrasound have been used in phonophoresis. Continuous ultrasound at an intensity great enough to produce thermal effects may induce a pro-inflammatory response.[39] If the goal is to decrease inflammation, pulsed ultrasound with low spatial-averaged temporal peak intensity may be the best choice.[51] If the treatment goal is to reduce pain, it has been demonstrated that whether or not pulsed phonophoresis was used, stretching, strengthening, and cryotherapy were significantly more effective in decreasing levels of perceived pain.[99]

USING ULTRASOUND IN COMBINATION WITH OTHER MODALITIES

In a sports medicine setting, it is not uncommon to combine modalities to accomplish a specific treatment goal. Ultrasound is frequently used with other modalities, including hot packs, cold packs, and electrical stimulating currents. Unfortunately there is very little documented evidence in the literature to substantiate the effectiveness of ultrasound and electrical currents; however, recent studies of cooling or heating the area prior to ultrasound application have produced interesting results.[24,34,108] In fact, it is possible that combining treatment modalities may actually interfere with the effectiveness of a treatment.[58]

Ultrasound and Hot Packs

Hot packs, like continuous or high intensity ultrasound, are used primarily for their thermal effects. Heat is effective in reducing muscle spasm and muscle guarding and is useful in pain reduction.

For these reasons heat and ultrasound used in combination can be effective for accomplishing these treatment goals. Two different studies have shown that a hot pack application prior to ultrasound had an additive heating effect.[32,63] It was suggested that the ultrasound treatment duration can be decreased by 3 to 5 minutes when tissues are preheated with hot packs.[28] However, it should be pointed out that since hot packs produce an increase in blood flow, particularly to the superficial tissues, creating a less dense medium for transmission of ultrasound, attenuation may be increased and the depth of penetration of ultrasound reduced.

Ultrasound and Cold Packs

Some authors have provided a rationale for ultrasound use immediately after ice. According to this premise, the application of a cold pack to human tissues initiates physiological responses, such as vasoconstriction and decreased blood flow. Thus, cooling the area not only results in decreased local temperature, but it may assist in temporarily increasing the density of the tissue to be heated. This occurs by decreasing superficial attenuation and facilitating transmission to deeper tissues and consequently improving the thermal effects of ultrasound.[34,77,108] Although this theory sounds good, two recent studies[34,108] appear to refute such claims. Whether an ice pack was applied for 5 minutes or 15 minutes, significant cooling took place in the muscle, reducing the rate and intensity of muscle temperature rise via ultrasound (Figure 5-18). It just doesn't make sense to cool something that you immediately want to heat.

When treating acute and postacute injuries, however, the combination of cold to reduce blood flow (i.e., swelling) and produce analgesia, and low intensity ultrasound for its nonthermal effects that promote soft tissue healing may be the treatment of choice. Cold packs are most often used for analgesia and to decrease blood flow acutely following injury. Because cold is such an effective analgesic, caution must be exercised when using ultrasound at higher intensities, which produce thermal ef-

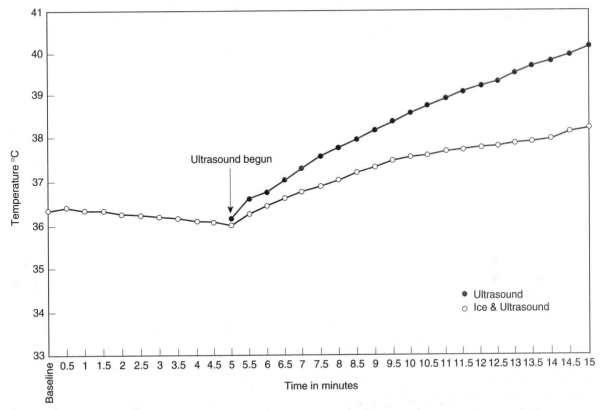

Figure 5-18   When an ice pack was applied for 5 minutes, it impeded the heat produced from ultrasound. The increase in muscle temperature was greater and faster during the ultrasound treatment (increase of 4° C) than during the ice/ultrasound treatment (increase of 1.8° C).

(From: Draper, DO, Schulthies, S, Sorvisto, P, and Hautala A: Temperature changes in deep muscles of humans during ice and ultrasound therapies: an in-vivo study, *J Orthop & Sports Phys Therapy* 21:153–157, 1995)

fects, since the patient's perception of temperature and pain are diminished. Pulsed ultrasound, however, could be used after ice application if the goal is pain reduction and healing in the acute stage.[13,14]

Ultrasound and Electrical Stimulating Currents

Ultrasound and electrical stimulating currents are frequently used in combination (Figure 5-19). Electrical stimulating currents are used for analgesia or producing muscle contraction. Ultrasound and electrical stimulating currents in combination have been recommended in the treatment of myofascial

trigger points.[54,74] Both modalities provide analgesic effects, and both have been shown to be effective in reducing the pain-spasm-pain cycle, although the specific mechanisms responsible are not clearly understood.

Electrical stimulating currents will be discussed in Chapters 7 and 8. When using ultrasound and electrical stimulating currents together, the ultrasound transducer serves as one electrode and thus delivers both acoustic energy and electrical energy. The electrical energy should be sufficient to cause a muscle contraction when the transducer passes over the trigger point, while the ultrasound should cause at least a moderate increase in tissue temperature. Since trigger points are found within the

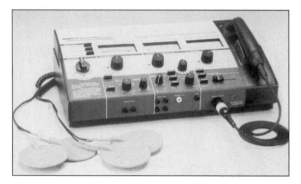

Figure 5-19 Ultrasound is frequently used in combination with electrical stimulating currents. (Courtesy Amrex)

muscle, it is likely that 3 MHz ultrasound will be more effective in reaching the deeper tissue. The transducer should be moved slowly (4cm/sec) in a small circular pattern over the trigger point. Stretching of the muscle during the application of ultrasound and an electrical stimulating current can also be helpful in treating a myofascial trigger point.

TREATMENT PRECAUTIONS AND CONSIDERATIONS

There are a number of treatment precautions to the use of therapeutic ultrasound. The use of continuous ultrasound with a high spatial-averaged temporal peak intensity should be avoided in acute and postacute conditions because of the associated thermal effects. Caution should be used when treating areas of decreased sensation particularly when there is a problem in perceiving pain and temperature. In areas of decreased circulation caution must be exercised due to excessive heat buildup, which can potentially damage tissues.

Individuals with vascular problems involving thrombophlebitis should not receive ultrasound because of the possibility of dislodging a clot and creating an embolus. Ultrasound should not be applied around the eye, since heat is not dissipated well, and both the lens and the retina may be damaged. Ultrasound should not be applied over reproductive organs, especially the testes, since

temporary sterility may result. Caution should be used in treating the abdominal region of the female during the reproductive years or immediately following menses. The use of ultrasound is contraindicated during pregnancy because of potential damage to the fetus. Some precaution should be used when treating areas around the heart due to potential changes in ECG activity. Ultrasound can certainly interfere with normal function of a pacemaker. Therapeutic ultrasound should not be used over malignant tissue since it has been suggested that this may cause cell detachment and metastasis. As previously mentioned, ultrasound should never be used over epiphyseal areas in young children.

Ultrasound may be used safely over metal implants since it has been shown that there is no increase in temperature of tissue adjacent to the implant because metal has high thermal conductivity, and thus heat is removed from the area faster than it can be absorbed. However, in cases of total joint replacement, the cement used (methyl methacrylate) absorbs heat rapidly and may be overheated damaging surrounding soft tissues. Table 5-8 provides a summary of the indications and contraindications for using therapeutic ultrasound.

GUIDELINES FOR THE SAFE USE OF ULTRASOUND EQUIPMENT

Currently, ultrasound units are the only therapeutic modality for which federal performance standards exist.[100] Ultrasound units produced since 1979 are required to indicate the magnitudes of ultrasound power and intensity with an accuracy of

■ **TABLE 5-8** Summary of Indications and Contraindications for Using Ultrasound

INDICATIONS	CONTRAINDICATIONS
Acute and postacute conditions (ultrasound with nonthermal effects)	Acute and postacute conditions (ultrasound with thermal effects)
Soft tissue healing and repair	Areas of decreased temperature sensation
Scar tissue	Areas of decreased circulation
Joint contracture	Vascular insufficiency
Chronic inflammation	Thrombophlebitis
Increase extensibility of collagen	Eyes
Reduction of muscle spasm	Reproductive organs
Pain modulation	Pelvis immediately following menses
Increase blood flow	Pregnancy
Soft tissue repair	Pacemaker
Increase in protein synthesis	Malignancy
Tissue regeneration	Epiphyseal areas in young children
Bone healing	Total joint replacements
Repair of nonunion fractures	Infection
Inflammation associated with myositis osificans	
Plantar warts	
Myofascial trigger points	

±20 percent and to accurately control treatment time. It is recommended that intensity output, pulse regime accuracy, and timer accuracy be checked at regular intervals by qualified personnel who have access to the appropriate testing equipment. The effective radiating area and the beam nonuniformity ratio of the transducer should be accurately provided by the manufacturer. The following treatment guidelines will help to ensure athletes safety:

1. Question athlete (contraindications/ previous treatments)
2. Position athlete (comfort, modesty)
3. Inspect part to be treated (check for rashes, infections, or open wounds)
4. Obtain appropriate soundhead size
5. Determine ultrasound frequency (1 MHz for deep, 3 MHz for superficial)
6. Set duty cycle (choose either continuous or pulsed setting)
7. Apply couplant to area
8. Set treatment duration (vigorous heat = 10 to 12 min at 1 MHz and 3 to 4 min at 3 MHz)
9. Maintain contact between the skin and the applicator (move at a rate of 4 cm/sec, for 2 era)
10. Adjust intensity to perception of heat (if this gets too hot, turn down the intensity, or move applicator slightly faster)
11. If goal is increased joint ROM, put part on stretch (for the last 2 to 3 minutes of insonation, and maintain stretch or friction massage 2 to 5 minutes after termination of treatment)
12. Terminate treatment (turn all dials to zero, clean gel from unit)
13. Assess treatment efficacy (inspect area, feedback from client)
14. Record treatment parameters

Note: Ultrasound units should be recalibrated every 6 to 12 months, depending on the frequency of use.

Summary

1. Ultrasound is defined as inaudible, acoustic vibrations of high frequency that may produce either thermal or nonthermal physiologic effects.
2. Ultrasound travels through soft tissue as a longitudinal wave at a therapeutic frequency of either 1 MHz or 3 MHz.
3. As the ultrasound wave is transmitted through the various tissues, there will be attenuation or a decrease in energy intensity due to either absorption of energy by the tissues or dispersion and scattering of the sound wave.
4. Ultrasound is produced by a piezoelectric crystal within the transducer, which converts electrical energy to acoustic energy through mechanical deformation via the piezoelectric effect.
5. Ultrasound energy travels within the tissues as a highly focused collimated beam with a nonuniform intensity distribution.
6. While continuous ultrasound is most commonly used when the desired effect is to produce thermal effects, pulsed ultrasound or continuous ultrasound at a low intensity will produce nonthermal or mechanical effects.
7. Therapeutic ultrasound when applied to biologic tissue may induce clinically significant responses in cells, tissues, and organs through both thermal effects, which produce a tissue temperature increase, and nonthermal effects, which include cavitation and microstreaming.
8. Recent research has provided answers to many of the contradictory results and conclusions of a number of previous laboratory and clinically based reports in the literature.
9. Therapeutic ultrasound is most effective when an appropriate coupling medium and technique using either direct contact, immersion, or a bladder is combined with a moving transducer.
10. Although there is relatively little documented evidence from the clinical community concerning the efficacy of ultrasound, it is most often used for soft tissue healing and repair, with scar tissue and joint contracture, for chronic inflammation, for bone healing, with plantar warts, and for placebo effects.
11. Phonophoresis is a technique in which ultrasound is used to drive molecules of a topically applied medication, usually either anti-inflammatories or anagelsics, into the tissues.
12. In a clinical setting, ultrasound is frequently used in combination with other modalities, including hot packs, cold packs, and electrical stimulating currents to produce specific treatment effects.
13. Although ultrasound is a relatively safe modality if used appropriately, the athletic trainer must be aware of the various contraindications and precautions.
14. For ultrasound to be effective, the athletic trainer must pay particular attention to correct parameters, such as intensity, frequency, duration, and treatment size.

Review Questions

1. What is therapeutic ultrasound, and what are its two primary physiologic effects?
2. How does an ultrasound wave travel through biologic tissues, and what happens to the acoustic energy within those tissues?
3. How does the transducer convert electrical energy into acoustic energy?
4. How does the frequency affect the ultrasound beam within the tissues?
5. What are the differences between continuous and pulsed ultrasound?
6. What are the potential thermal effects of ultrasound?
7. How can the nonthermal effects of ultrasound facilitate the healing process?
8. What is the relationship between treatment intensity and treatment duration in effecting a temperature increase in the tissues?

9. What are the various coupling agents and exposure techniques that may be used when treating an athlete with ultrasound?

10. What are the various clinical applications for using ultrasound in treating sport-related injuries?

11. What is the purpose of using a phonophoresis treatment?

12. How should ultrasound be used in combination with other therapeutic modalities?

 ## Self-Test Questions

T/F

1. Penetration and absorption are inversely related.
2. Three MHZ frequency ultrasound is absorbed deeper and faster than 1 MHz.
3. A low beam nonuniformity ratio (BNR) results in uneven heating.

Multiple Choice

4. The decrease in energy intensity of the ultrasound wave as it is scattered and dispersed while traveling through various tissues is known as which of the following?
   a. acoustic impedance
   b. attenuation
   c. rarefaction
   d. compression

5. A (n) _____ may develop when standing waves form at tissue interfaces and reflected energy meets transmitted energy, increasing the intensity.
   a. hot spot
   b. impedance
   c. rarefaction
   d. collimated beam

6. Which of the following is NOT a nonthermal effect of ultrasound?
   a. acoustic microstreaming
   b. cavitation
   c. increased collagen extensibility
   d. increased fibroblast activity

7. Which of the following is the LEAST effective ultrasound coupling method?
   a. massage lotion
   b. ultrasonic gel
   c. water immersion
   d. bladder technique

8. Ultrasound may be used to treat which of the following?
   a. bone fracture
   b. pain
   c. plantar warts
   d. all of the above

9. _____ uses ultrasound to drive molecules of medication into the skin.
   a. "combo therapy"
   b. iontophoresis
   c. phonophoresis
   d. none of the above

10. In order to increase tissue temperature 2° C, how long must the ultrasound treatment time be at a setting of 1 MHz and 1.0 W/cm^2?
    a. 5 minutes
    b. 10 minutes
    c. 7.5 minutes
    d. 15 minutes

Solutions to Clinical Decision-Making Exercises

5-1 The lower the frequency, the less the energy is absorbed in the superficial tissues, and thus the deeper it penetrates. The majority of the sound waves generated from the 3 MHz treatment would be absorbed in the muscle or tendon. Also, when treating subcutaneous structure, 3 MHz heats more rapidly and is more comfortable than 1 MHz.

5-2   The nonthermal effects of cavitation and microstreaming can be maximized while minimizing the thermal effects by using a spatial-averaged, temporal-averaged intensity of 0.1 to 0.2 W/cm^2 with continuous ultrasound. This range may also be achieved using a low temporal-averaged intensity by pulsing a higher temporal peak intensity of 1.0 W/cm^2 at a duty cycle of 20% to give a temporal-averaged intensity of 0.2 W/cm^2.

5-3   Since temperature increase is frequency dependent, at 1 MHz with an intensity of 1.5 W/cm^2, temperature will elevate at a rate of 0.3° C per minute. Therefore, a 10-minute treatment will be necessary.

5-4   When using a large sound head to treat over bony prominences, the immersion technique done in a plastic or rubber tub can be effective. Also the bladder technique could be used to make certain that there is consistent contact between the sound head and the coupling medium.

5-5   Phonophoresis would likely be a reasonable choice. The team physician could prescribe a topical anti-inflammatory medication that could be administered to the patient topically. In phonophoresis, ultrasound is used to enhance delivery of a medication into the tissues.

5-6   Since the athlete does not seem to be getting better, the athletic trainer might try combining ultrasound with an electrical stimulating current. Stretching during treatment is also recommended.

5-7   In this case, the best treatment choice is not to use ultrasound at all. A better decision would be to use either hydrocollator packs or diathermy, both of which are more useful in treating larger areas. If depth of penetration is a concern, then shortwave diathermy would be the treatment modality of choice.

References

1. Antich, TJ: Phonophoresis: the principles of the ultrasonic driving force and efficacy in treatment of common orthopedic diagnosis, *J Ortho Sport Phys Ther* 4(2):99–103, 1982.
2. Ashton, DF, Draper, DO, and Myrer, JW: Temperature rise in human muscle during ultrasound treatments using flex-all as a coupling agent, *Journal of Athletic Training* 33(2): 136–140, 1998.
3. Balmaseda, MT, Fatehi, MT, and Koozekanani, SH: Ultrasound therapy: a comparative study of different coupling medium, *Arch Phys Med Rehab* 67:147, 1986.
4. Benson, HAE, and McElnay, IC: Transmission of ultrasound energy through topical pharmaceutical products, *Physiotherapy* 74:587, 1988.
5. Bierman, W: Ultrasound in the treatment of scars, *Arch Phys Med Rehabil* 35:209, 1954.
6. Binder, A, Hodge, J, and Greenwood T: Is therapeutic ultrasound effective in treating soft tissue lesions? *Br Med J* 290: 512, 1985.
7. Black, K, Halverson, JL, Maierus, K, and Soderbere, GL: Alterations in ankle dorsiflexion torque as a result of continuous ultrasound to the anterior tibial compartment, *Phys Ther* 64(6):910–913, 1984.
8. Boone, L, Ingersol, CD, and Cordova, ML: Passive hip flexion does not increase during or following ultrasound treatment of the hamstring musculature, *Journal of Athletic Training* 34(2): S-70, 1999.
9. Byl, NN: The use of ultrasound as an enhancer for transcutaneous drug delivery: phonophoresis, *Physical Therapy* 75(6):89–95, 1995.
10. Bly, N, McKenzie, A, West, J, and Whitney, J: Low dose ultrasound effects on wound healing: a controlled study with Yucatan pigs, *Arch Phys Med Rehab* 73:656–664, 1992.
11. Brueton, RN, and Campbell, B: The use of geliperm as a sterile coupling agent for therapeutic ultrasound, *Physiotherapy* 73:653, 1987.
12. Cameron, M, and Monroe, L: Relative transmission of ultrasound by media customarily used for phonophoresis, *Physical Therapy* 72(2):142–148, 1992.
13. Castel, JC: *Electrotherapy application in clinical for neuromuscular stimulation and tissue repair.* Presented at the 46th Annual Clinical Symposium of the National Athletic Trainer's Association, June 16, 1995, Indianapolis.
14. Castel, JC: Therapeutic ultrasound, *Rehab and Therapy Products Review* Jan/Feb:22–32, 1993.
15. Chan, AK, Myrer, JW, Measom, G, and Draper, D: Temperature changes in human patellar tendon in response to therapeutic ultrasound, *Journal of Athletic Training* 33(2): 130–135, 1998.
16. Ciccone, C, Leggin, B, and Callamaro, J: Effects of ultrasound and trolamine salicylate phonophoresis on delayed-onset muscle soreness, *Physical Therapy* 71(9): 666–675, 1991.
17. Clarke, GR, and Stenner, L: Use of therapeutic ultrasound, *Physiotherapy* 62(6):85–190, 1976.

18. Craig, JA, Bradley, J, Walsh, DM, Baxter, GD, and Allen, JM: Delayed onset muscle soreness: lack of effect of therapeutic ultrasound in humans, *Archives of Physical Medicine & Rehab* 80(3): 318–23, 1999.

19. Currier, DP, and Kramer, IF: Sensory nerve conduction: Heating effects of ultrasound and infrared, *Physiotherapy Canada* 34:241, 1982.

20. Darrow, H, Schulthies, S, and Draper, D: Serum dexamethasone levels after decadron phonophoresis, *Journal of Athletic Training* 34(4): 338–341, 1999.

21. DeForest, RE, Henick, JF, and Janes, JM: Effects of ultrasound on growing bone: an experimental study, *Arch Phys Med Rehab* 34:21, 1953.

22. Delacerda, FG: Ultrasonic techniques for treatment of plantar warts in patients, *J Ortho Sports Phys Ther* 1:100, 1979.

23. Docker, MF: A review of instrumentation available for therapeutic ultrasound, *Physiotherapy* 73(4):154, 1987.

24. Docker, MF, Foulkes, DJ, and Patrick, MK: Ultrasound couplants for physiotherapy, *Physiotherapy* 68(4):124–125, 1982.

25. Downing, DS, and Weinstein, A: Ultrasound therapy of subacromial bursitis (abstr), *Phys Ther* 66:194, 1986.

26. Draper, DO: Guidelines to enhance therapeutic ultrasound treatment outcomes, *Athletic Therapy Today* 3(6):7–11, 28–29, 55, 1998.

27. Draper, DO: Ten mistakes commonly made with ultrasound use: current research sheds light on myths, *Ath Training: Sports Health Care Perspectives* 2:95–107, 1996.

28. Draper, DO: *The latest research on therapeutic ultrasound: clinical habits may need to be changed.* Presented at the 46th Annual Meeting and Clinical Symposium of the National Athletic Trainer's Association, June 16, 1995, Indianapolis.

29. Draper, DO: *Current research on therapeutic ultrasound and pulsed short-wave diathermy.* Presented at Physiotherapy Research Seminars Japan, Nov. 17, 1996, Sendai, Japan.

30. Draper, DO, Anderson, C, and Schulthies, SS: Immediate and residual changes in dorsiflexion range of motion using an ultrasound heat and stretch routine, *Journal of Athletic Training* 33(2):141–144, 1998

31. Draper, DO, Castel, JC, and Castel, D: Rate of temperature increase in human muscle during 1 Mhz and 3 Mhz continuous ultrasound, *J Orthop & Sports Phys Therapy*. 22:142–150, 1995.

32. Draper, DO, Harris, ST, and Schulthies, S: Hot pack and 1-MHz ultrasound treatments have an additive effect on muscle temperature increase, *Journal of Athletic Training* 33(1):21–24, 1998.

33. Draper, DO, and Ricard, MD: Rate of temperature decay in human muscle following 3 MHz ultrasound: the stretching window revealed, *J Ath Trng* 30:304–307, 1995.

34. Draper, DO, Schulthies, S, Sorvisto, P, and Hautala, A: Temperature changes in deep muscles of humans during ice and ultrasound therapies: an in-vivo study, *J Orthop & Sports Phys Therapy* 21:153–157, 1995.

35. Draper, DO, Sunderland, S, Kirkendall, DT, and Ricard, MD: A comparison of temperature rise in the human calf muscles following applications of underwater and topical gel ultrasound, *J Orthop & Sports Phys Therapy* 17:247–251, 1993.

36. Draper, DO, and Sunderland, S: Examination of the law of Grotthus-Draper: does ultrasound penetrate subcutaneous fat in humans? *J Ath Train* 28:246–250, 1993.

37. Dyson, M: The use of ultrasound in sports physiotherapy. In Grisogono, V, editor: *Sports injuries: International perspectives in physiotherapy*, Edinburgh, 1989, Churchill Livingstone.

38. Dyson, M: Mechanisms involved in therapeutic ultrasound, *Physiotherapy* 73(3):116–120, 1987.

39. Dyson, M: Therapeutic application of ultrasound. In Nyborg, WL, and Ziskin, MC, editors: *Biological effects of ultrasound*, Edinburgh, 1985, Churchill Livingstone.

40. Dyson, M, and Brookes, M: Stimulation of bone repair by ultrasound (abstr), *UItrasound Med Biol* 8(suppl 50):50, 1982.

41. Dyson, M, and Luke, DA: Induction of mast cell degranulation in skin by ultrasound. IEEE transactions and ultrasonics, ferroelectrics, and frequency control, *UFFC* 33:194. 1986.

42. Dyson, M, and Pond, JB: The effect of pulsed ultrasound on tissue regeneration, *Physiother* 64:105–108, 1970.

43. Echternach, JL: Ultrasound: An adjunct treatment for shoulder disability, *Phys Ther* 45:565, 1965.

44. EI Hag, M, Coghlan, K, and Christmas, P: The anti-inflammatory effects of dexamethasone and therapeutic ultrasound in oral surgery, *British J Oral and Maxillofacial Surg* 23:17, 1985.

45. Fahey, S, Smith, M, and Merrick, M: Intramuscular temperature does not differ among hydrocortisone preparations during exercise, *Journal of Athletic Training* 35(2): S-47, 2000.

46. Ferguson, BA: *A practitioners' guide to ultrasonic therapy equipment standard*, U.S. Dept. of Health and Human Services, Public Health Service, Food and Drug Administration, Rockville, Maryland, 1985.

47. Ferguson, HN: Ultrasound in the treatment of surgical wounds, *Physiotherapy* 67:12, 1981.

48. Frizell, LA, and Dunn, F: Biophysics of ultrasound and bio-effects of ultrasound. In Lehmann, JF, editor: *Therapeutic heat and cold*, ed. 3, Baltimore, 1982, Williams & Wilkins.

49. Fyfe, MC, and Bullock, M: Therapeutic ultrasound: some historical background and development in knowledge of its effects on healing, *Australian J Physiotherapy* 31(6): 220–224, 1985.

50. Fyfe, MC, and Chahl, LA: The effect of single or repeated applications of "therapeutic" ultrasound on plasma extravasation during silver nitrate induced inflammation of the rat hindpaw ankle joint, *Ultrasound Med Biol* 11:273, 1985.

51. Gann, N: Ultrasound: current concepts, *Clinical Management* 11(4):64–69, 1991.

52. Gatto, J, Kimura, IF, and Gulick, D: Effect of beam nonuniformity ratio of three ultrasound machines on tissue phantom temperature, *Journal of Athletic Training* 34(2): S-69, 1999.

53. Gersten, JW: Effect of ultrasound on tendon extensibility, *Am J Phys Med* 34:662, 1955.

54. Girardi, CQ, Seaborne, D, and Savard-Goulet, F: The analgesic effect of high voltage galvanic stimulation combined with ultrasound in the treatment of low back pain: a one group pretest/posttest study, *Physiotherapy Canada* 36(6): 327–333, 1984.

55. Gorkiewicz, R: Ultrasound for subacromial bursitis, *Phys Ther* 64:46, 1984.

56. Griffin, JE, Echternach, JL, and Price, RE: Patients treated with ultrasonic driven hydrocortisone and ultrasound alone, *Physical Therapy* 47:594–601, 1967.

57. Griffin, JE, and Karsalis, TC: *Physical agents for physical therapists*, Springfield, 1978, Charles C Thomas.

58. Gum, SL, Reddy, GK, Stehno-Bittel, L, and Enwemeka, CS: Combined ultrasound, electrical stimulation, and laser promote collagen synthesis with moderate changes in tendon biomechanics, *American Journal of Physical Medicine & Rehabilitation* 76(4):288–296, 1997

59. Harvey, W, Dyson, M, and Pond, JB: The simulation of protein synthesis in human fibroblasts by therapeutic ultrasound, *Rheumato Rehab* 14:237, 1975.

60. Hashish, I, Harvey, W, and Harris, M: Anti-inflammatory effects of ultrasound therapy: evidence for a major placebo effect, *British Journal of Rheumatology* 25:77, 1986.

61. Hecox, B, Mehreteab, TA, and Weisberg, J. *Physical agents: a comprehensive text for physical therapists*, East Norwalk, Conn., Appleton & Lange, 1994.

62. Hogan, RD, Burke, KM, and Franklin, TD: The effect of ultrasound on microvascular hemodynamics in skeletal muscle: effects during ischemia, *Microvasc Res* 23:370, 1982.

63. Holcomb, WR, Blank, C, and Davis, C: The effect of superficial pre-heating on the magnitude and duration of temperature elevation with 1 MHz ultrasound, *Journal of Athletic Training* 35(2): S-48, 2000.

64. Holdsworth, LK, and Anderson, DM: Effectiveness of ultrasound used with hydrocortisone coupling medium or epicondylitis clasp to treat lateral epicondylitis: pilot study, *Physiotherapy* 79(1):19–25, 1993.

65. Kahn, J: Iontophoresis and ultrasound for post-surgical temporomandibular trismus and paresthesia, *Physical Therapy* 60(3):307–308, 1980.

66. Kent, H: Plantar wart treatment with ultrasound, *Arch Phys Med Rehab* 40:15, 1959.

67. Kitchen, S, and Partridge, C: *A review of therapeutic ultrasound: part 1, background and physiological effects* 76(10): 593, 1990.

68. Kitchen, S, and Partridge, C: *A review of therapeutic ultrasound: part 2, the efficacy of ultrasound* 76(10):595–599, 1990.

69. Kleinkort, IA, and Wood, F: Phonophoresis with 1 percent versus 10 percent hydrocortisone, *Phys Ther* 55:1320, 1975.

70. Klucinec, B, Denegar, C, and Mahmood, R: The transducer pressure variable: its influence on acoustic energy transmission, *Journal of Sport Rehabilitation* 6(1):47–53, 1997.

71. Klucinec, B, Scheidler, M, and Denegar, C: Transmission of coupling agents used to deliver acoustic energy over irregular surfaes, *Journal of Orthopedic and Sports Physical Therapy* 30(5): 263–269, 2000.

72. Kramer, JF: Ultrasound: evaluation of its mechanical and thermal effects, *Arch Phys Med Rehab* 65:223, 1984.

73. Kremkau, F: In Nyborg, WL, and Ziskin, MC, editors: Transmission of ultrasound energy. *Biological Effects of Ultrasound*, Edinburgh, 1985, Churchill Livingstone.

74. Lee, JC, Lin, DT, and Hong, C: The effectiveness of simulataneous thermotherapy with ultrasound and electrotherapy with combined AC and DC current on the immediate pain relief of myofascial trigger points, *Journal of Musculoskeletal Pain* 5(1):81–90, 1997.

75. Lehmann, JF: Clinical evaluation of a new approach in the treatment of contracture associated with hip fracture after internal fixation, *Arch Phys Med Rehab* 42:95, 1961.

76. Lehmann, JF: Effect of therapeutic temperatures on tendon extensibility, *Arch Phys Med Rehab* 51:481, 1970.

77. Lehmann, JF, and De Lateur, BJ: Therapeutic heat. In Lehmann, JF, editor: *Therapeutic heat and cold*, ed 4, Baltimore, 1990, Williams & Wilkins.

78. Lehmann, JF, De Lateur, BJ, and Silverman, DR: Selective heating effects of ultrasound in human beings, *Arch Phys Med Rehab* 46:331, 1966.

79. Lehman, JF, DeLateur, BJ, Stonebridge, JB, and Warren, G: Therapeutic temperature distribution produced by ultrasound as modified by dosage and volume of tissue exposed, *Arch Phys Med Rehabil* 48:662–666, 1967.

80. Lehmann, JF, and Guy, AW: Ultrasound therapy. In Reid, J, and Sikov, MR, editors: *Interaction of ultrasound and biological tissues*, DHEW Pub (FDA) 73-8008, session 3(8): 141, 1971.

81. Lowden, A: Application of ultrasound to assess stress fractures, *Physiotherapy* 72(3):160–161 1986.

82. Lundeberg, T, Abrahamsson, P, and Haker, E: A comparative study of continuous ultrasound, placebo ultrasound and rest in epicondylalgia, *Scand Rehab Med* 20:99, 1988.

83. MacDonald, BL, and Shipster, SB: Temperature changes induced by continuous ultrasound, *South African J Physiotherapy* 37(1):13–15, 1981.

84. Makuloluwe, RT, and Mouzas, GL: Ultrasound in the treatment of sprained ankles, *Practitioner* 218:586–588, 1977.

85. Markham, DE, and Wood, MR: Ultrasound for Dupytren's contracture, *Physiotherapy* 66(2):55–58, 1980.

86. Merrick, MA: Ultrasound and range of motion examined, *Athletic Therapy Today* 5(3): 48–49, May, 2000.

87. Michlovitz, S: *Thermal agents in rehabilitation*, Philadelphia, 1996, FA Davis.

88. Mihaloyvov, MR, Roethmeier, JL, and Merrick, MA: Intramuscular temperature does not differ between direct ultrasound application and application with commercial gel packs, *Journal of Athletic Training* 35(2):S-47, 2000.

89. McDiarmid, T, and Burns, PN: Clinical applications of therapeutic ultrasound, *Physiotherapy* 73:155, 1987.

90. Middlemast, S, and Chatterjee, DS: Comparison of ultrasound and thermotherapy for soft tissue injuries, *Physiotherapy* 64:331, 1978.

91. Moll, MJ: A new approach to pain: lidocaine and decadron with ultrasound, *USAF Medical Service Digest*, May–June 8, 1977.

92. Munting, E: Ultrasonic therapy for painful shoulders, *Physiotherapy* 64:180, 1978.

93. Myrer, JW, Draper, DO, and Durrant, E: Contrast therapy and intramuscular temperature in the human leg, *J Ath Trng* 29:318–322, 1994.

94. Myrer, JW, Measom, G, and Fellingham, GW: Significant intramuscular temperature rise obtained when topical analgesics Nature's Chemist and Biofreeze were used as coupling agents during ultrasound treatment, *Journal of Athletic Training* 35(2):S-48, 2000.

95. Nwuga, VCB: Ultrasound in treatment of back pain resulting from prolapsed intervertebral disc, *Arch Phys Med Rehab* 64:88, 1983.

96. Oakley, EM: Application of continuous beam ultrasound at therapeutic levels, *Physiotherapy* 64(4):103–104, 1978.

97. Partridge, CJ: Evaluation of the efficacy of ultrasound, *Physiotherapy* 73(4):166–168, 1987.

98. Patrick, MK: Applications of pulsed therapeutic ultrasound, *Physiotherapy* 64(4):103–104, 1978.

99. Penderghest, C, Kimura, I, and Gulick, D: Double blind clinical efficacy study of pulsed phonophoresis on perceived pain associated with symptomatic tendinitis, *Journal of Sport Rehabilitation* (7):9–19, 1998.

100. *Performance Standards for Sonic, Infrasonic, and Ultrasonic Radiation Emitting Products*: 21 CFR 1050:10 Federal Register 43:7166, 1978.

101. Pilla, AA, Figueiredo, M, Nasser, P, Mont, M, Khan, S, Kaufman, JJ, and Siffert, RS: *Non-invasive low intensity pulsed ultrasound: a potent accelerator of bone repair*. Proceedings of the 36th Annual Meeting. Orthopaedic Research Society, New Orleans, 1990.

102. Plaskett, C, Tiidus, PM, and Livingston, L: Ultrasound treatment does not affect post exercise muscle strength recovery or soreness, *Journal of Sport Rehabilitation* 8(1):1–9, 1999.

103. Portwood, MM, Lieberman, SS, and Taylor, RG: Ultrasound treatment of reflex sympathetic dystrophy, *Arch Phys Med Rehab* 68:116, 1987.

104. Quade, AG, and Radzyminski, SF: Ultrasound in verruca plantaris, *J Am Podiatric Assoc* 56:503, 1966.

105. Rantanen, J, Thorsson, O, Wollmer, P, Hurme, T, and Kalimo, H: Effects of therapeutic ultrasound on the regeneration of skeletal myofibers after experimental muscle injury, *American Journal of Sports Medicine* 27(1):54–59, 1999.

106. Reed, B, Ashikaga, T, and Flemming, BC: Effects of ultrasound and stretch on knee ligament extensibility, *Journal of Orthopedic and Sports Physical Therapy* 30(6): 341–347, 2000.

107. Reid, DC, and Cummings, GE: Factors in selecting the dosage of ultrasound with particular reference to the use of various coupling agents, *Physiotherapy Canada* 63:255, 1973.

108. Rimington, S, Draper, DO, Durrant, E, and Fellingham, GW: Temperature changes during therapeutic ultrasound in the precooled human gastrocnemius muscle, *J Ath Trng* 29:325–327, 1994.

109. Rose, S, Draper, DO, Schulthies, SS, and Durrant, E. The stretching window part two: rate of thermal decay in deep muscle following 1 MHz ultrasound, *J Ath Trng* 31:139–143, 1996.

110. Sandler, V, and Feingold, P: The thermal effect of pulsed ultrasound, *South African J Physiotherapy* 37(1):10–12, 1951.

111. Smith, K, Draper, DO, Schulthies, SS, and Durrant E: *The effect of silicate gel hot packs on human muscle temperature*. Presented at the 46th Annual Meeting and Clinical Symposium of the National Athletic Trainer's Association, June 15, 1995, Indianapolis, Ind. Abstract published in *J Ath Trng* 30:S–33, 1995.

112. Snow, CJ, and Johnson, KA: Effect of therapeutic ultrasound on acute inflammation, *Physiotherapy Canada* 40:162, 1988.

113. Starkey, C: *Therapeutic modalities for athletic trainers*, Philadelphia, 1999, FA Davis.

114. Stein, T: Ultrasound: exploring benefits on bone repair, growth and healing, *Sports Medicine Update* 13(1): 1998, 22–23.

115. Summer, W, and Patrick, MK: *Ultrasonic therapy*, New York, 1964, American Elsevier.

116. Strapp, E, Guskiewicz, K, and Hackney, A: The cumulative effects of multiple phonophoresis treatments on dexamethasone and cortisol concentrations in the blood, *Journal of Athletic Training* 35(2):S-47, 2000.

117. Ter Haar, C: Basic physics of therapeutic ultrasound, *Physiotherapy* 73(3):110–113, 1987.

118. Ter Haar, G, and Hopewell, JW: Ultrasonic heating of mammalian tissue in vivo, *British J Cancer* 45(suppl V): 65–67, 1982.

119. Vaughn, DT: Direct method versus underwater method in treatment of plantar warts with ultrasound, *Phys Ther* 53:396, 1973.

120. Vaughen, IL, and Bender, LF: Effect of ultrasound on growing bone, *Arch Phys Med Rehab* 40:158, 1959.

121. Ward, AR: *Electricity fields and waves in therapy*, Marrickville, NSW, Australia, 1986, Science Press.

122. Werden, SJ, Bennell, KL, and McMeeken, JM: Can conventional therapeutic ultrasound units be used to accelerate fracture repair? *Physical Therapy Reviews* 4(2):117–126, 1999.

123. Williams, R: Production and transmission of ultrasound, *Physiotherapy* 73(3):113–116, 1987.

124. Williams, AR, McHale, I, and Bowditch, M: Effects of MHz ultrasound on electrical pain threshold perception in humans, *Ultrasound in Medicine and Biology* 13:249, 1987.

125. Wing, M: Phonophoresis with hydrocortisone in the treatment of temporomandibular joint dysfunction, *Physical Therapy* 62:32–33, 1982.

126. Woolf, N: *Cell, tissue and disease*, ed 2, London, 1986, Bailliere Tindall.

127. Zarod, AP, and Williams, AR: Platelet aggregation in vivo by therapeutic ultrasound, *Lancet* 1:1266, 1977.

128. Ziskin, M, McDiarmid, T, and Michlovitz, S: Therapeutic ultrasound. In Michlovitz, S, editor: *Thermal agents in rehabilitation*, Philadelphia, 1996, FA Davis.

Suggested Readings

Abramson, DI: Changes in blood flow, oxygen uptake and tissue temperatures produced by therapeutic physical agents. I. Effect of ultrasound, *Am J Phys Med* 39:51, 1960.

Aldes, IH, and Grabin, S: Ultrasound in the treatment of intervertebral disc syndrome, *Am J Phys Med* 37:199, 1958.

Allen, KGR, and Battye, CK: Performance of ultrasonic therapy instruments, *Physiotherapy* 64(6):174–179, 1978.

Antich, TJ: Physical therapy treatment of knee extensor mechanism disorders: comparison of four treatment modalities, *J Ortho Sports Physical Therapy* 8:255, 1986.

Aspelin, P, Ekberg, O, Thorsson, O, and Wilhelmsson, M: Ultrasound examination of soft tissue injury in the lower limb in patients, *Am J Sports Med* 20(5): 601–603, 1992.

Banties, A, and Klomp, R: Transmission of ultrasound energy through coupling agents, *Physiotherapy in Sport* 3:9–13, 1979.

Bare, A, McAnaw, M, and Pritchard, A: Phonophoretic delivery of 10% hydrocortisone through the epidermis of humans as determined by serum cortisol concentration, *Phys Ther* 76(7):738–749, 1996.

Bearzy, HJ: Clinical applications of ultrasonic energy in the treatment of acute and chronic subacromial bursitis, *Arch Phys Med Rehab* 34:228, 1953.

Behrens, BJ, and Michlovitz, SL: *Physical agents: theory and practice for the physical therapist assistant*, Philadelphia, 1966, FA Davis.

Benson, HA, McElnay, JC, and Harland, RL: Use of ultrasound to enhance percutaneous absorption of benzydamine, *Physical Therapy* 69(2):113–118, 1989.

Bickford, RH, and Duff, RS: Influence of ultrasonic irradiation on temperature and blood flow in human skeletal muscle, *Circ Res* 1:534, 1953.

Billings, C, Draper, D, Schulthies, S: Ability of the Omnisound 3000 Delta T to reproduce predictable temperature increases in human muscle, *J Ath Train* 31 supp: S-47, 1996.

Bondolo, W: Phenylbutazone with ultrasonics in some cases of anbrosynovitis of the knee, *Archives of Orthopaedics* 73: 532–540, 1960.

Borrell, RM, Parker, R, and Henley, EJ: Comparison of in vitro temperatures produced by hydrotherapy paraffin wax treatment and fluidotherapy, *Phys Ther* 60:1273–1276, 1984.

Brueton, RN, Blookes, M, and Heatley, FW: The effect of ultrasound on the repair of a rabbit's tibial osteotomy held in rigid external fixation, *Journal of Bone and Joint Surgery* 69B:494, 1987.

Buchan, JF: Heat therapy and ultrasonics, *The Practitioner* 208:130–131, 1972.

Buchtala, V: The present state of ultrasonic therapy, *Br J Phys Med* 15:3, 1952.

Bundt, FB: Ultrasound therapy in supraspinatus bursitis, *Phys Ther Rev* 38:826, 1958.

Burns, PN, and Pitcher, EM: Calibration of physiotherapy ultrasound generators, *Clinical Physics and Physiological Measurement* 5:37 (abstract), 1984.

Byl, N: The use of ultrasound as an enhancer for transcutaneous drug delivery: phonophoresis, *Phys Ther* 75(6):539–553, 1995.

Callam, MJ, Harper, DR, Dale, JJ, Ruckley, CV, and Prescott, R: A controlled trial of weekly ultrasound therapy in chronic leg ulceration, *Lancet* 2(8552):204, 1987.

Cerino, LE, Ackerman, E, and Janes, JM: Effects of ultrasound on experimental bone tumor, *Surg Forum* 16:466, 1965.

Cherup, N, Urben, J, and Bender, LF: The treatment of plantar warts with ultrasound, *Arch Phys Med Rehab* 44:602, 1963.

Chan, AK, Siealmann, RA, and Guy, AW: Calculations of therapeutic heat generated by ultrasound in fat-muscle-bone layers, Institution of Electrical and Electronic Engineers Transactions on Biomedical Engineering, *BME*-2t. 280–284, 1973.

Cline, PD: Radiographic follow-up of ultrasound therapy in calcific bursitis, *Phys Ther* 43:16, 1963.

Coakley, WT: Biophysical effects of ultrasound at therapeutic intensities, *Physiotherapy* 94(6):168–169, 1978.

Conger, AD, Ziskin, MC, and Wittels, H: Ultrasonic effects on mammalian multicellular tumor spheroids, *Clin Ultrasound* 9:167, 1981.

Conner-Kerr, T, Franklin, M, and Smith, S: Efficacy of using phonophoresis for the delivery of dexamethasone to human transdermal tissues, *JOSPT* 23(1):79, 1996.

Costentino, AB, Cross, DL, Harrineton, RJ, and Sodarberg, GL: Ultrasound effects on electroneuromyographic measures in sensory fibers of the median nerve, *Physical Therapy* 63(11): 1788–1792, 1983.

Creates, V: A study of ultrasound treatment to the painful perineum after childbirth, *Physiotherapy* 73:162, 1987.

Crumley, M, Nowak, P, and Merrick, M: Do ultrasound, active warm-up and passive motion differ on their ability to cause temperature and range-of-motion changes? *Journal of Athletic Training* 36(2 supp): S-92, 2001.

Currier, DF, Greathouse, D, and Swift, T: Sensory nerve conduction: effect of ultrasound, *Arch Phys Med Rehabil* 59:181, 1978.

DeDeyne, P, and Kirsh-Volders, M: In vitro effects of therapeutic ultrasound on the nucleus of human fibroblasts, *Phys Ther* 75(7):629–634, 1995.

Dilorio, A, Frommelt, T, and Svendsen, L: Therapeutic ultrasound effect on regional temperature and blood flow, *J Ath Train* 31 supp:S-14, 1996.

Duarte, LR: The stimulation of bone growth by ultrasound, *Archives of Orthopaedics and Trauma in Surgery* 101:153–159, 1983.

Dyson, M: The production of blood cell stasis and endothelial damage in the blood vessels of chick embryos treated with ultrasound in a stationary wave field, *Ultrasound Med Biol* 11:133, 1974.

Dyson, M: The stimulation of tissue regeneration by means of ultrasound, *Clin Sci* 35:273, 1968.

Dyson, M, and Pond, JB: The effect of pulsed ultrasound on tissue regeneration, *Physiotherapy* 56(6):134–142, 1970.

Dyson, M, and Suckling, J: Stimulation of tissue repair by ultrasound: a survey of mechanisms involved, *Physiotherapy* 64:105, 1978.

Dyson, M, and Ter Haar, GR: *The response of smooth muscle to ultrasound (abstr)*. In Proceedings from an International Symposium on Therapeutic Ultrasound. Winnipeg, Manitoba, September 10, 1981.

Dyson, M, Woodward, B, and Pond, JB: Flow of red blood cells stopped by ultrasound, *Nature* 232:572–573, 1971.

Edwards, MI: Congenital defects in guinea pigs: prenatal retardation of brain growth of guinea pigs following hyperthermia during gestation, *Teratology* 2:329, 1969.

Enwemeka, CS: The effects of therapeutic ultrasound on tendon healing, *American Journal of Physical Medicine and Rehabilitation* 68(6):283–287, 1989.

Falconer, J, Hayes, KW, and Ghang, RW: Therapeutic ultrasound in the treatment of musculoskeletal conditions, *Arthritis Care and Research* 3(2):85–91, 1990.

Farmer, WC: Effect of intensity of ultrasound on conduction of motor axons, *Physical Therapy* 48:1233–1237, 1968.

Faul, ED, and Imig, CJ: Temperature and blood flow studies after ultrasonic irradiation, *Am J Phys Med* 34:370, 1955.

Fieldhouse, C: Ultrasound for relief of painful episiotomy scars, *Physiotherapy* 65:217, 1979.

Forrest, G, and Rosen, K: Ultrasound: effectiveness of treatments given under water, *Arch Phys Med Rehab* 70:28, 1989.

Fountain, FP, Gersten, JW, and Sengu, O: Decrease in muscle spasm produced by ultrasound, hot packs and IR, *Arch Phys Med Rehab* 41:293, 1960.

Franklin, M, Smith, S, and Chenier, T: Effect of phonophoresis with dexamethasone on adrenal function, *JOSPT* 22(3):103–107, 1995.

Friedar, S: A pilot study: the therapeutic effect of ultrasound following partial rupture of achilles tendons in male rats, *J Ortho Sports Phys Ther* 10:39, 1988.

Fyfe, MC: A study of the effects of different ultrasonic frequencies on experimental oedema, *Australian J Physiotherapy* 25(5):205–207, 1979.

Fyfe, MC, and Bullock, M: Acoustic output from therapeutic ultrasound units, *Australian J Physiotherapy* 32(1):13–16, 1986.

Fyfe, MC, and Chahl, LA: The effect of ultrasound on experimental oedema in rats, *Ultrasound Med Biol* 6:107, 1980.

Gantz, S: Increased radicular pain due to therapeutic ultrasound applied to the back, *Arch Phys Med Rehab* 70:493–494, 1989.

Garrett, AS, and Garrett, M: Letters: Ultrasound for herpes zoster pain, *Journal of the Royal College of General Practice* Nov, 709, 1982.

Gersten, JW: Effect of metallic objects on temperature rises produced in tissues by ultrasound, *Am J Phys Med* 37:75, 1958.

Goddard, DH, Revell, PA, and Cason, J: Ultrasound has no anti-inflammatory effect, *Annals of Rheumatic Diseases* 42: 582–584, 1983.

Gracewski, SM, Wagg, RC, and Schenk, EA: High-frequency attenuation measurements using an acoustic microscope, *J of Acoustic Society of America* 83(6):2405–2409, 1988.

Grant, A, Sleep, J, McIntosh, J, and Ashurst, H: Ultrasound and pulsed electromagnetic energy treatment for peroneal trauma: a randomized placebo-controlled trial, *British J of Obstetrics and Gynecology* 96:434–439, 1989.

Grieder, A, et al.: An evaluation of ultrasonic therapy for temporomandibular joint dysfunction, *Oral Surg* 31:25, 1971.

Griffin, JE: Patients treated with ultrasonic driven cortisone and with ultrasound alone, *Phys Ther* 47:594, 1967.

Griffin, JE: Transmissiveness of ultrasound through tap water, glycerin, and mineral oil, *Phys Ther* 60:1010, 1980.

Griffin, JE, and Touchstone, JC: Low intensity phonophoresis of cortisol in swine, *Physical Therapy* 48(10):1336–1344, 1968.

Griffin, JE, and Touchstone, JC: Ultrasonic movement of cortisol into pig tissue: 1. Movement into skeletal muscle, *American J Physical Medicine* 42:77–85, 1962.

Griffin, JE, Touchstone, JC, and Liu, A: Ultrasonic movement of cortisol into pig tissues: II. Peripheral Nerve, *Am J Phys Med* 44:20, 1965.

Halle, JS, Scoville, CR, and Greathouse, DG: Ultrasound's effect on the conduction latency of superficial radial nerve in man, *Phys Ther* 61:345, 1981.

Halle, JS, Franklin, RJ, and Karalfa, BL: Comparison of four treatment approaches for lateral epicondylitis of the elbow, *J Ortho Sports Phys Ther* 8:62, 1986.

Hamer, J, and Kirk, JA: Physiotherapy and the frozen shoulder: a comparative trial of ice and ultrasound therapy, *New Zealand Medical Journal* 83(3):191, 1976.

Hansen, TI, and Kristensen, JH: Effects of massage, shortwave and ultrasound upon 133Xe disappearance rate from muscle and subcutaneous tissue in the human calf, *Scandinavian J Rehabilitation Medicine* 5:197, 1973.

Harris, S, Draper, D, and Schulthies, S: The effect of ultrasound on temperature rise in preheated human muscle, *J Ath Train* 30 supp: S-42, 1995.

Hashish, I, Hai, HK, Harvey, W, Feinmann, C, and Harris, M: Reduction of post-operative pain and swelling by ultrasound treatment, a placebo effect, *Pain* 33:303–311, 1988.

Hayes, B, Sandrey, M, and Merrick, M: The differences between 1 MHz and 3 MHz ultrasound in heating of subcutaneous tissue, *Journal of Athletic Training* 36(2 supp): S-92, 2001.

Hekkenberg, RT, Oosterbaan, WA, and van Beekum, WT: Evaluation of ultrasound therapy devices, *Physiotherapy* 72:390, 1986.

Hill, CR, and Ter Haar, G: Ultrasound and non-ionizing radiation protection. In Suess, MJ, editor: *WHO Regional Publication*, European Series No. 10. World Health Organization, Copenhagen, 1981.

Hogan, RD, Burke, KM, and Franklin, TD: The effect of ultrasound on microvascular hemodynamics in skeletal muscle: effects during ischemia, *Microvasc Res* 23:370, 1982.

Holcomb, W, and Joyce C: A comparison of the effectiveness of two commonly used ultrasound units, *Journal of Athletic Training* 36(2 supp): S-89, 2001.

Hone, C-Z, Liu, HH, and Yu, J: Ultrasound thermotherapy effect on the recovery of nerve conduction in experimental compression neuropathy, *Archives of Physical Medicine and Rehabilitation* 69:410–414, 1988.

Hustler, JE, Zarod, AP, and Williams, AR: Ultrasonic modification of experimental bruising in the guinea-pig pinna, *Ultrasound* 16:223–228, 1978.

Imig, CJ, Randall, BF, and Hines, HM: Effect of ultrasonic energy on blood flow, *American Journal of Physical Medicine* 53:100–102, 1954.

Inaba, MK, and Piorkowski, M: Ultrasound in treatment of painful shoulder in patients with hemiplegia, *Phys Ther* 52:737, 1972.

Jones, RI: Treatment of acute herpes zoster using ultrasonic therapy, *Physiotherapy* 70:94, 1984.

Klemp, P, Staberg, B, Korsgard, J, Veilsen, HV, and Crone, P: Reduced blood flow in fibromyotic muscles during ultrasound therapy, *Scandinavian J Rehab Medicine* 15:21–23, 1982.

Kramer, JF: Sensory and motor nerve conduction velocities following therapeutic ultrasound, *Australian J Physiotherapy* 33(4):235–243, 1987.

Kramer, JF: Effects of therapeutic ultrasound intensity on subcutaneous tissue temperature and ulnar nerve conduction velocity, *American Journal of Physical Medicine* 64:9, 1985.

Kramer, JF: Effect of ultrasound intensity on sensory nerve conduction velocity, *Physiotherapy Canada* 37:5–10, 1985.

Kuitert, JH, and Harr, ET: Introduction to clinical application of ultrasound, *Phys Ther Rev* 35:19, 1955.

Kuitert, JH: Ultrasonic energy as an adjunct in the management of radiculitis and similar referred pain, *Am J Phys Med* 33:61, 1954.

LaBan, MM: Collagen tissue: Implications of its response to stress in vitro, *Arch Phys Med Rehab* 43:461, 1962.

Lehmann, JF: Heating produced by ultrasound in bone and soft tissue, *Arch Phys Med Rehab* 48:397, 1967.

Lehmann, JF: Heating of joint structures by ultrasound, *Arch Phys Med Rehab* 49:28, 1968.

Lehmann, JF: Therapeutic temperature distribution produced by ultrasound as modified by dosage and volume of tissue exposed, *Arch Phys Med Rehab* 48:662, 1967.

Lehmann, JF: Ultrasound effects as demonstrated in live pigs with surgical metallic implants, *Arch Phys Med Rehab* 40:483, 1959.

Lehmann, JF, and Biegler, R: Changes of potentials and temperature gradients in membranes caused by ultrasound, *Arch Phys Med Rehab* 35:287, 1954.

Lehmann, JF, Brunner, GD, and Stow, RW: Pain threshold measurements after therapeutic application of ultrasound, microwaves and infrared, *Arch Phys Med Rehab* 39:560, 1958.

Lehmann, JF, Erickson, DJ, and Martin, GM: Comparative study of the efficiency of shortwave, microwave and ultrasonic diathermy in heating the hip joint, *Arch Phys Med Rehab* 40:510, 1959.

Lehmann, JR, and Henrick, JF: Biologic reactions to cavitation: a consideration for ultrasonic therapy, *Arch Phys Med Rehabil* 34:86, 1953.

Lehmann, JF, Stonebridge, JB, De Lateur, BJ, Warren, CG, and Halar, E: Temperatures in human thighs after hot pack treatment followed by ultrasound, *Archives of Physical Medicine and Rehabilitation* 59:472–475, 1978.

Lehmann, JF, Warren, CC, and Scham, SM: Therapeutic heat and cold, *Clinical Orthopaedics* 99:207–245,1974.

Leonard, J, Merrick, M, and Ingersoll, C: A comparison of ultrasound intensities on a 10 minute 1.0 MHz ultrasound treatment, *Journal of Athletic Training* 36 (2 supp): S-91, 2001.

Levenson, JL, and Weissberg, MP: Ultrasound abuse: a case report, *Archives of Physical Medicine and Rehabilitation* 64:90–91, 1983.

Lloyd, JJ, and Evans, JA: A calibration survey of physiotherapy equipment in North Wales, *Physiotherapy* 74(2):56–61, 1988.

Lota, MI, and Darling, RC: Change in permeability of the red blood cell membrane in a homogeneous ultrasonic field, *Arch Phys Med Rehab* 36:282, 1955.

Lyons, ME, and Parker, KJ: Absorption and attenuation in soft tissues II—Experimental results, *Institution of Electrical and Electronic Engineers Transactions on Ultrasonics, Ferroelectrics and Frequency Control* 35:4, 1988.

Madsen, PW, and Gersten, JW: Effect of ultrasound on conduction velocity of peripheral nerves, *Archives of Physical Medicine and Rehabilitation* 42:645–649, 1963.

Massoth, A, Draper, D, and Kirkendall, D: A measure of superficial tissue temperature during 1 MHz ultrasound treatments delivered at three different intensity settings, *J Ath Train* 28(2):166, 1993.

Maxwell, L: Therapeutic ultrasound and the metastasis of a solid tumor, *J Sport Rehab* 4(4):273–281, 1995.

Maxwell, L: Therapeutic ultrasound: its effects on the cellular and molecular mechanisms of inflammation and repair, *Physiotherapy* 78(6):421–425, 1992.

McDiarmid, T, Burns, PN, and Lewith, GT: Ultrasound and the treatment of pressure sores, *Physiotherapy* 71:661, 1985.

McLaren, J: Randomized controlled trial of ultrasound therapy for the damaged perineum, *Clinical Physics and Physiological Measurement* 5:40 (abstract), 1984.

Michlovitz, SL, Lynch, PR, and Tuma, RF: Therapeutic ultrasound: its effects on vascular permeability (abstr), *Fed Proc* 41:1761, 1982.

Mickey, D, Bernier, J, and Perrin, D: Ice and ice with nonthermal ultrasound effects on delayed onset muscle soreness, *J Ath Train* 31 (supp):S-19, 1996.

Miller, DL: A review of the ultrasonic bioeffects of microsonation, gas body activation and related cavitation-like phenomena, *Ultrasound in Medicine and Biology* 13(8): 443–470, 1987.

Mortimer, AJ, and Dyson, M: The effect of therapeutic ultrasound on calcium uptake in fibroblasts, *Ultrasound in Medicine and Biology* 14:499–508, 1988.

Mummery, CL: *The effect of ultrasound on fibroblasts in vitro.* Dissertation, London University, 1978.

Myrer, W, Measom, G, and Fellingham, G: Intramuscular temperature rises with topical analgesics used as coupling agents during therapeutic ultrasound, *Journal of Athletic Training* 36(1): 20–26, 2001.

National Council on Radiation Protection and Measurements (NCRP) Report No. 74. Biological effects of ultrasound, *Mechanisms and clinical applications,* NCRP, Bethesda, Maryland,197, 1983.

Newman, MK, Kill, M, and Frampton, G: Effects of ultrasound alone and combined with hydrocortisone injections by needle or hydrospray, *Am J Phys Med* 37:206, 1958.

Novak, EJ: Experimental transmission of lidocaine through intact skin by ultrasound, *Arch Phys Med Rehab* 45:231, 1964.

Oakley, EM: Evidence for effectiveness of ultrasound treatment in physical medicine, *British J Cancer* 45(suppl V):233–237, 1982.

Olson, S, Bowman, J, and Condrey, K: Transdermal delivery of hydrocortisone, lidocaine, and menthol in subjects with delayed onset muscle soreness, *JOSPT* 19(1):69, 1994.

Paaske, WP, Hovind, H, and Seyerson, P: Influence of therapeutic ultrasonic irradiation on blood flow in human cutaneous, subcutaneous and muscular tissues, *Scand J Clin Lab Invest* 31:389.

Paul, B: Use of ultrasound in the treatment of pressure sores in patients with spinal cord injury, *Arch Phys Med Rehab* 41:438, 1960.

Payne, C: Ultrasound for post-herpetic neuralgia, *Physiotherapy* 70:96, 1984.

Penderghest, C, Kimura, I, and Sitler, M: Double blind clinical efficacy study of dexamethasone-lidocaine pulsed phonophoresis on perceived pain associated with symptomatic tendinitis, *J Ath Train* 31 supp (supp):S-47, 1996.

Pesek, J, Kane, E, and Perrin, D: I-Prep ultrasound gel and ultrasound does not effect local anesthesia, *Journal of Athletic Training* 36(2 supp): S-89, 2001.

Popspisilova, L, and Rottova, A: Ultrasonic effect on collagen synthesis and deposition in differently localized experimental granulomas, *Acta Chirurgica Plastica* 19:148–157, 1977.

Reid, DC: Possible contra-indications and precautions associated with ultrasound therapy. In Mortimer, A, and Lee, N, editors: *Proceedings of the International Symposium on Therapeutic Ultrasound,* Canadian Physiotherapy Association, Winnipeg, 1981.

Reynolds, NL: Reliable ultrasound transmission (letter), *Physical Therapy* 72(8):611, 1992.

Roberts, M, Rutherford, JH, and Harris, D: The effect of ultrasound on flexor tendon repairs in the rabbit, *Hand* 14:17, 1982.

Robinson, S, and Buono, M: Effect of continuous-wave ultrasound on blood flow in skeletal muscle, *Phys Ther* 75(2):145–150, 1995.

Roche, C, and West, J: A controlled trial investigating the effects of ultrasound on venous ulcers referred from general practitioners, *Physiotherapy* 70(12):475–477, 1984.

Rowe, RJ, and Gray, IM: Ultrasound treatment of plantar warts, *Arch Phys Med Rehab* 46:273, 1965.

Shambereer, RC, Talbot, TL, Tipton, HW, Thibault, LE, and Brennan, MF: The effect of ultrasonic and thermal treatment of wounds, *Plastic and Reconstructive Surgery* 68(6):880–870, 1981.

Sicard-Rosenbaum, L, Lord, D, and Danoff, J: Effects of continuous therapeutic ultrasound on growth and metastasis of subcutaneous murine tumors, *Phys Ther* 75(1):3–12, 1995.

Smith, W, Winn, F, and Farette, R: Comparative study using four modalities in shinsplint treatments, *J Ortho Sports Phys Ther* 8:77, 1986.

Sokoliu, A: Destructive effect of ultrasound on ocular tissues. In Reid, JM, and Sikov, MR, editors: *Interaction of ultrasound and biological tissues,* DHEW Pub (FDA) 73–8008, 1972.

Soren, A: Evaluation of ultrasound treatment in musculoskeletal disorders, *Physiotherapy* 61:214–217, 1965.

Soren, A: Nature and biophysical effects of ultrasound, *J Occup Med* 7:375, 1965.

Stevenson, JH: Functional, mechanical, and biochemical assessment of ultrasound therapy on tendon healing in chicken toe, *Plastic and Reconstructive Surgery* 77:965, 1986.

Stewart, HF: Survey of use and performance of ultrasonic therapy equipment in Pinelles County, *Physical Therapy* 54:707, 1974.

Stewart, HF, Abzug, JL, and Harris, GF: Considerations in ultrasound therapy and equipment performance, *Phys Ther* 80(4):424–428, 1980.

Stoller, DW, Markholf, KL, Zager, SA, and Shoemaker SC: The effects of exercise ice and ultrasonography on torsional laxity of the knee joint, *Clinical Orthopaedics and Related Research* 174:172–150, 1983.

Stratford, PW, Cevy, DR, Gauldie, S, Miseferi, D, and Levy, K: The evaluation of phonophoresis and friction massage as treatments for extensor carpi radialis tendinitis: A randomized controlled trial, *Physiotherapy Canada* 41:93, 1989.

Stratton, SA, Heckmann, R, and Francis, RS: Therapeutic ultrasound: Its effect on the integrity of a nonpenetrating wound, *J Ortho Spors Phys Ther* 5:278, 1984.

Talaat, AM, El-Dibany, MM, and El-Garf, A: Physical therapy in the management of myofascial pain dysfunction syndrome, *Am Otol Rhinol Laryngol* 95:225, 1986.

Taylor, E, and Humphry, R: Survey of physical agent modality use, *American J Occupational Ther* 46(10):924–931, 1991.

Ter Haar, G: Basic physics of therapeutic ultrasound, *Physiotherapy* 64(4):100–103, 1978.

Ter Haar, C, Dyson, M, and Oakley, EM: The use of ultrasound by physiotherapists in Britain, 1985, *Ultrasound in Medicine and Biology* 13:659, 1987.

Ter Haar, G, and Wyard, SJ: Blood cell banding in ultrasonic standing waves: a physical analysis, *Ultrasound in Medicine and Biology* 4:111–123, 1978.

Van Levieveld, DW: Evaluation of ultrasonics and electrical stimulation in the treatment of sprained ankles: a controlled study, *Ugesrk-Laeger* 141(16):1077–1080, 1979, 1973.

Ward, A, Robertson, V: Comparison of heating of nonliving soft tissue produced by 45 KHz and 1 MHz frequency ultrasound machines, *JOSPT* 23(4):258–266, 1996.

Warren, CG, Lehmann, JF, and Koblanski, N: Heat and stretch procedures: an evaluation using rat tail tendon, *Arch Phys Med Rehab* 57:122, 1976.

Warren, CG, Koblanski, IN, and Sigelmann, RA: Ultrasound coupling media: their relative transmissivity, *Arch Phys Med Rehab* 57:218, 1976.

Wells, PN: *Biomedical ultrasonics*, London, 1977, Academic Press.

Wells, PE, Frampton, V, and Bowsher, D, editors: *Pain: management and control in physiotherapy*, London, 1988, Heinemann.

Williams, AR, McHale, I, and Bowditch, M: Effects of MHz ultrasound on electrical pain threshold perception in humans, *Ultrasound in Medicine and Biology* 13:249, 1987.

Williamson, JB, George, TK, Simpson, DC, Hannah, B, and Bradbury, E: Ultrasound in the treatment of ankle sprains, *Injury* 17:76–178, 1986.

Wilson, AG, Jamieson, S, and Saunders, R: The physical behavior of ultrasound, *New Zealand J Physiotherapy*, 12(1):30–31, 1984.

Wood, RW, and Loomis, AL: The physical and biological effects of high frequency waves of great intensity, *Philosoph Mag* 4:417, 1927.

Wright, ET, and Haase, KH: Keloid and ultrasound, *Arch Phys Med Rehab* 52:280, 1971.

Wyper, DJ, McNiven, DR, and Donnelly, TJ: Therapeutic ultrasound and muscle blood flow, *Physiotherapy* 64:321, 1978.

Zankei, HT: Effects of physical agents on motor conduction velocity of the ulnar nerve, *Archives of Phys Med and Rehab* 47:787–792, 1966.

CHAPTER **6**

Shortwave and Microwave Diathermy

William E. Prentice, David O. Draper, and Phillip B. Donley

Study Resources

Refer to the lab exercises in the accompanying Laboratory Manual, as well as eSims which simulates the athletic training certification exam at www.mhhe.com/esims. Also, check out the competency information found at www.mhhe.com/prentice11e. For more online study resources, visit our Health and Human Performance Website at www.mhhe.com/hhp/.

Following completion of this chapter, the student athletic trainer will be able to

- Evaluate how the diathermy may best be used in a clinical setting.

- Explain the physiologic effects of diathermy.

- Differentiate between capacitance and induction shortwave diathermy techniques and identify the associated electrodes.

- Compare treatment techniques for continuous shortwave and pulsed shortwave diathermy.

- Demonstrate the equipment setup and treatment technique for microwave diathermy.

- Discuss the various clinical applications and indications for using continuous shortwave, pulsed shortwave, and microwave diathermy.

- Identify the treatment precautions for using the diathermies.

- List the major differences between microwave and shortwave diathermy.

- Analyze the rate of heating and how long muscle retains the heat generated from a shortwave diathermy treatment.

- Compare and contrast diathermy and ultrasound as deep-heating agents.

Diathermy is the application of high-frequency electromagnetic energy that is primarily used to generate heat in body tissues. Heat is produced by resistance of the tissue to the passage of the energy. Diathermy may also be used to produce nonthermal effects. Diathermy as a therapeutic agent may be classified as two distinct modalities: shortwave diathermy and microwave diathermy. Shortwave diathermy may be either continuous or pulsed. Continuous shortwave diathermy has been used in the treatment of a variety of sports-related injuries for some time. Recently, pulsed shortwave diathermy has received renewed interest, and research documents its clinical efficacy.[4,8,19]

---

diathermy   The application of high-frequency electrical energy that is used to generate heat in body tissues as a result of the resistance of the tissue to the passage of energy. It may also be used to produce nonthermal effects.

139

- Diathermy can have both thermal and nonthermal effects.

- SWD (shortwave diathermy) can be continuous or pulsed

For the past 15 to 20 years, diathermy has not been widely used, particularly by athletic trainers. It is likely that many young athletic trainers have never even seen a diathermy unit. However, over the last 3 to 5 years, there seems to be renewed interest in this treatment modality due in large part to some newly published research-based information that has begun to appear in the professional literature. In addition there appears to be renewed efforts by equipment manufacturers who are once again beginning to market pulsed shortwave diathermy units. Shortwave diathermy is a relatively safe modality that can be very effectively incorporated into clinic use.

The effectiveness of a shortwave or microwave diathermy treatment depends on the athletic trainer's ability to tailor the treatment to the athlete's needs. This requires that the athletic trainer have an accurate evaluation or diagnosis of the athlete's condition and knowledge of the heating patterns produced by various electrodes or applicators.

The depth of penetration is greater than with any of the infrared modalities, yet many athletic trainers feel that neither shortwave nor microwave diathermy produces heating at the depths desired for the treatment of musculoskeletal injuries. However, it has recently been determined that pulsed shortwave diathermy produces the same magnitude and depth of muscle heating as 1 MHz ultrasound.[8,9]

PHYSIOLOGIC RESPONSES TO DIATHERMY

Thermal Effects

The diathermies are not capable of producing depolarization and contraction of skeletal muscle since the wavelengths are much too short in duration.[6] Thus, the physiologic effects of continuous shortwave and microwave diathermy are primarily thermal, resulting from high-frequency vibration of molecules.

The primary benefits of diathermy are those of heat in general, such as tissue temperature rise, increased blood flow, dilation of the blood vessels, increased filtration and diffusion through the different membranes, increased tissue metabolic rate, changes in some enzyme reactions, alterations in the physical properties of fibrous tissues (such as those found in tendons, joints, and scars), decreased joint stiffness, a certain degree of muscle relaxation, a heightened pain threshold, and enhanced recovery from injury.[2,3,10, 11,17,24,25,35,46,47]

Diathermy treatment doses are not precisely controlled, and the amount of heating the athlete receives cannot be accurately prescribed or directly measured. Heating occurs in proportion to the square of the current density and in direct proportion to the resistance of the tissue.

$$\text{heating} = \text{current density}^2 \times \text{resistance}$$

Lehmann[26] stated that temperature increases of 1° C can reduce mild inflammation and increase metabolism and that moderate heating—an increase of 2 to 3° C—will decrease pain and muscle spasm. Increasing tissue temperatures more than 3 to 4° C above baseline will increase tissue extensibility, thus enabling the clinician to treat chronic connective tissue problems.[26]

There are differing opinions regarding the desired temperature increases needed to enhance extensibility of collagen. Some[2] believe that optimal heating occurs when the tissue temperature rises above 38 to 40° C, while others believe that a tissue temperature increase of 3 to 4° C above baseline temperature is optimal.[1,20,26] Presently, no research can validate one opinion over another, but it is clear that the more vigorous the heating with diathermy, the greater chance there is for collagen elongation to occur.

Why certain pathologic conditions respond better to diathermy than other forms of deep heat is not well understood or documented. It probably is more directly related either to the skill of the clinician applying the modality or to some placebo effects associated with tissue temperature increase than it is to the specific effects of diathermy itself.

Nonthermal Effects

Pulsed shortwave diathermy has also been used for its nonthermal effects in the treatment of soft-tissue injuries and wounds that frequently occur in sports medicine.[21] The mechanism of its effectiveness has been theorized to occur at the cellular level, relating specifically to cell membrane potential.[22] Damaged cells undergo depolarization resulting in cell dysfunction which might include loss of cell division and proliferation and loss of regenerative capabilities. Pulsed shortwave diathermy has been said to repolarize damaged cells, thus correcting cell dysfunction.[33]

It has also been suggested that sodium tends to accumulate in the cell due to a decrease in activity of the sodium pump during the inflammatory process, creating a negatively charged environment. When a **magnetic field** is induced, the sodium pump is reactivated, thus allowing the cell to regain normal ionic balance.[40]

SHORTWAVE DIATHERMY

A shortwave diathermy unit is essentially a radio transmitter. The **Federal Communications Commission (FCC)** assigned three frequencies to shortwave diathermy units: the first is 27.12 MHz with a wavelength of 11 meters; the second is 13.56 MHz with a wavelength of 22 meters; and the third, although rarely used, is 40.68 MHz with a wavelength of 7.5 meters (see Figure 1-2).

magnetic field Created when current is passed through a coiled cable affecting surrounding tissues by inducing localized secondary currents, called eddy currents, within the tissues.

Federal Communications Commission (FCC) Federal agency charged with assigning frequencies for all radio transmitters, including diathermies.

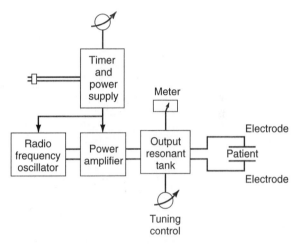

Figure 6-1 The component parts of a shortwave diathermy unit.

Shortwave Diathermy Generators

The shortwave diathermy unit consists of a power supply that provides power to a radio frequency oscillator (Figure 6-1). This radio frequency oscillator provides stable, drift-free oscillations at the required frequency. The power amplifier generates the power required to drive the different types of electrodes. The output resonant tank tunes in the athlete as part of the circuit and allows maximum power to be transferred to the athlete.

Figure 6-2 shows the control panel of a shortwave diathermy unit. The output intensity knob controls the percentage of maximum power transferred to the patient circuit. The tuning control adjusts the output circuit for maximum energy transfer

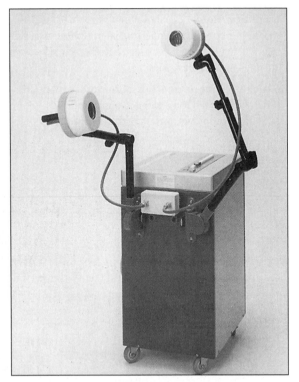

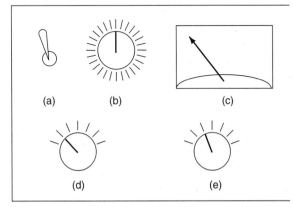

Figure 6-2 (top) Shortwave diathermy unit. (bottom) Control panel of a shortwave diathermy unit. (a) Power switch, (b) timer, (c) output power meter (monitors current drawn from power supply only and not in athlete circuit), (d) output intensity (controls the percentage of maximum power transferred to the athlete), (e) tuning control (tunes the output circuit for maximum energy transfer from radio frequency oscillator).

from the radio frequency oscillator. The power output meter monitors only the current that is drawn from the power supply and not the energy being delivered to the athlete. Thus, it is only an indirect measure of the energy reaching the patient.

The power output of a shortwave diathermy unit should produce sufficient energy to raise the tissue temperature into a therapeutic range. The **specific absorption rate (SAR)** represents the rate of energy absorbed per unit area of tissue mass. Most shortwave units have a power output of between 80 and 120 watts.

Some units are not capable of this level of power output, making them safe but ineffective. It is important to remember that the tissue temperature rise with diathermy units can be offset dramat-

specific absorption rate (SAR) Represents the rate of energy absorbed per unit area of tissue mass.

ically by an increase in blood flow, which has a cooling effect in the tissue being energized. Therefore, units should be able to generate enough power to provide for an excess of the SAR.

The patient's sensation provides the basis for recommendations of continuous shortwave diathermy dosage and thus varies considerably with different athletes.[27,40] The following dosage guidelines have been recommended:

Dose I (lowest): No sensation of heat
Dose II (low): Mild heating sensation

Dose III (medium): Moderate (pleasant) heating sensation

Dose IV (heavy): Vigorous heating which is tolerable below the pain threshold

Some older shortwave diathermy units have manual tuning, although the majority of newer models do have an automatic tuning device. If the machine is not an automatically tuning type, it is necessary to tune the athlete's circuit to resonance with the oscillating circuit of the unit. This is accomplished by placing the electrodes over the area to be treated and then setting the output intensity at 30% to 40%. Then the variable capacitor in the generator's circuitry can be adjusted by using the meter on the generator to determine the peak tuning readings. These readings should not be confused as an indication of the power received by the athlete. The tuning control should be adjusted down to patient tolerance, which is usually about 50% of maximum output. If more than 50% of the available power on the meter is used, then the athlete's setup is out of tune or out of resonance. Shortwave diathermy units with automatic tuning turn off the power when the patient circuit is out of tune.

A shortwave diathermy unit that generates a high-frequency electrical current will produce both an electrical field and a magnetic field in the tissues.[12] The ratio of the electrical field to the magnetic field depends on the characteristics of the different generators as well as on the characteristics of the electrodes or applicators. Shortwave units with a frequency of 13.56 MHz tend to produce a stronger magnetic field than does the frequency of 27.12 MHz, which produces a stronger electric field. The majority of the new pulsed shortwave diathermy units use a drum electrode and produce a stronger magnetic field.

Shortwave Diathermy Electrodes

Shortwave diathermy may be delivered to the athlete via either capacitance or induction techniques. Each of these techniques can effect different biologic tissues, and selection of the appropriate electrodes is essential for effective treatment.

■ **Analogy** *6-1*

A shortware diathermy generator functions much like a radio. The output intensity knob controls the percentage of maximum power transferred to the patient circuit. This is similar to the volume control on a radio. The tuning control adjusts the output circuit for maximum energy transfer from the radio frequency oscillator, which is similar to tuning in a station on a radio.

capacitor electrodes   Air space plates or pad electrode that creates a stronger electrical field than a magnetic field.

electrical field   The lines of force exerted on charged ions in the tissues by the electrodes that cause charged particles to move from one pole to the other.

The shortwave diathermy uses several types of applicators or electrodes, including air space plates, pad electrodes, cable electrodes, or drum electrodes.

Capacitor Electrodes.   The capacitance technique, using **capacitor electrodes,** creates a stronger electrical field than a magnetic field. As discussed in detail in Chapter 9, there are many free ions within the body that are positively or negatively charged. A positively charged electrode or plate will repel positively charged ions and attract negatively charged ions. Conversely, the negative electrode will repel negative ions and attract positive ions (Figure 6-3).

An **electrical field** is essentially the lines of force exerted on these charged ions by the electrodes, which causes charged particles to move from one pole to the other (Figure 6-4). The intensity of the electrical field is determined by the spacing of the electrodes and is greatest when they are close together. The center of this electrical field has a higher current density than regions at the periphery. When using capacitance electrodes, the athlete is placed between two electrodes or plates and becomes part of the circuit. Thus, the tissue between

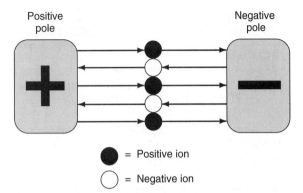

Positive pole   Negative pole

● = Positive ion

○ = Negative ion

Figure 6-3 A positively charged electrode or plate will repel positively charged ions and attract negatively charged ions. Conversely, the negative electrode will repel negative ions and attract positive ions.

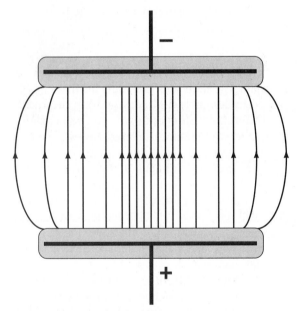

Figure 6-4 An electrical field is essentially the lines of force exerted on these charged ions by the electrodes, which causes charged particles to move from one pole to the other.

(Modified from Michlovitz, S: *Thermal agents in rehabilitation,* Philadelphia, 1990, FA Davis.)

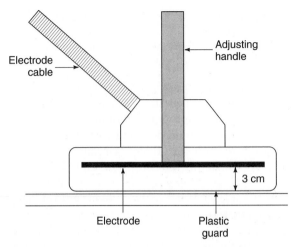

Electrode cable   Adjusting handle

3 cm

Electrode   Plastic guard

Figure 6-5 Air space plate electrodes consist of a metal plate enclosed in a glass or plastic plate guard. The metal plate may be adjusted approximately 3 cm within the plate guard, thus changing the distance from the skin.

> • Capacitor electrodes = strong electrical field

the two electrodes is in a series circuit arrangement (see Chapter 7).

As the electrical field is created in the biologic tissues, the tissue that offers the greatest resistance to current flow tends to develop the most heat. Tissues that have a high fat content tend to insulate and resist the passage of an electrical field. These tissues, particularly subcutaneous fat, tend to overheat when an electrical field is used, which is characteristic of a capacitance type of electrode application.

Air space plates. **Air space plates** are an example of a capacitance (strong electrical field) technique or a capacitor electrode. This type of electrode consists of two metal plates with a diameter of 7.5 to 17.5 cm surrounded by a glass or plastic plate guard. The metal plates may be adjusted approximately 3 cm within the plate guard, thus changing the distance from the skin[22] (Figure 6-5). Air space

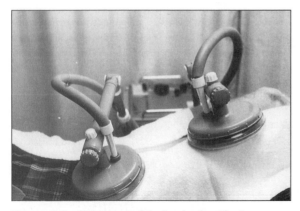

Figure 6-6 Treatment of the low back with air space plates. The athlete is in a series setup.

---

air space plate A capacitor-type electrode in which the plates are separated from the skin by the space in a glass case; used with shortwave diathermy.

pad electrodes Capacitor-type electrode used with shortwave diathermy to create an electrical field.

---

plates produce high-frequency oscillating current that is passed through each plate millions of times per second. When one plate is overloaded, it discharges to the other plate of the lower potential, and this is reversed millions of times per second.[15]

When air space plates are used, the area to be treated is placed between the electrode and becomes part of the external circuit (Figure 6-6). The sensation of heat tends to be in direct proportion to the distance of the plate from the skin. The closer the plate is to the skin, the better the energy transmission because there will be less reflection of the energy. However, it should be remembered that the closer plate will also generate more surface heat in the skin and the subcutaneous fat in that area (Figure 6-7). The greatest surface heat will be under the electrodes. Parts of the body that are low in subcutaneous fat content (e.g., hands, feet, wrists, and ankles) are best treated by this method. Athletes who have a very low subcutaneous fat content can be effectively treated in other body areas.[14] This technique is also very effective for treating the spine and the ribs.

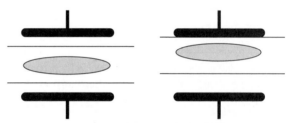

Figure 6-7 As the plate moves closer to the surface of the skin, the electrical field shifts, generating more surface heat in the skin and in the subcutaneous fat.

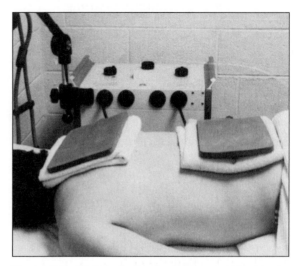

Figure 6-8 Pad electrodes showing correct placement and spacing.

Capacitor electrodes

- Air space plates
- pad electrodes

Pad electrodes. **Pad electrodes** are seldom used in the clinical setting; however, they may be available for some units. They are true capacitor electrodes, and they must have uniform contact pressure on the body part if they are to be effective in producing deep heat as well as in preventing skin burns (Figure 6-8). The athlete is part of the external circuit. Several layers of toweling are necessary to make sure that there is sufficient spacing between

■ **Clinical Decision-Making** *Exercise 6-1*

An athletic trainer is using pad electrodes to treat an athlete who has muscle guarding in the low back. What can be done with these electrodes to increase the depth of penetration without increasing output intensity?

• Induction electrodes = strong magnetic field

the skin and the pads. The pads should be separated such that they are at least as far apart as the cross-sectional diameter of the pads. In other words, if the pads are 15 cm across, then there should be at least 15 cm between the pads. The closer the spacing of the pads, the higher the current density in the superficial tissues. Increasing the spacing between the pads will increase the depth of penetration in the tissues (Figure 6-9). The part of the body to be treated should be centered between the pads.[13,15,18,25]

Induction Electrodes. The inductance technique using **induction electrodes** creates a stronger magnetic field than an electrical field. When the induction technique is used in shortwave diathermy, a cable or coil is either wrapped circumferentially around an extremity or it is coiled within an electrode. In either case, when current is passed through a coiled cable, a magnetic field is generated that can affect surrounding tissues by inducing localized secondary currents, called **eddy currents**, within the tissues[22] (Figure 6-10). Eddy currents are small circular electrical fields, and the intermolecular oscillation (vibration) of tissue contents causes heat generation.

In the induction technique, the athlete is in a magnetic field and is not part of the circuit. The tissues are in a parallel circuit (see Chapter 7); thus, the greatest current flow is through the tissues

induction electrodes Cable electrodes or drum electrodes that create a stronger magnetic field than electrical field.

eddy currents Small circular electrical fields induced when a magnetic field is created that result in intermolecular oscillation (vibration) of tissue contents causing heat generation.

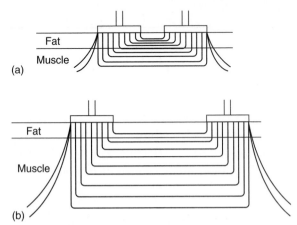

Figure 6-9 Pad electrodes should be separated by at least the diameter of the electrodes. (a) Electrodes placed close together produce more superficial heating. (b) As spacing increases, the current density increases in the deeper tissues.

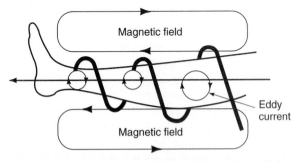

Figure 6-10 When current is passed through a coiled cable, a magnetic field is generated which can affect surrounding tissues by inducing localized secondary currents, called eddy currents, within the tissues. (Modified from Michlovitz, S: *Thermal agents in rehabilitation*, Philadelphia, 1990, FA Davis.)

■ Analogy 6-2

Eddy currents that are produced in a magnetic field are similar to eddy currents that occur in turbulent water, such as in rapids in a river. As the water flows over a rock, it produces a swirling effect so that the water flows backwards toward the rock. If you become trapped in one of these when whitewater rafting, it takes considerable effort to free the raft because of the power or energy that is being created by the swirling water.

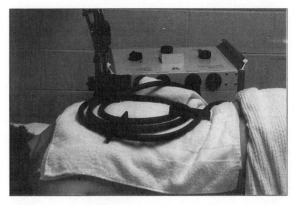

Figure 6-11 Pancake cable electrode.

with least resistance. When a magnetic field is used with an induction-type set up, the fat does not provide nearly as much resistance to the flow of the energy.

Therefore, tissues that are high in electrolytic content (i.e., muscle and blood) respond best to the magnetic field by producing heat. It is important to remember that if the energy is due primarily to generation of a magnetic field, heating may not be as obvious to the athlete because the magnetic field will not provide nearly as much sensation of warmth in the skin as an electrical field.

Cable electrodes. The **cable electrode** is an induction electrode that produces a magnetic field (Figure 6-11). There are two basic types of arrangements: the pancake coil and the wraparound coil. If a pancake coil is used, the size of the smaller circle should be greater than 6 inches in diameter. In either arrangement, there should be at least 1 cm of toweling between the cable and the skin. Stiff spacers should be used to keep the coils or the turns of the pancake or the wraparound coil between 5 and 10 cm between turns of the cable, thus providing spacing consistency. Both the pancake coils and the wraparound coils often provide more even heating because they both are more able to follow the contours of the skin than are the drum or the air space plates. It is important that the cables not touch each other because they will short out and cause excessive heat buildup. Diathermy units that operate on a frequency of 13.56 MHz are probably best suited to cable electrode-type applications. This is

cable electrodes An inductance-type electrode in which the electrodes are coiled around a body part, creating an electromagnetic field.

drum electrodes Induction electrodes that produce a strong magnetic field. Primarily used with pulsed shortwave diathermy.

primarily because the lower frequency provides better production of a magnetic field.[14]

Drum electrodes. The **drum electrode** also produces a magnetic field. The drum electrode is made up of one or more monoplaner coils that are rigidly fixed inside some kind of housing (Figure 6-12). If a small area is to be treated, particularly a small flat area, then a one-drum set up is fine. However, if the area is contoured, then two or more drums, which may be on a hinged apparatus or hinged arm, may be more suitable.

Penetration into the tissues tends to be on the order of 2 to 3 cm if the skin is no more than 1 to 2 cm away from the drum.[5] The magnetic field may be significant up to 5 cm away from the drum. A light towel must be kept in contact with the skin and between the drum and the skin. The towel is used to absorb moisture because an accumulation of water droplets would tend to overheat and cause hot spots on the surface. If there is

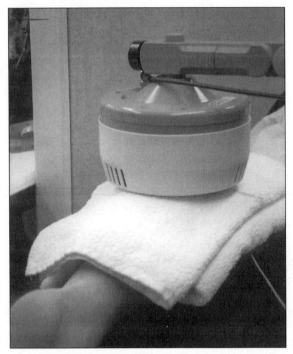

Figure 6-12 Drum electrode.

Induction electrodes

- Cable electrodes
- Drum electrodes

more than 2 cm of fat, there probably will be no great tissue temperature rise under the fat with a drum setup. The maximum penetration of short-wave diathermy with a drum electrode is 3 cm, provided there is no more than 2 cm of fat beneath the skin. For best absorption of energy, the housing of the drum should be in contact with the towel that is covering the skin.[14]

Pulsed Shortwave Diathermy

Pulsed shortwave diathermy, referred to in the literature as *pulsed electromagnetic energy (PEME)*, *pulsed electromagnetic field (PEMF)*, or *pulsed electromagnetic energy treatment (PEMET)*, is also a rela-

pulsed shortwave diathermy Created by simply interrupting the output of continuous shortwave diathermy at consistent intervals; it is used primarily for nonthermal effects.

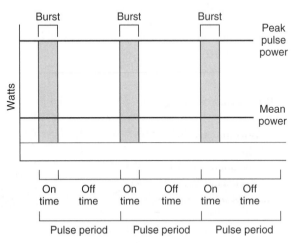

Figure 6-13 Pulsed diathermy is created by simply interrupting the output of continuous shortwave diathermy at consistent intervals.

tively new form of diathermy.[19] Pulsed diathermy is created by simply interrupting the output of continuous shortwave diathermy at consistent intervals (Figure 6-13). Energy is delivered to the athlete in a series of high-frequency bursts or pulse trains. Pulse duration is short, ranging from 20 to 400 microseconds, with an intensity of up to 1000 watts per pulse. The interpulse interval or off time depends on the pulse repetition rate, which ranges between 1 and 7000 Hz. The pulse repetition rate may be selected using the pulse-frequency control on the generator control panel.[22] Generally the off time is considerably longer than the on time. Therefore, even though the power output during the on time is sufficient to produce tissue heating, the long off-time interval allows the heat to dissipate. This reduces the likelihood of any significant tissue temperature increase and reduces the athlete's perception of heat.

Pulsed diathermy is claimed to have therapeutic value and to produce nonthermal effects with minimal thermal physiologic effects, depending on the intensity of the application. But pulsed shortwave diathermy can also have thermal effects.[37] When pulsed diathermy is used in intensities that create an increase in tissue temperature, its effects are no different from those of continuous shortwave diathermy. Successful treatments have largely resulted from the application of higher intensities and longer treatment times. Studies that use pulsed shortwave diathermy do not normally compare it with continuous shortwave diathermy but rather with a control group that has received no heat treatment.[25]

With pulsed shortwave diathermy, mean power provides a measure of heat production. Mean power may be calculated by dividing peak pulse power by the pulse repetition frequency to determine the pulse period (on time plus off time).

$$\text{pulse period} = \frac{\text{peak pulse power (watts)}}{\text{pulse repetition frequency (Hz)}}$$

The percentage on time is calculated by dividing the pulse duration by pulse period.

$$\text{percentage on time} = \frac{\text{pulse duration (milliseconds)}}{\text{pulse period (milliseconds)}}$$

The mean power is then determined by dividing the peak pulse power by the percentage on time.

$$\text{mean power} = \frac{\text{peak pulse power (watts)}}{\text{percentage on time}}$$

With pulsed shortwave diathermy, the highest mean power output is usually lower than the power delivered with continuous shortwave diathermy.

Generators that deliver pulsed shortwave diathermy typically use a drum type of electrode (Figure 6-14). As with continuous shortwave diathermy, the drum electrode is made of a coil wrapped in a flat circular spiral pattern and housed within a plastic case. The energy is induced in the treatment area via the production of a magnetic field.

■ **Clinical Decision-Making**   *Exercise 6-2*

A swimmer is complaining of an aching pain and tightness in the shoulder. In this case the athletic trainer decides that heating the joint with pulsed shortwave diathermy rather than ultrasound would be the best treatment choice. What are the potential advantages of using diathermy in this particular situation?

Pulsed shortwave diathermy

- Pulsed electromagnetic energy (PEME)
- Pulsed electromagnetic field (PEMF)
- Pulsed electromagnetic energy treatment (PEMET)

- Pulsed shortwave diathermy = nonthermal effects
- Pulsed shortwave diathermy uses drum electrodes

Treatment Time

Treatments lasting only 15 minutes have produced vigorous heating of the triceps surae muscle of humans.[8] A 20- to 30-minute treatment for one body area is probably all that is necessary to reach maximum physiologic effects.[14] The physiologic effects, particularly circulatory, seem to last about 30 minutes.

Treatments in excess of 30 minutes may create a circulatory rebound phenomenon in which the digital temperature may drop after the treatment because of reflex vasoconstriction. If an athletic trainer finds that a diathermy unit has been left on in excess of 30 minutes, it would be wise to check the temperature of the toes or the fingers, depending on which extremity has been treated. It was observed that pulsed shortwave diathermy administered to the

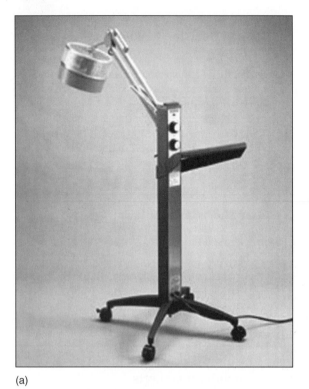

(a)

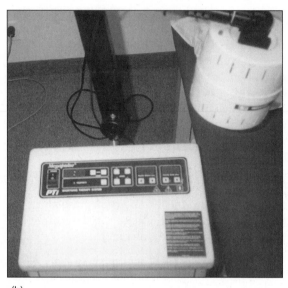

(b)

Figure 6-14 (a) The Magnatherm and (b) the Megapulse are examples of generators capable of producing pulsed shortwave diathermy. Energy is delivered to the athlete through a drum electrode.
(a, Courtesy of International Medical Electronics; b, Courtesy Physiotechnology, Inc.)

■ **Clinical Decision-Making** *Exercise 6-3*

The athletic trainer is treating a low back strain in a gymnast. What type of shortwave diathermy electrode would be the most appropriate choice when treating an area without a great deal of subcutaneous fat?

triceps surae resulted in peak heating at only 15 minutes into the treatment, and the temperature actually dropped 0.3° C from the 15 to 20 minute mark.[8] Perhaps this can be explained by the increase in blood flow created by the thermal effects of diathermy. The increase in temperature and blood flow engages the body's natural cooling mecha-

nism. Therefore, it may be more difficult to heat muscle tissue than the less vascular tendinous tissue. Perhaps tissue temperatures as high as 45° C, as postulated by other researchers, are too high for the body to tolerate.[8]

It is important to remember that as skin temperature goes up, impedance goes down. Therefore, the unit may need to be returned after 5 to 10 minutes of treatment.

MICROWAVE DIATHERMY

Microwave diathermy has two FCC-assigned frequencies in this country, 2456 MHz and 915 MHz. Microwave has a much higher frequency and a shorter wavelength than shortwave diathermy. Microwave diathermy units generate a strong electrical field and relatively little magnetic field.

intermolecular vibration   Movement between molecules that produces friction and thus heat.

applicator   The electrode used to transfer energy in microwave diathermy.

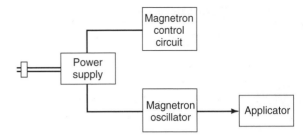

Figure 6-15   Component parts of a microwave diathermy unit.

With appropriate setup of the microwave diathermy unit, less than 10% of the energy is lost from the machine as it is applied to the athlete. The microwave applicator beams energy toward the athlete, creating the potential for much of the energy to be reflected. Heating is caused by the **intermolecular vibration** of molecules that are high in polarity.[20] If subcutaneous fat is greater than 1 cm, the fat temperature will rise to a level that is too uncomfortable before there is a tissue temperature rise in the deeper tissues.[15] This is less of a problem if the microwave diathermy is of the frequency of 915 MHz. However, there are very few commercial units operating on that frequency. Almost all of the older units have the higher frequency of 2456 MHz. If the subcutaneous fat is 0.5 cm or less, microwave diathermy can penetrate and cause a tissue temperature rise up to 5 cm deep in the tissue. Bone tends to absorb more shortwave and microwave energy than any type of soft tissue.

Microwave Diathermy Generators

The microwave diathermy generator consists of a power supply that energizes the magnetron and timing circuitry. The magnetron control regulates output power by varying the magnetron operating voltage. The magnetron oscillator uses a magnetic field to produce high-frequency currents (Figure 6-15).

Figure 6-16 represents the control panel of a microwave unit. The power output can be adjusted to athlete tolerance. The output meter indicates the relative output in watts or the amount of transmitted and unabsorbed energy. There are two indicator lamps: the amber lamp indicates

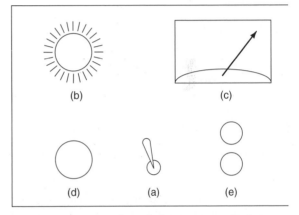

Figure 6-16   Control panel of a microwave diathermy unit. (a) Power switch. (b) Timer. (c) Output meter (indicates relative output in watts of transmitted energy). (d) Power output level. (e) Indicator lamps—amber: standby, magnetron accelerating, red: microwaves available for output.

that the machine is still warming up, and the red lamp indicates that the machine is ready to output energy.

Microwave Diathermy Applicators

Electrodes for microwave diathermy are called **applicators**. The microwave energy can only be beamed to one surface at a time. The contour of that surface must be very flat; otherwise there will be considerable reflection of the energy.

Those microwave diathermy units operating on the frequency 2456 MHz will have a specified air

Microwave diathermy applicators

- Circular
- Rectangular

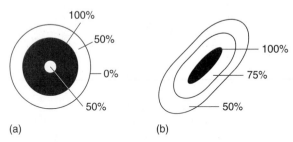

(a)   (b)

Figure 6-17 (a) Circular-shaped microwave electrode.
(b) Rectangular-shaped microwave electrode.

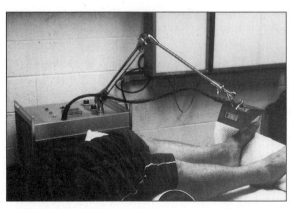

Figure 6-18 Typical microwave diathermy unit with rectangular applicator.

space required between the applicator and the skin. The manufacturer-suggested distances and power output should be followed closely. A directional antenna is attached to the applicator perpendicular to the face of the applicator to assure that spacing is correct and that the energy generated from the microwave unit is striking the target treatment area at the correct angle (cosine law). Units that operate on the higher frequency may have one or more applicators of various shapes and configurations.

There are two types of applicators that may be used with microwave diathermy: circular shaped and rectangular shaped. The circular-shaped applicators are either 4 or 6 inches in diameter. With circular-shaped electrodes, the maximum temperature is produced at the periphery of each radiation field (Figure 6-17a).

Rectangular-shaped applicators are either $41/2 \times 5$ inches or 5×21 inches and produce the maximum temperature at the center of the radiation field (Figure 6-17b).

In units that have a frequency of 915 MHz, the applicators are placed at a distance of 1 cm from the skin, and the air space between the antenna and the skin is built into the applicator, thus minimizing energy reflection.[25]

■ Analogy 6-3

Appropriate positioning of an applicator on a microwave diathermy unit is critical to ensure maximum absorption of energy in the treatment area. The energy should strike the surface at 90°. This is like being in the sun at the beach. At noon the sun is straight overhead and most of the energy will be absorbed by the skin. At 6 P.M. the sun is low, and a large portion of the energy will be reflected rather than absorbed.

Microwave Treatment Technique

Microwave diathermy units require a period of time to warm up. This is normally built into the circuitry so that the unit power cannot be turned on until the unit is sufficiently warmed. This warm-up time is a good time for the athletic trainer to position both the director and the athlete (Figure 6-18). The director should be located so that the maximum amount of energy will be penetrating at a right angle or perpendicular to the skin. Any angle greater or less than perpendicular will create reflection of the energy and significant loss of absorption (cosine law). Microwave diathermy is best used to treat conditions that exist in those areas of the body that are covered with low subcutaneous fat content. The tendons of the foot, hand, and wrist are well treated, as are the acromioclavicular and sternoclavicular joints, the patellar tendon, the distal tendons of the hamstrings, the Achilles tendon, and the costochondral joints and sacroiliac joints in lean individuals.

In review, there are some distinct differences between shortwave and microwave diathermy. Some of the major differences are as follows:

1. Microwave diathermy produces an electrical field that generates heat due to dipole response within the cell membrane. Most of the new shortwave diathermy generators produce magnetic fields.

2. Microwave diathermy does not penetrate as deep as shortwave diathermy.

3. Microwave diathermy cannot penetrate the fat layer as well as short wave diathermy (energy is collected by adipose tissue, rendering the effects at about one-third the depth of short wave diathermy).

4. No metal should be within 4 feet of microwave diathermy since it will interfere with the signal.

5. Spacing is required between the skin and applicator with microwave diathermy, whereas the applicator on a shortwave unit can be placed in contact with the treatment area.

6. It appears that shortwave diathermy is much safer than microwave diathermy.

CLINICAL APPLICATIONS FOR DIATHERMY

For the most part, the clinical applications for the diathermies are similar to those of other physical agents that are capable of producing thermal effects resulting in a tissue temperature increase.[41]

In addition to the diathermies, the infrared modalities discussed in Chapter 4 and ultrasound discussed in Chapter 5 are commonly used as heating modalities. As with pulsed shortwave diathermy, there have been nonthermal effects documented with microwave diathermy; however, there does not appear to be any evidence that these nonthermal effects have any significant role in the medical application of microwave diathermy.[16,27]

The diathermies have been used in the treatment of a variety of musculoskeletal conditions, including muscle strains, contusions, ligament sprains, tendinitis, tenosynovitis, bursitis, joint contractures, myofascial trigger points, and osteoarthritis.[34] Continuous shortwave and microwave diathermy are most often used for a variety of thermal effects, including inducing local relaxation by decreasing muscle guarding and pain,[25] selectively heating joint structures for the purpose of improving joint range of motion by decreasing stiffness and increasing the extensibility of the collagen fibers and the resilience of contracted soft tissues,[22,36] increasing circulation and improving blood flow to an injured area for the purpose of facilitating resolution of hemorrhage and edema as well as removal of the by-products of the inflammatory process,[25] and reducing both subacute and chronic pain.[31]

The majority of recent clinical studies relative to diathermy have focused primarily on the efficacy of pulsed shortwave diathermy in facilitating tissue healing, and to date results have been at best inconclusive.[32] Various claims have been made as to the specific mechanisms that facilitate healing, including an increase in the number and activity of the cells in the area, reduced swelling and inflammation, resorption of hematoma, increased rate of collagen deposition and organization, and increased nerve growth and repair. These claims are based on a limited number of clinical studies and even fewer experimental studies.[21]

There are a number of conditions that may potentially occur in a clinical setting that would make diathermy the treatment of choice:

1. If for any reason the skin or some underlying soft tissue is very tender and will not

tolerate the loading of a moist heat pack, or pressure from an ultrasound transducer, then diathermy should be used.

2. Both continuous shortwave and microwave diathermy are more capable of increasing temperatures to a greater tissue depth than any of the infrared modalities.

3. When the treatment goal is to increase tissue temperatures in a large area (i.e., throughout the entire shoulder girdle or in the low back region), the diathermies should be used.

4. In areas where subcutaneous fat is thick and deep heating is required, the induction technique using either cable or drum electrodes should be used to minimize heating of the subcutaneous fat layer. Both the capacitance technique with shortwave diathermy and microwave diathermy are more likely to selectively heat more superficial subcutaneous fat.

5. The athletic trainer should never underestimate the placebo effects that a treatment with any large machine may be capable of producing.

Athletic trainers should take the opportunity to examine several different types of diathermy units as well as the different applicators available with each unit. They should not only practice using the different applicators on healthy tissue, but they should also experience the sensation themselves. In particular, they should recognize or experience the difference between the energy flow with an induction-type application as opposed to the capacitor-type application.

DIATHERMY TREATMENT CONSIDERATIONS

There are probably more treatment precautions and contraindications for the use of shortwave— and especially microwave—diathermy than for any of the other physical agents used in a sports medicine setting.

A survey of more than 42,000 physical therapists found a modest increase in the risk of miscarriage of pregnant athletic trainers who were regularly exposed to microwave diathermy.[19] Regular exposure to shortwave diathermy during pregnancy, however, did not increase the risk of miscarriage. There are basic differences between microwave and shortwave diathermy, which could explain the difference in miscarriage risk. Shortwave diathermy uses high-frequency currents generated at 27.12 MHz and is applied using either a capacitive or inductive applicator, sometimes requiring the athlete to become part of the circuit. Microwave diathermy, however, uses higher frequencies of 2,450 MHz, and electromagnetic waves are beamed or transmitted into the body by a reflector.

Microwave diathermy does not require close contact between the applicator and the athletic trainer, allowing some stray emissions.[19] Until further research in this area is performed, it is suggested that the pregnant athletic trainer who treats athletes with microwave diathermy first set up the microwave application and then leave the immediate area until the treatment is completed. At this time, however, there is no known risk of miscarriage by pregnant athletic trainers who regularly employ shortwave diathermy.

Diathermy is known to produce a tissue temperature rise and may be contraindicated in any condition where this increased temperature may produce negative or undesired effects, including traumatic musculoskeletal injuries with acute bleeding,[12] acute inflammatory conditions,[26] areas with reduced blood supply (ischemia),[12] and areas with reduced sensitivity to temperature or pain.[22] It is important to keep in mind that the power meter on the diathermy units does not indicate the energy entering the tissues. Therefore, the athletic trainer must rely on the sensation of pain for a warning that the athlete's tolerance levels have been exceeded.[28]

Because diathermy selectively heats tissues that are high in water content, caution must be exercised when using diathermy over fluid-filled areas or organs. Joint effusion may be exacerbated by heating with diathermy. The increase in temperature may cause an increase in synovitis.[26] Because of the high fluid content, it should not be used around the eyes for any prolonged periods of time or for repeated treatments,[23] nor should it be used with contact lenses.[42]

In most cases, toweling should be used to absorb perspiration.[14] A single layer of toweling should be used with both the drum and with air space plates. However, with other types of applicators, such as pads and cables, the toweling should be more dense and thicker, up to 1 cm or more.[3] Toweling is not necessary with microwave diathermy. There should be no overlapping of skin surfaces. If the buttocks area is to be treated, then a towel should be placed in the cleavage between the buttocks. If the shoulder area is to be treated, a towel should be placed between the skin folds in the axilla.

If clothing is permitted in the exposed area, the treatment should be closely monitored. In most cases, however, pulsed shortwave diathermy can be applied over some clothing, such as a cotton T-shirt (Figure 6-19). Be aware that many of the synthetic fabrics worn today allow for no evaporation of moisture, serving as a vapor barrier, allowing moisture to accumulate. Similarly, moisture can accumulate in athletes taped with adhesive tape or wearing compressive wraps or supportive braces. This moisture can create extreme hot spots with diathermy treatments.[38] Diathermy should not be used over moist wound dressings again due to potential for rapid heating of moisture.[26]

Diathermy should not be applied to the pelvic area of the female who is menstruating since this can increase blood flow.[26] Exposure of the gonads to diathermy should be avoided.[45] The testes are more superficial and thus are more susceptible to injury from microwave treatment than the ovaries. Minimal evidence exists that diathermy may potentially cause damage to the human fetus, and since research in this area is impossible, it is recommended that caution be used in treating the pregnant female.[43]

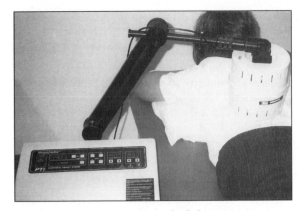

Figure 6-19   In most cases, pulsed shortwave diathermy can be applied over some clothing, such as a cotton T-shirt.

Caution should be used when using diathermy over boney prominences to avoid burning of the overlying soft tissue.[24] There should be no vigorous heating of the epiphysis in children.[26]

The athlete should not come in contact with any of the cables connecting the generator with the air space plates, pad, cable, or drum electrodes. There should be no crossover of the lead cables with any electrode set up. At no time should the antenna within the microwave applicator ever come in contact with skin, since this would cause a build up of energy sufficient to cause severe burns.

It is very important to use diathermy units at a safe distance from other types of medical electrical devices or equipment that is transistorized. Transcutaneous electrical nerve stimulation units and other low-frequency current units often have transistor-type circuits, and these can be damaged by the reflected or stray radiation that is produced by shortwave and microwave diathermy units.[26] Unshielded cardiac pacemakers may also be damaged by diathermy.[44]

There should be no metal chairs or metal tables used to support the athlete during treatment. The area being treated should also be free of metal implants. Women wearing intrauterine devices should not be treated in the low back or lower

■ **Clinical Decision-Making** *Exercise 6-5*

....

In treating a 2-day old rotator cuff strain what type of diathermy is best used during this time and why?

....

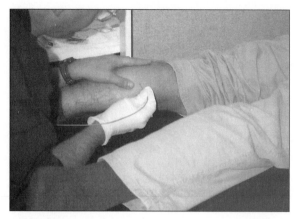

Figure 6-20 A 23-gauge thermistor is shown being inserted 3 cm below the skin's surface of the anesthetized left medial triceps surae muscle belly.

abdomen. There should be no watches or jewelry in the area because the electromagnetic energy will tend to magnetize the watch and may heat up the jewelry.[26] The athlete must remain in a reasonably comfortable position for the duration of the treatment so that the field does not change because of movement during treatment. The skin should be inspected before and after a diathermy treatment. It is recommended that the part being treated either be horizontal or elevated during treatment.

COMPARING SHORTWAVE DIATHERMY AND ULTRASOUND AS THERMAL MODALITIES

The use of therapeutic ultrasound was discussed in detail in Chapter 5. Ultrasound and pulsed shortwave diathermy are both clinically effective modalities for heating of both superficial and deep tissues; however, ultrasound is used much more frequently than shortwave diathermy. In surveys of physical therapists in both Canada[29] and Australia[30] only 0.6% and 8% of respondents, respectively, used shortwave diathermy daily, yet 94% and 93%, respectively, used ultrasound on a daily basis.

Recent research has demonstrated that shortwave diathermy may be more effective as a heating modality than ultrasound in treating certain conditions.[7,8] A study was done to determine the rate of temperature increase during pulsed shortwave diathermy, and the rate of temperature decay postapplication. A 23-gauge thermistor was inserted 3 cm below the skin's surface of the anesthetized left medial triceps surae muscle belly of 20 subjects (Figure 6-20). Diathermy was applied to the muscle belly for 20 minutes at 800 Hz,

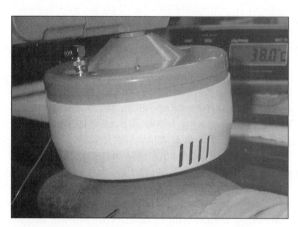

Figure 6-21 With the temperature probe in place, muscle temperature changes can be measured during shortwave diathermy treatments.
(Courtesy Sports Medicine Research Laboratory, Brigham Young University, Provo, Utah.)

a pulse width of 400 μsec, and an intensity of 150 watts. Temperature changes were recorded every 5 minutes during the treatment (Figure 6-21). The mean baseline temperature was 35.8° C and the temperature peaked at 39.8° C in 15 minutes, then dropped slightly (0.3° C) during the last 5 minutes of treatment. After the treatment terminated, intramuscular temperature dropped 1° C in 5 min-

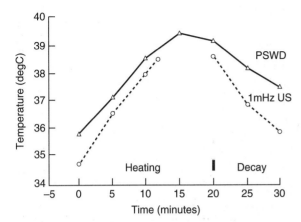

Figure 6-22   Intramuscular temperatures during heating and 10 minutes of decay resulting from 20 minutes of shortwave diathermy (PSWD: triangles) and 12 minutes of 1-MHz ultrasound (US: squares) application. Ultrasound data are from previous studies in our laboratory.[9,35] This illustrates that shortwave diathermy and 1-MHz ultrasound have similar heating rates, yet muscle heated with shortwave diathermy will retain its heat 2 to 3 times longer.

utes and 1.8° C by the tenth minute. Based on these findings, it appears that shortwave diathermy compares favorably with heating rates of 1 MHz ultrasound ($1 W/cm^2$ for 12 min = a 4° C temperature increase at 3 cms intramuscularly)[8] (Figure 6-22).

Shortwave diathermy, however, may be a better modality than ultrasound in some situations, and it appears that there are several advantages of diathermy use over ultrasound:

1. Since the surface of the shortwave applicator drum is 25 times larger than a typical ultrasound treatment area, it heats a much larger area (a standard drum heating area of the diathermy unit is 200 cm^2, or approximately 25 times that of ultrasound).

2. Unlike ultrasound, which causes a fluctuating tissue heating rate as the transducer is moved, diathermy's applicator is stationary so the heat applied to the area is more constant.

3. The rate of temperature decay is slower following diathermy application. Muscle

heated with pulsed shortwave diathermy will retain heat more than 60% longer than identical muscle depths heated with 1 MHz ultrasound.[9,39] This is important since it provides the athletic trainer more time for stretching, friction massage, and/or joint mobilization before the temperature drops to an ineffective level.

4. Application of diathermy doesn't require constant monitoring by the athletic trainer, whereas ultrasound application requires constant monitoring. Thus, an athletic trainer can work with another athlete while one is receiving diathermy treatment. This will enable the athletic trainer to be more efficient.

See Table 6-1 for a summary of indications and contraindications for shortwave and microwave diathermy.

GUIDELINES FOR THE SAFE USE OF DIATHERMY

Athletic trainers who are knowledgeable in the physics and biophysics of diathermy as well as its applications to a variety of cases tend to achieve good results. Athletic trainers who work with shortwave and microwave diathermy units must spend considerable time experimenting with equipment setup and the application of different types of electrodes on a variety of uninjured parts of the body if they are to develop the skills necessary to use diathermy safely and effectively on injured tissue. The following guidelines will help ensure the athlete's safety:

1. Question the athlete (contraindications/ previous treatments)
2. Position the athlete (comfort, modesty)
3. Inspect part to be treated (check for rashes, infections or open wounds)
4. If indicated, drape area with toweling
5. Place electrode drum on treatment area
6. Turn unit on
7. Set pulse duration
8. Set pulse frequency

■ **TABLE 6-1** Summary of Indications and Contraindications for Shortwave and Microwave Diathermy

INDICATIONS	CONTRAINDICATIONS
Postacute musculoskeletal injuries	Acute traumatic musculoskeletal injuries
Increased blood flow	Acute inflammatory conditions
Vasodilation	Areas with ischemia
Increased metabolism	Areas of reduced sensitivity to temperature or pain
Changes in some enzyme reactions	Fluid filled areas or organs
Increase collagen extensibility	Joint effusion
Decreased joint stiffness	Synovitis
Muscle relaxation	Eyes
Muscle guarding	Contact lenses
Increased pain threshold	Moist wound dressings
Enhanced recovery from injury	Malignancies
Joint contractures	Infection
Myofascial trigger points	Pelvic area during menstruation
Improving joint range of motion	Testes
Increasing the extensibility collagen	Pregnancy
Increasing circulation	Epiphyseal plates in adolescents
Reducing subacute and chronic pain	Metal implants
Resorption of hematoma	Unshielded cardiac pacemakers
Increased nerve growth and repair	Intrauterine devices
	Watches or jewelry

9. Adjust intensity
10. Set treatment time (15 to 30 minutes)
11. Press start button
12. Periodically ask athlete if heating is too vigorous
13. When timer shuts off, terminating the treatment, turn all dials to zero
14. Assess treatment efficacy (inspect area, feedback from athlete)
15. Record treatment parameters

Summary

1. Diathermy is the application of high-frequency electromagnetic energy that is primarily used to generate heat in body tissues. Diathermy as a therapeutic agent may be classified as two distinct modalities: shortwave diathermy and microwave diathermy. Shortwave diathermy may be continuous or pulsed.

2. The physiologic effects of continuous shortwave and microwave diathermy are primarily thermal, resulting from high-frequency vibration of molecules. Pulsed shortwave diathermy has been used for its nonthermal effects in the treatment of soft-tissue injuries and wounds.

3. A shortwave diathermy unit that generates a high-frequency electrical current will produce both an electrical field and a magnetic field in the tissues. The ratio of the electrical field to the magnetic field depends on the characteristics of the different units as well as on the characteristics of electrodes or applicators.

4. The capacitance technique, using capacitor electrodes (air space plates and pad electrodes), creates a strong electrical field, which is essentially the lines of force exerted on charged ions by the electrodes that cause charged particles to move from one pole to the other.

5. The inductance technique, using induction electrodes (cable electrodes and drum electrodes), creates a strong magnetic field when current is passed through a coiled cable affect surrounding tissues by inducing localized secondary currents, called eddy currents, within the tissues.

6. Pulsed diathermy is created by simply interrupting the output of continuous shortwave diathermy at consistent intervals. Generators that deliver pulsed shortwave diathermy typically use a drum type of electrode to induce energy in the treatment area via the production of a magnetic field.

7. Microwave diathermy units generate a strong electrical field and relatively little magnetic field through either circular-shaped and rectangular-shaped applicators that beam energy to the treatment area.

8. The diathermies have been used in the treatment of a variety of musculoskeletal conditions, including muscle strains, contusions, ligament sprains, tendinitis, tenosynovitis, bursitis, joint contractures, and myofascial trigger points.

9. There are probably more treatment precautions and contraindications for the use of microwave diathermy than for any of the other physical agents used in a clinical setting.

10. Effective treatments using the diathermies require practice in application and adjustment of techniques to the individual athlete.

11. Four advantages for the use of diathermy over ultrasound are larger heating area, more uniform heating, longer stretching window, and more clinician freedom.

Review Questions

1. What is diathermy, and what are the different types of diathermy?

2. What are the potential physiological effects of using continuous shortwave, pulsed shortwave, or microwave diathermy?

3. What determines ratio of the electrical field to the magnetic field in shortwave diathermy?

4. What are the differences between shortwave diathermy techniques that use capacitance or induction?

5. How is pulsed shortwave diathermy used, and what type of electrode is most typically used?

6. How should microwave diathermy be set up to achieve the most effective results?

7. What are the various clinical applications and indications for using continuous shortwave, pulsed shortwave, and microwave diathermy?

8. What are the most important treatment precautions for using the diathermies?

9. What are the major differences between microwave and shortwave diathermy?

10. What are the advantages and disadvantages of using diathermy or ultrasound as deep-heating modalities?

Self-Test Questions

T/F

1. Diathermy can create both thermal and nonthermal effects.

2. Microwave diathermy is more suited for use in areas with little subcutaneous fat.

3. Shortwave diathermy penetrates more superficially than microwave diathermy.

Multiple Choice

4. Shortwave capacitor electrodes are called which of the following?

a. air space plates
b. pad electrodes
c. Both a and b
d. Neither a nor b

5. The drum electrode is an example of a(n) _____ .

a. capacitor electrode
b. induction electrode
c. cable electrode
d. none of the above

6. Microwave diathermy units produce a strong _____ field and a weak _____ field.
   a. electrical field, magnetic field
   b. magnetic field, electrical field
   c. magnetic field, eddy currents
   d. eddy current, electrical field
7. What type of diathermy should be used to heat a large area on an athlete with thick subcutaneous fat?
   a. capacitance technique
   b. pulsed shortwave diathermy
   c. pad electrodes
   d. induction technique
8. Which of the following is a contraindication for diathermy?
   a. watches or jewelry

   b. improving range of motion
   c. muscle guarding
   d. increased blood flow
9. What conditions may be treated with diathermy?
   a. postacute muscle strain
   b. tendinitis
   c. joint contractures
   d. all of the above
10. Toweling must be used with thermal diathermy primarily to
   a. avoid contact with machine
   b. avoid moisture accumulation
   c. maintain patient modesty
   d. ensure even heating

Solutions to Clinical Decision-Making Exercises

6-1 The depth of penetration can be increased by simply moving the pad electrodes further apart. As the spacing is increased, the current density will be increased in the deeper tissues.

6-2 Pulsed shortwave diathermy is capable of heating a much larger area than ultrasound; the applicator is stationary so the heat applied to the area is more constant; the rate of temperature decay is slower following diathermy application, allowing more time for stretching; using diathermy doesn't require constant monitoring.

6-3 In areas where subcutaneous fat is minimal the capacitance technique using either airspace or pad electrodes should be used. The capacitance technique with shortwave diathermy is more likely to selectively heat

more superficial tissues that are not covered by fat.

6-4 Since an offensive lineman is likely to have a significant amount of subcutaneous fat in the abdominal area, shortwave diathermy, which heats using a magnetic field, would likely be more effective in penetrating the fat layer than would microwave diathermy, which produces electrical field heating.

6-5 Pulsed shortwave diathermy would likely be better then either continuous shortwave or microwave diathermy since the nonthermal effects of pulsed shortwave would assist in the healing process of the injured cell without causing any significant increase in temperature. Heating in this phase of the healing process would be contraindicated.

References

1. Abramson, DI, Burnett, C, Bell, Y, and Tuck, S: Changes in blood flow, oxygen uptake and tissue temperatures produced by therapeutic physical agents, *Am J Phys Med* 47:51–62, 1960.
2. Behrens, BJ, and Michlovitz, SL: *Physical agents: theory and practice for the physical athletic trainer assistant*, Philadelphia: FA Davis, 1996.
3. Brown, M, and Baker, RD: Effect of pulsed short wave diathermy on skeletal muscle injury in rabbits, *Phys Ther* 67(2):208–213, 1987.
4. Castel, JC, Draper, DO, Knight, K, Fujiwara, T, and Garrett, C: Rate of temperature decay in human muscle after treatments of pulsed short wave diathermy, *J Athletic Training* 32:S-34, 1997.

5. DeLateur, BJ, Lehmann, JF, Stonebridge, JB, Warren, CG, and Guy, AW: Muscle heating in human subjects with 915 MHz microwave contact applicator, *Arch Phys Med* 51:147–151, 1970.

6. Delpizzo, V, and Joyner, KH: On the safe use of microwave and shortwave diathermy units, *Australian Journal of Physiotherapy* 33(3):152–162, 1987.

7. Draper, DO: *Current research on therapeutic ultrasound and pulsed short-wave diathermy.* Presented at Physio Therapy Research Seminars Japan, Nov. 17, 1996, Sendai, Japan.

8. Draper, DO, Castel, JC, Knight, K, Fujiwara, T, and Darrow, H: Temperature rise in human muscle during pulsed short wave diathermy: does this modality parallel ultrasound, *J Athletic Training* 32:S-35, 1997.

9. Draper, DO, Castel, JC, and Castel, D: Rate of temperature increase in human muscle during 1 MHz and 3 MHz continuous ultrasound, *J Orthop Sports Phys Ther* 22:142–150, 1995.

10. Draper, D, Knight, KI, and Fujiwara, T: Temperature change in human muscle during and after pulsed shortwave diathermy, *Journal of Orthopedic and Sports Physical Therapy* (29)(1): 13–18, 1999.

11. Fenn, JE: Effect of pulsed electromagnetic energy (Diapulse) on experimental hematomas, *Can Med Ass J* 100:251, 1969.

12. Fischer, C, and Solomon, S: Physiologic responses to heat and cold. In Licht, S, editor: *Therapeutic heat and cold*, New Haven, 1965, Elizabeth Licht.

13. Griffin, JE: *Update on selected physical modalities.* Paper presented in Chicago, Dec. 1981.

14. Griffin, JE, and Karselis, TC: The diathermies. In *Physical agents for physical athletic trainers*, ed 2, Springfield, Illinois, 1982, Charles C Thomas.

15. Griffin, JE: Santiesleban, AJ, and Kloth, L: *Electrotherapy for instructors.* Paper presented in Lacrosse, Wisc., Aug. 1982.

16. Guy, AW, and Lehmann, JF: On the determination of an optimum microwave diathermy frequency for a direct contact applicator, *Inst. Electrical Electronics Engineers Transactions, Biomedical Engineering* 13:76–87, 1966.

17. Hansen, TI, and Kristensen, JH: Effect of massage, shortwave diathermy and ultrasound upon 133Xe disappearance rate from muscle and subcutaneous tissue in the human calf, *Scand J Rehabil Med* 5:179–182,1973.

18. *Health devices shortwave diathermy units.* Proceedings of the Emergency Care Research Institute, Meeting in Plymouth, Pa, June, 1979, 175–193.

19. Hellstrom, RO, and Stewart, WF: Miscarriages among female physical athletic trainers who report using radio- and microwave-frequency electromagnetic radiation, *Am J Epidemiol* 138(10):775–785, 1993.

20. Kitchen, S, and Partridge, C: A review of microwave diathermy, *Physiotherapy* 77(9):647–652, 1991.

21. Kitchen, S, and Partridge, C: Review of shortwave diathermy continuous and pulsed patterns, *Physiotherapy* 78(4):243–252, 1992.

22. Kloth, L, and Ziskin, M: Diathermy and pulsed electromagnetic fields. In Michlovitz, SL, editor: *Thermal agents in rehabilitation*, ed 2, Philadelphia, 1990, FA Davis.

23. Konarska, I, and Michneiwicz, L: Shortwave diathermy of diseases of the anterior portion of the eye, *Klin Oczna* 25:185, 1955.

24. Lehmann, JF: Comparison of relative heating patterns produced in tissues by exposure to microwave energy with exposures at 2450 and 900 megacycles, *Arch Phys Med Rehab* 46:307, 1965.

25. Lehmann, JF: Diathermy. In Krusen, FH, editor: *Handbook of physical medicine and rehabilitation*, Philadelphia, 1965, WB Saunders.

26. Lehmann, JF: *Therapeutic heat and cold*, ed 4, Baltimore, 1990, Williams & Wilkins.

27. Lehmann, JF, and DeLateur, BJ: Diathermy and superficial heat and cold. In Krusen, FH, editor: *Krusen's handbook of physical medicine & rehabilitation*, ed 3, Philadelphia, 1982, WB Saunders Co.

28. Lehmann, JF, Warren, CG, and Scham, SM: Therapeutic heat and cold, *Clin Ortho* 99:207, 1974.

29. Lindsay, DM, Dearness, J, and McGinley, CC: Electrotherapy usage trends in private physiotherapy practice in Alberta, *Physiother Can* 47(1):30–34, 1995.

30. Lindsay, DM, Dearness, J, Richardson, C, Chapman, A, and Cuskelly, G: A survey of electromodality usage in private physiotherapy practices, *Aust J Physiother* 36(4):249–256, 1990.

31. Low, JL: The nature and effects of pulsed electromagnetic radiations, *NZ Physiotherapy* 6:18, 1978.

32. Low, J: Dosage of some pulsed shortwave clinical trials, *Physiotherapy* 81(10):611–616, 1995.

33. Low, J, and Reed, A: *Electrotherapy explained: principles and practice*, London, 1990, Butterworth-Heinemann.

34. Marks, R, Ghassemi, M, Duarte, R, and Van Nguyen, JP: A review of the literature on shortwave diathermy as applied to osteo-arthritis of the knee, *Physiotherapy* 85(6):304–316, 1999.

35. Millard, JB: Effect of high frequency currents and infra-red rays on the circulation of the lower limb in man, *Ann Phys Med* 6:45, 1961.

36. Miner, L, Draper, D, and Knight, KL: Pulsed shortwave diathermy application prior to stretching does not appear to aid hamstring flexibility, *Journal of Athletic Training* 35(2):S-48, 2000.

37. Murray, CC, and Kitchen, S: Effect of pulse repetition rate on the perception of thermal sensation with pulsed shortwave diathermy, *Physiotherapy Research International* 5(2)73–84, 2000.

38. *Progress Report*, American Physical Therapy Association, June, 1980.

39. Rose, S, Draper, DO, Schulthies, SS, and Durrant, E: The stretching window part two: rate of thermal decay in deep muscle following 1 MHz ultrasound, *J Athl Train* 31: 139–143, 1996.

40. Sanseverino, EG: *Membrane phenomena and cellular processes under the action of pulsating magnetic fields.* Presented at the Second International Congress for Magneto Medicine, Rome, Italy, 1980.

41. Schliephake, E: Carrying out treatment. In Thom, H, editor: *Introduction to shortwave and microwave diathermy*, ed. 3, Springfield, Ill., 1966, Charles C Thomas.

42. Scott, BO: Effect of contact lenses on shortwave field distribution, *Br J Opthalmology* 40:696, 1956.

43. Smith, DW, Clarren, SK, and Harvey, MA: Hyperthermia as a possible teratogenic agent, *J Pediatrics* 92:878, 1978.

44. Smyth, H.: The pacemaker athlete and the electromagnetic environment, *JAMA* 227:1412, 1974.

45. Van Demark, NL, and Free, MJ: Temperature effects. In Johnson, AD, editor: *The testis*, vol.3, New York, 1973, Academic Press.

46. Wilson, DH: Treatment of soft tissue injuries by pulsed electrical energy, *Br Med J* 2:269, 1972.

47. Wright, GG: Treatment of soft tissue and ligamentous injuries in professional footballers, *Physiother* 59(12), 1973.

Suggested Readings

Abramson, DL, Bell, Y, Rejal, H, Tuck, S, Burnett, C, and Fleischer, CJ: Changes in blood flow, oxygen uptake and tissue temperatures produced by therapeutic physical agents, *American Journal of Physical Medicine* 39:87–95, 1960.

Abramson, DL, Chu, LSW, Tuck, S, Lee, SW, Richardson, G, and Levin, M: Effect of tissue temperature and blood flow on motor nerve conduction velocity, *Journal of the American Medical Association* 198:1082–1088, 1966.

Abramson, DI: Physiologic basis for the use of physical agents in peripheral vascular disorders, *Arch Phys Med Rehabil* 46:216, 1965.

Adey WR: Electromagnetic field effects on tissue, *Physiological Review* 61(3):436–514, 1981.

Adey, WR: Physiological signaling across cell membranes and co-operative influences of extremely low frequency electromagnetic fields. In Frohlich, H, editor: *Biological coherence and response to external stimuli*, Heidleberg, 1988, Springer Verlag.

Allberry, J: Shortwave diathermy for herpes zoster, *Physiotherapy* 60:386, 1974.

Aronofsky, D: Reduction of dental post-surgical symptoms using non-thermal pulsed high-peak-power electromagnetic energy, *Oral Surgery* 32(5):688–696, 1971.

Babbs, CF, and Dewitt, DP: Physical principles of local heat therapy for cancer, *Medical Instrumentation (USA)* 15: 367–373, 1981.

Balogun, J, and Okonofua, F: Management of chronic pelvic inflammatory disease with shortwave diathermy: a case report, *Phys Ther* 68(10):1541–1545, 1988.

Bansal, PS, Sobti, VK, and Roy, KS: Histomorphochemical effects of shortwave diathermy on healing of experimental muscle injury in dogs, *Indian Journal of Experimental Biology* 28: 766–770, 1990.

Barclay, V, Collier, RJ, and Jones, A: Treatment of various hand injuries by pulsed electromagnetic energy, *Physiotherapy* 69(6):186–188, 1983.

Barker, AT, Barlow, PS, Porter, J, Smith, ME, Clifton, S, Andrews, L, and O'Dowd, WJ: A double-blind clinical trial of lowpower pulsed shortwave therapy in the treatment of a soft tissue injury, *Physiotherapy* 71(12):500–504,1985.

Barnett, M.: SWD for herpes zoster, *Physiotherapy* 61:217, 1975.

Bassett. C: The development and application of pulsed electromagnetic fields (PEMFs) for un-united fractures and arthrodeses, *Orthopaedic Clinics of North America* 15(10): 61–89, 1984.

Benson, TB, and Copp, EP: The effect of therapeutic forms of heat and ice on the pain threshold of the normal shoulder, *Pheumatology and Rehabilitation* 13:101–104, 1974.

Bentall, RH, and Eckstein, HB: A trial involving the use of pulsed electromagnetic therapy on children undergoing orchidopexy, *Kinderchirugie* 17(4):380–389, 1975.

Brown, M, and Baker, RD: Effect of pulsed shortwave diathermy on skeletal muscle injury in rabbits, *Phys Ther* 67(2): 208–214, 1987.

Brown-Woodnan, PDC, Hadley, JA, Richardson, L, Bright, D, and Porter, D: Evaluation of reproductive function of female rats exposed to radio frequency fields (27.12 MHz) near a shortwave diathermy device, *Health Physics* 56(4):521–525, 1989.

Burr, B: *Heat as a therapeutic modality against cancer*, report 16, US National Cancer Institute, Bethesda, Maryland, 1974.

Cameron, BM: Experimental acceleration of wound healing, *American Journal of Orthopaedics* 3:336–343, 1961.

Chamberlain, MA, Care, G, and Gharfield, B: Physiotherapy in osteoarthrosis of the knee, *Annals of Rheumatic Diseases* 23:389–391, 1982.

Cole, A, and Eagleston, R: The benefits of deep heat: ultrasound and electromagnetic diathermy, *Physician Sportsmed* 22(2):76–78, 81–82, 84, 1994.

Constable, JD, Scapicchio, AP, and Opitz, B: Studies of the effects of diapulse treatment on various aspects of wound healing in experimental animals, *Journal of Surgical Research* 11: 254–257, 1971.

Coppell, R: Survey of stray electromagnetic emissions from microwave and shortwave diathermy equipment, *New Zealand Journal of Physiotherapy* 16(3):9–12, 14, 1988.

Currier, DP, and Nelson, RM: Changes in motor conduction velocity induced by exercise and diathermy, *Phys Ther* 49(2):146–152, 1969.

Daels, J: Microwave heating of the uterine wall during parturition, *J. Microwave Power* 11:166, 1976.

De la Rosette, J, De Wildt, M, and Alivizatos, G: Transurethral microwave thermotherapy (TUMT) in benign prostatic hyperplasia: placebo versus TUMT, *Urology* 44(1):58–63, 1994.

Department of Health Evaluation Report: Shortwave therapy units, *Journal of Medical Engineering and Technology* 11(6): 285–298, 1987.

Department of Health and Welfare (Canada): *Canada-wide survey of non-ionizing radiation-emitting medical devices,* 80-EHD-52, 1980.

Department of Health and Welfare (Canada): *Safety code 25— shortwave diathermy guidelines for limited radio frequency exposure,* 80-EHD-98, 1983.

Doyle, JR, and Smart, BW: Stimulation of bone growth by shortwave diathermy, *J Bone Joint Surg* 45A:15, 1963.

Engel, JP: The effects of microwaves on bone and bone marrow and adjacent tissues, *Arch Phys Med Rehabil* 31: 453, 1950.

Erdman, WJ: Peripheral blood flow measurements during application of pulsed high frequency currents, *American Journal of Orthopaedics* 2, 196–197, 1960.

Feibel, H, and Fast, H: Deep heating of joints: a reconsideration, *Arch Phys Med Rehabil* 57:513, 1976.

Fenn, JE: Effect of pulsed electromagnetic energy (diapulse) on experimental hematomas, *Canadian Medical Association Journal* 100:251–253, 1969.

Foley-Nolan, D, Barry, C, Coughlan, RJ, O'Connor, P, and Roden, D: Pulsed high frequency (27MHz) electromagnetic therapy for persistent neck pain, *Orthopaedics* 13(4): 445–451, 1990.

Foley-Nolan, D, Moore, K, and Codd, M: Low energy high frequency pulsed electromagnetic therapy for acute whiplash injuries: a double blind randomized controlled study, *Scand J Rehab Med* 24(1):51–59, 1992.

Foster, P: Diathermy burns, *Nursing RSA Verpleging* 2(10):4–5, 7–9, 1987.

Gibson, T, Grahame, R, Harkness, J, Woo, P, Blagrave, P, and Hills, R: Controlled comparison of shortwave diathermy treatment with osteopathic treatment in non-specific low back pain, *The Lancet* 1:1258–1261, 1985.

Ginsberg, AJ: Pulsed shortwave in the treatment of bursitis with calcification, *International Record of Medicine* 174(2):71–75, 1961.

Goldin, JH, Broadbent, NRG, Nancarrow, JD, and Marshall, T: The effect of diapulse on healing of wounds: a double blind randomized controlled trial in man, *Br J Plastic Surg* 34:267–270, 1981.

Grant, A, Sleep, J, McIntosh, J, and Ashurst, H: Ultrasound and pulsed electromagnetic energy treatment for peroneal trauma: a randomized placebo-controlled trial, *British Journal of Obstetrics and Gynaecology* 96:434–439, 1981.

Guy, AW: Biophysics of high frequency currents and electromagnetic radiation. In Lehmann, JF, editor: *Therapeutic heat and cold,* ed 4, Baltimore, 1990, Williams & Wilkins.

Guy, AW, Lehmann, JF, and Stonebridge, JB: Therapeutic applications of electromagnetic power, *Proceedings of the Institute Electrical and Electronic Engineers* 62:55–75, 1974.

Guy, AW, Lehmann, JF, Stonebridge, JB, and Sorensen, CC: Development of a 915 MHz direct contact applicator for therapeutic heating of tissues, *Inst. Electrical Electronics Engineers on Microwave Theory and Techniques* 26:550–556, 1978.

Guy, AW: Analyses of electromagnetic fields induced in biological tissues by thermographic studies on equivalent phantom models, *IEEE Trans. Microwave Theory Tech.* Vol MTT 19: 205, 1971.

Hall, E L: Diathermy generators, *Arch Phys Med Rehabil* 33:28, 1952.

Hansen, TI, and Kristensen, JH: Effect of massage, shortwave diathermy and ultrasound upon 133Xe disappearance rate from muscle and subcutaneous tissue in the human calf, *Scandinavian Journal of Rehabilitation Medicine* 5:179–182, 1973.

Harris, R: Effect of shortwave diathermy on radio-sodium clearance from the knee joint in the normal and in rheumatoid arthritis, *Phys Med Rehabil* 42:241, 1961.

Hayne, R: Pulsed high frequency energy: its place in physiotherapy, *Physiotherapy* 70(12):459–466, 1984.

Herrick, JF, and Krusen, FH: Certain physiologic and pathologic effects of microwaves, *Electrical Engineers* 72:239, 1953.

Herrick, JF, Jelatis, DG, and Lee, GM: Dielectric properties of tissues important in microwave diathermy, *Fed. Proc.* 9:60, 1950.

Hoeberlein, T, Katz, J, and Balogun, J: Does indirect heating using shortwave diathermy over the abdomen and sacrum affect peripheral blood flow in the lower extremities? *Phys Ther* 76(5):S-67, 1996.

Hollander, JL: Joint temperature measurement in evaluation of antiarthritic agents, *J Clin Invest* 30:701, 1951.

Hutchinson, WJ, and Burdeaux, BD: The effects of shortwave diathermy on bone repair, *J. Bone Joint Surg* 33A:155, 1951.

Johnson, CC, and Guy, AW: Nonionizing electromagnetic wave effects in biological materials and systems, *Proc. Institute of Electrical and Electronic Engineers* 66:692, 1972.

Jones, SL: Electromagnetic field interference and cardiac pacemakers, *Phys Ther* 56:1013, 1976.

Kantor, G, and Witters, DM: *The performance of a new 915 MHz direct contact applicator with reduced leakage—a detailed analysis,* HHS Publication (FDA) S3-8199, April 1983.

Kantor, G: Evaluation and survey of microwave and radio frequency applicators, *J Microwave Power* (2) 16:135, 1981.

Kaplan, EG, and Weinstock, RE: Clinical evaluation of diapulse as adjunctive therapy following foot surgery, *J American Pediatric Association* 58:218–221, 1968.

Kloth, LC, Morrison, M, and Ferguson, B: Therapeutic microwave and shortwave diathermy: a review of thermal effectiveness, safe use, and state-of-the-art-1984, *Center for Devices and Radiological Health* DHHS, FDA 85–8237, December, 1984.

Krag, C, Taudorf, U, Siim, E, and Bolund, S: The effect of pulsed electromagnetic energy (diapulse) on the survival of experimental skin flaps, *Scandinavian Journal of Plastic and Reconstructive Surgery* 13:377–380, 1979.

Lehmann, JF, McDougall, JA, Guy, AW, Warren, CG, and Esselman, PC: Heating patterns produced by shortwave diathermy applicators. In tissue substitute models, *Archives of Physical Medicine and Rehabilitation* 64:575–577, 1983.

Lehmann, JF, DeLateur, BJ, and Stonebridge, JB: Selective muscle heating by shortwave diathermy with a helical coil, *Arch Phys Med Rehabil* 50:117, 1969.

Lehmann, JF: *Review of evidence for indications, techniques of application, contraindications, hazards and clinical effectiveness for shortwave diathermy*, DHEW/FDA HFA510, 5600 Fischers Lane, Rockville, Md. 20852, 1974.

Lehmann, JF, Guy, AW, DeLateur, BJ, Stonebridge, JB, and Warren, CG: Heating patterns produced by shortwave diathermy using helical induction coil applicators, *Arch Phys Med* 49:193–198, 1968.

Lehmann, JF: Microwave therapy: stray radiation, safety and effectiveness, *Arch Phys Med Rehabil* 60:578, 1979.

Licht, S, editor: *Therapeutic heat and cold*, ed 2, New Haven, Conn., 1972, Elizabeth Licht.

Martin, C, McCallum, H, and Strelley, S: Electromagnetic fields from therapeutic diathermy equipment: a review of hazards and precautions, *Physiotherapy* 77(1):3–7, 1991.

McDowell, AD, and Lunt, MJ: Electromagnetic field strength measurements on megapulse units, *Physiotherapy* 77(12):805–809, 1991.

McGill, SN: The effect of pulsed shortwave therapy on lateral ligament sprain of the ankle, *New Zealand Journal of Physiotherapy* 10:21–24, 1988.

McNiven, DR, and Wyper, DJ: Microwave therapy and muscle blood flow in man, *J Microwave Power* 11:168–170, 1976.

Michaelson, SM: Effects of high frequency currents and electromagnetic radiation. In Lehmann, HF, editor: *Therapeutic heat and cold*, ed 4, Baltimore, 1990, Williams & Wilkins.

Millard, JB: Effect of high frequency currents and infrared rays on the circulation of the lower limb in man, *Annals of Physical Medicine* 6(2):45–65, 1961.

Morrissey, LJ: Effects of pulsed shortwave diathermy upon volume blood flow through the calf of the leg: plethysmography studies, *Journal of the American Physical Therapy Association* 46:946–952, 1966.

Mosley, H, and Davison, M: Exposure of physioathletic trainers to microwave radiation during microwave diathermy treatment, *Clin Phys Physiol Measl* no. 3, 2:217, 1981.

Nadasdi, M: Inhibition of experimental arthritis by athermic pulsing shortwave in rats, *American Journal of Orthopaedics* 2:105–107, 1960.

Nelson, AJM, and Holt, JAG: Combined microwave therapy, *Med. J. Aust.* 2:88–90, 1978.

Nicolle, FV, and Bentall, RM: The use of radio frequency pulsed energy in the control of post-operative reaction to blepharoplasty, *Anaesthetic Plastic Surgery* 6:169–171, 1982.

Nielson, NC, Hansen, R, and Larsen, T: Heat induction in copper bearing IUDs during shortwave diathermy, *Acta Obstetrica et Gynaecologica Scandinavica (Stockholm)* 58:495, 1972.

Nwuga, GB: *A study of the value of shortwave diathermy and isometric exercise in back pain management.* Proceedings of the IXth International Congress of the WCPT, Legitimerader Sjukgymnasters Riksforbund, Stockholm, Sweden, 1982.

Oliver, D: Pulsed electromagnetic energy—what is it? *Physiotherapy* 70(12): 458–459, 1984.

Osborne, SL, and Coulter, JS: Thermal effects of shortwave diathermy on bone and muscle, *Arch Phys Ther* 38:281–284, 1938.

Paliwal, BR: Heating patterns produced by 434 MHz erbotherm UHF69, *Radiology* 135:511, 1980.

Pasila, M, Visuri, T, and Sundholm A: Pulsating shortwave diathermy: value in treatment of recent ankle and foot sprains, *Archives of Physical Medicine and Rehabilitation* 59:383–386, 1978.

Patzold, J: Physical laws regarding distribution of energy for various high frequency methods applied in heat therapy, *Ultrasonics Bio. Med.* 2:58, 1956.

Peres, S, Draper, D, and Knight, K: Pulsed shortwave diathermy and prolonged stretch increases dorsiflexion range of motion more than prolonged stretch alone, *Journal of Athletic Training* 36 (2 supp): S-49, 2001.

Quirk, AS, Newman, RJ, and Newman, KJ: An evaluation of interferential therapy, shortwave diathermy and exercise in the treatment of osteo-arthrosis of the knee, *Physiotherapy* 71(2):55–57, 1985.

Rae, JW, Herrick, JF, Wakim, KG, and Krusen, FH: A comparative study of the temperature produced by MWD and SWD, *Arch Phys Med Rehabil* 30:199, 1949.

Raji, AM: An experimental study of the effects of pulsed electromagnetic field (diapulse) on nerve repair, *The Journal of Hand Surgery* 9B(2):105–112, 1984.

Reed, MW, Bickerstaff, DR, Hayne, CR, Wyman, A, and Davies, J: Pain relief after inguinal herniorrhaphy: ineffectiveness of pulsed electromagnetic energy, *British Journal of Clinical Practice* 41(6):782–784, 1987.

Religo, W, and Larson, T: Microwave thermotherapy: new wave of treatment for benign prostatic hyperplasia, *J American Academy Physician Assistants* 7(4):259–267, 1994.

Richardson, AW: The relationship between deep tissue temperature and blood flow during electromagnetic irradiation, *Arch Phys Med Rehabil* 31:19, 1950.

Rubin, A, and Erdman, W: Microwave exposure of the human female pelvis during early pregnancy and prior to conception, *Am J Phys Med* 38:219, 1959.

Ruggera, PS: Measurement of emission levels during microwave and shortwave diathermy treatments, *Bureau of Radiological Health Report*, HHS Publication (FDA), 80–8119, 1980.

Schwan, HP: Interaction of microwave and radio frequency radiation with biological systems. In Cleary, SF, editor: *Biological effects and health implications of microwave radiation*, US Department of Health, Education and Welfare, Washington, 1970.

Schwan, HP, and Piersol, GM: The absorption of electromagnetic energy in body tissues, part I, *Am J Phys Med* 33:371, 1954.

Schwan, HP, and Piersol, GM: The absorption of electromagnetic energy in body tissues, part II, *Am J Phys Med* 34:425, 1955.

Silverman, DR, and Pendleton, LA: A comparison of the effects of continuous and pulsed shortwave diathermy on peripheral circulation, *Archives of Physical Medicine and Rehabilitation* 49:429–436, 1968.

Stuchly, MA, Repacholi, MH, Lecuyer, DW, and Mann, RD: Exposure to the operator and athlete during shortwave diathermy treatments, *Health Physics* 42(3):341–366, 1982.

Svarcova, J, Trnavsky, K, and Zvarova, J: The influence of ultrasound, galvanic currents and shortwave diathermy on pain intensity in athletes with osteo-arthritis, *Scandinavian Journal of Rheumatology*, supplement 67:83–85, 1988.

Taskinen, H, Kyyronen, P, and Hemminki, K: The effects of ultrasound, shortwaves and physical exertion on pregnancy outcome in physioathletic trainers, *Journal of Epidemiology and Community Health* 44:96–201, 1990.

Thom, H: *Introduction to shortwave and microwave therapy*, ed 3, Springfield, Ill., 1966, Charles C Thomas.

Tzima, E, and Martin, C: An evaluation of safe practices to restrict exposure to electric and magnetic fields from therapeutic and surgical diathermy equipment, *Physiological Measurement* 15(2):201–216, 1994.

Van Ummersen, CA: The effect of 2450 mc radiation on the development of the chick embryo. In Peyton, MF, editor: *Biological effects of microwave radiation*, vol 1, New York, 1961, Plenum Press.

Vanharanta, H: Effect of shortwave diathermy on mobility and radiological stage of the knee in the development of experimental osteo-arthritis, *American Journal of Physical Medicine* 61(2):59–65, 1982.

Verrier, M, Falconer, K, and Crawford, JS: A comparison of tissue temperature following two shortwave diathermy techniques, *Physiotherapy Canada* 29(1):21–25, 1977.

Wagstaff, P, Wagstaff, S, and Downie, M: A pilot study to compare the efficacy of continuous and pulsed magnetic energy (shortwave diathermy) on the relief of low back pain, *Physiotherapy* 72(11):563–566, 1986.

Ward, AR: *Electricity fields and waves in therapy*, Science Press, Australia, 1980, NSW.

Wilson, D: Treatment of soft tissue injuries by pulsed electrical energy continuous and pulsed magnetic energy (shortwave diathermy) on the relief of low back pain, *Physiotherapy* 72(11):563–566, 1986.

Wilson, DH: Treatment of soft tissue injuries by pulsed electrical energy, *British Medical Journal* 2:269–270, 1972.

Wilson, DH: Comparison of shortwave diathermy and pulsed electromagnetic energy in treatment of soft tissue injuries, *Physiotherapy* 60(10):309–310, 1974.

Wilson, DH: The effects of pulsed electromagnetic energy on peripheral nerve regeneration, *Ann NY Acad Sci* 238:575, 1975.

Wise, CS: The effect of diathermy on blood flow, *Arch Phys Med Rehabil* 29:17, 1948.

Witters, DM, and Kantor, G: An evaluation of microwave diathermy applicators using free space electric field mapping, *Phys Med Biol* 26:1099, 1981.

Worden, RE: The heating effects of microwaves with and without ischemia, *Arch Phys Med Rehabil* 29:751, 1948.

Wyper, DJ, and McNiven, DR: Effects of some physiotherapeutic agents on skeletal muscle blood flow, *Physiotherapy* 63(3):83–85, 1976.

PART THREE

Electrical Modalities

CHAPTER 7

Basic Principles of Electricity

William E. Prentice

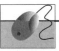
Study Resources

Refer to the lab exercises in the accompanying Laboratory Manual, as well as eSims which simulates the athletic training certification exam at www.mhhe.com/esims. Also, check out the competency information found at www.mhhe.com/prentice11e. For more online study resources, visit our Health and Human Performance Website at www.mhhe.com/hhp/.

Following completion of this chapter, the student athletic trainer will be able to

- Define potential difference, ampere, volt, ohm, and watt.

- Interpret Ohm's law and its mathematical expression.

- Differentiate between alternating, direct, and pulsitile currents.

- Categorize various waveforms and pulse characteristics.

- Contrast the various types of current modulation.

- Discriminate between series and parallel circuit arrangement.

- Explain current flow through various types of biologic tissue.

- Create a safe environment when using electrical equipment.

Many of the modalities discussed in this text may be classified as electrical modalities. These pieces of equipment have the capabilities of taking the electrical current flowing from a wall outlet and modifying that current to produce a specific, desired physiologic effect in human biologic tissue.

Understanding the basic principles of electricity is usually difficult, even for the athletic trainer who is accustomed to using electrical modalities on a daily basis. To understand how current flow affects biologic tissue, it is first necessary to become familiar with some of the principles that describe how electricity is produced and how it behaves in an electrical circuit.

The principles and concepts presented in this chapter can be applied to the use of all of the electrical modalities to be discussed in this text, including iontophoresis (Chapter 9), biofeedback (Chapter 13), the diathermies (Chapter 6), low-power laser (Chapter 14), ultraviolet (Chapter 15), and even ultrasound (Chapter 5), but are particularly applicable to Chapter 8, "Electrical Stimulating Currents."

COMPONENTS OF ELECTRICAL CURRENTS

All matter is composed of atoms that contain positively and negatively charged particles called **ions**. These charged particles possess electrical energy and thus have the ability to move about. They tend to move from an area of higher concentration to-

ion A positively or negatively charged particle.

electrical potential The difference between charged particles at a higher and lower potential.

electron Fundamental particle of matter possessing a negative electrical charge and very small mass.

electrical current The net movement of electrons along a conducting medium.

ampere Unit of measure that indicates the rate at which electrical current is flowing.

coulomb Indicates the number of electrons flowing in a current.

volt The electromotive force that must be applied to produce a movement of electrons.

voltage The force resulting from an accumulation of electrons at one point in an electrical circuit, usually corresponding to a deficit of electrons at another point in the circuit.

low-voltage current Current in which the waveform has an amplitude of less than 150 V.

high-voltage current Current in which the waveform has an amplitude of greater than 150 V with a relatively short pulse duration.

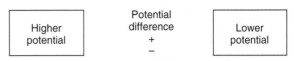

Figure 7-1 The difference between high potential and low potential is potential difference. Electrons tend to flow from areas of higher concentration to areas of lower concentration. A potential difference must exist if there is to be any movement of electrons.

The unit of measurement that indicates the rate at which electrical current flows is the **ampere** (amp). One amp is defined as the movement of 1 **coulomb** or 6.25×10^{18} electrons per second. Amperes indicate the rate of electron flow, while coulombs indicate the number of electrons. In the case of therapeutic modalities, current flow is generally described in milliamperes (1/1000 of an amp, denoted as mamp) or in microamperes (1/1,000,000 of an amp, denoted as μamp).

The electrons will not move unless an electrical potential difference in the concentration of these charged particles exists between two points. The electromotive force, which must be applied to produce a flow of electrons, is called a **volt** (V) and is defined as the difference in electron population (potential difference) between two points.[4]

Voltage is the force resulting from an accumulation of electrons at one point in an electrical circuit, usually corresponding to a deficit of electrons at another point in the circuit. If a suitable conductor connects the two points, the potential difference (difference in electron population) will cause electrons to move from the area of higher population to the area of lower population.

Commercial current flowing from wall outlets produces an electromotive force of either 115 V or 220 V. The electrotherapeutic devices used in injury rehabilitation modify voltages. Electrical generators are sometimes referred to as being either **low voltage** or **high voltage**. These terms are somewhat useless in meaning, although some older texts have referred to generators that produce less than 150 V as low volt and those that produce several hundred volts as high volt.[4]

ward an area of lower concentration. An electrical force is capable of propelling these particles from higher to lower energy levels, thus establishing **electrical potentials**. The more ions an object has, the higher its potential electrical energy. Particles with a positive charge tend to move toward negatively charged particles, and those that are negatively charged tend to move toward the positively charged particles (Figure 7-1).[12]

Electrons are particles of matter possessing a negative charge and very small mass. The net movement of electrons is referred to as an **electrical current**. The movement or flow of these electrons will always go from a higher potential to a lower potential.[21] An electrical force is oriented only in the direction of the applied force. This flow of electrons may be likened to a domino reaction.

■ **Analogy**   *7-1*

The flow of electrons may be likened to a domino reaction. As the first domino (electron) is knocked down, it causes the next domino to fall down and move slightly forward, thus moving the next and the next and so forth. Thus, energy is propagated along this chain of dominoes, just as electrical energy moves along a conducting medium.

conductors   Materials that permit this free movement of electrons.

conductance   The ease with which a current flows along a conducting medium.

insulators   Materials that resist current flow.

resistance   The opposition to electron flow in a conducting material.

electrical impedance   The opposition to electron flow in a conducting material.

ohm   A unit of measure that indicates resistance to current flow.

Ohm's law   The current in an electrical circuit is directly proportional to the voltage and inversely proportional to the resistance.

watt   A measure of electrical power. Mathematically, watts = volts × amperes.

Electrons can move in a current only if there is a relatively easy pathway to move along. Materials that permit this free movement of electrons are referred to as **conductors. Conductance** is a term that defines the ease with which current flows along a conducting medium. Metals (copper, gold, silver, aluminum) are good conductors of electricity, as are electrolyte solutions, because both are composed of large numbers of free electrons that are given up readily. Thus, materials that offer little opposition to current flow are good conductors. Materials that resist current flow are called **insulators**. Insulators contain relatively fewer free electrons and thus offer greater resistance to electron

■ **TABLE 7-1**   Electron Flow as Analogous to Water Flow

ELECTRON FLOW		WATER FLOW
Volt	=	Pump
Amperes	=	Gallons
Ohm (properties of conductor)	=	Resistance (length and distance of pipe)

flow. Air, wood, and glass are all considered insulators. The number of amps flowing in a given conductor is dependent both on the voltage applied and on the conduction characteristics of the material.[20]

The opposition to electron flow in a conducting material is referred to as **resistance** or **electrical impedance** and is measured in a unit known as an **ohm**. Thus, an electrical circuit that has high resistance (ohms) will have less flow (amps) than a circuit with less resistance and the same voltage.[2]

The mathematical relationship between current flow, voltage, and resistance is demonstrated in the formula:

$$\text{Current flow} = \frac{\text{Voltage}}{\text{Resistance}}$$

This formula is the mathematical expression of **Ohm's law**, which states that the current in an electrical circuit is directly proportional to the voltage and inversely proportional to the resistance. An analogy comparing the movement of water with the movement of electricity may help to clarify this relationship between current flow, voltage, and resistance (Table 7-1).

Electrical energy or power is a product of the voltage or electromotive force and the amount of current flowing. Electrical power is measured in a unit called a **watt**.

$$\text{watts} = \text{volts} \times \text{amperes}$$

Simply, the watt indicates the rate at which electrical power is being used. A watt is defined as the electrical power needed to produce a current flow of 1 amp at a pressure of 1 volt.

■ Analogy   7-2

The flow of electrical current along some conducting medium is similar to the flow of water in a pipe. For water to flow, some type of pump must create a force to produce water movement (the volt is the pump that produces the electron flow). The resistance to water flow is dependent on the length, diameter, and smoothness of the water pipe. The resistance to electrical flow depends on the characteristics of the conductor. The amount of water flowing is measured in gallons, while the amount of electricity flowing is measured in amperes. The amount of energy produced by flowing water is determined by two factors: (1) the number of gallons flowing per unit of time and (2) the pressure created in the pipe. The electrical energy or wattage produced is a function of amperage times voltage.

ELECTROTHERAPEUTIC CURRENTS

Electrotherapeutic devices generate three different types of current, which when introduced into biologic tissue are capable of producing specific physiologic changes. These three types of current are referred to as **alternating** (AC), **direct** (DC), or pulsitile (polyphasic). The therapeutic effects of these various types of electrical stimulating currents will be discussed in detail in Chapter 8.

Direct current, also referred to in some texts as *galvanic current*, has an uninterrupted, unidirectional flow of electrons toward the positive pole (Figure 7-2a). On most modern direct current devices, the polarity and thus the direction of current flow can be reversed.[21] Some generators have the capability of automatically reversing polarity, in which case the physiological effects will be similar to AC current.[19]

In an alternating current, the continuous flow of electrons constantly changes direction or, stated differently, reverses its polarity. Electrons flowing in an alternating current always move from the negative to positive pole, reversing direction when polarity is reversed (Figure 7-2b).

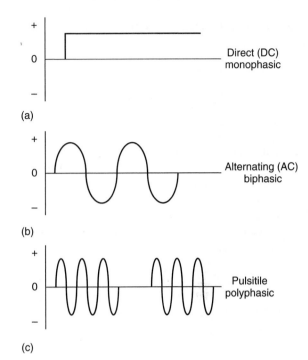

Figure 7-2   (a) Direct (DC) or monophasic current. (b) Alternating (AC) or biphasic current. (c) Pulsitile or polyphasic current.

alternating current   Current that periodically changes its polarity or direction of flow.

direct current   Galvanic current that always flows in the same direction and may flow in either a positive or a negative direction.

pulsitile (polyphasic) current   Current that contains three or more grouped phases in a single pulse and that is used in interferential and "Russian" currents.

Pulsitile currents usually contain three or more pulses grouped together (Figure 7-2c).[8] These groups of pulses are interrupted for short periods of time and repeat themselves at regular intervals. Pulsitile currents are used in interferential and so-called "Russian" currents that will be discussed in Chapter 8.[1,8]

Generators of Electrotherapeutic Currents

A great deal of confusion has developed relative to the terminology used to describe electrotherapeutic currents. All therapeutic electrical generators, regardless of whether they deliver AC, DC, or pulsitile currents through electrodes attached to the skin, are **transcutaneous electrical stimulators**. The majority of these are used to stimulate peripheral motor or sensory nerves and are correctly called **transcutaneous electrical nerve stimulators (TENS)**. Occasionally the terms **neuromuscular electrical stimulator (NMES)** or **electrical muscle stimulator (EMS)** are used interchangably with the term TENS to refer to any current that stimulates either nerve or muscle. Certainly NMES can be used for purposes such as muscle strengthening or to prevent disuse atrophy. However, these terms are perhaps most appropriate when the electrical current is being used to stimulate muscle directly, as would be the case with denervated muscle where peripheral nerves are not functioning. In recent years, a new type of transcutaneous electrical stimulator has gained popularity; it utilizes current intensities too small to excite peripheral nerves. The most common term used to describe these generators is **microcurrent electrical nerve stimulators (MENS)**. Most recently the term *MENS* has been replaced by the new term *Low Intensity Stimulation (LIS)*.[1,15,18]

There is no relationship between the type of current being delivered to the athlete by the generator and the type of current being used as a power source to drive the generator (i.e., a wall outlet or battery). Generators that produce electrotherapeutic currents may be driven by either alternating or direct currents. Devices that plug into the standard electrical wall outlet use alternating current. The commercially produced alternating current changes its direction of flow 120 times per second. In other words, there are 60 complete cycles per second. The number of cycles occurring in one second is called frequency and is indicated in Hertz (Hz), pulses per second (PPS), or cycles per second (CPS). The voltage of electromotive force

■ **Clinical Decision-Making**   *Exercise 7-1*

A student athletic trainer asks the clinical instructor the difference between a TENS unit and an NMES unit. How should the clinical instructor respond?

Commercial current

- 60 Hz either 120 V or 220 V

producing this alternating directional flow of electrons is set at a standard 120 V or 220 V. Thus, commercial alternating current is produced at 60 Hz with a corresponding voltage of either 120 V or 220 V.

Other electrotherapeutic devices are driven by batteries that always produce direct current, ranging between 1.5 and 9 V, although the devices driven by batteries may in turn produce modified types of current.

Components of Electrical Generators. To convert current coming from an AC power source to a DC current delivered to the athlete is accomplished by a series of electrical components within the stimulating unit: a **transformer**, a **rectifier**, a **filter**, a **regulator**, an **amplifier**, and an **oscillator**.[6,7] A transformer "steps down" or reduces the amount of voltage from the power sup-

transcutaneous electrical stimulator   All therapeutic electrical generators regardless of whether they deliver AC, DC, or pulsitile currents through electrodes attached to the skin.

transcutaneous electrical nerve stimulator (TENS)   A transcutaneous electrical stimulator used to stimulate peripheral nerves.

neuromuscular electrical stimulator (NMES)   Also called an electrical muscle stimulator (EMS), it is used to stimulate muscle directly as would be the case with denervated muscle where peripheral nerves are not functioning.

microcurrent electrical nerve stimulator (MENS)   Used primarily in tissue healing, the current intensities too small to excite peripheral nerves. (New term LIS.)

transformer   Reduces the amount of voltage from the power supply.

rectifier   Converts AC current to pulsating DC current.

filter   Changes pulsating DC current to smooth DC.

regulator   Produces a specific controlled voltage output.

oscillator   Used to produce and output a specific waveform, which may be different from that used to power or drive the stimulating unit.

output amplifier   Used to magnify or increase the amplitude of the voltage output of the generator and control it at a specific level.

waveform   The shape of an electrical current as displayed on an oscilloscope.

ply. The rectifier converts AC current to pulsating DC current. The filter changes the pulsating DC current to smooth DC. The regulator produces a specific controlled voltage output. An **output amplifier** within the stimulating unit is used to magnify or increase the amplitude of the voltage output of the generator and control it at a specific

■ **Clinical Decision-Making**   *Exercise 7-2*

An injured lacrosse player has a strain of the right quadriceps muscle group. The athletic trained has decided to use a high-volt electrical stimulator to induce a muscle contraction and is explaining how the electricity will do this when the athlete becomes fearful that there will be an electric shock. What should the athletic trainer explain about using electrical current to reassure the athlete?

Waveform shapes

- Sine
- Rectangular
- Square
- Spiked

level, regardless of the electrical impedance of the remainder of the circuit (including the electrodes and athlete). The oscillator is used to produce and output a specific waveform, which again may be different from that used to power or drive the stimulating unit.

WAVEFORMS

The term **waveform** indicates a graphic representation of the shape, direction, amplitude, duration, and pulse frequency of the electrical current being produced by the electrotherapeutic device, as displayed by an instrument called an oscilloscope (Figure 7-3).

Waveform Shape

Electrical currents may take on a *sine, rectangular, square,* or *spiked* waveform configuration, depending on the capabilities of the generator producing the current (Figure 7-4). Alternating, direct, and pulsitile currents may take on any of the waveform shapes.

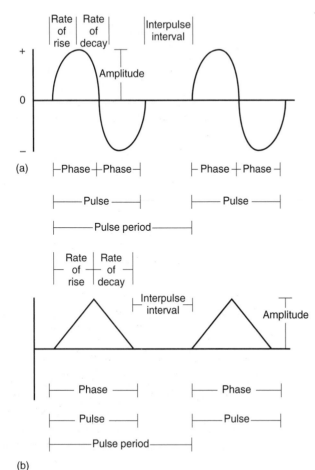

(a)

(b)

Figure 7-3   An individual waveform is referred to as a pulse. A pulse may contain either one or two phases, which is that portion of the pulse that rises above or below the baseline for some period of time. (a) Biphasic pulse. (b) Monophasic pulse.

Pulses versus Phases and Direction of Current Flow

On an oscilloscope, an individual waveform is referred to as a **pulse**. A pulse may contain either one or two **phases**, which is that portion of the pulse that rises above or below the baseline for some period of time. Direct current, also referred to as **monophasic current**, produces waveforms that have only a single phase in each pulse. Current flow

pulse   An individual waveform.

phases   That portion of the pulse that rises above or below the baseline for some period of time.

monophasic current   Another name for direct current, in which the direction of current flow remains the same.

biphasic current   Another name for alternating current, in which the direction of current flow reverses direction.

symetrical waveform   The size and shape of each phase of a waveform are identical.

asymetrical waveform   Either the size, or shape of a waveform is different in each phase of the waveform.

polyphasic current   Current that contains three or more grouped phases in a single pulse and that is used in interferential and "Russian" currents.

interpulse interval   The interruptions between individual pulses or groups of pulses.

intrapulse interval   The period of time between individual pulses.

is unidirectional, always flowing in the same direction toward either the positive or negative pole (Figure 7-3b). Conversely, alternating current, also referred to as **biphasic current**, produces waveforms that have two separate phases during each individual pulse. Current flow is bidirectional, reversing direction or polarity once during each pulse. Biphasic waveforms may be **symmetrical** or **asymmetrical.** If both phases of the waveform are symmetrical, the shape and size of each phase is identical (Figure 7-3a). Pulsitile current waveforms are called **polyphasic** and are representative of electrical current that is conducted as a series of pulses of short duration (μsec) followed by a short period of time when current is not flowing called the **interpulse interval** (msec). Single pulses may be interrupted by an **intrapulse interval** (see Figure 7-2c). Pulsitile current may flow in one direction as in DC current, or may reverse direction of flow as in AC current. With pulsed currents there is always some interruption of current flow.

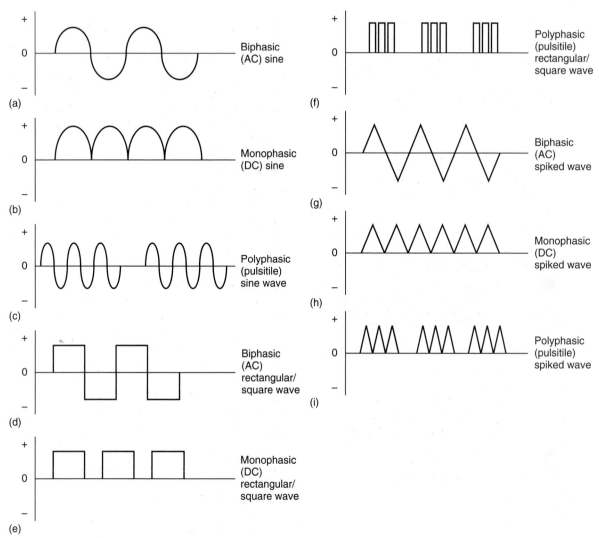

Figure 7-4   Waveforms of biphasic, monophasic, or polyphasic current may be sine, rectangular, square, or spiked in shape.

- Amplitude = Voltage = Current intensity

■ **Clinical Decision-Making**   *Exercise 7-3*

The athletic trainer is interested in producing a tetanic muscle contraction. What treatment parameter can be adjusted to produce this type of contraction?

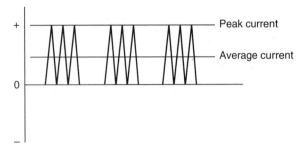

Figure 7-5 Average current is low compared to peak current amplitudes due to long interpulse intervals.

amplitude The intensity of current flow as indicated by the height of the waveform from baseline.

average current The amount of current flowing per unit of time.

pulse charge The total amount of electricity being delivered to the athlete during each pulse.

Pulse Amplitude

The **amplitude** of each pulse reflects the intensity of the current, the maximum amplitude being the tip or highest point of each phase (see Figure 7-3). The term *amplitude* is synonymous with the terms *voltage* and *current intensity*. The higher the amplitude, the greater the peak voltage or intensity. However, the peak amplitude should not be confused with the total amount of current being delivered to the tissues.

On electrical generators that produce short duration pulses, the total current produced (coulombs/sec) is low compared to peak current amplitudes because of long interpulse intervals that have current amplitudes of zero. Thus, the **average current**, or the amount of current flowing per unit of time, is relatively low, ranging from as low as 2mA (milliamps) to as high as 100 mA on some interferential generators. Average current can be increased by either increasing pulse duration or increasing pulse frequency or by some combination of the two (Figure 7-5).

rate of rise How quickly a waveform reaches its maximum amplitude.

decay time The time required for a waveform to go from peak amplitude to 0 V.

accommodation Adaptation by the sensory receptors to various stimuli over an extended period of time.

Pulse Charge

The term **pulse charge** refers to the total amount of electricity being delivered to the athlete during each pulse. With monophasic current, the phase charge and the pulse charge are the same, and it is always greater than zero. With biphasic current, the pulse charge is equal to the sum of the phase charges. If the pulse is symmetrical, the net pulse charge will be zero. In asymmetrical pulses, the net pulse charge is greater than zero, which by definition is a DC current.[1]

Pulse Rate of Rise and Decay Times

The **rate of rise** in amplitude or the rise time refers to how quickly the pulse reaches its maximum amplitude in each phase. Conversely, **decay time** refers to the time in which a pulse goes from peak amplitude to 0 V. The rate of rise is important physiologically because of the **accommodation** phenomenon, in which a fiber that has been subjected to a constant level of depolarization will become unexcitable at that same intensity or amplitude. Rate of rise and decay times are generally short, ranging

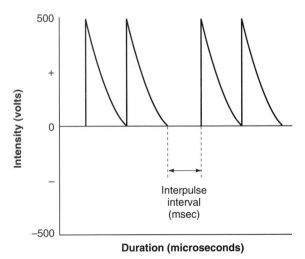

Figure 7-6   Most DC generators produce a twin-peak spiked pulse of short duration and high amplitude.

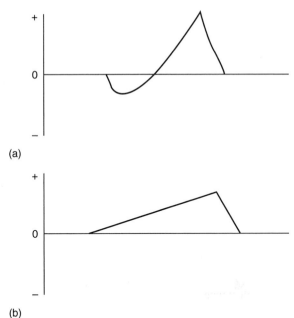

Figure 7-7   (a) Original faradic or asymmetric biphasic waveform. (b) Monophasic sawtooth or exponential waveform.

faradic current   An asymmetric biphasic waveform seldom used on modern electrical generators.

from nanoseconds (billionths of a second) to milliseconds (thousandths of a second) (see Figure 7-3).

By observing the three different waveforms, it is apparent that the sine wave has a gradual increase and decrease in amplitude for both alternating and direct currents (see Figure 7-4a,b,c). The rectangular wave has an almost instantaneous increase in amplitude, which plateaus for a period of time and then abruptly falls off (see Figure 7-4d,e,f). The triangular wave has a rapid increase and decrease in amplitude (see Figure 7-4g,h,i). The shape of these waveforms as they reach their maximum amplitude or intensity is directly related to the excitability of nervous tissue. The more rapid the increase in amplitude or the rate of rise, the greater the current's ability to excite nervous tissue.

Most modern DC generators make use of a twin-peak pulse of very short duration (1 to 70 microseconds) and peak amplitudes as high as 500 V (Figure 7-6). Combining high-peak intensity with short-phase duration produces a very comfortable type of current as well as an effective means of stimulating sensory, motor, and pain fibers.[22]

The effects of the various waveforms on biologic tissue will be discussed in Chapter 8.

Asymmetric Waveforms

Asymmetric biphasic waveforms have been used in the past but are seldom available on generators used by athletic trainers. Occasionally, manufacturers will indicate that their equipment is producing **faradic current**. However, the true faradic waveform is no longer used. The so-called faradic current is most likely a high-frequency (greater than 400 Hz) pulsed wave. The original faradic waveform (Figure 7-7a) could only have used alternating current because there was always a reversal of direction of current flow. The amplitude of the portion of the wave in the negative direction was not great enough to produce any physiologic response. Thus, the effects of this faradic wave would be similar to those of a direct current pulsed wave.[9]

In the monophasic sawtooth or exponential waveform (Figure 7-7b), the amplitude rises very

duration Sometimes referred to as pulse width. Indicates the length of time the current is flowing.

pulse period The combined time of the pulse duration and the interpulse interval.

frequency The number of cycles or pulses per second.

tetany Muscle condition that is caused by hyperexcitation and results in cramps and spasms.

bursts A combined set of three or more pulses; also referred to as packets or envelopes.

modulation Refers to any alteration in the magnitude or any variation in the duration of an electrical current.

gradually and then falls abruptly. Current that uses this waveform is used to stimulate denervated muscle without affecting normally innervated muscle, since the gradual rise in amplitude allows for accommodation of the normal muscle.[9]

Pulse Duration

The **duration** of each pulse indicates the length of time current is flowing in one cycle. With monophasic current, the *phase duration* is the same as the *pulse duration* and is the time from initiation of the phase to its end. With biphasic current, the *pulse duration* is determined by the combined *phase durations*. In some electrotherapeutic devices, the manufacturer presets the duration. Other devices have the capability of changing duration. The phase duration may be as short as a few microseconds or may be a long-duration direct current that flows for several minutes.

With pulsed currents, and in some instances with alternating and direct currents, the current flow is off for a period of time. The combined time of the pulse duration and the interpulse interval is referred to as the **pulse period** (see Figure 7-3).

Pulse Frequency

Pulse frequency indicates the number of pulses per second. Each individual pulse represents a rise and fall in amplitude. As the frequency of any waveform is increased, the amplitude tends to increase and decrease more rapidly. The muscular and nervous system responses depend on the length of time between pulses and on how the pulses or waveforms are modulated.[10] Muscle will respond with individual twitch contractions to pulse rates of less than 50 pulses per second. At 50 pulses per

second or greater, a **tetanic** contraction will result, regardless of whether the current is biphasic, monophasic, or polyphasic.

Stimulators have been clinically labeled as either low-, medium-, or high-frequency generators, and a great deal of misunderstanding exists over how these frequency ranges are classified.[1] Generally, all stimulating units are low-frequency electrical generators that deliver between one and several hundred pulses per second. Recently, a number of so-called medium-frequency generators have been developed that are claimed to have frequencies of 2500 to as high as 10,000 pulses per second. However, these high-frequency pulses are in reality groups of pulses combined as **bursts** that range in frequency from 1 to 200 pulses per second. These modulated bursts are capable of producing a physiologically effective frequency of stimulation only in this 1 to 200 pulse-per-second range, owing to the limitations of the absolute refractory period of nerve cell membranes. Therefore, many of the claims of equipment manufacturers relative to medium-frequency generators are inaccurate.[1]

Current Modulation

The physiologic responses to the various waveforms depend to a large extent on current **modulation**. Modulation refers to any alteration in the magnitude or any variation in duration of these pulses. Modulation may be *continuous, interrupted, burst,* or *ramped*.[1,11] The parameters of this modulation must be established according to various treatment goals.

Continuous Modulation. Continuous modulation means that the amplitude of current flow re-

medical galvanism   Creates either an acidic or alkaline environment that may be of therapeutic value.

iontophoresis   Uses continuous direct current to drive ions into the tissues.

Current modulation

- Continuous
- Interrupted
- Burst
- Ramped

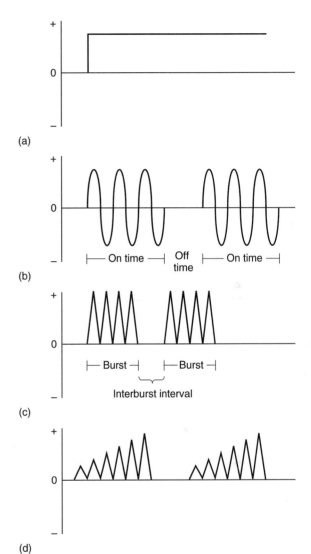

(a)

(b)

(c)

(d)

Figure 7-8   Current may be modulated using (a) continuous, (b) interrupted, (c) burst, or (d) ramped modes.

mains the same for several seconds or perhaps minutes. Continuous modulation is usually associated with long-pulse-duration direct current (Figure 7-8a). With direct current, flow is always in a uniform direction. In the discussion of physiologic responses to electrical currents, it was indicated that positive and negative ions are attracted toward poles or, in this case, electrodes of opposite polarity. This accumulation of charged ions over a period of time creates either an acidic or alkaline environment that may be of therapeutic value. This therapeutic technique has been referred to as **medical galvanism**. The technique of **iontophoresis** (Chapter 9) also uses continuous direct current to transport ions into the tissues. If the amplitude is great enough to produce a muscle contraction, the contraction will occur only when the current flow is turned on or off. Thus, with direct-current continuous modulation, there will be a muscle contraction both when the current is turned on and when it is turned off. Continuous modulation is also used with alternating current primarily for the purpose of eliciting muscle contractions.

Interrupted Modulation.   With interrupted modulation, current flows for some period of time called the *on time*, and is then periodically turned off during the *off time*. On most units, on time may be set between 1 and 60 seconds, while off time may

be set between 1 and 120 seconds. Interrupted modulation is used with monophasic or biphasic currents. Current with sine, rectangular, or spiral shaped waveforms may be interrupted. Interrupted modulation is used in sports medicine for muscle reeducation and strengthening and for improving range of motion (Figure 7-8b).

ramping Another name for surging modulation, in which the current builds gradually to some maximum amplitude.

circuit The path of current from a generating source through the various components back to the generating source.

series circuit A circuit in which there is only one path for current to get from one terminal to another.

parallel cricuit A circuit in which two or more routes exist for current to pass between the two terminals.

Burst Modulation. Burst modulation occurs when pulsed current flows for a short duration (milliseconds) and then is turned off for a short time (milliseconds) in a repetitive cycle. With polyphasic currents, sets of pulses are combined. These combined pulses are most commonly referred to in the literature as bursts but have also been called *packets, envelopes, pulse trains*, or *beats* (as is the case with interferential currents).[13] The interruptions between individual bursts are called interburst intervals (Figure 7-8c). The interburst interval is much too short to have any effect on a muscle contraction. Thus, the physiologic effects of a burst of pulses will be the same as with a single pulse.[1] Bursts may be used with monophasic and biphasic currents as well.

Ramping Modulation. In **ramping** modulation, also called surging modulation, current amplitude will increase or ramp up gradually to some preset maximum and may also decrease or ramp down in intensity (Figure 7-8d,e). Ramp-up time is usually preset at about one third of the time. The ramp-down option is not available on all machines. Most modern stimulators allow the athletic trainer to set the on time and the off time between 1 and 10 seconds. Ramping modulation is used in sports medicinally to elicit muscle contraction and is generally considered to be a very comfortable type of current since it allows for a gradual increase in the intensity of a muscle contraction.

ELECTRICAL CIRCUITS

The path of current from a generating power source through various components back to the generating source is called an electrical **circuit**. A *closed circuit* is one in which electrons are flowing, and in

an *open circuit* the current flow ceases. Electronic circuits are not ordinarily composed of single elements; they often encompass several branches or components with different resistances. The current in each branch may be easily calculated if the individual resistances are known and if the amount of voltage applied to the circuit is also known.[5]

With the development of the microelectronics industry, we all know that electrical circuits can be extremely complex. However, all electrical circuits have several basic components. There is a power source, which is capable of producing voltage. There is some type of conducting medium or pathway, along which current travels and which carries the flowing electrons. Finally, there is some component or group of components that are driven by this flowing current. These driven elements provide resistance to electrical flow.[5]

Series and Parallel Circuits

The components that provide resistance to current flow may be connected to one another in one of two different patterns: (1) a **series circuit** or (2) a **parallel circuit**. The main difference between these two is that in a series circuit, there is only one path for current to get from one terminal to another. In a parallel circuit, two or more routes exist for current to pass between the two terminals.

In a series circuit, the components are placed end to end (Figure 7-9). The number of amperes of an electrical current flowing through a series circuit is exactly the same at any point in that circuit. The resistance to current flow in this total circuit is equal to the resistance of all the components in the circuit added together.

$$R_T = R_1 + R_2 + R_3$$

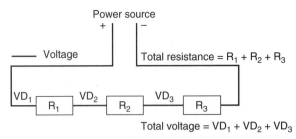

Figure 7-9 In a series circuit, the component resistors are placed end to end. The total resistance to current flow is equal to the resistance of all the components added together. There is a voltage decrease at each component such that the sum of the voltage decreases is equal to the total voltage.

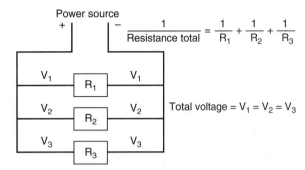

Figure 7-10 In a parallel circuit, the component resistors are placed side by side and the ends are connected. The current flow in each of the pathways is inversely proportional to the resistance of the pathway. The total voltage is the sum of the voltages at each component.

Electrical energy is required to force the current through the resistor, and this energy is dissipated in the form of heat. Consequently, there is a decrease in voltage at each component such that the total voltage at the beginning of the circuit is equal to the sum of the voltage decreases at each component.

$$V_T = VD_1 + VD_2 + VD_3$$

In a parallel circuit, the component resistors are placed side by side, and the ends are connected (Figure 7-10). Each of the resistors in a parallel circuit receives the same voltage. The current passing through each component depends on its resistance. So the total voltage will be exactly the same as the voltage at each component.

$$V_T = V_1 = V_2 = V_3$$

Each additional resistance added to a parallel circuit in effect decreases the total resistance. Adding an alternative pathway, regardless of its resistance to current flow, improves the ability of the current to get from one point to another. The current will, in general, choose the pathway that offers the least resistance. The formula for determining total resistance in a parallel circuit, according to Ohm's law, is

$$\frac{1}{R_T} = \frac{1}{R_1} + \frac{1}{R_2} + \frac{1}{R_3}$$

Thus, component resistors connected in a series circuit have a higher resistance and lower cur-

rent flow, and resistors in a parallel circuit have a lower resistance and a higher current flow.

The electrical modalities in general make use of some combination of both series and parallel circuits.[9] For example, to elicit a muscle contraction, the electrodes from an electrical stimulating unit are placed on the skin (Figure 7-11). The current from those electrodes must pass directly through the skin and fat. The total resistance to current flow seen by the electrical stimulating unit is equal to the combined resistances at each electrode. This passage of current through the skin is basically a series circuit.

After the current passes through the skin and fat, it comes into contact with a number of different

■ Analogy *7-3*

Series and parallel electrical circuits would be like obstacle courses set up for training military personnel. In one type of course (series circuit), the obstacles (component resistors) are set up end to end so that the soldier must go over or through each obstacle to complete the course. In the second type (parallel circuit), obstacles are set up side by side, and the soldier must choose the obstacle that is the easiest (offers the least resistance) so that he or she can finish the course quickly.

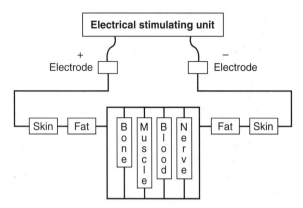

Figure 7-11 The electrical circuit that exists when electrons flow through human tissue is in reality a combination of a series and parallel circuit.

types of biologic tissue (i.e., bone, connective tissue, blood, muscle). The current has several different pathways through which it may reach the muscle to be stimulated. The total current traveling through these tissues is the sum of the currents in each different type of tissue, and since there are additional tissues through which current may travel, the total resistance is effectively reduced. Thus, in this typical application of a therapeutic modality, both parallel and series circuits are used to produce the desired physiologic effect.

CURRENT FLOW THROUGH BIOLOGIC TISSUES

As stated previously, electrical current tends to choose the path that offers the least resistance to flow or, stated differently, the material that is the best conductor.[22] The conductivity of the different types of tissue in the body is variable. Typically tissue that is highest in water content and consequently highest in ion content is the best conductor of electricity.

The skin has different layers that vary in water content, but generally the skin offers the primary resistance to current flow and is considered an insulator. Skin preparation for the purpose of reducing electrical impedance is of primary concern with electrodiagnostic apparatus (as discussed in

Chapter 13 on biofeedback), but it is also important with electrotherapeutic devices. The greater the impedance of the skin, the higher the voltage of the electrical current must be to stimulate underlying nerve and muscle. Chemical changes in the skin can make it more resistant to certain types of current. Thus, skin impedance is generally higher with direct current than with alternating current.

Blood is a biologic tissue that is composed largely of water and ions and is consequently the best electrical conductor of all of the tissues. Muscle is composed of about 75% water and depends on the movement of ions for contraction. Muscle tends to propagate an electrical impulse much more effectively in a longitudinal direction than transversely. Muscle tendons are considerably more dense than muscle, contain relatively little water, and are considered poor conductors. Fat contains only about 14% water and is thought to be a poor conductor. Peripheral nerve conductivity is approximately 6 times that of muscle. However, fat and a fibrous sheath, both of which are considered to be poor conductors, generally surround the nerve. Bone is extremely dense, contains only about 5% water, and is considered to be the poorest biologic conductor of electrical current. It is essential for the athletic trainer to understand that many biologic tissues will be stimulated by an electrical current. Selecting the appropriate treatment parameters is critical if the desired tissue response is to be attained.

Physiologic Responses to Electrical Current

The effects of electrical current passing through the various tissues of the body may be thermal, chemical, or physiologic.[3,19]

All electrical currents cause a rise in temperature in a conducting (tissue).[16] The tissues of the body possess varying degrees of resistance, and those of higher resistance should heat up more when electrical current passes through. As indicated in previous chapters, the diathermies generate a continuous high-frequency electrical current that is designed to produce a tissue temperature in-

Responses to electrical current

- Thermal
- Chemical
- Physiologic

■ **Clinical Decision-Making**   *Exercise 7-5*

When installing a whirlpool in the hydrotherapy area, the athletic trainer must always be concerned about the possibility of electrical shock. What measures can be taken to reduce the possibility of electrical shock?

crease. The electrical currents used for stimulation of nerve and muscle have a relatively low average current flow that produces minimal thermal effects.

Electrical currents are used to produce either muscle contractions or modification of pain impulses through effects on the motor and sensory nerves. This function is dependent to a great extent on selecting the appropriate treatment parameters based on the principles identified in this chapter.[16]

Electrical currents are also used to produce chemical effects. Most biologic tissue contains negatively and positively charged ions. A direct current flow will cause migration of these charged particles toward the pole of opposite polarity. At the positive pole the negatively charged particles cause an acid reaction in which there is coagulation of protein and hardening of the tissues. At the negative pole the positively charged particles produce an alkaline reaction, liquefying protein and causing softening of the tissues.

SAFETY IN THE USE OF ELECTRICAL EQUIPMENT

Electrical safety in the sports medicine setting should be of maximal concern to the professional athletic trainer. Too often there are reports of athletes being electrocuted as a result of faulty electri-

ground   A wire that makes an electrical connection with the earth.

cal circuits in whirlpools. This type of accident can be avoided by taking some basic precautions and acquiring some understanding of the power distribution system and electrical grounds.

The typical electrical circuit consists of a source producing electrical power, a conductor that carries the power to a resistor or series of driven elements, and a conductor that carries the power back to the power source.

Electrical power is carried from generating plants through high-tension power lines carrying 2200 V. The power is decreased by a transformer and is supplied in the wall outlet at 220 V or 120 V with a frequency of 60 Hz. The voltage at the outlet is alternating current, which means that one of the poles, the "hot" or "live" wire, is either positive or negative with respect to other neutral lines. Theoretically, the voltage of the neutral pole should be zero. Actually the voltage of the neutral line is about 10 V. Thus, both hot and neutral lines carry some voltage with respect to the earth, which has zero voltage. The voltage from either of these two leads may be sufficient to cause physiologic damage.

The two-pronged plug has only two leads, both of which carry some voltage. Consequently, the electrical device has no true ground. The term true **ground** literally means the electrical circuit is connected to the earth or the ground, which has the ability to accept large electrical charges without becoming charged itself. The ground will continually accept these charges until the electrical potential has been neutralized. Therefore, the ground almost immediately neutralizes any electrical charge that may be potentially hazardous (i.e., any electricity escaping from the circuit). If an individual were to come in contact with a short-circuited instrument that was not grounded, the electrical current would flow through that individual to reach the ground.

Electrical devices that have two-pronged plugs generally rely on the chassis or casing of the power source to act as a ground. The danger with the

- Electrical modalities use a combination of both series and parallel circuits to stimulate the tissues

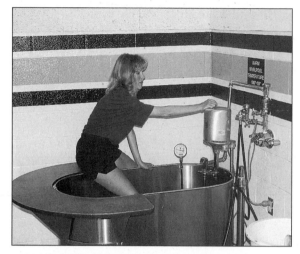

Figure 7-12 When a therapeutic device is not properly grounded, there is danger of electrical shock. This is a major problem in a whirlpool.

microshock An electrical shock that is imperceptible because of a leakage of current of less than 1 mA.

macroshock An electrical shock that can be felt and has a leakage of electrical current of greater than 1 mA.

two-pronged plug devices is that there is no true ground. So if an individual were to touch the casing of the instrument while in contact with some object or instrument that has a true ground, an electrical shock may result. With three-pronged plugs, the third prong is grounded directly to the earth and all excess electrical energy should theoretically be neutralized through this.

By far the most common mechanism of injury from therapeutic devices results when there is some damage, breakdown, or short circuit to the power cord. When this happens, the casing of the machine becomes electrically charged. In other words, there is a voltage leak, and in a device that is not properly grounded, electrical shock may occur (Figure 7-12).

The magnitude of the electrical shock is a critical factor in terms of potential health danger (Table 7-2). Shock from electrical currents flowing at one or less mamps will not be felt and is referred to as **microshock**. Shock from a current flow greater than 1 mamp is called **macroshock**. Currents that range between 1 and 15 mamps produce a tingling sensation or perhaps some muscle contraction. Currents flowing at 15 to 100 mamps cause a painful electrical shock. Currents between 100 and 200 mamps may result in fibrillation of cardiac muscle or respiratory arrest. When current flow is above 200 mamps, there is rapid burning and destruction of tissue.[14]

Most electrotherapeutic devices (e.g., muscle stimulators, ultrasound, and the diathermies) are generally used in dry environments. All new electrotherapeutic equipment being produced has three-pronged plugs and is thus grounded to the earth. However, in a wet or damp area, the three-pronged plug may not provide sufficient protection from electrical shock.

We know that the body will readily conduct electricity because of its high water content. If the body is wet or if an individual is standing in water, the resistance to electrical flow is reduced even more. Thus, if a short should occur, the shock could be as much as 5 times greater in this damp or wet environment. The potential danger that exists with whirlpools or tubs is obvious. The ground on the whirlpool will supposedly conduct all current leakage from a faulty motor or power cord to the earth. However, an individual in a whirlpool is actually a part of that circuit and is subject to the same current levels as any other component of the circuit. Small amounts of current can therefore be potentially harmful no matter how well the apparatus is grounded. For this reason, in 1981 the National Electrical Code required that all health care facilities

ground-fault interrupters (GFI) A safety device that automatically shuts off current flow and reduces the chances of electrical shock.

■ **TABLE 7-2** Physiologic Effects of Electrical Shock at Varying Magnitudes

INTENSITY	PHYSIOLOGIC EFFECTS
0–1 mA	Imperceptible
1–15 mA	Tingling sensation and muscle contraction
15–100 mA	Painful electrical shock
100–200 mA	Cardiac or respiratory arrest
> 200 mA	Instant tissue burning and destruction

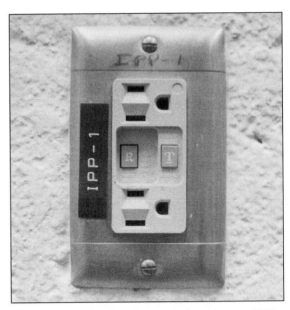

Figure 7-13 A typical ground-fault interrupter (GFI).

using whirlpools and tubs install **ground-fault interrupters (GFI)** (Figure 7-13). These devices constantly compare the amount of electricity flowing from the wall outlet to the whirlpool turbine with the amount returning to the outlet. If there is any leakage in current flow detected, the ground-fault circuit breaker will automatically interrupt current flow in as little as one fortieth of a second, thus shutting off current flow and reducing the chances of electrical shock.[17] These devices may be installed either in the electrical outlet or in the circuit breaker box.

Regardless of the type of electrotherapeutic device being used and the type of environment, the following safety practices should be considered:

1. The entire electrical system of the building or training room should be designed or evaluated by a qualified electrician. Problems with the electrical system may exist in older buildings or in situations where rooms have been modified to accommodate therapeutic devices (e.g., putting a whirlpool in a locker room where the concrete floor is always wet or damp).

2. It should not be assumed that all three-pronged wall outlets are automatically grounded to the earth. The ground must be checked.

3. The athletic trainer should become very familiar with the equipment being used and with any potential problems that may exist or develop. Any defective equipment should be immediately removed from the clinic.

4. The plug should not be jerked out of the wall by pulling on the cable.

5. Extension cords or multiple adaptors should never be used.

6. Equipment should be re-evaluated on a yearly basis and should conform to National Electrical Code guidelines. If a clinic or training room is not in compliance with this code, then there is no legal protection in a lawsuit.

7. Common sense should always be exercised when using electrotherapeutic devices. A situation that appears to be potentially dangerous may in fact result in injury or death.

Summary

1. Electrons move along a conducting medium as an electrical current.
2. A volt is the electromotive force that produces a movement of electrons; an ampere is a unit of measurement that indicates the rate at which electrical current is flowing.
3. Ohm's law expresses the relationship between current flow voltage and resistance. The current flow is directly proportional to the voltage and inversely proportional to the resistance.
4. Electrotherapeutic devices generate three different types of current: alternating (AC) or biphasic, direct (DC) or monophasic, or pulsitile or polyphasic, which, when introduced into biologic tissue, are capable of producing specific physiologic changes.
5. Confusion exists relative to the terminology used to describe electrotherapeutic currents, but all therapeutic electrical generators, regardless of whether they deliver AC, DC, or pulsitile currents through electrodes attached to the skin, are transcutaneous electrical stimulators.
6. The term *pulse* is synonymous with *waveform*, which indicates a graphic representation of the shape, direction, amplitude, duration, and pulse frequency of the electrical current being produced by the electrotherapeutic device, as displayed by an instrument called an oscilloscope.
7. Modulation refers to any alteration in the magnitude or any variation in duration of a pulse (or pulses) and may be continuous, interrupted, burst, or ramped.
8. The main difference between a series and a parallel circuit is that in a series circuit there is a single pathway for current to get from one terminal to another, and in a parallel circuit two or more routes exist for current to pass.
9. The electrical circuit that exists when electron flow is through human tissue is in reality a combination of both a series and a parallel circuit.
10. The effects of electrical current moving through biologic tissue may be chemical, thermal, or physiologic.
11. Electrical safety is critical when using electrotherapeutic devices. It is the responsibility of the athletic trainer to make sure that all electrical modalities conform to the National Electrical Code.

Review Questions

1. How are the following electrical terms defined: potential difference, ampere, volt, ohm, and watt?
2. What is the mathematical expression of Ohm's law and what does it represent?
3. What are the three different types of electrical current?
4. What is a transcutaneous electrical stimulator and how is it related to a TENS unit?
5. What are the different types of waveforms that may be produced by electrical stimulating generators?
6. What are the various pulse characteristics of the different waveforms?
7. How can electrical currents be modulated?
8. What are the differences between series and parallel circuits?
9. How does electrical current travel through various types of biologic tissue?
10. What steps can the athletic trainer take to ensure safety of the athlete when using electrical modalities?

Self-Test Questions

T/F
1. Electrons tend to flow from areas of low concentration to areas of high concentration.
2. Insulators resist current flow.
3. The greater the voltage, the greater the amplitude.

Multiple Choice
4. A particle of matter with very little mass and a negative charge is a(n)
   a. ion
   b. electron
   c. neutron
   d. proton
5. What is the name of the unit measuring the force necessary to produce electron movement?
   a. ampere (amp)
   b. coulomb (c)
   c. volt (V)
   d. watt (W)
6. In _____ current, electron flow constantly changes direction.
   a. alternating
   b. direct
   c. pulsitile
   d. galvanic

7. When the current increases gradually to a maximal amplitude, it is known as - _____ .
   a. burst
   b. ramping
   c. modulation
   d. galvanic
8. In _____ circuits, electrons have only one path to follow.
   a. galvanic
   b. parallel
   c. resistor
   d. series
9. Human response(s) to electrical current include
   a. thermal
   b. chemical
   c. physiologic
   d. all of the above
10. All whirlpools and tubs in a health care setting must have _____ .
    a. ground-fault interruptors
    b. a 3-prong outlet
    c. an insulated cord
    d. a waterproof motor

Solutions to Clinical Decision-Making Exercises

7-1   The terms TENS and NMES are for all intent and purposes interchangeable in terms of their physiologic effects. Both units can be used to stimulate peripheral motor or sensory nerves.

7-2   The athletic trainer should make it perfectly clear that even though the generator is producing a high-voltage current, the amperage is very small in the milliamp range and thus the total amount of electrical energy being output to the athlete is very small. It is important to explain exactly what the athlete will

feel, especially if this is the first time that he has experienced electrical stimulation.

7-3   The athletic trainer can simply increase current intensity sufficiently to produce a muscle contraction and then adjust the frequency to approximately 50 pulses per second. This will produce a tetanic contraction regardless of whether AC, DC, or pulsitile current is being used.

7-4   To accomplish both of the effects, only a long duration continuous DC current is capable of producing ion movement. Continuous DC current can also elicit a muscle contraction when the current is turned on and off.

7-5 The National Electrical Code requires that all whirlpools have ground-fault interruptors installed to automatically shut off current flow. In addition the athletic trainer should not allow the athlete to turn the whirlpool on and off. This is especially important when the athlete is already in contact with the water. Extension cords or multiple adaptors should never be used in the hydrotherapy area.

References

1. Alon, G: Principles of electrical stimulation. In Nelson, R, and Currier, D, editors: *Sports medicine electrotherapy*, Norwalk, Conn., 1991, Appleton-Lange.
2. Berqueld, F: *Electromedical instrumentation: a guide for medical personnel*, Cambridge, 1980, Cambridge University Press.
3. Carlos, J: Clinical electrotherapy part I: physiology and basic concepts, *PT—Magazine of Physical Therapy* 6(4):44–46, 48–57, 1998.
4. Chamishion, R: *Basic medical electronics*, Boston, 1964, Little, Brown & Co.
5. Cohen, H, and Brunilik, J: *Manual of electroneuromyography*, ed 2, New York, Harper & Row.
6. Cook, T, and Barr, J: Instrumentation. In Nelson, R, and Currier, D, editors: *Sports medicine electrotherapy*, Norwalk, Conn., 1991, Appleton-Lange.
7. Cromwell, J, Arditti, M, and Weibell, F: *Medical instrumentation for health care*, Englewood Cliffs, N.J., 1976, Prentice Hall.
8. DeDomenico, G: *Basic guidelines for interferential therapy*, Sydney, Australia, 1981, Theramed.
9. Griffin, J, and Karselis, T: *Physical agents for physical athletic trainers*, Springfield, Ill., 1988, Charles C Thomas.
10. Holcomb, WR: A practical guide to electrical therapy, *Journal of Sport Rehabilitation* 6(3):272–282, 1997.
11. Kloth, L, and Cummings, J: *Electrotherapeutic terminology in physical therapy*, Alexandria, Va., 1990. Section on sports medicine electrophysiology and the American Physical Therapy Association.
12. Licht, S: *Therapeutic electricity and ultraviolet radiation*, vol. IV, ed 2, Baltimore, 1969, Waverly.
13. McLoda, TA, and Carmack, JA: Optimal burst duration during a facilitated quadriceps femoris contraction, *Journal of Athletic Training* 35(2):145–150, 2000.
14. Myklebust, B, and Kloth, L: Electrodiagnostic and electrotherapeutic instrumentation: characteristics of recording and stimulation systems and principles of safety. In Gersh, MR, ed: *Electrotherapy in rehabilitation*, Philadelphia, 1992, FA Davis.
15. Myklebust, B, and Robinson, A: Instrumentation. In Snyder-Mackler, L, and Robinson, A: *Sports medicine electrophysiology, electrotherapy and electrotherapy and electrophysiologic testing*, Baltimore 1989, Williams and Wilkins.
16. Nalty, T, and Sabbaki, M: *Electrotherapy clinical procedures manual*, Boston, 2000, McGraw-Hill.
17. Porter, M, and Porter, J: Electrical safety in the training room, *Athletic Training* 16(4):263–264, 1981.
18. Robinson, A: Basic concepts and terminology in electricity. In Snyder-Mackler, L, and Robinson, A: *Clinical electrophysiology, electrotherapy and electrotherapy and electrophysiologic testing*, Baltimore 1989, Williams and Wilkins.
19. Shriber, W: *A manual of electrotherapy*, ed 4, Philadelphia, 1975, Lea & Febiger.
20. Stillwell, G: *Therapeutic electricity and ultraviolet radiation*, ed 3, Baltimore, 1983, Williams & Wilkins.
21. Watkins, A: *A manual of electrotherapy*, ed 3, Philadelphia, 1968, Lea & Febiger.
22. Wolf, S: *Electrotherapy: clinics in physical therapy*, vol. 2, New York, 1981, Churchill Livingstone.

Suggested Readings

Alon, G: *High voltage stimulation: a monograph*, Chattanooga, Tenn., 1984, Chattanooga Corporation.

Alon, G: Electrical stimulators, Chattanooga, Tenn., 1985, Chattanooga Corporation (video presentation).

Alon, G, Allin, J, and Inbar, G: Optimization of pulse duration and pulse charge during TENS, *Aust. J. Physiother.* 29:195, 1983.

Baker, L, McNeal, D, and Benton, L: *Neuromuscular Electrical stimulation: a practical guide*, Downey, Calif., 1993, Rancho Los Amigos Hospital.

Benton, L, Baker, L, and Bowman, B: *Functional electrical stimulation: a practical sports medicine guide*, Downey, Calif., 1980, Rancho Los Amigos Hospital.

Binder, S: In Wolf, S, editor: *Electrotherapy*, New York, 1981, Churchill Livingstone.

Bowman, B, and Baker, L: Effects of waveform parameters on comfort during transcutaneous neuromuscular electrical stimulation, *Ann Bioned Eng* 13:59–74, 1985.

Brown, I: *Fundamentals of electrotherapy*, course guide, Madison, Wis., 1963, University of Wisconsin Press.

Campbell, J: A critical appraisal of the electrical output characteristics of ten TENS units, *Clin. Phys. Physiol. Meas.* 3:141, 1982.

Geddes, L: A short history of electrical stimulation of excitable tissue, *Physiologist* 27:1, 1984.

Geddes, L, and Baler, L: *Applied biomedical instrumentation*, New York, 1975, John Wiley.

Kahn, J: *Principles and practice of electrotherapy*, New York, 1994, Churchill Livingstone.

Kottke, F: *Handbook of physical medicine and rehabilitation*, ed 3, Philadelphia, 1982, WB Saunders.

Lane, J: Electrical impedances of superficial limb tissues, epidermis, dermis, and muscle sheath, *Ann. N.Y. Acad. Sci.* 238: 812, 1974.

Licht, S: *Electrodiagnosis and electromyography*, vol. 1, ed 3, Baltimore, 1971, Waverly.

Mannheimer, J, and Lampe, G: *Sports medicine transcutaneous electrical nerve stimulation*, Philadelphia, 1984, FA Davis.

Nelson, R, and Currier, D: *Sports medicine electrotherapy*, Norwalk, Conn., 1987, Appleton-Lange.

Newton, R: *Electrotherapy: selecting wave form parameters*. Paper presented at the American Physical Therapy Association Conference, Washington, D.C., 1981.

Newton, R: *Electrotherapeutic treatment: selecting appropriate wave form characteristics*, Clinton, N.J., 1984, Preston.

Reismann, M.: A comparison of electrical stimulators eliciting muscle contraction, *Phys Ther* 64:751, 1984.

Scott, P: *Clayton's electrotherapy and actinotherapy*, eds 5 and 7, Baltimore, 1965 and 1975, Williams & Wilkins.

Sunderland, S: *Nerves and nerve injuries*, Baltimore, 1968, Williams & Wilkins.

Wadsworth, H, and Chanmugan, A: *Electrophysical agents in physical therapy*, Marickville, Australia, 1983, Science Press.

Ward, A: *Electricity waves and fields in therapy*. Marickville, Australia, 1980, Science Press.

CHAPTER 8

Electrical Stimulating Currents

Daniel N. Hooker

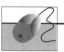

Study Resources

Refer to the lab exercises in the accompanying Laboratory Manual, as well as eSims which simulates the athletic training certification exam at www.mhhe.com/esims. Also, check out the competency information found at www.mhhe.com/prentice11e. For more online study resources, visit our Health and Human Performance Website at www.mhhe.com/hhp/.

Following completion of this chapter, the student athletic trainer will be able to

- Explain muscle and nerve responses to electrical stimulation.

- Describe nonexcitatory cell and tissue responses to electrical stimulation.

- Articulate the uses of electrically stimulated muscle contractions.

- Establish the various treatment parameters that must be considered with electrical stimulating currents.

- Determine the effect of noncontractable stimulation on edema.

- Compare techniques for the modulation of pain through the use of electrical stimulating currents.

- Differentiate between specialized electrical current generators in relation to physiologic changes and benefits.

- Identify problems that might respond to electrical stimulation.

Often the athletic trainer uses electrical stimulating currents for treatment in an effort to create a quick cure for the physical problems suffered by his or her athletes. Although electrical treatments can provide dramatic results at times, this is the exception rather than the rule. The use of electricity in treating an injury can be beneficial, but the athletic trainer must base the use of electricity on facts about the effects of electricity on biologic tissues. The treatment program must be tailored toward influencing the problems identified in the evaluation. Electrical therapy should not be used in a "shotgun" approach if we are to maximize the effectiveness of this modality.

The clinical use of electrotherapy has changed as the changing technology has enabled the equipment manufacturers to design and promote their latest product lines. Modern electronics has opened the doors to electronic equipment that could conceivably generate any electrical output desired. Wave shapes, amplitudes, and frequencies all can be manipulated so that any combination might be possible.

The research is, as usual, lagging behind commercial development. Of the research that has been and will be conducted, experts will continue to disagree with or challenge the interpretations of the results. Researchers in the biologic responses find it difficult to isolate one variable for experimentation and maintain control of all the other variables that

....

bioelectromagnetics   The study of biologic tissues' electrical and magnetic properties.

....

could affect their results. Deciding whether the results of a study are significant for cause and effect or are merely a chance happening or are significant but not directly caused by the manipulation of the experimental variable becomes very difficult for the clinician. There are still more questions than answers in this field of research.

Electrotherapy of the future is moving toward attempts at controlling cellular and tissue function with externally generated electrical currents. The athletic trainer will need the concepts of **bioelectromagnetics**, the study of biologic tissues' electrical and magnetic properties, to apply and understand the therapeutic outcomes of the next generation of electrical modalities. Knowledge of the electric properties of cells, intercellular, intracellular communication, bioelectric potentials, tissue currents, strain generated electric potentials, and the biologic effects of other nonionizing energy will be essential for the expert clinician to use present and future electrical modalities for maximum therapeutic benefit.[23,24]

PHYSIOLOGIC RESPONSE TO ELECTRICAL CURRENTS

Electricity will have an effect on each cell and tissue that it passes through.[23,24,112] The type and extent of this response are dependent on (1) the type of tissue and its response characteristics (for example, how it normally functions and how it grows or changes under normal stress); and (2) the nature of the current applied (that is, direct or alternating, intensity, duration, voltage, and density). The tissue should respond to electrical energy in a manner similar to that in which it normally functions or grows. These statements are true within a certain range of current parameters, but current density above critical levels can cause coagulation and tissue destruction.[2] Clinically,

■ **TABLE 8-1**   Summary of Indications and Contraindications for Electrical Stimulating Currents

....

INDICATIONS

modulation of acute, postacute, and chronic pain
muscle contraction
stimulating contraction of denervated muscle
muscle re-education
retardation of atrophy
muscle strengthening
increasing range of motion
decreasing edema
decreasing muscle spasm
decreasing muscle guarding
stimulate the healing process
wound healing
fracture healing
tendon healing
ligament healing
stimulate nerve regeneration
stimulate peripheral nervous system function
change membrane permeability
protein synthesis
stimulate fibroblasts and osteoblasts
tissue regeneration
increase circulation through muscle pumping
   contractions

CONTRAINDICATIONS

pacemakers
infection
malignancies
pregnancy
musculoskeletal problems where muscle contraction
   would exacerbate the condition

....

athletic trainers use electrical currents for the following (see Table 8-1):

1. Creating muscle contraction through nerve or muscle stimulations.
2. Stimulating sensory nerves to help in treating pain.

Therapeutic uses of electricity

- Muscle contraction
- Sensory stimulation

Physiologic responses

- Excitatory
- Nonexcitatory

3. Creating an electrical field in biologic tissues to stimulate or alter the healing process.[20]
4. Creating an electrical field on the skin surface to drive ions beneficial to the healing process into or through the skin.

As electricity moves through the body's conductive medium, changes in the physiologic functioning can occur at various levels of the total system. Four levels can be readily identified from the functional standpoint:

I. Cellular
II. Tissue
III. Segmental
IV. Systematic

As in all classification systems there is some overlap, and assignment to one level may be a bit arbitrary. The effects can be defined as follows:

Cellular level—can be broken down into 5 major effects

1. excitation of nerve cells
2. changes in cell membrane permeability
3. protein synthesis
4. stimulation of fibroblast, osteoblast
5. modification of microcirculation

Tissue level—this requires multiple cellular events

1. skeletal muscle contraction
2. smooth muscle contraction
3. tissue regeneration

Segmental level—involves a regional effect of the previous two level activities

1. modification of joint mobility
2. muscle pumping action to change circulation and lymphatic activity
3. an alteration of the microvascular system not associated with muscle pumping
4. an increased movement of charged proteins into the lymphatic channels with subsequent oncotic force bringing increases in fluid to the lymph system; lymphatic contraction increases as a result and more fluid is moved centrally
5. transcutaneous electrical stimulation cannot directly stimulate lymph smooth muscle or the autonomic nervous system without also stimulating a motor nerve; it is possible that sensory stimulation may have indirectly activated the autonomic system, and the autonomic system may have released an adrenergic substance that would enhance the lymph smooth muscle contraction

Systematic effects—throughout the entire system

1. analgesic effects as endogenous pain suppressors are released and act at different levels to control pain
2. analgesic effects from the stimulation of certain neurotransmitters to control neural activity in the presence of pain stimuli.[4]

These responses can be broken into direct and indirect effects. There is always a direct effect along the lines of current flow and under the electrodes. Indirect effects occur remote to the area of current flow and are usually the result of stimulating a natural physiologic event to occur.[4,27]

If a certain effect is desired from stimulation, goals must be established to achieve a specific physiologic response as a goal of your treatment. These responses can be grouped into two basic physiologic responses: nonexcitatory and excitatory.

The excitatory is the most obvious and the one that has been used the most often in the past in treating our athletes. In the clinical setting we spend most of our time trying to get the excitatory response from the nerve cells and muscle tissue. Athletes perceive excitatory responses as electric sensation, muscle contraction, and electric pain.

Physiologically, the nerves that affect these perceptions fire in that order as the stimulus intensity is increased gradually. Nerves have very little discriminatory ability. They can tell only if there is electricity in sufficient magnitude to cause a depolarization of the nerve membrane. They have very little regard for the different shape and polarities of waveforms. To the nerve cell, electricity is electricity. As in all things dealing with higher level organisms, there is a big range of responses to the same stimulus depending on the environmental and systemic factors.

All perception is a product of the brain's activity of receiving the signal that a nerve has been stimulated electrically. This further enlarges the broad range of systemic effects that occur in response to the electric stimulation.

Stimulation events will change the body's perception. As the strength of the current increases and/or the duration of the current increases, more nerve cells will fire. As the strength of the stimulus increases and these events occur, certain quality judgments about the electric stimuli are made. Is the current pleasant or unpleasant? Is the intensity of the stimulus weak or strong? The broad range of individual responses to these quality judgments has a significant impact on the beneficial effects of this therapy.

Muscle and Nerve Responses to Electrical Currents

Presently, the major therapeutic uses of electricity center on muscle contraction, or sensory stimulation, or both. Let us look in a general way at the physiologic effects of electricity on nerve and muscle tissue. Specific currents or frequencies will be discussed later in the chapter.

Nerves and muscles are both excitable tissues. This excitability is dependent on the cell membrane's **voltage sensitive permeability**. The nerve or muscle cell membrane regulates the interchange of substances between the inside of the cell and the environment outside the cell. This voltage sensitive permeability produces an unequal distri-

voltage sensitive permeability   The quality of some cell membranes that makes them permeable to different ions based on the electric charge of the ions. Nerve and muscle cell membranes allow negatively charged ions into the cell while actively transporting some positively charged ions outside the cell membrane.

resting potential   The potential difference between the inside and outside of a membrane.

bution of charged ions on each side of the membrane, which in turn creates a potential difference between the charge of the interior of the cell and the exterior of the cell. The membrane then is considered to be polarized. The potential difference between the inside and outside is known as the **resting potential**, because the cell tries to maintain this electrochemical gradient as its normal homeostatic environment.[23]

Both electrical and chemical gradients are established along the cell membrane with a greater concentration of diffusable positive ions on the outside of the membrane than on the inside. Using the continuous activity of the sodium pumps in the nerve cell membrane, the nerve cell continually moves Na+ from inside the cell to outside the cell membrane while voltage activated potassium channels allow K+ to move into the cell. This maintains the larger concentration of K+ on the inside of the cell membrane. The overall charge difference between the inside and the outside of the membrane creates an electrical gradient at its resting level of −70mV to −90mV (Figure 8-1). As explained by Guyton, "The potential is proportional to the difference in tendency of the ions to diffuse in one direction versus the other direction." Two conditions are necessary for the membrane[52] potential to develop: (1) the membrane must be semipermeable, allowing ions of one charge to diffuse through the pores more readily than ions of the opposite charge; (2) the concentration of the diffusible ions must be greater on one side of the membrane than on the other side.[23,52]

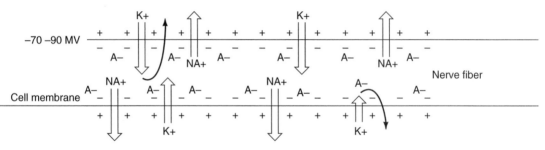

Figure 8-1 Nerve cell membrane with active transport mechanisms maintaining the resting membrane potential.

action potential A recorded change in electrical potential between the inside and outside of a nerve cell, resulting in muscular contraction.

depolarization Process or act of neutralizing the cell membrane's resting potential.

anode Positively charged electrode in a direct current system.

cathode Negatively charged electrode in a direct current system.

indifferent or dispersive electrode Large electrode used to spread out electrical charge and decrease current density at that electrode site.

- Negative electrode = cathode
- Positive electrode = anode

The resting membrane potential is generated because the cell is an ionic battery whose concentration of ions inside and outside the cell are maintained by regulatory NA^+/K^+ pumps within the cell wall. In addition to the ability of the nerve and muscle cell membranes to develop and maintain the resting potential, the membranes are excitable.[23,52]

To create transmission of an impulse in the nerve tissue, resting membrane potential must be reduced below a threshold level. Changes in the membrane's permeability may then occur. These changes create an **action potential** that will propagate the impulse along the nerve in both directions from the location of the stimulus. An action potential created by a stimulus from chemical, electrical, thermal, or mechanical means always creates the same result, membrane **depolarization**.

Not all stimuli are effective in causing an action potential and depolarization. To be an effective agent, the stimulus must have an adequate intensity and last long enough to equal or exceed the membrane's basic threshold for excitation. The stimulus must alter the membrane so that a number of ions are pushed across the membrane, exceeding the ability of the active transport pumps to

maintain the resting potentials. A stimulus of this magnitude forces the membrane to depolarize and results in an action potential.[52,124]

Depolarization. As the charged ions move across the nerve fiber membranes beneath the **anode** and **cathode**, membrane depolarization occurs. The cathode usually is the site of depolarization (Figure 8-2a). As the concentration of negatively charged ions increases, the membrane's voltage potential becomes low and is brought toward its threshold for depolarization (Figure 8-2b). The anode makes the nerve cell membrane potential more positive, increasing the threshold necessary for depolarization (Figure 8-2c). The cathode in this example becomes the active electrode; the anode becomes the **indifferent** or **dispersive electrode**. The anode and cathode may switch

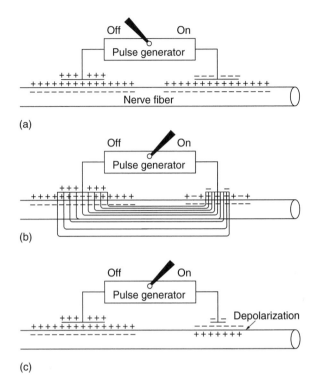

(a)

(b)

(c)

Figure 8-2   Depolarization of nerve cell membrane.

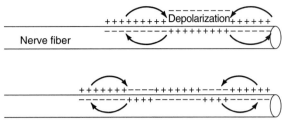

Figure 8-3   Propagation of a nerve impulse.

---

absolute refractory period   Brief time period (.5 μ sec) following membrane depolarization during which the membrane is incapable of depolarizing again.

twitch muscle contraction   A single muscle contraction caused by one depolarization phenomenon.

■ Analogy   *8-1*

The propagation of a nerve fiber depolarization impulse is similar to the movement of a wave in the ocean. A "wave" of relative polarity change on the inside of the cell membrane relative to the outside of the cell membrane moves along through the nerve. The difference is that the wave travels in both directions along the nerve fiber.

active and indifferent roles under other circumstances.[4,12,124] The number of ions needed to exceed the membrane pump's ability to maintain the normal membrane resting potential is tissue dependent.

Depolarization Propagation.   Following excitement and propagation of the impulse along the nerve fiber, there is a brief period during which the nerve fiber is incapable of reacting to a second stim-

ulus. This is the **absolute refractory period**, which lasts about 0.5 μ sec. Excitability is restored gradually as the nerve cell membrane repolarizes itself. The nerve then is capable of being stimulated again. The maximum number of possible discharges of a nerve may reach 1000 per second, depending on fiber type.[9,12,52,124]

The difference in electrical potential between the depolarized region and the neighboring inactive region causes a small electric current to flow between the two regions. This forms a complete local circuit and makes the depolarization self-propagating as the process is repeated all along the fiber in each direction from the depolarization site. Energy released by the cell keeps the intensity of the impulse uniform as it travels down the cell.[9,12,52,124] This process is illustrated in Figure 8-3.

Depolarization Effects.   As the nerve impulse reaches its effector organ or another nerve cell, the impulse is transferred between the two at a motor end plate or a synapse. At this junction, a transmitter substance is released from the nerve, rather than the impulse jumping from one to another. This transmitter substance causes the other excitable tissue to discharge (Figure 8-4).[12,124]

In terms of muscle excitation, a **twitch muscle contraction** results. This contraction, initiated by

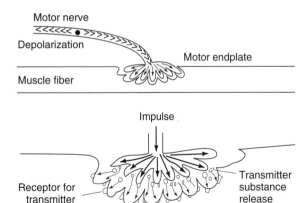

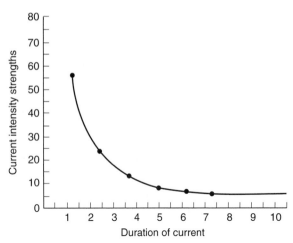

Figure 8-4   Change of electrical impulse to transmitter substance at the motor end plate. When activated, the muscle cell membrane will depolarize and contraction will occur.

Figure 8-5   Strength-duration curve.

an electrical stimulus, is the same as a twitch contraction coming from voluntary activity. Voluntary muscular activity is different only in the rate and synchrony (simultaneous response) of the muscle fiber contractions.[12,94] A graphic illustration of this threshold and propagation and contraction is the **strength-duration curve** (Figure 8-5).

As illustrated, there is a nonlinear relationship between current duration and current intensity, in which shorter duration stimuli require increasing

---

strength-duration curve   A graphic illustration of the relationship between current intensity and current duration in causing depolarization of a nerve or muscle membrane.

rheobase   The intensity of current necessary to cause observable tissue excitation, given a long current duration.

chronaxie   The duration of time necessary to cause observable tissue excitation, given a current intensity of two times rheobasic current.

---

intensities to reach the threshold of the nerve or muscle. Nerve and muscle membrane thresholds differ significantly. Different sizes and types of nerve fibers also have different thresholds. The strength-duration curves for different classes of nerve and muscle tissue illustrate the different thresholds of excitability of these tissues. The curves are symmetric, but the intensity of current necessary to reach the membrane's threshold for excitation differs for each tissue (Figure 8-6).[52,93,124,129]

Strength-Duration Curve.   Three important concepts are represented in the strength-duration (SD) curve. These terms and ideas are used frequently in discussions on the effects of electrical currents on the nerve cellular level.[57,124]

1.   The shape of the curve relates the intensity of the electrical stimulus and the length of time (duration) necessary to cause the tissue to depolarize.

2.   The **rheobase** describes the minimum intensity of current necessary to cause tissue excitation when applied for a maximum duration (Figure 8-7).

3.   **Chronaxie** describes the length of time (duration) required for a current of twice the intensity of the rheobase current to produce tissue excitation (Figure 8-7).

If you look at the SD curve and wish to get maximum sensory or motor response, you must use a stimulus with a high intensity and short duration. Equipment manufacturers use the strength-duration curve in choosing their preset pulse durations to be

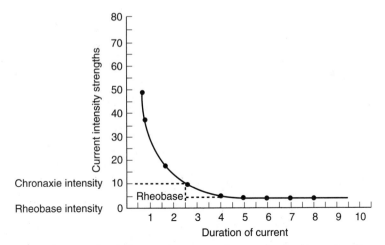

Figure 8-6   Excitation time of nerve cell membrane. Chronaxie is 2 times rheobase intensity. Chronaxie duration is 0.25.

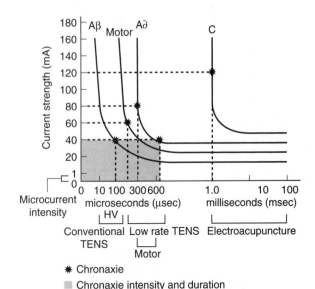

Figure 8-7   Strength duration curves Aβ sensory, motor, A∂ sensory, and pain nerve fibers. Durations of several electrical stimulators are indicated along the lower axis. Corresponding intensities would be necessary to create a depolarizing stimulus for any of the nerve fibers. Microcurrent intensity is so low that the nerve fibers will not depolarize. This current travels through other body tissues to create effects.

all-or-none response   The depolarization of nerve or muscle membrane is the same once a depolarizing intensity threshold is reached; further increases in intensity do not increase the response. Stimuli at intensities less than threshold do not create a depolarizing effect.

effective in creating action potentials. Most are in the area defined as chronaxie. The intensity is high enough to easily stimulate nerve tissue (Figure 8-6). Electrical engineers have designed some units to maximize this effect. But as the charge increases and more and more nerve fibers fire, the brain becomes more and more involved in the perceptual part of the experience.

Muscular Responses to Electrical Current. Stimulation of the motor nerve is the method used in most clinical applications of electrical muscular contractions. In the absence of innervation, muscle contraction can be stimulated by an electrical current that causes the muscle membrane to depolarize. This will create the same muscle contraction as a natural stimulus.

The **all-or-none response** is another important concept in applying electrical current to nerve or muscle tissue. Once a stimulus reaches a depolarizing threshold, the nerve or muscle membrane depolarizes, and propagation of the impulse or muscle contraction occurs. This reaction remains the same regardless of increases in the strength of the stimulus used. Either the stimulus causes depolarization—the all—or it does not cause depolarization—the none. There is no gradation of response; the response of the single nerve or muscle fiber is maximal or nonexistent.[12,94,124]

This all-or-none phenomenon does not mean that muscle fiber shortening and overall muscle activity cannot be influenced by changing the intensity, pulses per second, or duration of the stimulating current. Adjustments in current parameters can cause changes in the shortening of the muscle fiber and in the overall muscle activity.

The Effects of Electrical Stimulation on Nonexcitable Tissue and Cells

The nonexcitatory cells respond to electric current in ways that are consistent with their cell type and tissue function. To understand the theory of stimulating these nonexcitatory cells, a good understanding of the cell as a part of the body's bioelectric system is needed.

Cellular Electrical Circuits.

The Cell Membrane. The basic cell—with cell membrane, nucleus, organelles, and so on—acts like an ionic battery with the inside of the cell electrically negative and the outside electrically positive. The cell's plasma membrane is responsible for maintaining this electrochemical gradient as well as sending and receiving messages. The membrane is made up of phospholipid molecules studded with several types of proteins that project into and or through the phospholipid layers. These proteins support, transport things in and out, receive specific molecules that alter cell functions, and promote reactions on the surface of the cell (Figure 8-8a).

General cell electrical gradients are similar to those described for nerve cells but contain four electrical zones. The central cytoplasm area is negative and is surrounded by a narrow band of positively

---

dipoles Molecules whose ends carry opposite charge.

---

charged potassium ions along the inside of the cell membrane. The outer wall of the cell membrane is positively charged with sodium ions and potassium ions, and this is surrounded by a negative zone composed of sialic acid molecules (Figure 8-8a, b, c, d).

The difference in potential across the membrane is maintained as described previously for nerve cell membranes with the sodium and potassium pumps in the cell membrane doing the work. Any ionic fluctuations in the cytoplasm cause the ion pumps in the membrane to activate and return the equilibrium of the cell. There are also passive ionic channels in the wall that allow passive ion movement along the electrochemical gradients (Figure 8-8c).

The only difference between excitable and nonexcitable cell membranes is the presence of voltage-gated sodium ion channels. In the excitatory cells, these ion channels generate the action potentials once a depolarizing stimulus causes the membrane to become more permeable to the outside NA^+. The NA^+ channels are triggered to open, and NA^+ ions move into the cell, causing a brief reversal of charge. The charge reversal causes these ion channels to close, and the normal membrane potential returns.

The cell membrane is not just an outside covering but is also intimately involved with internal cell structures as an intercellular membrane—it surrounds organelles and supports the internal structure of the cell. This intercellular membrane can then exercise control of the movement of substances out from the cytoplasm or into the cytoplasm from the organelles. This movement is controlled by the same type electrochemical gradients and selective ions channels as is used in maintaining the cell wall[23,24] (Figure 8-8a, b, c, d).

Intercellular Structures. The internal cell structure is also made up of a dense network of hollow microtubules. These microtubules can be built and dismantled by the cell relatively rapidly and are **dipoles** with the negatively charged end directed

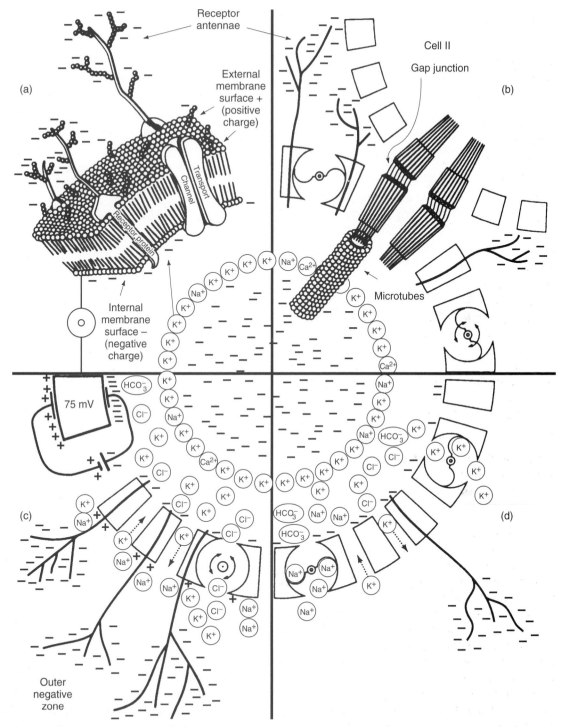

Figure 8-8 The electric cell with a central negative zone and inner positive zone; the cell membrane with an outer positive zone and an outer negative zone. (a) Three-dimensional model of the cell membrane with transmembrane receptor proteins, receptor antennae, the outer positive surface charge, and inner negative surface charge. (b) Gap junctions connect one cell to another and allow direct communication between cells. Receptors connect to microtubes within the cell. (c) Cell membrane pumps and passive ion channels act as ion balancers to preserve equilibrium of the cell. (d) Total electrochemical equilibrium acts as an ion battery creating a resting potential across the cell membrane.

centrally and the positive end directed peripherally. The microtubes are very active in cell function, moving materials like neurotransmitters along the surface of the cell, and making cilia move, moving organelles around within the cell, acting as sensors of the extracellular environment. The microtubes also form the mitotic spindle in the cell division process (Figure 8-8b). Because of their ability to change rapidly and help in cell movement and intercellular movement, the microtubes are probably significant factors in the organization of the cells during wound healing and regeneration.

Normal cells are signaled and respond to changes when messages contact the outer projections of the cell wall. Likewise, messages from within the cell can be sent outside the cell. The message can be chemical, like hormones, or possibly be an electromagnetic energy-coded message. Once the message is received, the signal is conveyed across the membrane to the cell's interior. The message is then transferred to another message system or switchboard that activates the cell's response to the message. The message may speed the cell up, make it move, stimulate production of extracellular proteins, or increase the secretions of that cell[23] (Figure 8-8 a, b).

Electrical Circuits in Tissue. Many cells are physically united with neighboring cells of like structure and collectively perform as one tissue. The cell membranes are bound together by junctions between the outer projections of each cell membrane. These specialized junctions allow direct communication between adjacent cells. These specialized junction areas are called **gap junctions** and contain channels for ionic, electrical, and small molecule signaling. The cells connected by gap junctions can then act together when one cell receives an extracellular message; the tissue can be coordinated in its response by the gap junction's internal message system. Embryonic and regenerating tissues are particularly rich in gap junctions, and they probably play a significant role in tissue growth and differentiation (Figure 8-8b).

Cells are surrounded by a bonding medium of collagen, elastin, and hyaluronic acid gel. This extracellular matrix can also interact with the adja-

gap junctions Specialized junction areas connecting cells of like structure that contain channels for ionic, electrical, and small molecule signaling that passes messages from cell to cell.

electrets Insulators carrying a permanent charge similar to a permanent magnet.

piezoelectric activity Changing electric surface charges of a structure forces the structure to change shape.

electropiezo activity Changing electric surface charges of a structure forces the structure to change shape.

strain-related potentials Tissue-based electric potentials generated in response to strain for the tissue.

cent cell surface receptors to modify cell function, orientation and alignment, shape, movement, metabolic rate, and differentiation.[23]

Strain-Related Potentials. The previous discussion on cell structure points out that every cell surface carries a charge. Every support structure within the cell, membranes, or microtubes are dipoles. In effect, cell structures have similar properties to **electrets** (insulators carrying a permanent charge, similar to a permanent magnet). Electrets are capable of **piezoelectric activity**, in which mechanical deformation of the structure causes a change in the surface electrical charge of the structure. They are also capable of **electropiezo activity**, in which changing an electric surface charge would force the electret to change shape. This becomes important when considering the piezoelectric effect of bone and connective tissue and how this change in electrical surface activity may guide or stimulate growth and/or healing.

Most connective tissues also generate a tissue based electrical potential in response to strain of the tissue. Tension on surfaces or distraction on the surface create these **strain-related potentials** (SRP). Where there is compression, the strain-related potentials are negative. Where there is tension these SRPs are positive. Functionally, these strain-

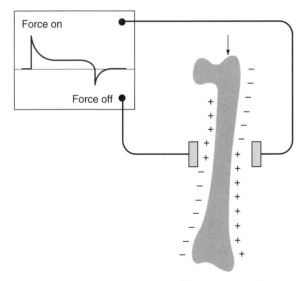

Figure 8-9   Electrical response of boney tissue to the momentary deforming stress of weight bearing.

related potentials have helped provide an electro-mechanical explanation for Wolff's law governing bone's growth in response to mechanical stress. The controlling mechanism for these events is most likely some form of the intrinsic electrochemical responses discussed earlier in this chapter, as no specific hormonal or neurologic controls have been discovered. The stress-generated potential must signal the membranes of the osteoblast, osteocytes, and osteoclasts to add or take away bone in areas of compression or tension. The cells have the necessary mechanisms to receive and decode the strain information, and intrinsically the cells can respond appropriately to maintain the integrity of the tissue[8,18,23] (Figure 8-9).

Cells are grouped together into tissues creating segmental units, which combine into a whole system. Each cell, considered an ionic battery when added together with other cells, can collectively summate the influence and generate potential differences across the surface of the body or between different areas of the same tissue. These endogenous currents with their polarity gradients seem to play a key role in guiding the development, growth,

regeneration, and repair of the cells, tissues, and segments of our body.[23]

Normal Bioelectric Fields.   Becker demonstrated a direct-current bioelectric field that could be measured in salamanders and other animals. The spatial configuration of this field coincided with the arrangement of their central nervous systems, with the positive areas being located near the major nerve cell accumulations—i.e., brain, brachial, and lumbar plexus areas. The negative areas were near the major peripheral nerve outflows from these areas.[9,10,11,23,24]

This bioelectric field has been measured in other animals and has also been recorded for humans. The skin surface also is always negative relative to the dermis, so there is a permanent electrical gradient through the skin tissue.[10,11,25] Potential difference gradients also exist on long bones with the midpoints more positive than the ends, and areas of increased cellular activity, (i.e., epiphyseal plate area) more negative than other areas. This direct current seems to be in a continuous circuit along the length of the bone and will vary in strength according to local differences in metabolism[23] (Figure 8-10).

Bioelectric Activity in Skin Wounds.   When skin is damaged, a steady current will move from the relatively positively charged dermis into the wound area and re-enter the skin just below the stratum corneum. The wound currents also generate a lateral potential difference from outside the normal area to the wound edge, forming a lateral electrical gradient. This lateral gradient appears to stimulate epithelial cells in the wound edge to regenerate and begin to grow across the wound. Once the wound edges approximate, the surface integrity is re-established, and the lateral gradient disappears. If the wound dries out, these currents will also drop because of increased resistance to electrical flow. The skin thickness is re-established as cell layering returns to normal and the increased electric potentials also return to normal[23,47] (Figure 8-11).

Bioelectric Field Changes in Response to Injury.   Becker's experiments with salamander limb injury showed that the bioelectric field gradient reversed immediately when a salamander limb was

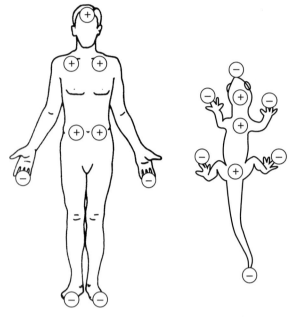

Figure 8-10 The bioelectric field. Skin potentials in man and salamander.

....

current of injury A bioelectric current produced by any type of cellular trauma that plays a key role in stimulating healing.

....

amputated. The normal current was −10 millivolts, and at amputation it jumped to a +20 millivolts current. Gradually as healing started to take place, this current returned to a highly negative current −30 millivolts and then gradually returned to baseline values as limb regeneration occurred[10,11] (Figure 8-12).

In the frog, a nonregenerating cousin of the salamander, this bioelectric current behaved similarly upon amputation but never jumped back to a negative current. Instead, it gradually moved back to the normal negative baseline values as the stump scarred over and healing became complete. Becker found this **current of injury** was produced by any type of cellular trauma and suggested that this cur-

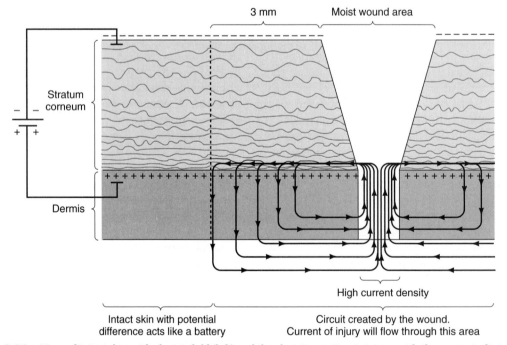

Figure 8-11 Normal intact skin with electric field (left) and the electric reaction to injury with the current of injury path through the skin wound (right).

rent of injury plays a key role in stimulating the healing and regeneration of tissue.[9,10,11]

Regeneration is more and more limited as we move up the phylogenetic ladder. Regeneration is also greatest in younger animals. Regeneration in humans is certainly limited, but certain tissues have some capacity to respond (muscle, nerve, bone, skin, and connective tissue). Becker felt there were three essential ingredients for regeneration.[9] The first was a powerful initial current of injury— first a positive current, then becoming strongly negative as the wound blastema formed and gradually returned to baseline value as the limb regenerated. The second was that a high tissue versus innervation density was a critical factor, and if innervation density is below a critical level, regeneration will not occur. The third ingredient was the presence of peripheral nerves in the wound area and the growth of these nerves to reinervate the epithelial ingrowth at the amputation site. These neuro-epidermal junctions form at about 7 to 8 days in the wound blastema. This event seems to play a significant role in the sudden reversal of the current of injury from positive to negative[11,23] (Figure 8-12).

Becker and others have stimulated regeneration in nonregenerating species (frogs and rats) by applying a direct current to the amputation site that mimics the high negative current found in salamander regeneration during the blastema stage of growth, approximately 7 to 10 days post injury. The electrode must also stay at the growing tip throughout regeneration.[9,10,11,23,60]

This artificial current of injury apparently caused the proliferating cells in the injured area to differentiate to a more primitive cell type and then to differentiate into the appropriate cell types needed to continue the regeneration of the limb. The overall progression of the limb orientation and alignment is also probably guided by the bioelectric field with the distal electrode being negative (Figure 8-12).

Becker after several subsequent experiments concluded that the bioelectric field of animals was a function of DC circuits that originated in the CNS and returned to the CNS, indicating that there is a constant flow of DC current present in neural tissue and that the amplitude and direction of

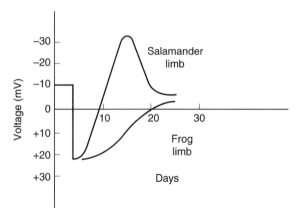

Figure 8-12   Voltage changes in amputated salamander and frog limbs during regeneration and healing.

current flow are dependent upon central nervous system activity.[11,23]

Electrical Stimulation Influence on Cellular and Tissue Activity

Cell behavior can be influenced by having extracellular molecules lock into receptor sites on the cell membrane, which activate the message relay and action system within the cell (see Figure 8-8). The recognition of receptor sites and the guiding of the extracellular molecule to that destination is caused by an interaction of the electric fields from the receptor site and the extracellular molecule. Electrical stimulation of the appropriate frequency and amplitude may also be able to activate the cellular receptor site and stimulate the same cellular changes as the naturally occurring chemical molecular stimulation.

The cell functions by incorporating a multitude of chemical reactions into a living process. Enzymatic activity accelerates these reactions, and each cell contains approximately 3000 enzymes. The enzymatic activity of the cell depends on the availability of specific charged sites on the intracellular membrane surfaces. These sites may be made more or less available for enzymatic reactions by changes in shape or configuration of the surface. These changes usually occur in response to a messenger

---

frequency window selectivity Cellular responses may be triggered by a certain electrical frequency range.

---

molecule, but it is conceivable that the appropriate electrical signal could also create more specific sites for enzymatic activity, thereby changing or stimulating cell function[23] (see Figure 8-8).

The microtubules system may selectively receive and transmit electromagnetic signals through the cell. As the energy travels along the microtube, the signal may stimulate organelles to activate their routine functions. The microtubule system could transmit this energy wave from cell to cell through the tight cell-to-cell contact areas at the gap junctions. This transmission could create cells working together to respond as a tissue and could also allow a very small amperage current to move quickly over the length of the tissue (see Figure 8-8).

Cells seem responsive to steady direct current gradients. The cells either move or grow toward one pole and away from the other. The electric field created by the DC current may help guide the healing process and/or the regenerative capabilities of injured or developing tissues.[23,76]

Cells may also respond to a particular frequency of current. The cell may be selectively responsive to certain frequencies and unresponsive to other frequencies. Some researchers claim that specific genes for protein manufacture can be activated by a certain shaped electrical impulse. This frequency could change in certain ways according to the cellular state. This phenomenon has been termed the **frequency window selectivity** of the cell.[23]

Overall, we see that small amplitude direct currents are intrinsic to the ways the body works to grow and repair. Clinically, if we can duplicate some of these same signals, we may be successful in using electrotherapy in the most effective efficient manner. The secrets to this type of use are only beginning to be uncovered.

After reading this review of cell biology slanted toward the electrical components, it is hoped that the magnitude of the cellular electrical activity and its potential to influence cell function become apparent. Many of the unexplained phenomena surrounding electrotherapy may become more understandable as more research promotes better understanding of the normal electrical activity at the cellular and tissue levels.

In this discussion of how electrical current influences nonexcitatory cells and tissue, we must start to rely on theory more than on well-proven researched ideas. The student must understand that theories are projections on what might take place to explain observed behavior, and the authors expect changes in these theories to occur. So beware and believe cautiously as you incorporate these theories into your clinical practice.[58]

ELECTRICAL CONCEPTS: EFFECTS OF CHANGES IN CURRENT PARAMETERS AND THEIR EFFECT ON TREATMENT PROTOCOLS

When using any of the treatment protocols aimed at the electrical stimulation of muscle or nerve tissue, several concepts must be understood for athletic trainers to accomplish their goals:

1. Alternating versus direct current
2. Tissue impedance
3. Current density
4. Frequency of wave or pulse
5. Intensity of wave or pulse
6. Duration of wave or pulse
7. Polarity of electrodes
8. Electrode placement

Changes in these parameters affect how the electrical current changes the physiology of the body part being treated. The waveform used gives us a graphic way to measure and quantify these parameters.[130]

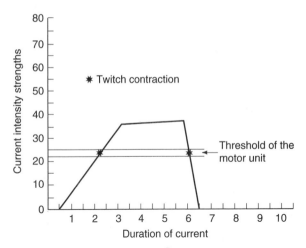

Figure 8-13   Direct current influence on a motor unit.

Alternating versus Direct Current

To further understand electrically stimulated muscle contractions, we must think in terms of multiple stimuli rather than a simple direct current response. The motor nerves are not stimulated by a steady flow of direct current. The nerve repolarizes under the influence of the current and will not depolarize again until a sudden change in current intensity occurs.

If continuous direct current were the only current mode available, we would get a muscle contraction only when the current intensity rose to a stimulus threshold. Once the membrane repolarized, another change in the current intensity would be needed to force another depolarization and contraction (Figure 8-13).

The biggest difference in the effects of alternating and direct currents is the ability of direct current to cause chemical changes. Chemical effects from using direct current usually occur only when the stimulus is continuous and is applied over a period of time. These chemical changes become measurable when the duration of the stimulus reaches the 1-minute mark, but the effect is cumulative over the total treatment time. This type of current is available in most low-voltage equipment. The duration of the current in most high-voltage stimulators

impedance   The resistance of the tissue to the passage of electrical current.

current density   Amount of current flow per cubic area.

> • Chemical changes occur only with long-duration continuous current

is nonadjustable and is too short to create any chemical effect, unless treatment time in excess of 1 hour is used.[96,124]

One theory on using direct high-volt current in treatment of edema proposes that the direct current enhances the movement of charged proteins into the lymphatic channels. The electric field causes the charged proteins to increase their movement and migrate into the lymph channels.[33]

Tissue Impedance

Impedance is the resistance of the tissue to the passage of electrical current. Bone and fat are high-impedance tissues; nerve and muscle are low-impedance tissues. If a low-impedance tissue is located under a large amount of high-impedance tissue, the current will never become high enough to cause a depolarization.[12,124]

Current Density

The **current density** (amount of current flow per cubic volume) at the nerve or muscle must be high enough to cause depolarization. The current density is highest where the electrodes meet the skin and diminishes as the electricity penetrates into the deeper tissues (Figure 8-14).[12,124] If there is a large fat layer between the electrodes and the nerve, the electrical energy may not have a high enough density to cause depolarization (Figure 8-15).

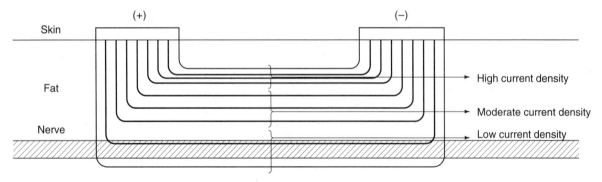

Figure 8-14 Current density using equal size electrodes spaced close together.

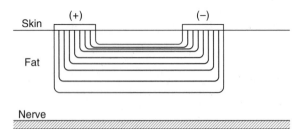

Figure 8-15 Equal size electrodes spaced close together on body part with thick fat layers. Thus, the electrical current does not reach the nerve.

If the electrodes are spaced closely together, the area of highest current density is relatively superficial (Figure 8-16a). If the electrodes are spaced farther apart, the current density will be higher in the deeper tissues, including nerve and muscle (Figure 8-16b).

Electrode size will also change current density. As the size of one electrode relative to another is decreased, the current density beneath the smaller electrode is increased. The larger the electrode, the larger the area over which the current is spread, decreasing the current density (Figure 8-17).[2,4,12,94,124]

Using a large *dispersive electrode* remote from the treatment area while placing a smaller **active electrode** as close as possible to the nerve or muscle motor point will give the greatest effect at the small electrode. The large electrode disperses the current over a large area; the small electrode con-

---

active electrode Electrode at which greatest current density occurs.

---

centrates the current in the area of the motor point (Figure 8-17).

Electrode size and placement are key elements that the athletic trainer controls that will have great influence on the results. High-current density close to the neural structure you want to stimulate makes it more certain that you will be successful with the least amount of current. Electrode placement is probably one of the biggest causes of poor results from electrical therapy.[58]

Frequency

The amount of shortening of the muscle fiber and the amount of recovery allowed the muscle fiber is a function of the frequency. The mechanical shortening of the single muscle fiber response can be influenced by stimulating again as soon as the tissue membrane repolarizes. Only the membrane has the absolute refractory period; the contractile mechanism operates on a different timing sequence and is just beginning to contract. When the second stimulus is received by the muscle membrane, the myofilaments are already overlapping, and the second stimulus causes an increased mechanical shortening of the muscle fiber. This process of superimposing one

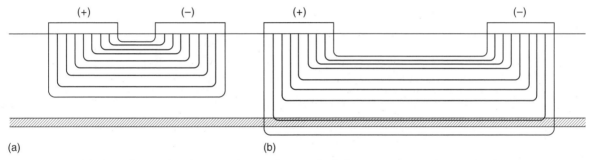

Figure 8-16   (a) Electrodes are very close together, producing a high-density current in the superficial tissues. (b) Increasing the distance between the electrodes increases the current density in deeper tissues.

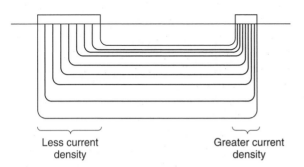

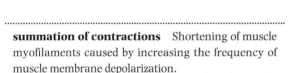

Figure 8-17   The greatest current density is under the small or active electrode.

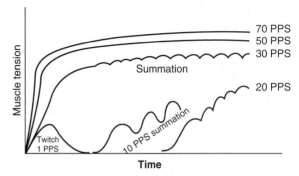

Figure 8-18   Summation of contractions and tetanization.

---

summation of contractions   Shortening of muscle myofilaments caused by increasing the frequency of muscle membrane depolarization.

tetanization   When individual muscle-twitch responses can no longer be distinguished and the responses force maximum shortening of the stimulated muscle fiber.

---

twitch contraction on another is called **summation of contractions**. As the number of twitch contractions per second increases, single twitch responses cannot be distinguished, and **tetanization** of the muscle fiber is reached (Figure 8-18). The tension developed by a muscle fiber in tetany is much greater than the tension from a twitch contraction. This muscle fiber tetany is strictly a function of the fre-

- Muscle contraction = negative active electrode

quency of the stimulating current; it is not dependent on the intensity of the current.[12,94] In general, a higher frequency can be used to produce an increase in muscle tension due to the summative effects, whereas a lower frequency is more often used for muscle pumping and edema reduction.

The primary difference between electrically induced muscle contraction and voluntary muscle contraction is the asynchrony of firing of motor units under voluntary control versus the synchronous firing of electrically stimulated motor units.

Each time the electrical stimulus is applied, the same motor units respond. This may lead to greater fatigue in the electrically stimulated muscles. Normal firing in voluntary muscle contraction varies from one movement to the next because some motor units are contracting while others are inactive. Voluntary contractions do not lead to muscular fatigue as early in the exercise period as do electrical contractions. This synchrony of contraction may also be important in training the muscle to use more synchronous contractions to improve muscular strength.[12,94]

Intensity

Increasing the intensity of the electrical stimulus in Figure 8-19a to that in Figure 8-19b causes the current to reach deeper into the tissue. Depolarization of more fibers then is accomplished by two methods: (1) higher threshold fibers within the range of the first stimulus (Figure 8-19a) are depolarized by the higher intensity stimulus, and (2) fibers with the same threshold but deeper in the structure are depolarized by the deeper spread of the current. High-voltage stimulators are capable of deeper penetration into the tissue than low-voltage stimulators and may be desirable when stimulating deep muscle tissue. This is one of the most significant differences between high-voltage and low-voltage generators.[4,94]

Duration

We also can stimulate more nerve fibers with the same intensity current by increasing the length of time (duration) that an adequate stimulus is available to depolarize the membranes (Figure 8-19c). Greater numbers of nerve fibers then would react to the same intensity stimulus, because the current would be available for a longer period of time.[12,59,124] This method requires the use of a stimulator with an adjustable duration. The low-voltage stimulators usually are available with this parameter, whereas the high-voltage stimulators usually have a preset pulse duration.

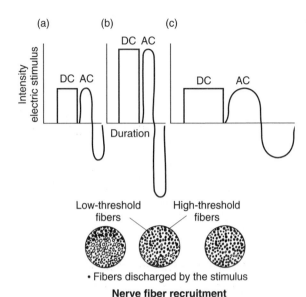

Figure 8-19 Recruitment of nerve fibers. (a) A stimulus pulse at a duration intensity just above threshold will excite the closest and largest fibers. Each electrical pulse of the same intensity at the same location will cause the same fibers to fire. (b) Increasing the intensity will excite smaller fibers and those farther away. (c) Increasing the duration will also excite smaller fibers and those farther away.

Polarity

During the use of any stimulator, an electrode that has a greater level of electrons is called the negative electrode or the cathode. The other electrode in this system has a lower level of electrons and is called the positive electrode or the anode. The negative electrode attracts positive ions and the positive electrode attracts negative ions and electrons. With AC waves, these electrodes change polarity with each current cycle.

With a direct current generator, the athletic trainer can designate one electrode as the negative and one electrode as the positive, and for the duration of the treatment the electrodes will provide that polar effect. The polar effect can be thought of in terms of three characteristics: (1) chemical effects, (2) ease of excitation, and (3) direction of current flow.[11,12,81,94,101,124]

Chemical Effects.   Changes in pH under each electrode, a reflex vasodilation, and the ability to facilitate movement of oppositely charged ions through the skin into the tissue (iontophoresis) are all thought of as chemical effects. A tissue-stimulating effect is ascribed to the negative electrode. To create these effects, longer pulse durations (greater than 1 minute) are required.[11,46,96,101] The bacteriostatic effect was achieved at either the anode or cathode with intensities in the 5 mA to 10 mA range. While at 1 mA or below, the greatest bacteriostatic effect was found at the cathode.[52] Another study using treatment times exceeding 30 minutes found some bacteriostatic effect of high-voltage pulsed currents.[67]

Ease of Excitation of Excitable Tissue. The polarity of the active electrode usually should be negative when the desired result is a muscle contraction because of the greater facility for membrane depolarization at the negative pole. However, current density under the positive pole can be increased rapidly enough to create a depolarizing effect. Using the positive electrode as the active electrode is not as efficient, because it will require more current intensity to create an action potential. This may cause the athlete to be less comfortable with the treatment. In treatment programs requiring muscle contraction or sensory nerve stimulation, athlete's comfort should dictate the choice of positive or negative polarity. Negative polarity usually is the most comfortable in this instance.[94,124]

Direction of Current Flow.   In some treatment schemes, the direction of current flow is also considered important. Generally speaking, the negative electrode is positioned distally and the positive electrode proximally. This arrangement tries to replicate the naturally occurring pattern of electrical flow in the body.[11,84]

The direction of current flow could also influence shifting of the water content of the tissues and movement of colloids (fluid suspension of the intracellular fluid). Neither of these phenomena is well documented or understood, and further study is needed before clinical treatments are designed around these concepts.[91,103,124]

- Cathode = distal
- Anode = proximal

True polar effects can be substantiated when they occur close to the electrodes, through which the current is entering the tissue. In laboratory situations in physics and physical therapy, polar effects occur in very close proximity to the electrode. To cause these effects, the current must flow through a medium. If the tissue to be treated is centrally located between the two electrodes, results cannot be assigned to polar effects.[11,58] Clinically, polar effects are an important consideration in iontophoresis, stimulating motor points or peripheral nerves, and in the biostimulative effect on nonexcitatory cells.

Electrode Placement

When using any of the treatment protocols aimed at the electrical stimulation of sensory nerves for pain suppression, there are several guidelines that will help the athletic trainer select the appropriate sites for electrode placement. Transcutaneous electrical nerve stimulation (TENS) uses similar-sized electrodes placed according to a pattern and moved in a trial-and-error pattern until pain is decreased. The following patterns may be used:

1. Electrodes may be placed on or around the painful area.
2. Electrodes may be placed over specific dermatomes, myotomes, or sclerotomes that correspond to the painful area.
3. Electrodes may be placed close to the spinal cord segment that innervates an area that is painful.
4. Peripheral nerves that innervate the painful area may be stimulated by placing electrodes over sites where the nerve becomes superficial and can be easily stimulated.
5. Vascular structures contain neural tissue as well as ionic fluids that would transmit

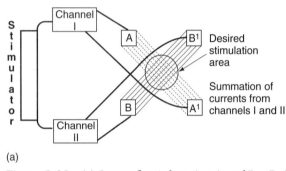

(a)   (b)

Figure 8-20   (a) Current flow is from A to A, and B to B. As the currents cross the area of stimulation, they summate in intensity. (b) Typical crossing pattern for electrodes.

electrical stimulating currents and may be most easily stimulated by electrode placement over superficial vascular structures.

6. Electrode placement over trigger point locations.[122]

7. Both acupuncture and trigger points have been conveniently mapped out and illustrated. A reference on acupuncture and trigger areas is included in Appendix A. The athletic trainer should systematically attempt to stimulate the points listed as successful for certain areas and types of pain. If they are effective, the athlete will have decreased pain. These points also can

be identified using an ohm meter point locator to determine areas of decreased skin resistance.

8. Combinations of any of these preceding systems and bilateral electrode placement can also be successful.[71,72,81,129]

9. Crossing patterns, also referred to as an interferential technique, involve electrode application such that the electrical signals from each set of electrodes add together at some point in the body and the intensity accumulates. The electrodes are usually arranged in a criss-cross pattern around the point to be stimulated (Figure 8-20). If

there is a specific superficial area (i.e., medial collateral acromioclavicular joint) that you wish to stimulate, your electrodes should be relatively close together. They should be located so the area to be treated is central to the location of the electrodes. If there is poorly localized pain (general shoulder pain) that seems to be deeper in the joint or muscle area, spread your electrodes farther apart to give more penetration to the current.

The athletic trainer should not be limited to any one system but should evaluate electrode placement for each athlete. The effectiveness of sensory stimulation is closely tied in with proper electrode placement. As in all trial-and-error treatment approaches, a systematic, organized search is always better than a "shotgun," hit-and-miss approach. Numerous articles have identified some of the best locations for common pain problems, and these may be used as a starting point for the first approach.[71] If the treatment is not achieving the desired results, the electrode placement should be reconsidered.

THERAPEUTIC USES OF ELECTRICALLY INDUCED MUSCLE CONTRACTION

A variety of therapeutic gains can be made by electrically stimulating a muscle contraction:

1. Muscle re-education
2. Muscle pump contractions
3. Retardation of atrophy
4. Muscle strengthening
5. Increasing range of motion
6. Reducing edema

Any electrical stimulator—high voltage, low voltage, alternating current, **hybrid current**, or transcutaneous electrical nerve stimulators (TENS)—may be used to cause muscle contraction. Following the protocols as closely as possible with the available equipment can increase the efficiency and effectiveness of treatment.

hybrid currents   Currents that have wave forms containing parameters that are not classically alternating or direct.

■ **Clinical Decision-Making**   *Exercise 8-1*

How should an athletic trainer go about setting up a conventional TENS treatment for a sore biceps muscle?

Muscle fatigue should be considered when deciding on treatment parameters. The variables that have an influence on muscle fatigue are

1. intensity—combination of the pulse stimulus's amplitude intensity and the pulse duration
2. the number of pulses or bursts per second
3. on time
4. off time

Muscle force is varied by changing the intensity to recruit more or less motor units. Muscle force can also be varied to a certain degree by increasing the summating quality of the contraction with high burst or pulse rates. The greater the force, the greater the demands on the muscle, the greater the occlusion of muscle blood flow, the greater the fatigue. If high muscle forces are not required, the intensity and frequency can be adjusted to desired levels but fatigue can still be a factor. To minimize fatigue associated with forceful contractions, a combination of the lowest frequency and the higher intensity will keep the force constant and is the most fatigue resistant.[14]

If high force levels are desired, then higher frequencies and intensities can be used. To keep the muscle fatigue as low as possible, the rest time between contractions should be at least 60 seconds for each 10 seconds of contraction time. A variable frequency train in which a high-frequency then a low-frequency stimulus is used will also help minimize fatigue in repetitive functional electric stimulation.[14]

■ **Clinical Decision-Making** *Exercise 8-2*

....

An athletic trainer is using an electrical stimulator to induce a muscle contraction of the rectus femoris. The active electrode is placed over the motor point of the muscle and the dispersive electrode is placed under the leg. What changes in the setup of the electrodes and/or changes in current parameters can be made to reach the threshold of depolarization for this muscle?

Neuromuscular induced contractions at the higher torques are associated with athlete perceptions of pain, either from the current used or the intensity of the contraction. This is often a limiting factor in the success of any of the following protocols. Each athlete needs supervision and good athletic trainer-athlete confidence for the most effective compliance with the treatment goals.[14,37,58]

When using electrical stimulation for muscle contraction, motor point stimulation can give the best individual muscle contraction. To find the motor point of a muscle, a probe electrode should be used to stimulate the muscle. Stimulation should be started in the approximate location of the desired motor point. (See Appendix A for motor point chart.) The intensity should be increased until contraction is visible, and the current intensity should be maintained at that level. The probe should be moved around until the best visible contraction for that current intensity is found; this is the motor point.[12,123] By choosing this location for stimulation, the current density can be increased in an area where numerous motor nerve fibers can be affected, maximizing the muscular response from the stimulation.

Muscle Re-Education

Muscular inhibition after surgery or injury is the primary indication for muscle re-education. If the neuromuscular mechanisms of a muscle have not been damaged, then central nervous system inhibition of this muscle usually is a factor in loss of control. The atrophy of synaptic contacts that remain unused for long periods is theorized as a source of this sensorimotor alienation. The addition of electrical stimulation of the motor nerve provides an artificial use of the inactive synapses and helps restore a more normal balance to the system as the ascending sensory information will be reintegrated into the athlete's movement control patterns. A muscle contraction usually can be forced by electrically stimulating the muscle. Forcing the muscle to contract causes an increase in the sensory input from that muscle. The athlete feels the muscle contract, sees the muscle contract, and can attempt to duplicate this muscular response.[12,35,42,93] The object here is to re-establish control, not to create a strengthening contraction.

Protocols for muscle re-education do not list specific parameters to make this treatment more efficient, but the following criteria are essential for effective electrical stimulation:

1. Current intensity must be adequate for muscle contraction but comfortable for the athlete.

2. Pulse duration should be set as close as possible to chronaxie for motor neurons (300 μsec–600 μsec).

3. Pulses per second should be high enough to produce a tetanic contraction (35 to 55 pulses per second), but adjusted so that muscle fatigue is minimized. Higher rates may be more fatigue producing than rates in the midrange of tetanic contraction.

4. On/off cycles should be based on the equipment parameters available and the athletic trainer's preference in teaching the athlete to regain control of his/her muscle. Currents that ramp up or down will require longer on times so the effective current is on for 2 to 3 seconds. Off times can either be a 1:1 contraction to recovery ratio or 1:4 or 5, depending on the athletic trainer's preference or the athlete's attention span and/or level of fatigue.

5. Interrupted or surged current must be used.

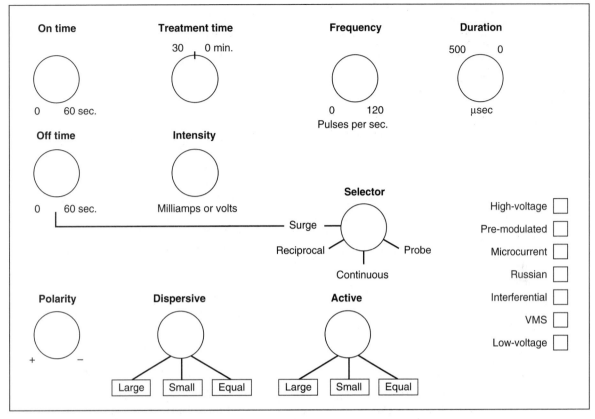

Figure 8-21   Electrical stimulator control panel.

6. The athlete should be instructed to allow just the electricity to make the muscle contract, so the athlete can feel and see the response desired. Next, the athlete should alternate voluntary muscle contractions with current-induced contractions.

7. Total treatment time should be about 15 minutes, but this can be repeated several times daily.

8. High-voltage pulsed or medium-frequency alternating current may be most effective (Figure 8-21).[12,35,42]

Muscle Pump Contractions

Electrically induced muscle contractions can be used to duplicate the regular muscle contractions that help stimulate circulation by pumping fluid and blood through venous and lymphatic channels back into the heart. A discussion of edema formation is included in the chapter on intermittent compression. Using sensory level stimulation has also been found to decrease edema in sprain and contusion injuries in animals. That discussion is included in Chapter 11.

Electrical stimulation of muscle contractions in the affected extremity can help in re-establishing the proper circulatory pattern while keeping the injured part protected. It has been demonstrated that vasodilation occurs with both voluntary and electrically induced muscle contractions, but electrically induced vasodilation appears to last longer.[90]

The following criteria must be satisfied for the electrical treatment to be successful in helping to reduce swelling:

1. Current intensity must be high enough to provide a strong, comfortable muscle contraction.
2. Pulse duration is preset on most of the therapeutic generators. If adjustable, it should be set as close as possible to the duration needed for chronaxie (300–600 μsec) of the motor nerve to be stimulated.
3. Pulses per second should be in the beginnings of tetany range (35–50 pulses per second).
4. Interrupted or surged current must be used.
5. On time should be 5 to 10 seconds.
6. Off time should be 5 to 10 seconds.
7. The part to be treated should be elevated.
8. The athlete should be instructed to allow the electricity to make the muscles contract. Active range of motion may be encouraged at the same time if it is not contraindicated.
9. Total treatment time should be between 20 and 30 minutes; treatment should be repeated two to five times daily.
10. High-voltage pulsed or medium-frequency alternating current may be most effective[35,42,97,100,113] (see Figure 8-21).
11. Use this protocol in addition to the normal I.C.E. for best effect.[44,91]

Retardation of Atrophy

Prevention or retardation of atrophy has traditionally been a reason for treating athletes with electrically stimulated muscle contraction. The maintenance of muscle tissue, after an injury that prevents normal muscular exercise, can be accomplished by

....

maximum voluntary isometric contraction
Peak torque produced by a muscular contraction.

....

substituting an electrically stimulated muscle contraction. The electrical stimulation reproduces the physical and chemical events associated with normal voluntary muscle contraction and helps to maintain normal muscle function.[5]

Again, no specific protocols exist. In designing a program, the practitioner should try to duplicate muscle contractions associated with normal exercise routines. The following criteria can be used as guidelines in developing effective treatment protocols:

1. Current intensity should be as high as can be tolerated by the athlete. This can be increased during the treatment as some sensory accommodation takes place. The contraction should be capable of moving the limb through the antigravity range or of achieving 25% or more of the normal **maximum voluntary isometric contraction** (MVIC) torque for the muscle. The higher torque readings seem to have the best results.
2. Pulse duration is preset on most of the therapeutic generators. If it is adjustable, it should be set as close as possible to the duration needed for chronaxie (300–600 μsec) of the motor nerve to be stimulated.
3. Pulses per second should be in the tetany range (50 to 85 pulses per second).
4. Interrupted or surge type current should be used.
5. On time should be between 6 and 15 seconds.
6. Off time should be at least 1 minute.
7. The muscle should be given some resistance, either gravity or external resistance provided by the addition of weights or by fixing the joint so that the contraction becomes isometric.

8. The athlete can be instructed to work with the electrically induced contraction, but voluntary effort is not necessary for the success of this treatment.

9. Total treatment time should be 15 to 20 minutes, or enough time to allow a minimum of 10 contractions; some protocols have been successful with 3 sets of 10 contractions. The treatment can be repeated two times daily. Some protocols using battery-powered rather than line-powered units have advocated longer bouts with more repetitions probably because of low contractions force.

10. A medium-frequency alternating current stimulator is the machine of choice (see Figure 8-21).[14,35-37,42,93,105,108,109]

Muscle Strengthening

Muscle strengthening from electrical muscle stimulation has been used with some good results in athletes with weakness or denervation of a muscle group.[5] The protocol is better established for this use, but more research is needed to clarify the procedures and to allow us to generalize the results to other athlete problems. The following summarizes the protocols used successfully:

1. Current intensity should be high enough to make the muscle develop 60% of the torque developed in a maximum voluntary isometric contraction (MVIC).

2. Pulse duration is preset on most therapeutic generators. If adjustable, it should be set as close as possible to the duration needed for chronaxie (300–600 μsec) of the motor nerve to be stimulated. In general, longer pulse durations should include more nerves in response.

3. Pulses per second should be in the tetany range (70 to 85 pulses per second).

4. Surged or interrupted current with a gradual ramp to peak intensity is most effective.

5. On time should be in the 10 to 15 second range.

■ **Clinical Decision-Making**   *Exercise 8-3*

An athletic trainer is using electrical stimulation for muscle strengthening following a hamstring muscle strain. What treatment parameters will likely be most effective in improving strength?

6. Off time should be in the 50 seconds to 2 minute range.

7. Resistance usually is applied by immobilizing the limb. The muscle is then given an isometric contraction torque equal to or greater than 25% of the MVIC torque. The greater the percentage of torque produced, the better the results.

8. The athlete can be instructed to work with the electrically induced contraction, but voluntary effort is not necessary for the success of the treatment.

9. Total treatment time should include a minimum of 10 contractions, but mimicking normal active resistive training protocols of 3 sets of 10 contractions can also be productive. Fatigue is a major factor in this setup. Electrical stimulation bouts should be scheduled at least three times weekly. Generally, strength gains will continue over the treatment course, but intensities may need to increase to keep pace with the most current maximum voluntary contraction torques.

10. A medium-frequency alternating current stimulator is the machine of choice (see Figure 8-20).[14,35-37,42,93,105,108,109]

Increasing Range of Motion

Increasing the range of motion in contracted joints is also a possible and documented use of electrical muscle stimulation. Electrically stimulating a muscle contraction pulls the joint through the limited range. The continued contraction of this muscle group over an extended time appears to make the contracted joint and muscle tissue modify and lengthen. Reduction of contractures in athletes with hemiplegia has been reported, although no studies have reported this type of use in contracted joints from athletic injuries or surgery. The protocol needed to affect joint contracture is the following:

1. Current intensity must be of sufficient intensity and duration to make a muscle contract strongly enough to move the body part through its antigravity range. Intensity should be increased gradually during treatment.

2. Pulse duration is preset on most of the therapeutic generators. If it is adjustable, it should be set as close as possible to the duration needed for chronaxie (300–600 μsec) of the motor nerve to be stimulated.

3. Pulses per second should be at the beginning of the tetany range (40 to 60 pulses per second).

4. Interrupted or surged current should be used.

5. On time should be between 15 and 20 seconds.

6. Off time should be equal to or greater than on time; fatigue is a big consideration.

7. The stimulated muscle group should be antagonistic to the joint contracture, and the athlete should be positioned so the joint will be moved to the limits of the available range.

8. The athlete is passive in this treatment and does not work with the electrical contraction.

9. Total treatment time should be 90 minutes daily. This can be broken into three 30-minute treatments.

10. High-voltage pulsed or medium-frequency alternating current stimulators are the best choices (see Figure 8-21).

The Effect of Noncontractile Stimulation on Edema

Ion movement within biologic tissues is a basic theory in the electrotherapy literature. This is clearly seen in the action potential model of nerve cell depolarization. The effects of sensory level stimulation on edema has been theorized to work on this principle. Research has not documented the effectiveness of this type of treatment, and the athletic trainer should continue to use other, more proven mechanisms to decrease edema. See Chapter 11 on intermittent compression for a discussion of edema formation.

Since 1987, numerous studies using rat and frog models have helped to more clearly define the effects of electrical stimulation on edema formation and reduction. The muscle pumping theory has seemed the most viable way to affect this problem. Most of the recent studies have focused on a sensory level stimulation. Early theory supported the use of sensory level direct current as a driving force to make the charged plasma protein ions in the interstitial spaces move in the direction of the oppositely charged electrode. Cook, Tepper et al. demonstrated an increase in lymphatic uptake of labeled albumin with rats treated with sensory level high-volt stimulation.[32] There was, however, no significant reduction in the limb volume. They hypothesized that the electric field introduced into the area of edema facilitated the movement of the charged proteins into the lymphatic channels. When the lymphatic channel volume increased, the contraction rate of the smooth muscle in the lymphatics increased; they also hypothesized that simulation of sensory neurons may cause an indirect activation of the autonomic nervous system. This might cause release of adrenergic substances, which would also increase the rate of lymph smooth muscle contraction and lymph circulation. Treatment considerations include:

1. Extended treatment times: 1 hour

2. Direct current stimulation with polarity arranged in correct fashion

3. Electrodes arranged to pull or push plasma proteins into the lymphatic system and be

moved back into the circulatory system via the thoracic duct

Another proposed mechanism is that a microamp stimulation of the local neurovascular components in an injured area may cause a vasoconstriction and reduce the permeability of the capillary walls to limit the migration of plasma proteins into the interstitial spaces. This would retard the accumulation of plasma proteins and the associated fluid dynamics of the edema exudate. In a study on the histamine stimulated leakage of plasma proteins, animals treated with small doses of electrical current produced less leakage. The underlying mechanisms were a reduced pore size in the capillary walls and reduced pooling of blood in the capillaries, which could have been initiated by hormonal, neural, mechanical, or electrochemical factors.

Theory on the exact mechanism of edema control from these methods remains cloudy and contradictory, but we do not have enough research findings to support trying an edema control electrical stimulation trial clinically. The following is an edema control sensory stimulation protocol:

1. Most effective current intensity is 30V to 50V, or 10% less than needed to produce a visible muscle contraction.
2. Preset short-duration currents on the high-voltage equipment are effective.
3. High-pulse frequencies (120 pps) are most effective.
4. Interrupted DC currents are most effective. Biphasic currents showed increases in volume.
5. The animals treated with a negative distal electrode had a significant treatment effect. The animals with a positive distal electrode showed no change.
6. Time of treatment after injury: the best results were reported when treatment began immediately after injury. Treatment started after 24 hours showed an effect on the accumulation of new edema volume but showed no effect on the existing edema volume.

denervated muscle Muscle that has lost its peripheral nerve supply.

7. A 30-minute treatment showed good control of volume for 4 to 5 hours.
8. The water immersion electrode technique was effective, but using surface electrodes was not effective.
9. High-voltage pulsed generators were effective; low-voltage generators were not effective.[4,13,19,33,43,44,51,65,67,74,87,89,92,119,120]

STIMULATION OF DENERVATED MUSCLE

Electrical currents may be used to produce a muscle contraction in **denervated muscle**. Although denervation of a muscle is relatively uncommon in a sports medicine setting, there are situations where this does occur. For example, a severe contusion of the shoulder might tear the axillary nerve, thus denervating the deltoid and teres minor. A muscle that is denervated is one that has lost its peripheral nerve supply. The primary purpose for electrically stimulating denervated muscle is to help minimize the extent of atrophy during the period while the nerve is regenerating. Following denervation, the muscle fibers experience a number of progressive anatomic, biochemical, and physiological changes that lead to a decrease in the size of the individual muscle fibers and in the diameter and weight of the muscle. Consequently, there will be a decrease in the amount of tension that can be generated by that muscle and an increase in the time required for the muscle to contract.[29,34] These degenerative changes progress until the muscle is reinnervated by axons regenerating across the site of the lesion. If reinnervation does not occur within 2 years, it is generally accepted that fibrous connective tissue will have replaced the contractile elements of the muscle, and recovery of muscle function is not possible.[34]

A review of the literature indicates that the majority of studies support the use of electrical stimulation of denervated muscle. These studies generally indicate that muscle atrophy can be retarded,[55] loss of both muscle mass and contractile strength can be minimized,[30] and muscle fiber size can be maintained[54] by the appropriate use of electrical stimulation. Electrically stimulated contractions of denervated muscle may limit edema and venous stasis, thus delaying muscle fiber fibrosis and degeneration.[34] However, there also seems to be general agreement that electrical stimulation has little or no effect on the rate of nerve regeneration or muscle reinnervation.

A few studies have suggested that electrical stimulation of denervated muscle may actually interfere with reinnervation, thus delaying functional return.[76,106] These studies propose that the muscle contraction disrupts the regenerating neuromuscular junction retarding reinnervation[55,76] and that electrical stimulation may traumatize denervated muscle since it is more sensitive to trauma than normal muscle.[34]

Treatment Parameters for Stimulating Denervated Muscle

The following treatment parameters have been recommended for stimulating denervated muscle:

1. A current with an asymmetric, biphasic (faradic) waveform with a pulse duration < 1 ms may be used during the first 2 weeks.[69]
2. After 2 weeks, either an interrupted square-wave direct current or a progressive exponential-wave direct current, each with a long pulse duration of greater than 10 ms, or a sine wave alternating current with a frequency lower than 10 Hz will produce a twitch contraction.[34] The length of the pulse should be as short as possible but long enough to elicit a contraction.[121]
3. The current waveform should have a pulse duration equal to or greater than the chronaxie of the denervated muscle. (To determine chronaxie see page 197).
4. The amplitude of the current, along with the pulse duration, must be sufficient to stimulate a denervated muscle with a prolonged chronaxie (15 to 40 MAmp) while producing a moderately strong contraction of the muscle fibers.
5. The pause between stimuli should be 1: 4 or 5 times longer (about 3 to 6 seconds) than the stimulus duration to minimize fatigue.[121]
6. Either a monopolar or bipolar electrode set-up can be used with the small-diameter active electrode placed over the most electrically active point in the muscle. This may not be the motor point since the muscle is not normally innervated.
7. Stimulation should begin immediately following denervation, using 3 stimulation treatments per day involving 3 sets of between 5 and 20 repetitions, which can be varied according to fatiguability of the muscle.[34]
8. The contraction needs to create muscle tension so joints may need to be fixed or isotonic contraction for end range positions may be needed.

THERAPEUTIC USES OF ELECTRICAL STIMULATION OF SENSORY NERVES

Clinically, efforts are made to stimulate the sensory nerves to change the athlete's perception of a painful stimulus coming from an injured area. To understand how to maximally affect the perception of pain through electrical stimulation, it is necessary to understand pain perception. The gate control theory, the descending or central biasing theory, and the opiate pain control theory are the theoretical bases for pain reduction phenomena. These theories are covered in depth in Chapter 3.

Gate Control Theory

Electrically stimulating the large sensory fibers when there is pain in a certain area will force the central nervous system to make the brain's recognition area aware of the electrical stimuli. As long as the stimuli are applied, the perception of pain is diminished. Electrical stimulation of sensory nerves will evoke the gate control mechanism and diminish awareness of painful stimuli. As long as the stimulation is causing firing of the sensory nerves, the gate to pain should be closed. If accommodation to the electrical stimulus occurs or if the stimulus stops, the gate is then open, and pain returns to perception.[15,18,71,72,73,84,85,104,105,109,124]

The physical dominance, enkephalin-release model is used in treating pain from acute injuries, problems with the musculoskeletal system, or postoperative pain. The following criteria can be used as guidelines in developing effective treatment protocols:

1. Current intensity should be adjusted to tolerance but should not cause a muscular contraction; the higher, the better.
2. Pulse duration (pulse width) should be 75 to 150 μ sec or maximum possible on the machine.
3. Pulses per second should be 80 to 125 or as high as possible on the machine.
4. A transcutaneous electrical stimulator waveform should be used.
5. On time should be continuous mode.
6. Total treatment time should correspond to fluctuations in pain; the unit should be left on until pain is no longer perceived, turned off, then restarted when pain begins again.
7. If this treatment is successful, you will have some pain relief within the first 30 minutes of treatment.
8. If it is not successful, but you feel this is the best theoretical or most clinically applicable approach, change the electrode placements and try again. If this is not successful, then using a different theoretical approach may offer more help.
9. Any stimulator that can deliver this current is acceptable. Portable units are better for 24-hour pain control[71,72,80] (see Figure 8-21).

---

central biasing   The use of hyperstimulation analgesia to bias the central nervous system against transmitting painful stimuli to the sensory recognition area. This occurs through hormonal influences created by brain stem stimulation.

Descending Pain Control (Central Biasing Theory)

Intense electrical stimulation of the smaller fibers (C fibers or pain fibers) at peripheral sites (trigger and acupoint) for short time periods causes stimulation of descending neurons, which then affect transmission of pain information by closing the gate at the spinal cord level[22] (see Figure 3-5).

The **central biasing** set-up is used on sharp chronic pain or severe pathological pain. Changing the bias of the central nervous system and increasing the descending influences on the transmission of pain are best accomplished with the following protocols:

1. Current intensity should be very high, approaching a noxious level; muscular contraction is not desirable.
2. Pulse duration should be 10 msec.
3. Pulses per second should be 80.
4. On time should be 30 seconds to 1 minute.
5. Stimulation should be applied over trigger or acupuncture points.
6. Selection and number of points used varies according to the part treated.
7. A low-frequency, high-intensity generator is the stimulator of choice for central biasing[22] (see Figure 8-20).
8. If this treatment is successful, pain will be relieved shortly after the treatment.
9. If this treatment is not successful, try different electrode setups by expanding the treatment points used.

■ **Clinical Decision-Making**   *Exercise 8-4*

The athletic trainer is treating a myofascial trigger point in the upper trapezius. He decides to use a point stimulator for the purpose of pain modulation. What treatment technique will likely be most effective?

Opiate Pain Control Theory

Electrical stimulation of sensory nerves may stimulate the release of enkephalin from local sites throughout the central nervous system and the release of β-endorphin from the pituitary gland into the cerebral spinal fluid. The mechanism that causes the release and then the binding of enkephalin and β-endorphin to some nerve cells is still unclear. It is certain that a diminution or elimination of pain perception is caused by applying an electrical current to areas close to the site of pain or to acupuncture or trigger points, both local and distant to the pain area.[22,28,68,78,85,86,105,110,128]

To use the influence of hyperstimulation analgesia and β-endorphin release, a point stimulation setup must be used. A large dispersive pad and a small pad or handheld, probe-point electrode are utilized in this approach. The point electrode is applied to the chosen site, and the intensity is increased until it is perceived by the athlete. The probe is then moved around the area, and the athlete is asked to report relative changes in perception of intensity. When a location of maximum-intensity perception is found, the current intensity is increased to maximum tolerable levels. This is much the same as finding a motor point, as described earlier.[22,98]

β-endorphin stimulation may offer better relief for the deep aching or chronic pain similar to overuse injury's pain. β-endorphin production may be stimulated using the following protocols:

1. Current intensity should be high, approaching a noxious level; muscular contraction is acceptable.

2. Pulse duration should be 200 μ to 10 msec.
3. Pulses per second should be between 1 and 5.
4. High-voltage pulsed current should be used.
5. On time should be 30 to 45 seconds.
6. Stimulation should be applied over trigger or acupuncture points.
7. Selection and number of points used varies according to the part and condition being treated.
8. A high-voltage pulsed current or a low-frequency, high-intensity machine is best for this effect[22,85,86] (see Figure 8-21).
9. If stimulation is successful, you should know at the completion of the treatment. The analgesic effect should last for several (6 to 7) hours.
10. If not successful, try expanding the number of stimulation sites. Add the same stimulation points on the opposite side of the body, add auricular (ear) acupuncture points, and add more points on the same limb.

A combination of intense point stimulation and transcutaneous electrical nerve stimulation may be used. The transcutaneous electrical nerve stimulation applications should be used as much as needed to make the athlete comfortable, and the intense point stimulation should be used on a periodic basis. Periodic use of intense point stimulation gives maximal pain relief for a period of time and allows some gains in overall pain suppression. Daily intense point stimulation may eventually bias the central nervous system and decrease the effectiveness of this type of stimulation.[59]

Placebo Effects of Electrical Stimulation

All three of these theories of sensory electrical stimulation produce their effects on the transmission lines of pain by interrupting or slowing the flow of pain information to the brain. The brain is the reception and interpretation center for these pain messages, and incorporating this area into your treatment can enhance the treatment's effects. This is crucial to a successful treatment because the athletic trainer is trying to alter the athlete's pain perception. This perceptual change is influenced by many factors at the cognitive and affective levels.

There is a big placebo effect in all that we do in providing any therapy to our athletes. This placebo effect is a basic and extremely important tool to help us achieve the best results. Our attitude toward the athlete and our presentation of the therapy to him are crucial. When the athletic trainer demonstrates a sincere interest in the athlete's problems, the athlete uses that interest to add to his own conviction and motivation to get well.

When these factors are active, real physiologic changes occur that assist in the healing process. The athletic trainer should not intentionally deceive the athlete with a sham treatment but should use the treatment to have the best impact on the athlete's perception of his problem and the treatment's effectiveness.

The treatment will work better if the athlete has a profound belief in the treatment's ability to change the problem. To gain the most from this effect, the athlete needs to be intimately involved with his or her treatment. We must educate, encourage, and empower the athlete to get better. Giving the athlete the knowledge and ability to feel some control and to be self determined in healing reduces the stress of injury and enhances the recovery powers of the athlete. In stressful situations, any measure of control lessens the extent of the stress and results in the improvement of disease resistance or injury recovery factors that will improve treatment outcomes.[59]

CLINICAL USES OF LOW-VOLTAGE CONTINUOUS DIRECT CURRENT

Medical Galvanism

The application of continuous low-voltage direct current causes several physiologic changes that can be used therapeutically. The therapeutic benefits are related to the polar and vasomotor effects and to the acid reaction around the positive pole and the alkaline reaction at the negative pole. The athletic trainer must be concerned with the damaging effects of this variety of current. Acidic or alkaline changes can cause severe skin reactions.[124] These reactions occur only with low-voltage continuous direct current and are not likely with the high-voltage pulsed generators. The pulse duration of the high-voltage pulsed generators is too short to cause these chemical changes.[96]

There is also a vasomotor effect on the skin, increasing blood flow between the electrodes. The benefits from this type of direct current are usually attributed to the increased blood flow through the treatment area.[124]

The following protocols for continuous, low-voltage direct current can be used to give the greatest vasomotor effects:

1. Current intensity should be to the athlete's tolerance; it should be increased as accommodation takes place. This intensity is in the milliamp range.
2. Continuous direct current should be used.
3. Pulses per second should be 0.
4. A low-voltage, direct-current stimulator is the machine of choice.
5. Treatment time should be between a 15-minute minimum and a 50-minute maximum.
6. Equal-sized electrodes are used over gauze that has been soaked in saline solution and lightly squeezed.
7. Skin should be unbroken[64,94,98] (see Figure 8-21).

Iontophoresis

Direct current has been used for many years to drive ions from the heavy metals into and through the skin for treatment of skin infections or for a counterirritating effect. Iontophoresis is discussed in detail in Chapter 9.

Treatment Precautions with Continuous Direct Currents

Skin burns are the greatest hazard of any continuous, direct-current technique. These burns result from excessive electrical density in any area, usually from direct metal contact with skin or from setting the intensity too high for the size of the active electrode. Both these problems cause a very high density of current in the area of contact.[94,98]

LOW-INTENSITY STIMULATORS (LIS)

Another type of low-voltage equipment is the low-intensity stimulator (LIS). The characteristic that distinguishes this type of generator is that the intensity of the stimulus is limited to 1000 microamps or less in LIS, while the intensity of the standard low-voltage equipment can be increased into the milliamp range.

Generators that produce low-intensity stimulation are among the newer electrical therapy units available to today's athletic trainer. These units were originally called microcurrent electrical neuromuscular stimulators (MENS).[116] However, the stimulation pathway is not the usual neural pathway and they are not designed to stimulate a muscle contraction. Consequently, this type of generator was subsequently referred to as a microcurrent electrical stimulator (MES).[116] Low-intensity stimulator is the most recent and currently used term in an ongoing evolution of terminology relative to this type of stimulator.

Perhaps the most important point to emphasize is that currents generated by these devices are not substantially different from the currents discussed previously.[88] These currents still have a direction, and both AC and DC waveforms are available. The currents also have amplitude (intensity), pulse duration, and frequency.

LIS currents are defined as those currents of less than 1 milliamp or 1000 microamps. The generators can generate a variety of waveforms from modified monophasic to biphasic square waves

- LIS<1mA

with frequencies from .3 HZ to 50 HZ. The pulse durations are also variable and may be prolonged at the lower frequencies from 1 to 500 milliseconds. This varies as the frequency changes or is preset when pulsed currents are used. Many of these devices are made with an impedance-sensitive voltage that adapts the current to the impedance to keep the current constant as selected.[100]

If the current generator can be adjusted to allow increases of intensity above 1000 microamps, the current becomes like those previously described in this text. If the current provokes an action potential in a sensory or motor nerve, the results on that tissue will be the same as previously described for other currents sensation or muscle contraction.

Most of the literature on microcurrents and subsequently on low-intensity stimulators has been generated by researchers interested in stimulating the healing process in fractures and skin wounds. Subsequent research is aimed at identifying why and how microcurrents work. The best-researched areas of application of LIS type currents is in the stimulation of bone formation in delayed union or nonunion of fractures of the long bones. Most of this research was done using implanted rather than surface electrodes, and most have used low-intensity direct current (LIDC) with the negative pole placed at the fracture site.[4,10,36] We are in danger of generalizing treatments for all problems based on success in this one area. These applications were intended to mimic the normal electrical field created during the injury and healing process.[3,43] At present these electrical changes are poorly understood, and the effects of adding additional electric current to the normal electrical activity created by the injury and healing process are still being investigated.

As can be seen in the previous sections on the bioelectric properties of cells and tissues, there are

■ **LIS effects**
···

- Analgesia
- Fracture healing
- Wound healing
- Ligament and tendon healing

several possible theories that might explain the biostimulative effects of LIS currents and give the athletic trainer some guidance in developing clinical protocols.

The current of injury, stress-generated potentials, cell metabolism stimulation, and bioelectric fields guiding growth are all natural events that low-intensity stimulation may augment, stimulate, or artificially replace.[23,24]

Low-intensity stimulation has been used for two major effects:

1. Analgesia of the painful area and
2. Biostimulation of the healing process either for enhancing the process or for acceleration of its stages

Analgesic Effects of LIS

The mechanism of analgesia created by LIS current does not fit into our present theoretical framework, as sensory nerve excitation is a necessary component of all three models of electroanalgesia stimulation. At best, LIS can create or change the constant direct current flow of the neural tissues that may have some way of biasing the transmission of the painful stimulus. LIS may also make the nerve cell membrane more receptive to neurotransmitters that will block transmission. The exact mechanism has not yet been established. The research is not supportive of the effectiveness of LIS for pain reduction. This lack of consensus and disagreement in the research gives the athletic trainer limited security in devising an effective protocol. Most of the research uses delayed onset muscle soreness (DOMS) or cold-induced pain models, and results show no significant difference between LIS and placebo treatments.[1,7,19,40,48,62,70,83,102,104,125,127,132]

Promotion of Wound Healing

Low-intensity direct current has been used to treat skin ulcers that have poor blood flow. The treated ulcers show accelerated healing rates when compared with untreated skin ulcers.

The following protocol was used to promote wound healing:

1. Current intensity was 200 to 400 μ amp for normal skin and 400 to 800 μ amp for denervated skin.
2. Long pulse durations or continuous uninterrupted currents can be used.
3. Maximum pulse frequency.
4. Monophasic direct current is best, but biphasic direct current is acceptable. Low-intensity stimulators can be used, but other generators with intensities adjusted to subsensory levels can also be effective. A battery-powered portable unit is most convenient.
5. Treatment time was 2 hours followed by a 4-hour rest time.
6. Two to three treatment bouts per day.
7. The negative electrode is positioned in the wound area for the first 3 days. The positive electrode should be positioned 25 cm proximal to the wound.
8. After 3 days, the polarity is reversed, and the positive electrode is positioned in the wound area.
9. If infection is present, the negative electrode should be left in the wound area until the signs of infection are not evident. The negative electrode remains in the wound for 3 days after the infection clears.
10. If the wound size decrease plateaus, then return the negative electrode to the wound area for 3 days.

Other protocols have been successful using the anode in the wound area for the entire time. High-volt stimulation has also been used in a manner similar to the negative-positive model presented. The intensity was adjusted to give a microamp current.

The mechanism by which LIS stimulates healing is elusive, but cells are stimulated to increase their normal proliferation, migration, motility, DNA synthesis, and collagen synthesis. Receptor levels for growth factor has also shown a significant increase when wound areas are stimulated.[3,25,26,46,47,50,60,75,93,123,126,131] The naturally occurring electrical potential gradients are enhanced following electrical stimulation.[48]

Promotion of Fracture Healing

The use of low-intensity direct current may be an adjunctive modality in the treatment of fractures, especially fractures prone to nonunion. Fracture healing may be accelerated by passing a direct current through the fracture site. Getting the current into the bony area without an invasive technique is difficult.[11,18,22,23,31,36,61,99,118]

Using a standard transcutaneous electrical nerve stimulation unit, Kahn reported favorable results in the electrical stimulation of callus formation in fractures that had nonunions after 6 months.[64] This information is based on a case study. Results of a more extensive population of nonunions have not been documented. Kahn used the following protocol:

1. Current intensity was just perceptible to the athlete.
2. Pulse duration was the longest duration allowed on the unit (100 to 200 msec).
3. Pulses per second were set at the lowest frequency allowed on the unit (5 to 10 pps).
4. Standard monophasic or biphasic current in the transcutaneous electrical stimulating units were used.
5. Treatment time was from 30 minutes to 1 hour, three to four times daily.
6. A negative electrode was placed close to but distal to the fracture site. A positive electrode was placed proximal to the immobilizing device.
7. If four pads were used, the interferential placement described earlier was used.
8. Results were reassessed at monthly intervals[64] (see Figure 8-20).

Promotion of Healing in Tendon and Ligament

There are only a few research studies on the biostimulative effect of electrical stimulation on tendon or ligament healing. Both tissues have been found to generate strain-generated electric potentials naturally in response to stress. These potentials help signal the tissue to grow in response to the stress, according to Wolff's law.

In an experimental study on partial division of dog patellar tendons, treated with 20 μ amp cathodal stimulation, the stimulated tendons showed 92% recovery of normal breaking strength at 8 weeks.[112]

Tendon stimulated in vitro in a culture medium showed increased fibroblastic cellular activity, tendon cellular proliferation, and collagen synthesis. The rate at which stimulated tendons demonstrated histologic repair at the injury site was also significantly accelerated over the control group.[96] Litke and Dahners studied rat medial collateral ligament (MCL) injuries treated with electrical simulation. The treated group showed statistical significance in the rupture force, stiffness and energy absorbed, and laxity.[76]

As can be seen by the previous sections, LIS current can be a valuable addition to the clinical armamentarium of the athletic trainer, but they are untested clinically.

This is a case where more may not be better. For electricity to produce these effects

1. Cells must be current sensitive
2. Correct polarity orientation may be necessary
3. Correct amounts of current will cause the cells to be more active in the healing process

If results are not going correctly, then reduce the current and/or change polarity. Weak stimuli may increase physiologic activity while very strong stimuli abolish or inhibit activity.

Most generators in use today are capable of low-intensity current. Simply turn the machine on but do not increase the intensity to threshold levels. This can also be a function of current density using electrode size and placement as well as intensity to keep current in the microamp range.

The athletic trainer is certainly entitled to be very skeptical of the manufacturers' claims until more research is reported. Existing protocols for use are not well established, which leaves the athletic trainer with an insecure feeling about this modality.

RUSSIAN CURRENTS (MEDIUM-FREQUENCY CURRENT GENERATORS)

This class of current generators was developed in Canada and the United States after the Russian scientist Yadou M. Kots presented a seminar on the use of electrical muscular stimulators to augment strength gain. The stimulators developed after this presentation were termed **Russian current** generators. These stimulators have evolved and presently deliver a medium (2000 to 10,000 Hz) frequency polyphasic AC wave form.[57,114] The pulse can be varied from 50 to 250 μ sec; the phase duration will be one half of the pulse duration or 25 to 125 μ sec. As the pulse frequency increases, the pulse duration decreases.[24,43,49] There are two basic waveforms: a sine wave and a square wave cycle with a fixed intrapulse interval.

The sine wave is produced in a burst mode, which has a 50% duty cycle. According to strength-duration curve data, to obtain the same stimulation effect as the duration of the stimulus decreases, the intensity must be increased. The intensity associated with this duration of current could be considered as painful.

McLoda has shown that a burst duty cycle of 10% was the most efficient ratio of burst duration to interburst interval for eliciting the strongest muscle contraction.[82]

To make this intensity of current tolerable, it is generated in 50-burst-per-second envelopes with an interburst interval of 10 msec. This slightly reduces the total current but allows enough of a peak current intensity to stimulate muscle very well (Figure 8-22). If the current continued without the burst effect, the total current delivered would equal the lightly shaded area in Figure 8-23. When generated with the burst effect, the total current is

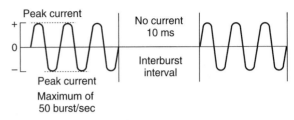

Figure 8-22   Russian current with polyphasic AC waveform and 10 ms interburst interval.

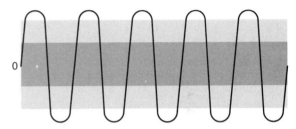

Figure 8-23   Russian current without an interburst interval. The lightly shaded area is equal to the total current.

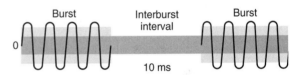

Figure 8-24   Russian current with an interburst interval. Darkly shaded area represents total current, and light shading indicates total current without the interburst interval.

Russian current   A medium-frequency (2000 to 10,000 Hz) polyphasic AC wave generated in 50 burst-per-second envelopes.

---

decreased. Here the total current would equal the darkly shaded area in Figure 8-24. This allows tolerance of greater current intensity by the athlete. The other factor affecting athlete comfort is the effect that frequency will have on the impedance of the tissue. Higher frequency currents reduce the

Specialized currents

- LIS
- Russian current
- Interferential current

resistance to the current flow, again making this type of waveform comfortable enough that the athlete may tolerate higher intensities. As the intensity increases, more motor nerves are stimulated, increasing the magnitude of the contraction. Because it is a fast oscillating AC current, as soon as the nerve repolarizes, it is stimulated again, producing a current that will maximally summate muscle contraction.[56]

The frequency (pulses per second or, in this case, bursts per second) is also a variable that can be controlled. This would make the muscle respond with a twitch rather than a gradually increasing mechanical contraction. Gradually increasing the numbers of bursts interrupts the mechanical relaxation cycle of the muscle and causes more shortening to take place[94,114] (see Figure 8-18).

INTERFERENTIAL CURRENTS

The research and use of interferential currents (IFC) has taken place primarily in Europe. An Austrian scientist, Ho Nemec, introduced the concept and suggested its therapeutic use. Nemec's concept resulted in the creation of a type of electrical generator that is difficult to understand, not because the theory is so complex, but because electrical engineers added so many options to the generator that the current can be modified substantially while still maintaining its basic waveform.

The theories and behavior of electrical waves are part of basic physics. This behavior is easiest to understand when continuous sine waves are used as an example.

With only one circuit, the current behaves as described earlier; if put on an oscilloscope, it looks like generator 1 in Figure 8-25. If a second generator is brought into the same location, the currents may interfere with each other. This interference can be summative—that is, the amplitudes of the electric

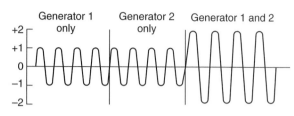

Figure 8-25 Sine wave from generator 1 and sine wave from generator 2 showing a constructive interference pattern.

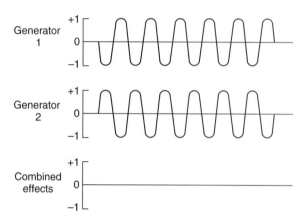

Figure 8-26 Sine wave from generator 1 and sine wave from generator 2 showing a destructive interference pattern.

constructive interference The combined amplitude of two distinct circuits increases the amplitude.

destructive interference Combined amplitude of two distinct circuits decreases the amplitude.

wave are combined and increase (Figure 8-25). Both waves are exactly the same; if they are produced in phase or originate at the same time, they combine. This is called **constructive interference**.

If these waves are generated out of sync, generator 1 starts in a positive direction at the same time that generator 2 starts in a negative direction; the waves then will cancel each other out. This is called **destructive interference**; in the summation, the waves end up with an amplitude of 0 (Figure 8-26).

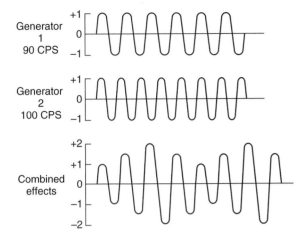

Figure 8-27   Sine wave from generator 1 at 90 CPS and sine wave from generator 2 at 100 CPS showing the heterodyne, or beating pattern, of interference.

....

beat   Distinct wave pattern created by combining two distinct circuit electrical waves that blend into a gradual rising and falling wave.

heterodyne   Cyclic rising and falling wave form of interferential current.

....

To make this a bit more complex, assume that one generator has a slightly slower or faster frequency and that the generators begin producing current simultaneously. Initially, the electric waves will be constructively summated; however, because the frequencies of the two waves differ, they gradually will get out of phase and become destructively summated. When dealing with sound waves, we hear distinct beats as this phenomenon occurs. We borrow the term **beat** when describing this behavior.[57] When any waveforms are out of phase but are combined in the same location, the waves will cause a beat effect. The blending of the waves is caused by the constructive and destructive interference patterns of the waves and is called **heterodyne** (Figure 8-27).[43,45,115]

The heterodyne effect is seen on an oscilloscope as a cyclic, rising and falling waveform. The

■ **Clinical Decision-Making**   *Exercise 8-5*

....

When using interferential current to treat muscle guarding in the low back, how should the electrodes be placed?

_____

■ Analogy   *8-2*

....

When using interferential current, an electric field is created that resembles a four-petaled flower, with the center of the flower located where the two currents cross and the petals falling between the electric current force lines. The maximum interference effect takes place near the center, with the field gradually decreasing in strength as it moves toward the points of the petal.

peaks or beat frequency in this heterodyne wave behavior occur regularly, according to the difference of each current; for example, 100 pps − 90 pps = 10 pps beat frequency. In electric currents, this beat frequency is, in effect, the stimulation frequency of the waveform because the destructive interference negates the effects of the other part of the wave. The intensity (amplitude) will be set according to sensations created by this peak.[43] When using an interference current for therapy, the athletic trainer should select the frequencies to create a beat frequency corresponding to his or her choices of frequency when using other stimulators 20 to 50 pps for muscle contraction, 50 to 120 pps for pain management, 1 pps for acustim pain relief.

When the electrodes are arranged in a square alignment and interferential currents are passed through a homogeneous medium, a predictable pattern of interference will occur.[115] In this pattern, an electric field is created where the two currents cross between the lines of electric current flow. The maximum interference effect takes place near the center, with the field gradually decreasing in strength as it moves away from the center (Figure 8-28).[43]

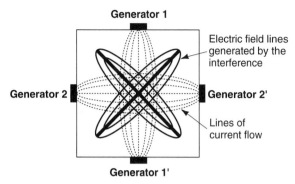

Figure 8-28 Square electrode alignment and interference pattern of current in a homogeneous medium.

■ **Clinical Decision-Making** *Exercise 8-6*
....

How can the athletic trainer make adjustments in the electrode placement to increase the current density in the deeper tissues?

Because the body is not a homogeneous medium, we cannot predict the exact location of this interference pattern; we must rely on the athlete's perception. If the athlete has a localized structure that is painful, locating the stimulation in the correct location is relatively easy. The athletic trainer moves the electrode placement until the athlete centers the feeling of the stimulus in the problem area.[43,45] When an athlete has poorly localized pain, the task becomes more difficult. See the discussion in the electrode placement section for a general discussion on the effect of electrode movement. The engineers added features to the generators and created a scanning interferential current that moves the flower petals of force around while the treatment is taking place. This enlarges the effective treatment area. Additional technology and another set of electrodes create a three-dimensional flower effect when one looks at the electrical field. This is called a stereodynamic interference current.[43,45]

All these alterations and modifications are designed to spread the heterodyne effect throughout the tissue. Because it is controlled by a cyclic electrical pattern, however, we actually may be decreasing the current passed through the structures we are trying to treat. The machines seem complex but lack the versatility to do much more than the conventional TENS treatment.[94,111]

Nikolova[97] has used IFC for a variety of clinical problems and found them effective in dealing with pain problems (e.g., joint sprains with swelling, restricted mobility, and pain; neuritis; retarded callus formation following fractures; and pseudarthrosis). These claims are supported by other researchers. Each of these researchers used slightly different protocols in treating the different clinical problems. To be successful in achieving the desired results with interferential currents, the athletic trainer must thoroughly review existing protocols and acquire a good working knowledge of the application techniques.

The world of electrical therapy is constantly changing, owing to the advances in research, engineering, and technology and because of the competitive pressures of the marketplace. Equipment manufacturers will develop a different machine and try to market it on the basis of a single feature of their product. The old adage "let the buyer beware" is certainly good advice. The more understanding of electrical currents the athletic trainer has, the less likely he or she is to be "snowed" or confused by the salesperson's spiel. Even more important, the greater the understanding, the easier it becomes to manipulate the treatment protocols for each athlete to optimize the results.[59]

Summary

1. When an electrical system is applied to muscle or nerve tissue, the result will be tissue membrane depolarization, provided that the current has the appropriate intensity, duration, and waveform to reach the tissue's excitability threshold.

2. Nerve function and muscle contraction are the same regardless of the stimulation mechanism (i.e., natural or electrical).

3. Muscle and nerve tissue respond in an all-or-none fashion; there is no gradation of response.

4. Muscle contraction will change according to changes in current. As the frequency of the electrical stimulus increases, the muscle will develop more tension as a result of the summation of the contraction of the muscle fiber through progressive mechanical shortening. Increases in intensity spread the current over a larger area and increase the number of motor units activated by the current. Increases in the duration of the current also will cause more motor units to be activated.

5. Electrically stimulated muscle contractions are used clinically to help with muscle reeducation, muscle contraction for muscle pumping action, reduction of swelling, prevention or retardation of atrophy, muscle strengthening, and increasing range of motion in tight joints.

6. Sensory level stimulation may retard edema accumulation in traumatic injuries.

7. Constant direct current has several major influences. The primary uses involve polar effects (acid or alkaline), increased blood flow, bacteriostatic effects (negative electrode), and migration and alignment of cellular building blocks in the healing processes.

8. Nonexcitatory cells and tissues respond to electric current and contain continuous direct currents circuits.

9. The body responds to injury by producing changes in the local electric circuits that may guide and assist the healing process.

10. To stimulate a given muscle, location of the muscle's motor point, size and spacing of electrodes, and impedance of the tissue between the electrodes and the motor points must be selected and adjusted to provide the most effective therapy.

11. Electrically stimulated discharges of sensory nerves help decrease pain perceptions.

12. The pain gating effect of electrical stimulation may occur at different levels in the central nervous system, depending on the type of electrical current used. Types of current similar to that used in transcutaneous electrical nerve stimulation will be gated at the spinal cord level. Hyperstimulation analgesia will stimulate central biasing with inhibitory influences descending from the brain and brain stem levels. Noxious stimuli to acupuncture or trigger areas will cause production of β-endorphin in the spinal cord and brain, with a resultant analgesic effect.

13. Specialized current waveforms (low-intensity stimulation, "Russian," interferential, and so on) all have physiologic responses that can be attributed to the characteristics of their waveforms. The differences in the waveforms and the physiologic response of each have particular effects that can be used therapeutically.

Review Questions

1. What are the physiological responses that can be elicited by using electrical stimulating currents?
2. Explain the concept of depolarization of muscle and nerve in response to electrical stimulation.
3. What do the strength-duration curves represent?
4. What are the effects of electrically stimulating nonexcitatory cells and tissues?
5. What are the various treatment parameters that must be considered when setting up a treatment using electrically stimulating currents?
6. What are the various therapeutic uses of electrically stimulated muscle contractions?
7. How should electrical stimulating currents be used with denervated muscle?
8. How can electrical stimulating currents be used to modulate pain?
9. What are the clinical applications for using low-voltage direct currents?
10. What are the various physiologic effects of using low-intensity stimulation (LIS)?
11. Are there advantages to using interferential currents as opposed to other types of electrical stimulating currents?

Self-Test Questions

T/F

1. The cathode is the negatively charged electrode in a direct current system.
2. Chronaxie refers to the minimum current intensity needed for tissue excitation if applied for a maximum time.
3. The electrode with the greatest current density is the active electrode.

Multiple Choice

4. During the absolute refractory period the cell is not capable of _____ .
   a. depolarization
   b. an action potential
   c. twitch muscle contraction
   d. all of the above
5. The part of the cell responsible for transmitting messages to other cells via ionic, electrical, or small molecule signals is _____ .
   a. electrets
   b. gap junctions
   c. dipoles
   d. cell membrane pump
6. To _____ current density in deeper tissue, the electrodes must be placed _____ .
   a. increase, closer
   b. increase, further apart
   c. decrease, closer
   d. decrease, further apart

7. Electrical stimulation may release enkephalin and β-endorphin to cause pain relief. What is the name of this pain control method?
   a. gate control theory
   b. central biasing theory
   c. opiate pain control theory
   d. placebo effects
8. Two currents combine and the amplitude decreases. This is called _____ .
   a. destructive interference
   b. constructive interference
   c. heterodyne current
   d. beat current
9. Which of the following currents is a polyphasic AC wave, generated in bursts, designed to create muscle contraction?
   a. low-intensity stimulation
   b. iontophoresis
   c. interferential current
   d. Russian
10. Increased blood flow between electrodes is an effect of which of the following?
    a. interferential current
    b. function electrical stimulation
    c. low-intensity stimulation
    d. medical galvanism

Solutions to Clinical Decision-Making Exercises

8-1   In a conventional TENS treatment, the goal is to provide as much sensory cutaneous input as possible. Thus, both the frequency and the pulse duration should be set as high as the unit will allow. The intensity should be increased until a muscle contraction is elicited, then decreased slightly until the athlete feels only a tingling sensation. If using a portable unit, the treatment may continue for several hours if necessary or until the pain subsides.

8-2   The current density under the active electrode could be increased by using a smaller electrode. The current intensity or the current duration or a combination of the two may be increased to cause a depolarization.

8-3   A medium-frequency alternating current stimulator should be used. Frequency should be set at 20 to 30 Hz using an interrupted or surge modulation. On time should be set at about 20 sec with off time also set at 20 sec. On most generators of this type, pulse duration is preset. Intensity should be increased to elicit a strong muscle contraction that moves the lower leg through its antigravity range. The athlete should be instructed to simultaneously produce a voluntary muscle contraction.

8-4   In treating both trigger points and acupuncture points, the athletic trainer should use a DC current with the frequency set between 1 to 5 Hz, pulse duration between 220 microseconds and 10 msec; intensity should be increased to the point where there is a muscle contraction, then increased further until it is somewhat painful. The point should be stimulated for 45 sec.

8-5   The four electrodes should be set up in a square pattern with the target muscle in the center of the square so that the maximum interference will take place where the electric field lines cross at the center of the pattern.

8-6   The size of the active electrode can be decreased, which will increase current density under that electrode. The active electrodes can be moved further apart. The current intensity can be increased, and the current duration may also be increased.

References

1. Allen, JD, Mattacola, CG, and Perrin, DH: Effect of microcurrent stimulation on delayed-onset muscle soreness: a double-blind comparison, *Journal of Athletic Training* 34(4):334–337, 1999.
2. Alon, G: High voltage stimulation: effects of electrode size on basic excitatory responses, *Phys. Ther.* 65:890, 1985.
3. Alon, G: "Microcurrent" stimulation: a progress report 1998, *Athletic Therapy Today* 3(6): 15–17, 28–29, 55, 1998.
4. Alon, G, and DeDomeico, G: *High-voltage stimulation: an integrated approach to clinical electrotherapy*, Chattanooga, Tenn., 1987, Chattanooga Corp.
5. Alon, G, Kantor, G, and Smith, GV: Peripheral nerve excitation and plantar flexion force elicited by electrical stimulation in males and females, *Journal of Orthopaedic & Sports Physical Therapy* 29(4):208–217, 1999.
6. American Physical Therapy Association: *Electro therapeutic terminology in physical therapy*, APTA Publications, Alexandria, VA. 1990.
7. Ansoleaga, E, and Wirth, V: Microcurrent electrical stimulation may reduce clinically induced DOMS, *Journal of Athletic Training* 34(2):S-67, 1999.
8. Baker, L, McNeal, D, and Benton, L: *Neuromuscular electrical stimulation*, Downey, Calif., 1993, Rancho Los Amigos Medical Center.
9. Becker, R: The bioelectric factors in amphibian-limb regeneration, *J.B.J.S.*: 43-A:643–656, 1961.
10. Becker, R, Bachman, C, and Friedman, H: The direct current control system, *NY State J of Medicine* 62:1169–1176, 1962.
11. Becker, R, and Selden, G: *The body electric*, New York, 1985, William Morrow & Co.
12. Benton, L, Baker, L, and Bowman, B: *Functional electrical stimulation: a practical clinical guide*, Downey, Calif., 1980. Rancho Los Amigos Hospital.
13. Bettany, J: Influence of high-voltage pulsed current on edema formation following impact injury, *Phys Ther* 70:219–224, 1990.
14. Binder-MacLeod, S, and Snyder-Mackler, L: Muscle fatigue: clinical implications for fatigue assessment and neuromuscular electrical stimulation, *Phys Ther* 73:902–910, 1993.
15. Bishop. B: Pain: its physiology and rationale for management, *Phys Ther* 60:13–37, 1980.

16. Bogataj, U, Gros, N, and Kljajic, M: The rehabilitation of gait in patients with hemiplegia: a comparison between conventional therapy and multichannel functional electrical stimulation therapy, *Phys Ther* 75(6):490–502, 1995.

17. Bonacci, JA, and Higbie, EJ: Effects of microcurrent treatment on perceived pain and muscle strength following eccentric exercise, *Journal of Athletic Training* 32(2): 119–223, 1997.

18. Brighton, C: Bioelectric effects on bone and cartilage, *Clin Orthop* 124:2–4, 1977.

19. Brown, S: The effect of microcurrent on edema, range of motion, and pain in treatment of lateral ankle sprains, Abstract. *JOSPT* 19:55, 1994.

20. Butterfield, DL, Draper, DO, and Ricard, M: The effect of high-volt pulsed current electrical stimulation on delayed-onset muscle soreness, *Journal of Athletic Training* 32(1):15–20, 1997.

21. Carley, P, and Wainapel, S: Electrotherapy for the acceleration of wound healing: low-intensity direct current, *Arch Phys Med Rehab* 66:443–446, 1985.

22. Castel, J: *Pain management with acupuncture and transcutaneous electrical nerve stimulation techniques and photo simulation (laser).* Symposium on Pain Management, Walter Reed Army Medical Center, Nov. 13, 1982.

23. Charman, R: Bioelectricity and electrotherapy—towards a new paradigm? Part 1: the cell; Part 2: cellular reception and emission of electromagnetic signals, *Physiotherapy* 76:502–518; Part 3: bioelectric potentials and tissue currents, *Physiotherapy* 76:643–654; Part 4: strain-generated potentials in bone and connective tissue, *Physiotherapy* 76:725–730; Part 5: exogenous currents and fields—experimental and clinical applications, *Physiotherapy* 76:743–750, 1990.

24. Charman, R: Bioelectricity and electrotherapy—towards a new paradigm? Part 6: environmental current and fields—the natural background, *Physiotherapy* 77:8–13; Part 7: environmental currents and fields—manmade, *Physiotherapy* 77:129–140; Part 8: grounds for a new paradigm? *Physiotherapy* 77:211–221, 1991.

25. Chreng, N. Van Houf, H, and Bockx, E: The effects of electric current on ATP generation, protein synthesis and membrane transport in rat skin, *Clin. Orthop. Relat. Res.* 171:264–272, 1982.

26. Chu, C: Weak direct current accelerates split thickness graft healing on tangentially excised second-degree burns, *J. Burn Care Rehab* 12:285–293, 1991.

27. Clements, F: Effect of motor neuromuscular electrical stimulation on microvascular perfusion of stimulated rat skeletal muscle, *Phys Ther* 71:397–406, 1991.

28. Clement-Jones, V: Increased β-endorphin but not metenkephalin levels in human cerebrospinal fluid after acupuncture for recurrent pain, *Lancet* Nov 1, 8:946–948, 1980.

29. Clemente, F, and Barron, K: Transcutaneous neuromuscular electrical stimulation effect on the degree of microvascular perfusion in autonomically denervated rat skeletal muscle, *Arch Phys Med Rehab* 77(2):155–160, 1996.

30. Cole, B, and Gardiner, P: Does electrical stimulation of denervated muscle continued after reinnervation, influence recovery of contractile function? *Exp Neuro* 85:52, 1984.

31. Connolly, J, Hahn, H, and Jardon, O: The electrical enhancement of periosteal proliferation in normal and delayed fracture healing, *Clin. Orthop.* 124:97–105, 1977.

32. Cook, H, et al.: Effect of electrical stimulation on lymphatic flow and limb volume in the rat, *Phys Ther* 74:1040–1046, 1994.

33. Cosgrove, K, and Alon, G: The electrical effect of two commonly used clinical stimulators on traumatic edema in rats, *Phys Ther* 72:227–233, 1992.

34. Cummings, J: Electrical stimulation of denervated muscle, In Gersch, M, editor: *Electrotherapy in rehabilitation*, Philadelphia, 1992, FA Davis.

35. Currier, D, Lehman, J, and Lightfoot, P: Electrical stimulation in exercise of the quadriceps femoris muscle, *Phys Ther* 59: 1508–1512, 1979.

36. Currier, D, and Mann, R: Muscular strength development by electrical stimulation in healthy individuals, *Phys Ther* 63:915–921, 1983.

37. Dallmann, S: Preference for low versus medium frequency electrical stimulation at constant induced muscle forces, Abstract R345, *Phys Ther* 725:5107, 1992.

38. Delitto, A: A study of discomfort with electrical stimulation, *Phys Ther* 72:410–424, 1992.

39. Denegar, C: The effects of low-volt microamperage stimulation on delayed onset muscle soreness, *J. Sport Rehabil* 1:95–102, 1993.

40. Denegar, C: Influence of transcutaneous electrical nerve stimulation on pain, range of motion, and serum cortisol concentration in females experiencing delayed onset muscle soreness, *JOSPT* 11:100–103, 1989.

41. DeVahl, J: Neuromuscular electrical stimulation (NMES) in rehabilitation. In Gersh, M, editor: *Electrotherapy in rehabilitation*, Philadelphia, 1992, FA Davis.

42. Eriksson, E, and Haggmark, T: Comparison of isometric muscle training and electrical stimulation supplement, isometric muscle training in the recovery after major knee ligament surgery, *Am. J. Sports Med.* 7:169–171, 1979.

43. Fish, D: Effect of anodal high-voltage pulsed current on edema formation in frog hind limbs, *Phys Ther* 71:724–733, 1991.

44. Flicker, MT: *An analysis of cold intermittent compression with simultaneous treatment of electrical stimulation in the reduction of post acute ankle lymphedema.* Unpublished master's thesis, University of North Carolina, Chapel Hill, NC, May, 1993.

45. Franklin, ME: Effect of varying the ration of electrically induced muscle contraction time to rest time on serum creatini kinase and perceived soreness, *JOSPT* 13:310–315, 1991.

46. Gault, W, and Gatens, P: Use of low intensity direct current in management of ischemic skin ulcers, *Phys Ther* 56:265–269, 1976.

47. Gentzkow, G: Electrical stimulation to heal dermal wounds, *J. Derm Surg Oncol* 19:753–778, 1993.

48. Gersh, MR: Microcurrent electrical stimulation: putting it in perspective, *Clinical Management* 9(4):51–54, 1990.

49. Goodgold, J, and Eberstein, A: *Electrodiagnosis of neuromuscular diseases*, Baltimore, 1972, Williams & Wilkins.

50. Griffin, J: Efficacy of high voltage pulsed current for healing of pressure ulcers in patients with spinal cord injury, *Phys Ther* 71:433–444, 1991.

51. Griffin, J: Reduction of chronic posttraumatic hand edema: a comparison of high-voltage pulsed current, intermittent pneumatic compression, and placebo treatments, *Phys Ther* 70:279–286, 1990.

52. Guyton, A: *Textbook of medical physiology*, ed 2, Philadelphia, 1961, WB Saunders Co.

53. Guffey, J, and Asmussen, M: In vitro bactericidal effects of high-voltage pulsed current versus direct current against staphylococcus aureus, *J. Clin. Electrophysiol* 1:5–9, 1989.

54. Guttman E, and Guttman, L: Effect of electrotherapy on denervated and reinnervated muscles in rabbits, *Lancet* 1:169, 1942.

55. Herbison, G, Jaweed, M, and Ditunno, J: Acetylcholine sensitivity and fibrillation potentials in electrically stimulated crush-denervated rat skeletal muscle, *Arch Phys Med Rehab* 64:217, 1983.

56. Holcomb, WR, Golestani, S, and Hill, S: AQ comparison of knee extension force production with biphasic versus Russian current, *Journal of Athletic Training* 34(2):S-17, 1999.

57. Holcomb, WR: A practical guide to electrical therapy, *Journal of Sport Rehabilitation* 6(3):272–282, 1997.

58. Hooker, Daniel N: Personal communication, January 30, 1994.

59. Howson, D: *Report on neuromuscular reeducation*, Minneapolis, 1978, Medical General.

60. Howson, DC: Peripheral neural excitability, *Phys Ther* 58:1467–1473, 1978.

61. *Instruction manual for electrostim:* 180–182, 1989, Promatek, Canada.

62. Jeter, J, and Valcenta, D: The effects of microcurrent electrical nerve stimulation on delayed onset muscle soreness and peak torque deficits in trained weight lifters, abstract PO-RO65-M. *Phys Ther* 735:5–24, 1993.

63. Kagaya, H, and Shimada, Y: Restoration and analysis of standing-up in complete paraplegia utilizing functional electrical stimulation, *Arch Phys Med Rehab* 76(9): 876–881, 1995.

64. Kahn, J: *Low voltage technique*, ed 4, Syossett, N.Y., 1983, Joseph Kahn.

65. Karnes, J: Effects of low-voltage pulsed current on edema formation in frog hind limbs following impact injury, *Phys Ther* 72:273–278, 1992.

66. Karnes, J: Influence of high-voltage pulsed current on diameters of anterioles during histamine-induced vasodilation, abstract R341, *Phys Ther* 725:5105, 1992.

67. Kincaid, C, Lavoie, K: Inhibition of bacterial growth in vitro following stimulation with high-voltage monophasic pulsed current, *Phys Ther* 69:651–655, 1989.

68. Kono, T, Ingersoll, CD, and Edwards, JE: A comparison of acupuncture, TENS, and acupuncture with TENS for pain relief during DOMS, *Journal of Athletic Training* 34(2): S-67, 1999.

69. Kosman A, Osborne, S, and Ivey, A: Comparative effectiveness of various electrical currents in preventing muscle atrophy in rat, *Arch Phys Med Rehab* 28:7, 1947.

70. Kulig, K: Comparison of the effects of high-velocity exercise and microcurrent neuromuscular stimulation on delayed onset muscle soreness, abstract R284, *Phys Ther* 715:5115, 1991.

71. Lampe, G: A clinical approach to transcutaneous electrical nerve stimulation in the treatment of chronic and acute pain, Minneapolis, July, 1978, Med. General.

72. Lampe, G: Introduction to the use of transcutaneous electrical nerve stimulation devices, *Phys Ther* 58: 1450–1454, 1978.

73. Laughman, R, Youdes, J, and Garrett, T: Strength changes in the normal quadriceps femoris muscle as a result of electrical stimulation, *Phys Ther* 63:494–499, 1983.

74. Lea, J: The effect of electrical stimulation on edematous rat hind paws, abstract R379, *Phys Ther* 725:5116, 1992.

75. Leffmann, D: The effect of subliminal transcutaneous electrical stimulation on the rate of wound healing in rats, abstract R166, *Phys Ther* 725:567, 1992.

76. Litke, D, and Dahners, L: Effect of different levels of direct current on early ligament healing in a rat model, *J. Orthopaedic Research* 12:683–688, 1994.

77. Malizia, E: Electroaccupuncture and Peripheral β-Endorphin and ACTH Levels, *Lancet* Sept 8:535–536, 1979.

78. Malezic, M, and Hesse, S: Restoration of gait by functional electrical stimulation in paraplegic patients: a modified programme of treatment, *Paraplegia* 33(3):126–131, 1995.

79. Mannheimer, J, and Lampe, G: *Clinical transcutaneous electrical nerve stimulation*, Philadelphia, 1984, FA Davis.

80. Marino, A, and Becker, R: Biologic effects of extremely low frequency electric and magnetic fields: a review, *Phys. Chem. Physics* 9:131–143, 1977.

81. Maurer, C: The effectiveness of microelectrical neural stimulation on exercise-induced muscle trauma, abstract R200, *Phys Ther* 725:574, 1992.

82. McLoda, TA, and Carmack, JA: Optimal burst duration during a facilitated quadriceps femoris contraction, *Journal of Athletic Training* 35(2):145–150, 2000.

83. Melzack, R: *The puzzle of pain*, New York, 1973, Basic Books.

84. Melzack, R: Prolonged relief of pain by brief, intense transcutaneous electrical stimulation, *Pain* 1(4):357–373, 1975.

85. Melzack, R, Stillwell, D, and Fox, E: Trigger points and acupuncture points for pain: correlations and implications, *Pain* 3(1):3–23, 1977.

86. Mendel, F: High-voltage pulsed current using surface electrodes: effect on acute edema formation after hyperflexion injury in frogs, *JOSPT* 16:140–144, 1992.

87. Mendel, F: Influence of high-voltage pulsed current on edema formation following impact injury in rats, *Phys Ther* 72:668–673, 1992.

88. Merrick, MA: Research digest. Unconventional modalities: microcurrent. *Athletic Therapy Today*, 4(5):53–54, 1999.

89. Michlovitz, S: Ice and high-voltage pulsed stimulation in treatment of acute lateral ankle sprains, *JOSPT* 9:301–304, 1988.

90. Miller, BF, Gruben, KG, and Morgan, BJ: Circulatory responses to voluntary and electrically induced muscle contractions in humans, *Physical Therapy* 80(1):53–60, 2000.

91. Mohr, T. Akers, T. and Landry, R: Effect of high-voltage stimulation on edema reduction in the rat hind limb, *Phys Ther* 67:1703–1707, 1987.

92. Mulder, G: Treatment of open-skin wounds with electric stimulation, *ARCH Phys Med Rehabil* 72:375–377, 1991.

93. Lomo, T, and Slater, C: Control of acetylcholine sensitivity and synapse formation by muscle activity, *J Physiol* 275:391, 1978.

94. Nelson, R, and Currier, D: *Clinical electrotherapy*, Norwalk, Conn., 1987, Appleton and Lange.

95. Nessler, J, and Mass, P: Direct current electrical stimulation of tendon healing in vitro, *Clin Ortho Relat. Research* 217:303–312, 1987.

96. Newton, R, and Karselis, T: Skin pH following high-voltage pulsed galvanic stimulation, *Phys Ther* 63:1593–1596, 1983.

97. Nikolova, L: *Treatment with interferential current*, New York, 1987, Churchill Livingstone.

98. Notes on low-volt therapy: White Plains, N.Y., 1966, TECA Corporation.

99. Pettine, K: External electrical stimulation and bracing for treatment of spondylolysis—a case report, *Spine* 188:436–439, 1993.

100. Picker, R: Current trends: low-volt pulsed microamp stimulation, Part 1 and Part 2, *Clinical Management* 9:11–14; 9(3):28–33, 1990.

101. Randall, B, Imig, C, and Hines, HM: Effect of electrical stimulation upon blood flow and temperature of skeletal muscles, *Arch. Phys. Med.* 33:73–78, 1952.

102. Rapaski, D: Microcurrent electrical stimulation: comparison of two protocols in reducing delayed onset muscle soreness, abstract R286, *Phys Ther* 715:5116, 1991.

103. Reed, B: Effect of high-voltage pulsed electrical stimulation on microvascular permeability to plasma proteins: a possible mechanism in minimizing edema, *Phys Ther* 68:491–495, 1988.

104. Rolle, W, Alon, G, and Nirschl, R: Comparison of subliminal and placebo stimulation in the management of elbow epicondylitis, abstract R280, *Phys Ther* 715:5114, 1991.

105. Salar, G: Effect of transcutaneous electrotherapy on CSF β-endorphin content in patients without pain problems, *Pain* 10:169–172, 1981.

106. Schimrigk, K, Mclaughlen, J, and Gruniger, W: The effect of electrical stimulation on the experimentally denervated rat muscle, *Scand J Rehab Med* 9:55, 1977.

107. Selkowitz, D: High-frequency electrical stimulation in muscle strengthening. *AM J Sport Med.* 17:103–111, 1989.

108. Selkowitz, D: Improvement in isometric strength of the quadriceps femores muscle after training with electrical stimulation, *Phys Ther* 65:186–196, 1985.

109. Siff, M: Applications of electrostimulation in physical conditioning: a review. *J. Appl. Sport Sci. Research* 4:20–26, 1990.

110. Synder-Mackler, L, Garrett, M, and Roberts, M: A comparison of torque generating capabilities of three different electrical stimulating currents, *JOSPT* 10:297, 301, 1989.

111. Snyder, S: Opiate receptors and internal opiates, *Sci. Am.* 236:44–56, 1977.

112. Stanish, W, and Gunnlaugson, B: Electrical energy and soft tissue injury healing, *Sport Care and Fitness* Sept/Oct:12–14, 1988.

113. Stillwell, G: *Therapeutic electricity and ultraviolet radiation*, Baltimore, 1983, Williams & Wilkins.

114. Stone, JA: Prevention and rehabilitation: "Russian" electrical stimulation, *Athletic Therapy Today* 2(3):27, 1997.

115. Stone, JA: Prevention and rehabilitation: interferential electrical stimulation, *Athletic Therapy Today* 2(2):27, 1997.

116. Stone, JA: Prevention and rehabilitation: microcurrent electrical stimulation, *Athletic Therapy Today* 2(6):15, 1997.

117. Svacina, L: Modified interferential technique, *Pain Control* April 1978, pp. 1–2, Staodynamics, Inc.

118. Szabo, G, and Illes, T: Experimental stimulation of osteogenesis induced by bone matrix, *Orthopaedics* 14:63–67, 1991.

119. Taylor, K: Effect of electrically induced muscle contraction on post-traumatic edema formation in frog hind limbs, *Phys Ther* 72:127–132, 1992.

120. Taylor, K: Effect of a single 30–minute treatment of high-voltage pulsed current on edema formation in frog hind limbs, *Phys Ther* 72:63–68, 1992.

121. Thom, H: Treatment of paralysis with exponentially progressive current, *Br J Phys Med* 20:49. 1957.

122. Travell, J, and Simon, D: Myofascial pain and dysfunction: *The trigger point manual*, Baltimore, 1983, Williams & Wilkins.

123. Unger, P: A randomized clinical trial of the effects of HVPC on wound healing, abstract R294, *Phys Ther* 715:5118, 1991.

124. Watkins, A: *A manual of electrotherapy*, ed 3, Philadelphia, 1968, Lea & Febiger.

125. Weber, W: The effect of MENS on pain and torque deficits associated with delayed onset muscle soreness, abstract R034, *Phys Ther* 715:535, 1991.

126. Weiss, D, Kirsner, R, and Eaglstein, W: Electrical stimulation and wound healing, *ARCH Derm* 126:222–225, 1990.

127. Wolcot, C: A comparison of the effects of high-voltage and microcurrent stimulation on delayed onset muscle soreness, abstract R287, *Phys Ther* 715:5116, 1991.

128. Wolf, S: Perspectives on central nervous system responsiveness to transcutaneous electrical nerve stimulation, *Phys Ther* 58: 1443–1449, 1978.

129. Wolf, S: *Electrotherapy*, New York, 1981, Churchill Livingstone.

130. Wolf, S, Gersh, M, and Kutner, M: Relationship of selected clinical variables to current delivered during transcutaneous electrical nerve stimulation, *Phys Ther* 58:1478–1483, 1978.

131. Wood, J: A multicenter study on the use of pulsed low-intensity direct current for healing chronic stage II and stage III decubitus ulcers, *ARCH Dermatol* 129:999–1009, 1993.

132. Young, S: Efficacy of interferential current stimulation alone for pain reduction in patients with osteoarthritis of the knee: a randomized placebo control clinical trail abstract R088, *Phys Ther* 715:552, 1991.

Suggested Readings

Akyuz, G: Transcutaneous electrical nerve stimulation (TENS) in the treatment of postoperative pain and prevention of paralytic ileus, *Clin Rehab* 7(3):218–221, 1993.

Allen, J, Mattacola, C, and Perrin, D: Microcurrent stimulation effect on delayed onset muscle soreness, *J Ath Train* 31:S-47, 1996.

Alon, G, Allin, and Inbar, G: Optimization of pulse duration and pulse charge during transcutaneous electrical stimulation, *Aust. J. Physiother.* 29:195, 1983.

Alon, G, Bainbridge, J, and Croson, G: High-voltage pulsed direct current effects on peripheral blood flow, *Phys Ther* 61:678, 1981.

Alon, G: High-voltage stimulation: effects of electrode size on basic excitatory responses, *Phys Ther* 65:890, 1985.

Alon, G, Kantor, G, and Ho, H: Effects of electrode size on basic excitatory responses and on selected stimulus parameters, *JOSPT* 20(1):29–35, 1994.

Andersson, S, Hansson, G, and Holmgren, E: Evaluation of the pain suppression effect of different frequencies of peripheral electrical stimulation in chronic pain conditions, *Acta Orthop. Scand.* 47:149, 1979.

Andersson, S: Pain control by sensory stimulation. In Bonica, J J, et al., editors: *Advances in pain research and therapy*, New York, 1979, Raven, vol. 3, 569–584.

Aubin, M, and Marks, R: The efficacy of short-term treatment with transcutaneous electrical nerve stimulation for osteoarthritic knee pain, *Physiotherapy* 81(11):669–675, 1995.

Baker, L: Neuromuscular electrical stimulation in the restoration of purposeful limb movements. In Wolf, SL, editor: *Electrotherapy-clinics in physical therapy*, New York, 1981, Churchill Livingstone.

Balogun, J, and Onilari, O: High voltage electrical stimulation in the augmentation of muscle strength: effects of pulse frequency, *Arch Phys Med Rehab* 74(9):910–916, 1993.

Bending, J: TENS relief of discomfort, *Physiotherapy* 79(11):773–774, 1993.

Berlandt, S: Method of determining optimal stimulation sites for transcutaneous nerve stimulation, *Phys Ther* 64:924, 1984.

Binder-Macleod, S, and McDermond, L: Changes in the force-frequency relationship of the human quadriceps femoris muscle following electrically and voluntarily induced fatigue, *Phys Ther* 72(2):95–104, 1992.

Brown, M, Cotter, M, and Hudlicka, O: Metabolic changes in long-term stimulated fast muscles. In Howland, H, and Poortmans, JR, editors: *Metabolic adaptation to prolonged physical exercise*, Basel, 1975, Birkhauser.

Brown, M, Cotter, M, and Hudlicka, O: The effects of long-term stimulation of fast muscles on their ability to withstand fatigue, *J. Physiol.* (London) 238:47, 1974.

Burr, H, Taffel, M, and Harvey, S: An electrometric study of the healing wound in man, *Yale J. Biol. Med.* 12:483, 1940.

Burr, H, and Harvey, S: Bio-electric correlates of wound healing, *Yale J. Biol. Med.* 11:103, 1938–1939, 1939.

Buxton, B, Okasaki, E, and Hetzler, R: Self-selection of transcutaneous electrical nerve stimulation parameters for pain relief in injured patients, *J Ath Train* 29(2): 178, 1994.

Byl, N, McKenzie, A, and West, J: Pulsed microamperage stimulation: a controlled study of healing of surgically induced wounds in Yucatan pigs, *Phys Ther* 74(3): 201–211, 1994.

Caggiano, E, Emrey, T, and Shirley, S: Effects of electrical stimulation or voluntary contraction for strengthening the quadriceps femoris muscles in an aged male population *JOSPT* 20(1):22–28, 1994.

Campbell, J: A critical appraisal of the electrical output characteristics of ten transcutaneous nerve stimulators, *Clin. Phys. Physiol. Meas.* 3:141, 1982.

Carlos J, Jr: Clinical electrotherapy, Part I: physiology and basic concepts, *PT—Magazine of Physical Therapy*, 6(4):44–46, 48–57, 1998.

Carmick, J: Clinical use of neuromuscular electrical stimulation for children with cerebral palsy, Part 1: lower extremity, *Phys Ther* 73(8): 505–513, 1993.

Carmick, J: Clinical use of neuromuscular electrical stimulation for children with cerebral palsy, Part 2: upper extremity, *Phys Ther* 73(8): 514–522, 1993.

Chan, C, and Chow, S: Electroacupuncture in the treatment of post-traumatic sympathetic dystrophy (Sudek's atrophy), *Br. J. Anesth.* 53:899, 1981.

Chase, J: Elicitation of periods of inhibition in human muscle by stimulation of cutaneous nerves, *J. Bone Joint Surg. (Am.)* 54:173–177, 1972.

Cook, H, Morales, M, and La Rosa, E: Effects of electrical stimulation on lymphatic flow and limb volume in the rat, *Phys Ther* 74(11): 1040–1046, 1994.

Cooperman, A: Use of transcutaneous electrical stimulation in the control of post operative pain: results of a prospective, randomized, controlled study, *Am. J. Surg.* 133:185, 1977.

Curico, F, and Berweger, R.: A clinical evaluation of the pain suppressor TENS, Fairleigh Dickenson University School of Dentistry, 1983. *Current Opinion in Orthopaedics.* 4(6): 105–109, 1993.

Currier, D, and Mann, R: Muscular strength development by electrical stimulation in healthy individuals, *Phys Ther* 63:915, 1983.

Currier, D, and Mann, R: Pain complaint: comparison of electrical stimulation with conventional isometric exercise, *JOSPT* 5:318, 1984.

Currier, D, Petrilli, C, and Threlkeld, A: Effect of medium-frequency electrical stimulation on local blood circulation to healthy muscle, *Phys Ther* 66:937, 1986.

Currier, D, Ray, J, and Nyland, J: Effects of electrical and electromagnetic stimulation after anterior cruciate ligament reconstruction, *JOSPT* 17(4):177–184, 1993.

DeGirardi, C, Seaborne, D, and Goulet, F: The analgesic effect of high-voltage galvanic stimulation combined with ultrasound in the treatment of low back pain: a one-group pre-test/post-test study, *Physiother. Can.* 36:327, 1984.

Dimitrijevic, M: Mesh-glove 1: a method for whole-hand electrical stimulation in upper motor neuron dysfunction, *Scand J Rehab Med* 26(4):183–186, 1994.

Dimitrijevic, M: Mesh-glove 2: modulation of residual upper limb motor control after stroke with whole-hand electric stimulation. *Scand J Rehab Med* 26(4):187–190, 1994.

Draper, V., Lyle, L., and Seymour, T: EMG biofeedback versus electrical stimulation in the recovery of quadriceps surface EMG, *Clinical Kinesiology* 51(2):28–32, 1997.

Eisenberg, B, and Gilal, A: Structural changes in single muscle fibers after stimulation at a low frequency, *J. Gen. Physiol.* 74:1, 1979.

Eriksson, E., Haggmark, T, and Kiessling, KH: Effect of electrical stimulation on human skeletal muscle, *Int. J. Sports Med.* 2:18, 1981.

Ersek, R: Transcutaneous electrical neurostimulation—a new modality for controlling pain, *Clin. Orthop. Relat. Res.* 128:314, 1977.

Finlay, C: TENS: an adjunct to analgesia, *Canadian Nurse* 88(8):24–26, 1992.

Fleischli, JG, and Laughlin, TJ. Electrical stimulation in wound healing, *Journal of Foot & Ankle Surgery* 36(6):457–461, 474–476, 1997.

Fourie, JA, and Bowerbank, P. Stimulation of bone healing in new fractures of the tibial shaft using interferential currents, *Psysiotherapy Research* International 2(4): 255–268, 1997.

Fox, F, and Melzack, R: Transcutaneous electrical stimulation and acupuncture: comparison of treatment for low back pain, *Pain* 2:141, 1976.

Frank, C, Schachar, N, and Dittrich, D: Electromagnetic stimulation of ligament healing in rabbits, *Clin. Orthop. Relat. Res.* 175:263, 1983.

Geddes, L: A short history of the electrical stimulation of excitable tissue, *Physiologist* 27(suppl):1, 1984.

Godfrey, C, Jayawardena, H, and Quance, T: Comparison of electro-stimulation and isometric exercise in strengthening the quadriceps muscle, *Physiother. Can.* 31:265, 1979.

Gotlin, R, and Hershkowitz, S: Electrical stimulation effect on extensor lag and length of hospital stay after total knee arthroplasty, *Arch Phys Med Rehab* 75(9):957–959, 1994.

Gould, M, Donnermeyer, D, and Gammon, GG: Transcutaneous muscle stimulation to retard disuse atrophy after open meniscectomy, *Clin. Orthop. Rel. Res.* 178: 190, 1983.

Granat, M: Functional electrical stimulation and hybrid orthosis systems, *Paraplegia* 34(1):24–29, 1996.

Greathouse, D, Nitz, A, and Matullonis, D: Effects of electrical stimulation on ultrastructure of rat skeletal muscles, *Phys Ther* 64:755, 1984.

Gum, SL, Reddy, GK, Stehno-Bittel, L, and Enwemeka, CS. Combined ultrasound, electrical stimulation, and laser promote collagen synthesis with moderate changes in tendon biomechanics, *American Journal of Physical Medicine & Rehabilitation*, 76(4):288–296, 1997.

Halback, J, and Straus, D: Comparison of electromyostimulation to isokinetic training in increasing power of the knee extensor mechanism, *JOSPT* 2:20, 1980.

Holcomb, W, Mangus, B, and Tandy, R: The effect of icing with the Pro-Stim Edema Management System on cutaneous cooling, *J Ath Train* 31(2):126–129, 1996.

Ignelzi, R, and Nyquist. J: Excitability changes in peripheral nerve fibers after repetitive electrical stimulation: implications in pain modulation, *J. Neurosurg.* 61:824, 1979.

Indergand, H, and Morgan, B: Effects of high-frequency transcutaneous electrical stimulation on limb blood flow in healthy humans, *Phys Ther* 74(4):361–367, 1994.

Indergand, H, and Morgan, B: Effect of interference current on forearm vascular resistance in asymptomatic humans, *Phys Ther* 75(5), 306–312, 1995.

Johnson, MI: The mystique of interferential currents when used to manage pain, *Physiotherapy* 85(6):294–297, 1999.

Johnson, MI, Penny, P, and Sajawal, MA: Clinical technical note: an examination of the analgesic effects of microcurrent electrical stimulation (MES) on cold-induced pain in healthy subjects, *Physiotherapy Theory & Practice*, 13(4):293–301, 1997.

Johnson, MI, and Tabasam, G: A double-blind placebo controlled investigation into the analgesic effects of inferential currents (IFC) and transcutaneous electrical nerve stimulation (TENS) on cold-induced pain in healthy subjects, *Physiotherapy Theory & Practice*, 15(4):217–233, 1999.

Jones, D, Bigland-Ritchie, B, and Edwards, R: Excitation and frequency and muscle fatigue: mechanical responses during voluntary and stimulated contractions, *Exper. Neurol.* 64:401, 1979.

Kahn, J: *Low-volt technique*, Syosset, N.Y., 1973, Joseph Kahn.

Karmel-Ross, K, and Cooperman, D: The effect of electrical stimulation on quadriceps femoris muscle torque in children with spina bifida, *Phys Ther* 72(10):723–730, 1992.

Karnes, JL, Mendel, FC, and Fish, DR: High-voltage pulsed current: its influence on diameters of histamine-dilated arterioles in hamster cheek pouches, *Archives of Physical Medicine and Rehabilitation* 76(4):381–386, 1995.

Kostov, A, Andrews, B, and Popovic, D: Machine learning in control of functional electrical stimulation systems for locomotion, *IEEE Transactions Biomedical Engineering*, 42(6):541–551, 1995.

Kramer, J, and Mendryk, S: Electrical stimulation as a strength improvement technique: a review, *J. Orthop. Sports Phys. Ther.* 4:91, 1982.

Kues, J, and Mayhew, T: Concentric and eccentric force-velocity relationships during electrically induced submaximal contractions, *Phys Ther* 76(5): S-17, 1996.

Lainey, C, Walmsley, R, and Andrew, G: Effectiveness of exercise alone versus exercise plus electrical stimulation in strengthening the quadriceps muscle, *Physiother. Can.* 35:5, 1983.

Lampe, G: Introduction to the use of transcutaneous electrical nerve stimulation devices, *Phys Ther* 58:1450, 1978.

Lane, J: Electrical impedances of superficial limb tissue, epidermis, dermis and muscle sheath, *Ann. N.Y. Acad. Sci.* 238:812, 1974.

Latash, M, Yee, M, and Orpett, C: Combining electrical muscle stimulation with voluntary contraction for studying muscle fatigue, *Arch Phys Med Rehab* 75(1):29–35, 1994.

Laughman, R, Youdas, J, and Garrett, T: Strength changes in the normal quadriceps femoris muscle as a result of electrical stimulation, *Phys Ther* 63:494, 1983.

LeDoux, J, and Quinones, M: An investigation of the use of percutaneous electrical stimulation in muscle re-education, *Phys Ther* 61: 678, 1981.

Leffman, D, Arnall, D, and Holmgren, P: Effect of microamperage stimulation on the rate of wound healing in rats: a histological study, *Phys Ther* 74(3):195–200, 1994.

Levin, M, and Hui-Chan, C: Conventional and acupuncture-like transcutaneous electrical nerve stimulation excite similar afferent fibers, *Arch Phys Med Rehab* 74(1):54–60, 1993.

Licht, S: History of electrotherapy. In Stillwell, GK, editor: *Therapeutic electricity and ultraviolet radiation*, ed 3, Baltimore, Md, 1983, Williams & Wilkins.

Litke, D, and Dahners, L: Effects of different levels of direct current on early ligament healing in a rat model, *J. Orthopedic Research* 12:683–688.

Livesley, E: Effects of electrical neuromuscular stimulation on functional performance in patients with multiple sclerosis. *Physiotherapy* 78(12):914–917, 1992.

Loeser, J: Nonpharmacologic approaches to pain relief. In Ng, L, and Bonica, J, editors: *Pain, discomfort and humanitarian care*, New York, 1980, Elsevier.

Loesor, J, Black, R, and Christman, A: A relief of pain by transcutaneous stimulation, *J. Neurosurg.* 42:308, 1975.

Long, D: Cutaneous afferent stimulation for relief of chronic pain, *Clin. Neurosurg.* 21:257, 1974.

Macdonald, A, and Coates, T: The discovery of transcutaneous spinal electroanalgesia and its relief of chronic pain, *Physiotherapy* 81(11):653–661, 1995.

Mannneimer, C, and Carlsson, C: The analgesic effect of transcutaneous electrical nerve stimulation (TNS) in patients with rheumatoid arthritis: a comparative study of different pulse patterns, *Pain* 6:329, 1979.

Mannheimer, J: Electrode placements for transcutaneous electrical nerve stimulation, *Phys Ther* 58:1455, 1978.

Mannheimer, C, Lund, S, and Carlsson, C: The effect of transcutaneous electrical nerve stimulation (TENS) on joint pain in patients with rheumatoid arthritis, *Scand. J. Rheumatol.* 7:13, 1978.

Mao, W, Ghia, J, and Scott, D: High versus low intensity acupuncture analgesic for treatment of chronic pain: effects on platelet serotonin, *Pain* 8:331, 1980.

Markov, M: Electric current and electromagnetic field effects on soft tissue: implications for wound healing, wounds, *A Compendium of Clinical Research & Practice* 7(3):94–110, 1995.

Marvie, K: A major advance in the control of post-operative knee pain, *Orthopedics* 2:129, 1979.

Massey, B, Nelson, R, and Sharkey, B: Effects of high frequency electrical stimulation on the size and strength of skeletal muscle, *J. Sports Med. Phys. Fit.* 5:136, 1965.

Matsunaga, T, Shimada, Y, and Sato, K: Muscle fatigue from intermittent stimulation with low- and high-frequency electrical pulses, *Archives of Physical Medicine & Rehabilitation*, 80(1):48–53, 1999.

Mattison, J: Transcutaneous electrical nerve stimulation in the management of painful muscle spasm in patients with multiple sclerosis, *Clin Rehab* 7(1):45–48, 1993.

McMiken, D, Todd-Smith, M, and Thompson, C: Strengthening of human quadricep muscles by cutaneous electrical stimulation, *Scand. J. Rehab. Med.* 15:25, 1983.

McQuain, M, Sinaki, M, and Shibley, L: Effect of electrical stimulation on lumbar paraspinal muscles, *Spine* 18(13):1787–1792, 1993.

Meyer, G, and Fields, H: Causalgia treated by selective large fibre stimulation of peripheral nerve, *Brain* 95:163, 1972.

Milner-Brown, H, and Stein, R: The relation between the surface electromyogram and muscular force, *J. Physiol.* 246:549, 1975.

Mohr, T, Carlson, B, and Sulentic, C: Comparison of isometric exercise and high-volt galvanic stimulation on quadriceps, femoris muscle strength, *Phys Ther* 65:606, 1985.

Mostowy, D: An application of transcutaneous electrical nerve stimulation to control pain in the elderly, *J Gerontological Nurs* 22(2):36–38, 1996.

Munsat, T, McNeal, D, and Waters, R: Preliminary observations on prolonged stimulation of peripheral nerve in man, *Arch. Neurol.* 33:608, 1976.

Myklebust, J, editor: *Neural stimulation*, Boca Raton, Fla. 1985, CRC Press.

Naess, K, and Storm-Mathison, A: Fatigue of sustained tetanic contractions, *Acta Physiol. Scand.* 34:351, 1955.

Owens, J, and Malone, T: Treatment parameters of high frequency electrical stimulation as established on the electro stim 180, *JOSPT* 4.162, 1983.

Pert, V: TENS for pain in multiple sclerosis, *Physiotherapy* 77(3):227–228, 1991.

Picaza, J, Cannon, B, and Hunter, S: Pain suppression by peripheral stimulation, Part I: Observations with transcutaneous stimuli, *Surg. Neurol.* 4:105, 1975.

Procacci, P, Zoppi, M, and Maresca, M: Transcutaneous electrical stimulation in low back pain: a critical evaluation, *Acupunct. Electro-ther. Res.* 7:1, 1982.

Qin, L, Appell, H, Chan, K, and Maffulli, N: Electrical stimulation prevents immobilization atrophy in skeletal muscle of rabbits, *Archives of Physical Medicine & Rehabilitation*, 78(5):512–517, 1997.

Rabischong, E, Doutrelot, P, and Ohanna, F: Compound motor action potentials and mechanical failure during sustained contractions by electrical stimulation in paraplegic, *Paraplegia* 33(12):707–714, 1995.

Rack, P, and Westbury, D: The effects of length and stimulus rate on tension in the isometric cat soleus muscle, *J. Physiol.* 204:443, 1969.

Ray, R, and Samuelson, A: Microcurrent versus a placebo for the control of pain and edema, *J Ath Train* 31:S-48, 1996.

Reddana, P, Moortly, C, and Govidappa, S: Pattern of skeletal muscle chemical composition during in vivo electrical stimulations, *Ind. J. Physiol. Pharmacol.* 25:33, 1981.

Rieb, L, and Pomeranz, B: Alterations in electrical pain thresholds by use of acupuncture-like transcutaneous electrical nerve stimulation in pain-free subjects, *Phys Ther* 72(9):658–667, 1992.

Rochester, L: Influence of electrical stimulation of the tibialis anterior muscle in paraplegic subjects: contractile properties, *Paraplegia* 33(8):437–449, 1995.

Roeser, W, Meeks, L, Venis, R, and Strideland, G: The use of transcutaneous nerve stimulation for pain control in athletic medicine: a preliminary report, *Am. J. Sports Med.* 4(5):210, 1976.

Romero, J, Sanford, T, and Schroeder, R: The effects of electrical stimulation of normal quadriceps on strength and girth, *Med. Sci. Sports Exerc.* 14:194, 1982.

Rosenberg, M, Vutyid, L, and Bourbe, D: Transcutaneous electrical nerve stimulation for the relief of post-operative pain, *Pain* 5:129, 1978.

Rowley, B, McKenna, J, and Chase, G: The influence of electrical current on an infecting microorganism in wounds, *Ann. N.Y. Acad. Sci.* 238:543, 1974.

Schmitz, R, Martin, D, and Perrin, D: The effects of interferential current of perceived pain and serum cortisol in a delayed onset muscle soreness model, *J Ath Train* 29(2):171, 1994.

Seib, T, Price, R, and Reyes, M: The quantitative measurement of spasticity: effect of cutaneous electrical stimulation, *Arch Phys Med Rehab* 75(7):746–750, 1994.

Selkowitz, D: Improvement in isometric strength of the quadricep femoris muscle after training with electrical stimulation, *Phys Ther* 65.186, 1985.

Shealey, C, and Maurer, D: Transcutaneous nerve stimulation for control of pain, *Surg. Neurol.* 2:45, 1974.

Simmonds, M, Wessel, J, and Scudds, R: The effect of pain quality on the efficacy of conventional TENS, *Physiotherapy Canada* 44(3):35–40, 1992.

Sjolund, B, and Eriksson, M: The influence of naloxone on analgesia produced by peripheral conditioning stimulation, *Brain. Res.* 173:295, 1979.

Sjolund, B, Terenius, L, and Eriksson, M: Increased cerebrospinal fluid levels of endorphin after electro acupuncture, *Acta Physiol. Scand.* 100:382, 1977.

Smith, B, Betz, R, and Mulcahey, M: Reliability of percutaneous intramuscular electrodes for upper extremity functional neuromuscular stimulation in adolescents with C5 injury, *Arch Phys Med Rehab* 75(9):939–945, 1994.

Smith, B, Mulcahey, M, and Betz, R: Quantitative comparison of grasp and release abilities with and without functional neuromuscular stimulation in adolescents with tetraplegia, *Paraplegia* 34(1):16–23, 1996.

Snyder-Mackler, L, Delitto, A, and Stralka, S: Use of electrical stimulation to enhance recovery of quadriceps femoris muscle force production in patients following anterior cruciate ligament reconstruction, *Phys Ther* 74(10): 901–907, 1994.

Standish, W, Valiant, G, and Bonen, A: The effects of immobilization and of electrical stimulation on muscle glycogen and myofibrillar ATPase, *Can. J. Appl. Sports Sci.* 7:267, 1982.

Szehi, E, and David, E: The stereodynamic interferential current—a new electrotherapeutic technique, *Electromedica* 48:13, 1980.

Szuminsky, N, Albers, A, and Unger, P: Effect of narrow pulsed high voltages on bacterial viability, *Phys Ther* 74(7): 660–667, 1994.

Tan, G, Monga, T, and Thornby, J: Electromedicine: efficacy of microcurrent electrical stimulation on pain severity, psychological distress, and disability, *American Journal of Pain Management*, 10(1):35–44, 2000.

Taylor, K, Mendel, FC, and Fish, DR: Effect of high-voltage pulsed current and alternating current on macromolecular leakage in cheek pouch microcirculation, *Phys Ther* 77(12):1729–1740, 1997.

Taylor, M, Newton, R, and Personius, W: The effects of interferential current stimulation for the treatment of subjects with recurrent jaw pain, abstract, *Phys Ther* 66:774, 1986.

Taylor, P, Hallet, M, and Flaherty, L: Treatment of osteoarthritis of the knee with transcutaneous electrical nerve stimulation, *Pain* 11:233, 1981.

Terezhalmy. G, Ross, G, and Holmes-Johnson, E: Transcutaneous electrical nerve stimulation treatment of TMJMPDS patients, *Ear Nose Throat J.* 61:664, 1982.

Thornton, RM, Mendel, FC, and Fish, DR: Effects of electrical stimulation on edema formation in different strains of rats, *Phys Ther* 78(4):386–394, 1998.

Thorsteinsson, G, and Stonnington, H: The placebo effect of transcutaneous electrical stimulation, *Pain* 5:31, 1978.

Walsh, D, Foster, N, and Baxter, G: Transcutaneous electrical nerve stimulation parameters to neurophysiological and hypoalgesic effects, *Phys Ther* 76(5), 552, 1996.

Weber, M, Servedio, F, and Woddall, W: The effects of three modalities on delayed-onset muscle soreness, *JOSPT* 20(5):236–242, 1994.

Wheeler, P, Wolcott, L, and Morris, J: Neural considerations in the healing of ulcerated tissue by clinical electrotherapeutic application of weak direct current: findings and theory. In Reynolds, D, and Sjoberg, A, editors: *Neuroelectric research*, Springfield, Ill. 1971, Charles C Thomas, 83–96.

Windsor, R, and Lester, J: Electrical stimulation in clinical practice. *Phys Sports medicine* 21(2):85–86, 89–90, 91–92, 1993.

Wolf, S, Gersh, M, and Rao, V: Examination of electrode placements and stimulating parameters in treating chronic pain with conventional transcutaneous nerve stimulation (TENS), *Pain* 11:37, 1981.

Wong, R, and Jette, D: Changes in sympathetic tone associated with different forms of transcutaneous electrical nerve stimulation in healthy subjects, *Phys Ther* 64:478, 1984.

Yarkony, G, Roth, E, and Cybulski, J: Neuromuscular stimulation in spinal cord injury II: prevention of secondary complications, Part 2, *Arch Phys Med Rehab* 73(2):195–200, 1992.

Yarkony, G, and Roth, E: Neuromuscular stimulation in spinal cord injury: restoration of functional movement of the extremities, Part 1, *Arch Phys Med Rehab* 73(1):78–86, 1992.

Zecca, L, Ferrario, P, and Furia, G: Effects of pulsed electromagnetic field on acute and chronic inflammation, *Trans. Biol. Repair Growth Soc.* 3:72, 1983.

CHAPTER **9**

Iontophoresis

William E. Prentice

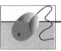

Study Resources

Refer to the lab exercises in the accompanying Laboratory Manual, as well as eSims which simulates the athletic training certification exam at www.mhhe.com/esims. Also, check out the competency information found at www.mhhe.com/prentice11e. For more online study resources, visit our Health and Human Performance Website at www.mhhe.com/hhp/.

Following completion of this chapter, the student athletic trainer will be able to

- Differentiate between iontophoresis and phonophoresis.

- Explain the basic mechanisms of ion transfer.

- Establish specific iontophoresis application procedures and techniques.

- Identify the different ions most commonly used in iontophoresis.

- Choose the appropriate clinical applications for using an iontophoresis technique.

- Establish precautions and concerns for using iontophoresis treatment.

iontophoresis   A therapeutic technique that involves the introduction of ions into the body tissues by means of a direct electrical current.

ions   Positively or negatively charged particles.

ion transfer   A technique of transporting chemicals across a membrane using an electrical current as a driving force.

I ontophoresis is a therapeutic technique that involves the introduction of **ions** into the body tissues by means of a direct electrical current.[12,76] Originally referred to as **ion transfer**, it was first described by LeDuc in 1903 as a technique of transporting chemicals across a membrane using an electrical current as a driving force.[49] Since that time there have been increases and decreases in the popularity and use of iontophoresis as a therapeutic technique. Recently new emphasis has been placed on iontophoresis, and it has become a commonly used technique in athletic training settings. Iontophoresis has several advantages as a treatment technique in that it is a painless, sterile, noninvasive technique for introducing specific ions into the tissue that have been demonstrated to have a positive effect on the healing process.[17]

The athletic trainer using iontophoresis as a treatment modality must be aware that the majority of the medications used require a physician's perscription.

IONTOPHORESIS VERSUS PHONOPHORESIS

It is critical to point out the difference between iontophoresis and phonophoresis since the two techniques are often confused and the two terms are occasionally erroneously interchanged. It is true that both techniques are used to deliver chemicals to various biologic tissues.[66] Phonophoresis, which is discussed in detail in Chapter 15, involves the use of acoustic energy in the form of ultrasound to carry whole molecules across the skin into the tissues, whereas iontophoresis uses an electrical current to transport ions into the tissues.

BASIC MECHANISMS OF ION TRANSFER

Pharmacokinetics of Iontophoresis

In an ideal drug delivery system, the goal is to maximize the therapeutic effects of a drug while minimizing adverse effects and simultaneously providing a high degree of patient compliance and acceptability.[72] Transdermal iontophoresis delivers medication at a constant rate so that the effective plasma concentration remains within a therapeutic window for an extended period of time. The *therapeutic window* refers to the plasma concentrations of a drug, which should fall between a minimum concentration necessary for a therapeutic effect and the maximum effective concentration above which adverse effects may possibly occur.[72] Iontophoresis is able to facilitate the delivery of charged and high molecular weight compounds that cannot be effectively delivered by simply applying them to the skin. Iontophoresis is useful because it appears to overcome the resistive properties of the stratum corneum to charged ions.[72]

Iontophoresis decreases the absorption lag time while increasing the delivery rate when compared with passive skin application. A primary advantage of iontophoresis is the ability to provide both a spiked

ionization   A process by which soluble compounds, such as acids, alkaloids, or salts, dissociate or dissolve into ions that are suspended in some type of solution.

electrolytes   Solutions in which ionic movement occurs.

and sustained release of a drug, thus reducing the possibility of developing a tolerance to the drug. The rate at which an ion may be delivered is determined by a number of factors, including the concentration of the ion, pH of the solution, molecular size of the solute, current density, and duration of the treatment.

It appears that mechanisms of absorption of drugs administered by iontophoresis are similar to administration of drugs via other methods.[72] However, there are advantages of taking medication via transdermal iontophoresis relative to taking oral medications since the medication is concentrated in a specific area, and it does not have to be absorbed within the gastrointestinal tract. Additionally, transdermal administration is safer than administering a drug through injection.

The Movement of Ions in Solution

As defined in Chapter 7, ions are positively or negatively charged particles. Through the process of **ionization**, soluble compounds such as acids, alkaloids, or salts dissociate or dissolve into ions that are suspended in some type of solution.[13] The resulting solutions are called **electrolytes**; in these solutions, ionic movement occurs. Ions will move or migrate within this solution according to the electrically charged

electrophoresis The movement of ions in solution.

> • Anode = positive electrode
> • Cathode = negative electrode

alkaline reaction The accumulation of positive ions under the negative electrode, which produces sodium hydroxide.

acidic reaction The accumulation of negative ions under the positive pole, which produces hydrochloric acid.

> • Negative ions = acidic reaction
> • Positive ions = alkaline reaction

currents acting on them. The term **electrophoresis** refers to the movement of ions in solution.

At any given instant, the electrode that has the greatest concentration of electrons is negatively charged and is referred to as the negative electrode or cathode. Conversely, the electrode with a lower concentration of electrons is called the positive electrode or anode. Negatively charged ions will be repelled from the negative electrode, and thus they move toward the positive electrode, creating an acidic reaction. Positively charged ions will tend to move toward the negative electrode and away from the positive electrode, resulting in an alkaline reaction.

The manner in which ions move in solution forms the basis for iontophoresis. Positively charged ions are carried into the tissues from the positive pole, and negatively charged ions are introduced by the negative pole. Once they enter the tissues, the ions are picked up by the body's own charged ions, and electrolytes pick up the electrons and transport them, allowing flow of current between active and dispersive electrodes. Thus, knowing the correct ion polarity and matching it with the appropriate electrode polarity is of critical importance in using iontophoresis.

The Movement of Ions Through Tissue

The force that acts to move ions through the tissues is determined by both the strength of the electrical field and the electrical impedance of tissues to current flow. The strength of the electrical field is determined by the current density. The difference in current density between the active and inactive or dispersive electrodes establishes a gradient of potential difference that produces ion migration within the

electrical field. (*In Chapter 8 the active electrode was defined as the smaller of the two electrodes, which has the greatest current density. When using iontophoresis the active electrode is defined as the one that is being used to carry the ion into the tissues.*) Current density may be altered either by increasing or decreasing current intensity or by changing the size of the electrode. Increasing the size of the electrode will decrease current density under that electrode. It has been recommended that the current density be reduced at the cathode or negative electrode. The accumulation of positively charged ions in a small area creates an **alkaline reaction**, which is more likely to produce tissue damage than an accumulation of negatively charged ions, which produces an **acidic reaction**. Thus, it has been recommended that the negative electrode should be larger, perhaps twice the size of the positive electrode, to reduce current density.[13,47] This size relationship should remain the same even when the negative electrode is the active electrode. However, it should be added that on most modern iontophoresis units the commercially produced electrodes tend to be the same size (Figure 9-1).

Skin and fat are poor conductors of electrical current, offering greater resistance to current flow. Higher current intensities are necessary to create ion movement in areas where the skin and fat layers are thick, further increasing the likelihood of burns, particularly around the negative electrode. However, the presence of sweat glands decreases impedance, thus facilitating the flow of direct cur-

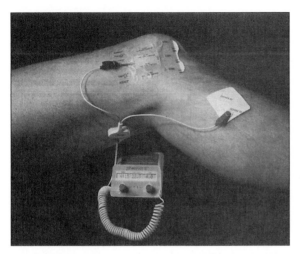

Figure 9-1   The Phoresor® is an example of a generator which produces continuous direct current specifically used for iontophoresis.

rent as well as ions. The sweat ducts are the primary paths by which ions move through the skin.[38] As the skin becomes more saturated with an electrolyte and blood flow increases to the area during treatment, overall skin impedance will decrease under the electrodes.[13]

Iontophoresis should be considered a relatively superficial treatment with the medication penetrating no more than 1.5 cm over a 12 to 24 hour period but only 1–3 mm during the duration of the average treatment.

The quantity of ions transferred into the tissues through iontophoresis is determined by the intensity of the current or the current density at the active electrode, the duration of the current flow, and the concentration of ions in solution.[13] The number of ions absorbed is directly proportional to the current density. In addition, the longer the current flows, the greater the number of ions transferred to the tissues. Therefore, increasing the intensity and duration of the treatment may increase ion transfer. Unfortunately, as treatment duration increases, the skin impedance decreases, thus increasing the likelihood of burns. Although ion concentration effects ion transfer, concentrations greater than 1 to 2 percent are not more effective than medications at lower concentrations.[55,56]

■ **Analogy** *9-1*

The delivery of ions into the tissues occurs when like charges repel one another, as would be the case with two magnets. One and of each magnet is negatively charged, while the other is positively charged. If you try to place the negatively charged ends together, the magnets will feel as if they are pushing each other away. Similarly, if you place a positively charged ion under the positively charged electrode, the ion will be driven away and into the skin.

Once the ions have passed through the skin, they recombine with existing ions and free radicals floating in the bloodstream, thus forming the necessary new compounds for favorable therapeutic interactions.[47]

IONTOPHORESIS TECHNIQUES

Type of Current Required

Continuous direct current has traditionally been used for iontophoresis. Direct current ensures the unidirectional flow of ions that cannot be accomplished using a bidirectional or alternating current. However, a recent study has shown that drugs can be delivered by AC iontophoresis. Iontophoresis using alternating current avoids electrochemical burns and delivery of the drug increases with duration of application.[34] Neither high-voltage direct currents nor interferential currents may be used for iontophoresis since the current is interrupted and the current duration is too short to produce significant ion movement. We should add, however, that modulated pulsed currents have been used with some success in *in vivo* and *in vitro* studies on laboratory animals for transdermal delivery of drugs.[2,68,74]

Iontophoresis Generators

There are a variety of current generators available on the market that produce continuous direct current and are specifically used for iontophoresis (see Figure 9-1). We should emphasize that any generator that has the capability of producing continuous direct current may be used for iontophoresis.

• Iontophoresis generators produce continuous DC current

Some generators are driven by batteries, others by alternating current. Many generators produce current at a constant voltage that gradually reduces skin impedance, consequently increasing current density and thus increasing the risk of burns. The generator should deliver a constant voltage output to the athlete by adjusting the output amperage to normal variations that occur in tissue impedance, thereby reducing the likelihood of burns. For safety purposes the generator should automatically shut down if the skin impedance decreases to some preset limit.

The generator should have some type of current intensity control that can be adjusted between 1 and 5 mA (milliamps). There should also be an adjustable timer that can be set for up to 25 minutes. Polarity of the terminals should be clearly marked, and a polarity reversal switch is desirable. The lead wires connecting the electrodes to the terminals should be well insulated and should be checked regularly for damage or breakdown.

Current Intensity

Low amperage currents appear to be more effective as a driving force than currents with higher intensities.[36,47,53] Higher intensity currents tend to reduce effective penetration into the tissues. Recommended current amplitudes used for iontophoresis range between 3 and 5 mA.[6,14,29,47] When initiating the treatment, the current intensity should always be increased very slowly until the athlete reports feeling a tingling or prickly sensation. If pain or a burning sensation is elicited, the intensity is too great and should be decreased. Likewise, when terminating the treatment, current intensity should be slowly decreased to zero before the electrodes are disconnected.[46]

The recommended maximum current intensity should be determined by the size of the active electrode[54] (Figure 9-2). Current amplitude is usually set so that the current density falls between 0.1 and 0.5 mA/cm^2 of the active electrode surface.[13]

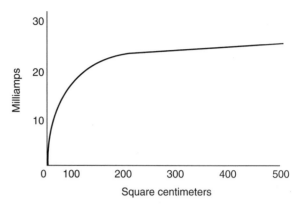

Figure 9-2 The maximum current intensity should be determined by the size of the active electrode. Current amplitude is usually set so that the current density falls between 0.1 and 0.5 mA/cm^2 of the active electrode surface.

Treatment Duration

Recommended treatment durations range between 10 and 20 minutes, with 15 minutes being an average. During this 15-minute treatment, the athlete should be comfortable, with no reported or visible signs of pain or burning. The athletic trainer should check the athlete's skin every 3 to 5 minutes during treatment, looking for signs of skin irritation. Since skin impedance usually decreases during the treatment, it may be necessary to decrease current intensity to avoid pain or burning.

It should be added that the medicated electrode can be left in place for 12 to 24 hours to enhance the initial treatment.

Dosage of Medication

An iontophoresis dose of medication delivered during treatment is expressed in milliampere-minutes (mA-min). A mA/min is a function of current and time. The total drug dose delivered (mA-min) = current × treatment time. For example:

40mA-min dose = 4.0mA current × 10 minutes treatment time

OR

30mA-min dose = 2.0mA current × 15 minutes treatment time

A typical iontophoretic drug delivery dose is 40mA/min, but can vary from 0 to 80 mA-min depending on the medication.

Electrodes

The continuous direct electrical current must be delivered to the athlete through some type of electrode. Many different electrodes are available to the athletic trainer, ranging from those "borrowed" from other electrical stimulators to those that are commercially manufactured, ready-to-use, disposable electrodes made specifically for iontophoresis.[6,30]

The more traditional electrodes are made of tin, copper, lead, aluminum, or platinum, backed by rubber and completely covered by a sponge, towel, or gauze that is in contact with the skin. The absorbent material is soaked with the ionized solution to be driven into the tissues. If the ions are contained in an ointment, it should be rubbed into the skin over the target zone and covered by some absorbent material soaked in water or saline before the electrode is applied.

The commercially produced electrodes are sold with most iontophoresis systems. These electrodes have a small chamber that is covered by some type of semipermeable membrane that contains the ionized solution. The electrode self-adheres to the skin (Figure 9-3). This type of electrode eliminates the mess and hassles that have been associated with electrode preparation for iontophoresis in the past.

Regardless of the type of electrode used, to ensure maximum contact of the electrodes, the skin should be shaved and cleaned prior to their attachment. Care should be taken not to excessively abrade the skin during cleaning, since damaged skin has a lower resistance to the current and a burn may more easily occur. Also, caution should be used when treating areas that, for one reason or another, have reduced sensation.

Once this electrode has been prepared, it then becomes the active electrode, and the lead wire to the generator is attached such that the polarity of the wire is the same as the polarity of the ion in so-

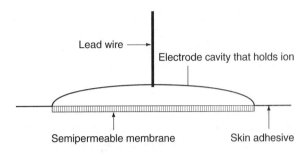

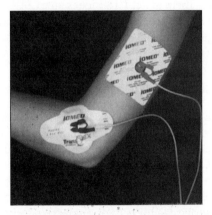

Figure 9-3   The commercially produced, self-adhering electrodes used with most iontophoresis systems have a small chamber that is covered by some type of semipermeable membrane that contains the ionized solution.
(Courtesy Iomed)

lution. A second electrode, the dispersive electrode, is prepared with water, gel, or some other conductive material as recommended by the manufacturer. Both electrodes must be securely attached to the skin such that uniform skin contact and pressure is maintained under both electrodes to minimize the risk of burns. Electrodes via the lead wires should not be connected to the generator unless both the generator and the amplitude or intensity control are turned off. At the end of the treatment the intensity control should be returned to zero and the generator turned off before the electrodes are detached from the athlete.

The size and shape of the electrodes can cause a variation in current density and can affect the size of the area treated.[24] Smaller electrodes have a higher current density and should be used to treat a specific lesion. Larger electrodes should be used when the target treatment area is not well defined.

Recommendations for spacing between the active and dispersive electrodes seem to be variable. They should be separated by at least the diameter of the active electrode. One source has recommended spacing them at least 18 inches apart.[13] As spacing between the electrodes increases, the current density in the superficial tissues will be decreased, perhaps minimizing the potential for burns.

Selecting the Appropriate Ion

While most of the ions used with iontophoresis are prescription medications that must be prescribed by the team physician, there are other ions used in a sports medicine setting that are not. Therefore, it is critical that the athletic trainer be knowledgeable in the selection of the most appropriate ions for treating specific conditions. For a compound to penetrate a membrane such as the skin, it must be soluble in both fat and water. It must be water-soluble if it is to remain in an ionized state in solution. However, since human skin is relatively impervious to water, ions that are soluble only in water do not diffuse in the tissues.[8] They must be fat soluble to permeate the tissues of the body.[30] Penetration is relatively superficial and is generally less than 1 mm.[29] The majority of the ions deposited in the tissues are found primarily at the site of the active electrode, where they are stored as either a soluble or insoluble compound. They may be used locally as a concentrated source or transported by the circulating blood, producing more systemic effects.[47] The tendency of some ions to form insoluble precipitates as they pass into the tissues inhibits their ability to penetrate. This is particularly true with heavy metal ions, including iron, copper, silver, and zinc.[18]

Negative ions accumulating at the positive pole or anode produce an acidic reaction through the formation of hydrochloric acid. Negative ions are scle-

■ **Clinical Decision-Making** *Exercise 9-2*

A field hockey player is getting her first iontophoresis treatment for patellar tendonitis. Dexamethasone has been prescribed for a dose of 40 mA-min. What can the athletic trainer do to minimize the chances of an adverse sensitivity to this medication during this first-time treatment?

■ **Clinical Decision-Making** *Exercise 9-3*

The athletic trainer gets a prescription from the team physician for using dexamethasone, an anti-inflammatory, to treat Achilles tendonitis. What considerations and treatment parameters are important for preparing the athlete for this iontophoresis treatment?

rotic and produce hardening of the tissues by increasing protein density. In addition, some negative ions can also produce an analgesic effect (salicylates).

The majority of the ions used for iontophoresis are positively charged. Positive ions that accumulate at the negative pole produce an alkaline reaction with the formation of sodium hydroxide. Positive ions are sclerolytic; thus, they produce softening of the tissues by decreasing protein density. This is useful in treating scars or adhesions.

Table 9-1, modified from a list compiled by Kahn,[44] lists the ions most commonly used with iontophoresis.

CLINICAL APPLICATIONS FOR IONTOPHORESIS

A relatively long list of conditions for which iontophoresis is an appropriate treatment technique has been cited in literature.[5] Clinically, iontophoresis is most often used in the treatment of inflammatory musculoskeletal conditions.[17,41] It may also be

■ **TABLE 9-1**   Recommended Ions for Use by the Athletic Trainer

....

POSITIVE

Antibiotics Gentamycin Sulfate (+), 8 mg/ml, for suppurative ear chondritis.

Calcium (+), from calcium chloride, 2% aqueous solution, believed to stabilize the irritability threshold in either direction, as dictated by the physiologic needs of the tissues. Effective with spasmodic conditions, tics, and "snapping fingers" (joints).

Copper (+), from a 2% aqueous solution of copper sulfate crystals; fungicide, astringent, useful with intranasal conditions, e.g., allergic rhinitis ("hay fever"), sinusitis, and also dermatophytosis ("athlete's foot").

Hyaluronidase (+), from Wydase crystals in aqueous solution as directed; for localized edema.

Lidocaine (+), from XYLOCAINE 5% ointment, anesthetic/analgesic, especially with acute inflammatory conditions, e.g., bursitis, tendinitis, tic doloreux, and TMJ pain.

Lithium (+), from lithium chloride or carbonate, 2% aqueous solution, effective as an exchange ion with gouty tophi and hyperturicemia.*

Magnesium (+), from magnesium sulfate ("Epsom Salts"), 2% aqueous solution, and excellent muscle relaxant, good vasodilator, and mild analgesic.

Mecholyl (+), familiar derivative of acetylcholine, 0.25% ointment, is a powerful vasodilator, good muscle relaxant and analgesic. Used with discogenic low back radiculopathies and sympathetic reflex dystrophy.

Priscoline (+), from benzazoline hydrochloride, 2% aqueous solution, reported effective with indolent ulcers.

Zinc (+), from zinc oxide ointment 20%, a trace element necessary for healing, especially effective with open lesions and ulcerations.

NEGATIVE

Acetate (−), from acetic acid, 2% aqueous solution; dramatically effective as a sclerolytic exchange ion with calcific deposits.+

Chlorine (−), from sodium chloride, 2% aqueous solution, good sclerolytic agent. Useful with scar tissue, keloids, and burns.

Citrate (−), from potassium citrate, 2% aqueous solution, reported effective in rheumatoid arthritis.

Dexamethasone (−) from Decadron, used for treating musculoskeletal inflammatory conditions.

Iodine (−), from "Iodex" ointment, 4.7%, an excellent sclerolytic agent, as well as bacteriocidal, fair vasodilator. Used successfully with adhesive capsulitis ("frozen shoulder"), scars, etc.

Salicylate (−), from "Iodex with methyl salicylate," 4.8% ointment, a general decongestant, sclerolytic, and anti-inflammatory agent. If desired without the iodine, may be obtained from MYOFLEX ointment (trolamine salicylate 10%) or a 2% aqueous solution of sodium salicylate powder. Used successfully with frozen shoulder, scar tissue, warts, and other adhesive or edematous conditions.

EITHER

Ringer's solution (+/−), with alternating polarity for open decubitus lesions.

Tap water (+/−), usually administered with alternating polarity and sometimes with glycopyrronium bromide in hyperhidrosis.

....

*The lithium ion replaces the weaker sodium ion in the insoluble sodium urate tophus, converting it to soluble lithium urate.
+The acetate radical replaces the carbonate radical in the insoluble calcium carbonate calcific deposit, converting it to soluble calcium acetate.
From Kahn, J: Non-Steroid Iontophoresis, *Clin Manage Phys Ther* 7(1):14–15, 1987.

used for analgesic effects, scar modification, wound healing, and in treating edema, calcium deposits, and hyperhydrosis.[4] Many of these published studies are case reports that attempt to establish the clinical efficacy of iontophoresis in treating various conditions.[24] Table 9-2 provides a list of studies that have treated various conditions using iontophoresis.

TREATMENT PRECAUTIONS AND CONSIDERATIONS

Problems that might potentially arise from treating an athlete using iontophoresis techniques may for the most part be avoided if the athletic trainer (1) has a good understanding of the existing condition that is to be treated, (2) uses the most appropriate ions to accomplish the treatment goal, and (3) uses appropriate treatment parameters and equipment setup. Poor treatment technique on the part of the athletic trainer is most often responsible for adverse reactions to iontophoresis.

Treatment Burns

Perhaps the single most common problem associated with iontophoresis is a chemical burn, which usually occurs as a result of the direct current itself and not because of the ion being used in treatment.[54] Passing a continuous direct electrical current through the tissues creates migration of ions, which alters the normal pH of the skin.[27] The normal pH of the skin is between 3 and 4. In an acidic reaction, the pH falls below 3, while in an alkaline reaction, the pH is greater than 5. Although chemical burns may occur under either electrode, they most typically result from the accumulation of sodium hydroxide at the cathode. The alkaline reaction causes sclerolysis of local tissues. Initially, the burn lesion is pink and raised but within hours becomes a grayish, oozing wound.[47] Decreasing current density by increasing the size of the cathode relative to the anode can minimize the potential for chemical burn.

Thermal burns may occur as a result of high resistance to current flow created by poor contact of the electrodes with the skin. Poor contact results

■ **Clinical Decision-Making** *Exercise 9-4*

After having an iontophoresis treatment, the athlete comes into the training room the next day with an area of skin that is red and tender. It is apparent that the treatment has produced a mild burn. What can the athletic trainer do to minimize the likelihood of a reoccurrence?

when the electrodes are not moist enough, when there are wrinkles in the gauze or paper towels impregnated with the ionic solution, or when there is space between the skin and electrode around the perimeter of the electrode. The athlete should not be treated with body weight resting on top of the electrode since this is likely to create some ischemia (reduced circulation) under the electrode. Instead, the electrode should be held firmly in place with adhesive tape, elastic bands, or lightweight sand bags. Both chemical burns and heat burns should be treated with sterile dressings and antibiotics.[47]

Sensitivity Reactions to Ions

Sensitivity reactions to ions rarely occur, however, they may potentially be very serious. (Table 9–3) The athletic trainer should routinely question the athlete about known drug allergies prior to initiating iontophoresis treatment. During the treatment, the athletic trainer should closely monitor the athlete, looking for either abnormal localized reactions of the skin or systemic reactions.

Athletes who have sensitivity to aspirin may have a reaction when using salicyates. Hydrocortisone may adversely affect individuals with gastritis or an active stomach ulcer. In cases of asthma, mecholyl should be avoided. Athletes who are sensitive to metals should not be treated with copper, zinc, or magnesium. Iodine iontophoresis should not be used with individuals who have allergies to seafood or those who have had a bad reaction to intravenous pyelograms.[47]

■ TABLE 9-2   Conditions Treated with Iontophoresis

CONDITION	IONS USED IN TREATMENT	CONDITION	IONS USED IN TREATMENT
Inflammation		**Hyperhydrosis**	
Bertolucci 1982[6]	Hydrocortisone, salicylate	Kahn 1973[47]	Tap water
Kahn 1982[45]	Dexamethasone	Levit 1968[50]	
Chantraine et al. 1986[10]		Abell et al. 1974[1]	
Harris 1982[29]		Shrivastava, Sing 1977[71]	
Hasson 1991[31]		Grice et al. 1972[25]	
Hasson et al. 1992[32]		Hill 1976[33]	
Delacerda 1982[14]		Stolman 1987[73]	
Glass et al. 1980[23]		**Fungi**	
Zawislak et al. 1996[78]		Kahn 1985[40]	Copper
McEntaffer et al. 1996[51]		Haggard 1939[28]	
Banta 1995[5]		**Open Skin Lesions**	
Petelenz et al. 1992[60]			
Panus et al 1999[57]	Ketoprofen	Cornwall 1981[11]	Zinc
Analgesia		Jenkinson et al. 1974[37]	
		Balogun et al. 1990[3]	
Schaeffer et al. 1971[69]	Lidocaine, magnesium	**Herpes**	
Russo et al. 1980[67]			
Gangarosa 1974[19]		Gangarosa et al. 1989[21]	
Gangarosa 1993[20]		**Allergic Rhinitis**	
Garzione 1978[22]			
Pellecchia et al. 1994[58]		Kahn 1991[48]	Copper
Reid et al. 1993[64]		**Gout**	
Spasm			
		Kahn 1982[43]	Lithium
Kahn 1975[44]	Calcium, magnesium	**Burns**	
Kahn 1985[48]			
Ischemia		Rapperport et al. 1965[63]	Antibiotics
		Rigano et al. 1992[65]	
Kahn 1991[40]	Magnesium, mecholyl, iodine	Driscoll et al. 1999[16]	
Edema		**Reflex Sympathetic Dystrophy**	
Kahn 1991[40]	Magnesium, mecholyl, hyaluronidase, salicylate	Bonezzi et al. 1994[7]	Guanethidine
		Lateral Epicondylitis	
Boone 1969[9]			
Magistro 1964[52]		Demirtas, et al. 1998[15]	Sodium salicilate
Schwartz 1955[70]			Sodium diclofenac
Calcium Deposits		**Plantar Fasciitis**	
Weider 1992[77]	Acetic acid	Gudeman et al. 1997[26]	Dexamethasone
Kahn 1977[42]		**Patellar Tendinitis**	
Psaki 1955[62]			
Kahn 1996[39]		Huggard et al. 1999[35]	Dexamethasone
Perron et al. 1997[59]		**Rotator Cuff**	
Scar Tissue			
		Preckshot 1999[61]	Dexamethasone
Tannenbaum 1980[75]	Chlorine, iodine, salicylate		Lidocaine
Kahn 1985[48]			

■ **TABLE 9-3** Summary of Indications and Contraindications for Iontophoresis

INDICATIONS	CONTRAINDICATIONS
Inflammation	Skin sensitivity reactions
Analgesia	Sensitivity to aspirin (salicylates)
Muscle Spasm	Gastritis or active stomach ulcer (hydrocortisone)
Ischemia	Asthma (mecholyl)
Edema	Sensitivity to metals (zinc, copper, magnesium)
Calcium deposits	Sensitivity to seafood (iodine)
Scar tissue	
Hyperhydrosis	
Fungi	
Open skin lesions	
Herpes	
Allergic rhinitis	
Gout	
Burns	
Reflex sympathetic dystrophy	

Summary

1. Iontophoresis is a therapeutic technique that involves the introduction of ions into the body tissues by means of a direct electrical current.
2. The manner in which ions move in solution forms the basis for iontophoresis. Positively charged ions are driven into the tissues from the positive pole, and negatively charged ions are introduced by the negative pole.
3. The force that acts to move ions through the tissues is determined by both the strength of the electrical field and the electrical impedance of tissues to current flow.
4. The quantity of ions transferred into the tissues through iontophoresis is determined by the intensity of the current or the current density at the active electrode, the duration of the current flow, and the concentration of ions in solution.
5. Continuous direct current must be used for iontophoresis, thus ensuring the unidirectional flow of ions, which cannot be accomplished using a bidirectional or alternating current.
6. Electrodes may be either reusable or commercially produced, that is a self-adhering, prepared electrode that must be securely attached to the skin.
7. It is critical that the athletic trainer be knowledgeable in the selection of the most appropriate ions for treating specific conditions.
8. Clinically, iontophoresis is used in the treatment of inflammatory musculoskeletal conditions; for analgesic effects, scar modification, and wound healing; and in treating edema, calcium deposits, and hyperhydrosis.
9. Perhaps the single most common problem associated with iontophoresis is a chemical burn, which usually occurs as a result of the direct current itself and not because of the ion being used in treatment.

Review Questions

1. What is iontophoresis, and how may it be used in the athletic population?
2. What is the difference between iontophoresis and phonophoresis?
3. How do ions move in solution?
4. What determines the quantity of ions transferred through the tissues during iontophoresis?
5. Why must continuous direct current be used for iontophoresis?
6. What types of electrodes can be used with iontophoresis and how should they be applied?
7. What characteristics should be considered when selecting the appropriate ion for an iontophoresis treatment?
8. What are the various clinical uses for iontophoresis in athletic training?
9. What treatment precautions must be taken when using iontophoresis?

 ## Self-Test Questions

T/F
1. Ionization is the movement of ions in solution.
2. The dispersive electrode contains the ions.
3. pH reactions of greater than 5 are alkaline.

Multiple Choice
4. Which type of current does iontophoresis produce?
   a. biphasic
   b. continuous DC
   c. polyphasic
   d. AC
5. What is the recommended range for iontophoresis current amplitude?
   a. 3–5 mA
   b. 5–10 mA
   c. 50–100 mA
   d. 100–150 mA
6. Chemical burn is often associated with iontophoresis and may be attributed to _____ .
   a. allergic reaction
   b. poor electrode contact
   c. the medication
   d. continuous direct current
7. Which of the following is NOT an ion used to treat inflammation?
   a. hydrocortisone
   b. salicylate
   c. lidocaine
   d. dexamethasone
8. Skin impedance usually decreases during treatment, meaning _____ should be decreased to avoid pain and burning.
   a. current intensity
   b. electode size
   c. treatment time
   d. ion dosage
9. What problem do areas of thick fat and skin present?
   a. decreased ion absorption
   b. increased ion absorption
   c. decreased resistance
   d. increased resistance
10. Which of the following is a contraindication for iontophoresis?
   a. inflammation
   b. analgesia
   c. asthma
   d. muscle spasm

Solutions to Clinical Decision-Making Exercises

9-1   The hydrocortisone could come in a eucerine-based cream preparation or in solution. The athletic trainer should use phonophoresis with the cream preparation to deliver whole molecules. Iontophoresis is more appropriate when ions are suspended in solution and can be carried into the tissues by an electrical current.

9-2   The safest choice is to reduce the intensity of the treatment while increasing the duration. For example, a normal dosage may be delivered at 4 mA for 10 minutes. A setting of 2 mA with a treatment time of 20 minutes would deliver the same dosage at a safer intensity.

9-3   The dexamethasone should be placed under the negative electrode since it is a negatively charged ion. Current intensity should be set between 3 and 5 mA. Treatment time should be 15 minutes. The athletic trainer should check the skin every 3 to 5 minutes for a reaction.

9-4   By increasing the size of the cathode relative to the anode, the current density can be decreased. Also, increasing the spacing between the electrodes will decrease current intensity, thus minimizing the chances of a chemical burn.

References

1. Abell, E, and Morgan, K: Treatment of idiopathic hyperhydrosis by glycopyrronium bromide and tap water iontophoresis, *Br J Dermatol.* 91:87, 1974.

2. Bagniefski, T, and Burnette, R: A comparison of pulsed and continuous current iontophoresis, *J Controlled Release* 11:113–122, 1990.

3. Balogun, J, Abidoye, A, and Akala, E: Zinc iontophoresis in the management of bacterial colonized wounds: a case report, *Physiotherapy Canada* 42(3):147–151, 1990.

4. Banga, AK, and Panus, PC: Clinical applications of iontophoretic devices in rehabilitation medicine, *Critical Reviews in Physical & Rehabilitation Medicine* 10(2): 147–179, 1998.

5. Banta, C: A prospective nonrandomized study of iontophoresis, wrist splinting, and anti-inflammatory medication in the treatment of early mild carpal tunnel syndrome, *JOSPT* 21(2):120, 1995.

6. Bertolucci L: Introduction of anti-inflammatory drugs by iontophoreses: a double-blind study. *JOSPT* 4(2):103, 1982.

7. Bonezzi, C, Miotti, D, and Bettagilo, R: Electromotive administration of guanethidine for treatment of reflex sympathetic dystrophy, *J Pain Symptom Manag* 9(1):39–43, 1994.

8. Boone, D: Applications of iontophoresis. In Wolf, S, editor: *Electrotherapy*, New York, 1981, Churchill Livingstone.

9. Boone, D: Hyaluronidase iontophoresis, *J Am Phys Ther Assoc* 49:139–145, 1969.

10. Chantraine, A, Lundy, J, and Berger, D: Is cortisone iontophoresis possible? *Arch Phys Med Rehab* 67:380, 1986.

11. Cornwall, M: Zinc oxide iontophoresis for ischemic skin ulcers, *Phys Ther* 61(3):359, 1981.

12. Costello, C, and Jeske, A: Iontophoresis:applications in transdermal medication delivery, *Phys Ther* 75(6): 554–563, 1995.

13. Cummings, J: Iontophoresis. In Nelson, RM, and Currier, DP, editors: *Clinical Electrotherapy*, Norwalk, Conn., 1991, Appleton & Lange.

14. Delacerda, F: A comparative study of three methods of treatment for shoulder girdle myofascial syndrome, *JOSPT* 4(1):51–54, 1982.

15. Demirtas, RN, and Oner, C: The treatment of lateral epicondylitis by iontophoresis of sodium salicylate and sodium diclofenac, *Clinical Rehabilitation* 12(1):23–29, 1998.

16. Driscoll, JB, Plunkett, K, and Tamari, A: The effect of potassium iodide iontophoresis on range of motion and scar maturation following burn injury, *Physical Therapy Case Reports* 2(1):13–18, 1999.

17. Federici, P: Injury management update: treating iliotibial band friction syndrome using iontophoresis, *Athletic Therapy Today* 2(5):22–23, 1997.

18. Gadsby, P: Visualization of the barrier layer through iontophoresis of ferric ions, *Med Instrum.* 13:281, 1979.

19. Gangarosa, L. Iontophoresis for surface local anesthesia, *J Am Dent Assoc.* 88:125, 1974.

20. Gangarosa, L: Iontophoresis in pain control, *Pain Digest* 3:162–174, 1993.

21. Gangarosa, L, Payne, L, and Hayakawa, K: Iontophoretic treatment of herpetic whitlow, *Arch Phys Med Rehab* 70(4):336–340, 1989.

22. Garzione, J: Salicylate iontophoresis as an alternative treatment for persistent thigh pain following hip surgery, *Phys Ther* 58(5):570–571, 1978.

23. Glass, J, Stephen, R, and Jacobsen, S: The quantity and distribution of radiolabeled dexamethasone delivered to tissues by iontophoresis, *Int J Dermatol.* 19:519, 1980.

24. Glick, E, and Synder-Mackler, L: Iontophoresis. In Snyder-Mackler, L, and Robinson, A, editors: *Clinical electrophysiol-*

ogy and electrophysiologic testing, Baltimore, 1989, Williams and Wilkins.

25. Grice, K, Sattar, H, and Baker, H: Treatment of idiopathic hyperhidrosis with iontophoresis of tap water and poldine methosulphate, *Br J Dermatol.* 86:72, 1972.

26. Gudeman, SD, Eisele, SA, Heidt, RS, Jr., Colosimo, AJ, and Stroupe, AL: Treatment of plantar fasciitis by iontophoresis of 0.4% dexamethasone: a randomized, double-blind, placebo-controlled study, *American Journal of Sports Medicine* 25(3):312–316, 1997.

27. Guffey, JS, Rutherford, MJ, Payne, W, and Phillips, C: Skin pH changes associated with iontophoresis, *Journal of Orthopaedic & Sports Physical Therapy* 29(11):656–660, 1999.

28. Haggard, H, Strauss, M, and Greenberg, L: Fungous infections of hand and feet treated by copper iontophoresis, *JAMA* 112:1229, 1939.

29. Harris, P: Iontophoresis: clinical research in musculoskeletal inflammatory conditions, *J Ortho Sports Phys Ther* 4(2):109–112, 1982.

30. Harris, R: Iontophoresis. In Licht, S, editor: *Therapeutic electricity and ultraviolet radiation*, Baltimore, 1967, Waverly.

31. Hasson, S: Exercise training and dexamethsone iontophoresis in rheumatoid arthritis: a case study, *Physiotherapy Canada* 43:11, 1991.

32. Hasson, S, Wible, C, and Reich, M: Dexamethasone iontophoresis: effect on delayed muscle soreness and muscle function, *Can J Sport Sci* 17:8–13, 1992.

33. Hill, B: Poldine iontophoresis in the treatment of palmar and plantar hyperhidrosis, *Aust J Dermatol.* 17:92, 1976.

34. Howard, J, Drake, T, and Kellogg, D: Effects of alternating current iontophoresis on drug delivery, *Arch Phys Med Rehab* 76(5):463–466, 1995.

35. Huggard, C, Kimura, I, and Mattacola, C: Clinical efficacy of dexamethasone iontophoresis in the treatment of patellar tendinitis in college athletes: a double blind study, *Journal of Athletic Training* 34(2): S-70, 1999.

36. Jacobson, S, Stephen, R, and Sears, W: *Development of a new drug delivery system (iontophoresis)*, University of Utah, Salt Lake City, 1980.

37. Jenkinson, D, McEwan, J, and Walton, G: The potential use of iontophoresis in the treatment of skin disorders, *Vet Rec* 94:8–12, 1974.

38. Johnson, C, and Shuster, S: The patency of sweat ducts in normal looking skin, *Br J Dermatol.* 83:367, 1970.

39. Kahn, J: Acetic acid iontophoresis, *Phys Ther* 76(5):S-68, 1996.

40. Kahn, J: *Practices and principles of electrotherapy*, New York, 1991, Churchill Livingstone.

41. Kahn, J: Non-steroid iontophoresis, *Clin Manage Phys Ther* 7(1):14–15, 1987.

42. Kahn, J: A case report: lithium iontophoresis for gouty arthritis, *J Orthop Sports Phys Ther* 4:113, 1982.

43. Kahn, J: Acetic acid iontophoresis for calcium deposits, *JAPTA* 57(6):658, 1977.

44. Kahn, J: Calcium iontophoresis in suspected myopathy, *JAPTA* 55(4):276, 1975.

45. Kahn, J: Iontophoresis with hydrocortisone for Peyronie's disease, *JAPTA* 62(7):995, 1982.

46. Kahn, J: Iontophoresis: practice tips, *Clin Management* 2(4):37, 1982.

47. Kahn, J: *Tap-water iontophoresis for hyperhidrosis.* Reprinted in Medical Group News, August 1973.

48. Kahn, J: *Clinical electrotherapy*, ed 4, Syosset, N.Y., 1985, J. Kahn.

49. LeDuc, S: *Electric ions and their use in medicine*, Liverpool, 1903, Rebman.

50. Levit, R: Simple device for treatment of hyperhidrosis by iontophoresis, *Arch Dermatol* 98:505–507, 1968.

51. McEntaffer, D, and Sailor, M: The effects of stretching and iontophoretically delivered dexamethasone on plantar fascitis, *Phys Ther* 76(5):S-68, 1996.

52. Magistro, C: Hyaluronidase by iontophoresis in the treatment of edema: a preliminary clinical report, *Phys Ther* 44:169, 1964.

53. Mandleco, C: *Research: iontophoresis*. University of Utah Institute for Biomedical Engineering, Salt Lake City, 1978.

54. Molitor, H: Pharmacologic aspects of drug administration by ion transfer, *The Merck Report* 22–29, January 1943.

55. Murray, W, Levine, L., and Seifter, E: The iontophoresis of C2 esterified glucocorticoids: preliminary report, *Phys Ther* 43:579, 1963.

56. O'Malley, E, and Oester, Y: Influence of some physical chemical factors on iontophoresis using radio-isotopes, *Arch Phys Med Rehabil* 36:310, 1955.

57. Panus, PC, Ferslew, KE, Tober-Meyer, B, and Kao, RL: Ketoprofen tissue permeation is swine following cathodic iontophoresis, *Phys Ther* 79(1):40–49, 1999.

58. Pellecchia, G, Hamel, H, and Behnke, P: Treatment of infrapatellar tendinitis: a combination of modalities and transverse friction massage versus iontophoresis, *J Sport Rehab* 3(2):135–145, 1994.

59. Perron, M, and Malouin, F: Acetic acid iontophoresis and ultrasound for the treatment of calcifying tendinitis of the shoulder: a randomized control trial, *Archives of Physical Medicine & Rehabilitation* 78(4):379–384, 1997.

60. Petelenz, T, Buttke, J, and Bonds, C: Iontophoresis of dexamethasone: laboratory studies, *J Controlled Release* 20:55–66, 1992.

61. Preckshot, J: Iontophoresis with lidocaine and dexamethasone for treating rotator cuff injury in a hockey player, *International Journal of Pharmaceutical Compounding* 3(6):441, 1999.

62. Psaki, C, and Carol, J. Acetic acid ionization: a study to determine the absorptive effects upon calcified tendinitis of the shoulder, *Phys Ther Rev* 35:84, 1955.

63. Rapperport, A: Iontophoresis—a method of antibiotic administration in the burn athlete, *Plast Reconstr Surg* 36(5):547–552, 1965.

64. Reid, K, Sicard-Rosenbaum, L, and Lord, D: Iontophoresis with normal saline versus dexamethasone and lidocaine in the treatment of athletes with internal disc derangement of the temporomandibular joint, *Phys Ther* 73(6):S-20, 1993.

65. Rigano, W, Yanik, M, and Barone, F: Antibiotic iontophoresis in the management of burned ears, *J Burn Care REHAB* 13(4):407–409, 1992.

66. Roberts, D: Transdermal drug delivery using iontophoresis and phonophoresis, *Orthopaedic Nursing* 18(3):50–54, 1999.

67. Russo J, Lipman, A, and Comstock, T: Lidocane anesthesia: comparison of iontophoresis, injection and swabbing, *Am J Hosp Pharm* 37:843–847, 1980.

68. Sabbahi, M, Costello, C, and Emran, A: A method for reducing skin irritation from iontophoresis, *Phys Ther* 74: S-156, 1994.

69. Schaeffer, M, Bixler, D, and Yu, P: The effectiveness of iontophoresis in reducing cervical hypersensitivity, *J Peridontol* 42:695, 1971.

70. Schwartz, M: The use of hyaluronidase by iontophoresis in the treatment of lymphedema, *Arch Intern Med* 95:662, 1955.

71. Shrivastava, S, and Sing, G: Tap water iontophoresis in palm and plantar hyperhidrosis, *Br J Dermatol* 96:189, 1977.

72. Singh, P, and Maibach, H: Transdermal iontophoresis: pharmacokinetic considerations, *Clinical Pharmacokinetics* 26:327–334, 1994.

73. Stolman L: Treatment of excess sweating of the palms by iontophoresis, *Arch Dermatol* 123:893, 1987.

74. Su, M, Srinivasan, V, and Ghanem, A: Quantitative in vivo iontophoretic studies, *J Pharm Sci* 83:12–17, 1994.

75. Tannenbaum, M: Iodine iontophoresis in reduction of scar tissue, *Phys Ther* 60 (6): 792, 1980.

76. Van Hern, G: Iontophoresis: a review of the literature, *New Zealand Journal of Physiotheraphy* 25(2):16–17, 1997.

77. Wieder, D: Treatment of traumatic myositis ossificans with acetic acid iontophoresis, *Phys Ther* 72(2): 133–137, 1992.

78. Zawislak, D, Rau, C, and Lee, M: The effects of dexamethasone iontophoresis on acute inflammation using a sports model of treatment, *Phys Ther* 76(5):S-17, 1966.

PART FOUR

Mechanical Modalities

CHAPTER 10

Therapeutic Sports Massage

William E. Prentice and Clairbeth Lehn

Study Resources

Refer to the lab exercises in the accompanying Laboratory Manual, as well as eSims which simulates the athletic training certification exam at www.mhhe.com/esims. Also, check out the competency information found at www.mhhe.com/prentice11e. For more online study resources, visit our Health and Human Performance Website at www.mhhe.com/hhp/.

Following completion of this chapter, the student athletic trainer will be able to

- Discuss the physiologic effects of sports massage, differentiating between reflexive and mechanical effects.

- Apply specific treatment guidelines and considerations when administering sports massage.

- Demonstrate the various strokes involved with classic Hoffa massage.

- Summarize connective tissue massage.

- Explain how acupressure massage is most effectively used, and identify the relationship between acupuncture and trigger points.

- Explain how myofascial release can be used to restore normal functional movement patterns.

- Contrast special massage techniques, including Rolfing® and Tragering.®

THE EVOLUTION OF MASSAGE AS A TREATMENT MODALITY

The earliest available medical records seem to indicate that massage has played an important role in the treatment of sick and injured people.[25] A natural reaction when a part of the body hurts is to rub the injured area with a hand.

In early writings pertaining to medical treatments, little difference is shown between massage, as we know it, and general exercise of the body. In fact, although there are very detailed descriptions of techniques, one has a great deal of difficulty in making a determination as to exactly what is meant because the terminology is unfamiliar. Language changes with time.

In Europe during the Middle Ages, the influence of the Church of Rome and its religious teachings discouraged the use of massage as a healing practice. This brought the art to somewhat of a halt until enlightened individuals strove to bring medical knowledge into the forefront and scholars in the medical fields started to delve again into how and why the body functions as it does.

The word *massage* is derived from two sources. One is the Arabic verb *mass*, "to touch," and the other is the Greek word *massein*, "to knead." However, history shows that this was not an art exclusive to the Greeks and Arabs. The general knowledge of massage was also known and practiced by the Egyptians, Romans, Japanese, Persians, and Chinese.

In Sweden in the early part of the nineteenth century, Peter H. Ling (1776–1839), the acknowledged founder of curative gymnastics, used massage as a branch of gymnastics. He appears to be the founder of modern day massage techniques, with some incorporation of French massage techniques into his system.[13]

Massage techniques have changed dramatically in the past 50 years. They are based on the research and teachings of Albert Hoffa (1859–1907), James B. Mennell (1880–1957), and Gertrude Beard (1887–1971). Medical practitioners of the twentieth century added a scientific basis to massage, along with additional techniques and terms.[9] In modern day preventative and rehabilitative therapy, massage is a widely used therapeutic modality that seems to be gaining renewed interest.[9,33]

In the late 1980s, a number of professional associations of massage therapists were organized, the most notable of these being the American Massage Therapy Association. In 1992, the National Certification Examination for Therapeutic Massage and Bodywork was created to set minimal entry-level standards for practicing massage professionals. A number of states currently license massage therapists, as the profession struggles to gain acceptance among the health professions.

PHYSIOLOGIC EFFECTS OF MASSAGE

Massage is a mechanical stimulation of the tissues by means of rhythmically applied pressure and stretching.[62] Over the years many claims have been made relative to the therapeutic benefits of massage in the athletic population, although few are based on well-controlled and designed studies.[1,7,52,53,60] Athletes have used massage to increase flexibility and coordination as well as to increase pain threshold;[5,24] to decrease neuromuscular excitability in the muscle being massaged;[45,56] to stimulate circulation, thus improving energy transport to the mus-

massage   The act of rubbing, kneading, or stroking the superficial parts of the body with the hand or with an instrument for the purpose of modifying nutrition, restoring power of movement, or breaking up adhesions.

effleurage   To stroke; any stroke that glides over the skin without attempting to move the deep muscle masses. The hand is molded to the part, stroking with more or less constant pressure, usually upward. Any degree of pressure may be applied, varying from the lightest possible touch to very deep pressure.

Physiologic effects of massage

- Reflexive
- Mechanical

cle;[35] to facilitate healing and restore joint mobility;[29] and to remove lactic acid, thus alleviating muscle cramps.[34] Conclusive evidence of the efficacy of massage as an ergogenic aid in the athletic population is lacking.[24]

How these effects may be accomplished is determined by the specific approaches used with massage techniques and how they are applied. Generally, the effects of massage may be either *reflexive* or *mechanical*.[12] The effect of massage on the nervous system will differ greatly according to the method employed, pressure exerted, and the duration of applications. Through the reflex mechanism, sedation is induced. Slow, gentle, rhythmical, and superficial **effleurage** may relieve tension and soothe, rendering the muscles more relaxed. This indicates an effect on sensory and motor nerves locally and some central nervous system response. The mechanical approach seeks to make mechanical or histological changes in myofascial structures through direct force applied superficially.[12]

Reflexive Effects

The first approach in massage therapy involves a reflexive mechanism. The reflexive approach attempts to exert its effects through the skin and superficial connective tissues.[45] Mobilization of soft tissue stimulates sensory receptors in the skin and superficial fascia.[12] If hands are passed lightly over the skin, a series of responses occur as a result of the sensory stimulus of cutaneous receptors. This reflex mechanism is believed to be an autonomic nervous system phenomenon.[4] The reflex stimulus can occur alone (i.e., unaccompanied by the mechanical mechanism). Mennell[73] calls this the "reflex effect." In itself, it is not an effect but the cause of an effect (i.e., causes sedation, relieves tension, and increases blood flow).

Effects on Pain. The effect of massage on pain is probably regulated by both the gate control theory and through the release of endogenous opiads (see Chapter 3). In gate control, cutaneous stimulation of large-diameter afferent nerve fibers effectively blocks transmission of pain information carried in small-diameter nerve fibers. Stimulation of painful areas in the skin or myofascia can facilitate the release of β-endorphins and enkephalin, which essentially effect the transmission of pain associated information in descending spinal tracts.

Effects on Circulation. The effect of massage on the circulation of the blood, according to Pemberton,[47] takes place through a reflex influence on blood vessels from a sympathetic division in the nervous system. He believes that vessels in the muscular system are emptied during massage not only by being squeezed but also by this reflex action. Very light massage (effleurage) produces an almost instantaneous reaction through transient dilation of lymphatics and small capillaries. Heavier pressure brings about a more lasting dilation. If capillary dilation occurs, blood volume and blood flow will increase producing an increase in temperature in the area being massaged.[18]

Massage increases lymphatic flow.[20] In the lymphatic system, movement of fluid depends on forces outside of the system. Such factors as gravity,

■ Analogy   *10-1*

Massage is effective in pain reduction, most likely taking advantage of the gate control mechanism of pain relief. If someone walks up to you and punches you in the shoulder, the first thing you do to make it feel better is to rub it. Creating sensory cutaneous input will help to override the pain associated with the punch.

Reflexive effects

- Pain
- Circulation
- Metabolism

muscle contraction, movement, and massage can affect the flow of lymph. Increased lymphatic flow will assist in the removal of edema.[11] When administering massage to an edematous part, elevation will also help to increase lymph flow.

It has been proposed that massage can promote lactate clearance following exercise. However, evidence suggests that increases in blood flow that occur from massage have little or no effect on lactate metabolism and its subsequent clearance from blood and tissues.[21,26,41]

Effects on Metabolism. Massage does not alter general metabolism appreciably.[47] There is no change in acid-base equilibrium of blood. Massage does not appear to have any significant effects on the cardiovascular system.[8] Massage metabolically augments a chemical balance. The increased circulation means increased dispersion of waste products and an increase of fresh blood and oxygen. The mechanical movements may assist in the removal and hasten the resynthesis of lactic acid.

Mechanical Effects

The second approach to massage is mechanical in nature. Techniques that stretch a muscle, elongate fascia, or mobilize soft-tissue adhesions or restrictions are all mechanical techniques. The mechanical effects are always accompanied by some reflex effects. As the mechanical stimulus becomes more effective, the reflex stimulus becomes less effective. Mechanical techniques should be performed after reflexive techniques. This is not to imply that mechanical techniques are more aggressive forms of massage. However, mechanical techniques are most often directed at deeper tissues, such as adhesions or restrictions in muscle, tendons, and fascia.

Effects on Muscle.   The basic goal of massage on muscle tissue is to "maintain the muscle in the best possible state of nutrition, flexibility, and vitality so that after recovery from trauma or disease the muscle can function at its maximum."[56,62] Muscle massage is done either for mechanical stretching of the intramuscular connective tissue or to relieve pain and discomfort associated with myofascial trigger points. Massage has been shown to increase blood flow to skeletal muscle[17,63] and thus to increase venous return. It has also been shown to retard muscle atrophy following injury.[55] Massage has also been shown to increase the range of motion in hamstring muscles due to the combined decrease in neuromuscular excitability and stretching of muscle and scar tissue.[15] Massage does not increase strength or bulk of muscle, nor does it increase muscle tone.

Effects on Skin.   Effects of massage on the skin include an increase in skin temperature, possibly as a result of direct mechanical effects, and indirect vasomotor action. It has also been found that increased sweating and decreased skin resistance to galvanic current also resulted from massage.

If skin becomes adherent to underlying tissues, and scar tissue is formed, friction massage can usually be used to mechanically loosen the adhesions and to soften the scar. Massage toughens yet softens the skin. It acts directly on the surface of the skin to remove dead cells that result from prolonged casting of 6 to 8 weeks.

The effect of massage on scar tissue is that it stretches and breaks down the fibrous tissue. It can break down adhesions between skin and subcutaneous tissue and stretch contracted or adhered tissue.[46]

PSYCHOLOGIC EFFECTS OF MASSAGE

Psychologic effects of massage can be as beneficial to some athletes as the physiologic effects. The "hands-on" effect helps athletes feel as if someone is helping them. A general sedative effect can be most beneficial for the athlete. Massage has been shown to lower psycho-emotional and somatic arousal, such as tension and anxiety.[36] It has been suggested that massage performed in water further enhances relaxation.[5] The athletic trainer's approach should inspire a feeling of confidence in the athlete, and the athlete should respond with a feeling of well-being—a feeling of being helped.

MASSAGE TREATMENT CONSIDERATIONS AND GUIDELINES

The athletic trainer must have the basic essential knowledge of anatomy and of the particular area being treated. The physiology of the area to be treated and the total function of the athlete must be considered. There should be an understanding of the existing pathology so that the process by which repair occurs is known. The athletic trainer needs a thorough knowledge of massage principles and skillful techniques as well as manual dexterity, coordination, and concentration in the use of massage techniques. The athletic trainer also needs to exhibit such traits as patience, a sense of caring for the athlete's welfare, and courteousness both in speech and manner.

Perhaps the most important tools in massage therapy are the hands of the clinician. They must be clean, warm, dry, and soft. The nails must be short and smooth. Washing of the hands before and after treatment must take place for sanitary reasons. If the athletic trainer's hands are cold, they should be placed in warm water for a short period. Rubbing them together briskly helps to warm them too.

Positioning is also important for the clinician. Correct positioning will allow relaxation, prevent fatigue, and permit free movement of arms, hands,

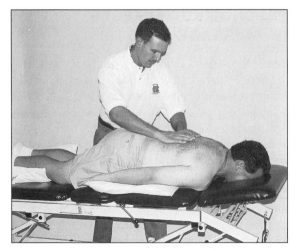

Figure 10-1 Position of athletic trainer for stroking.

- Hands are the most important tool in massage

and the body. Good posture will also help prevent fatigue and backache. The weight should rest evenly on both feet with the body in good postural alignment. When massaging a large area, the weight should shift from one foot to the other. You must be able to fit your hands to the contour of the area being treated. A good position is required to allow the correct application of pressure and rhythmic strokes during the procedure (Figure 10-1).

These points are important to consider when administering massage:

1. Pressure regulation should be determined by the type and amount of tissue present. It must also be governed by the athlete's condition and which tissues are to be affected. The pressure must be delivered from the body, through the soft parts of the hands, and it is adjusted to the contours of the athlete's body parts.
2. Rhythm must be steady and even. The time for each stroke and time between successive strokes should be equal.

■ Analogy *10-2*

When using massage to help reduce swelling in an extremity it is suggested that you begin proximally. The rationale for this is that you are first "uncorking the bottle" so that when you begin to "pour" the swelling from the extremity by using a massage technique, the lymphatic channels are clear, and the edema has some place to move to.

3. Duration depends on the pathology, size of the area being treated, speed of motion, age, size, and condition of the athlete. One also should observe the response of the athlete to determine duration of the procedure. Massage of the back or the neck area might take 15 to 30 minutes. Massage of a large joint (such as a hip or shoulder) may require less than 10 minutes.
4. If swelling is present in an extremity, treatment should begin with the proximal part. The purpose of this is to help facilitate the lymphatic flow proximally. The subsequent effects of distal massage in removing fluid or edema will be more efficient since the proximal resistance to lymphatic flow will be reduced. This technique has been referred to as the "uncorking effect."
5. Massage should never be painful, except possibly for friction massage, nor should it be given with such force that it causes ecchymosis (discoloration of the skin resulting from contusion).
6. In general, the direction of forces should be applied in the direction of the muscle fibers (Figure 10-2).
7. During a session, one should begin and end with effleurage. The maneuvers should increase progressively to the greatest energy possible and end by decreasing energy maneuvers.
8. The athletic trainer must consider the position in which massage can best be given and be sure the athlete is warm and in a comfortable, relaxed position.

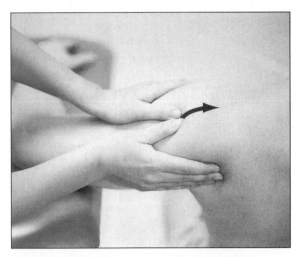

Figure 10-2   In the application of massage, forces should be applied in the direction of muscle fibers.

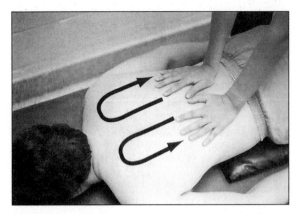

Figure 10-4   Massage pressure should be in line of venous flow followed by a return stroke without pressure.

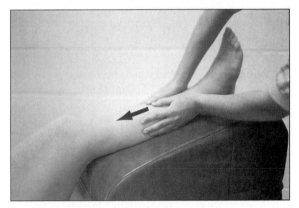

Figure 10-3   The part being massaged should be elevated, especially when the part is swollen.

9. The body part may be elevated if necessary and possible (Figure 10-3).
10. The athletic trainer should be in a position in which the whole body, as well as hands and arms, can be relaxed and the procedure accomplished without strain (see Figure 10-1).
11. Sufficient lubricant should be used so that the athletic trainer's hands will move smoothly along the skin surface (except in

friction). The use of too much lubricant should be guarded against.
12. Massage should begin with superficial stroking; this stroke is used to spread the lubricant over the part being treated.
13. Each stroke should start at the joint or just below the joint (unless massage over joints is contraindicated) and finish above the joint so that strokes will overlap.
14. The pressure should be in line with venous flow followed by a return stroke without pressure. The pressure should be in the centripetal direction (Figure 10-4).
15. Care should be used over body areas. Hands should be relaxed and pressure adjusted to fit the contour of the area being treated.
16. Bony prominences and painful joints should be avoided if possible.
17. All strokes should be rhythmic. The pressure strokes should end with a swing off, in a small half circle, in order that the rhythm will not be broken by an abrupt reversal.

Equipment SetUp

Table.   A firm table, easily accessible from both sides, is most desirable. The height of the table should be reasonably comfortable for the athletic trainer; leaning over or reaching up to perform the

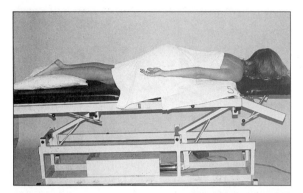

Figure 10-5 Draping of prone athlete. Towels are used for removal of lubricants, sheets are used for draping, and pillows are placed under hips and ankles for athlete comfort.

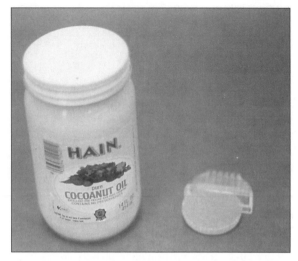

Figure 10-6 Example of lubricant to be used, beeswax and coconut oil.

required movements should not be necessary. An adjustable table is almost a must in this situation. To facilitate cleaning and disinfecting, a washable plastic surface is much preferred. There should be a storage area close by for linens and lubricant. If the table is not padded, a mattress or foam pad should be used for the comfort of the athlete.

Linens and Pillows. The athlete should be draped with a sheet, so only that part to be massaged is uncovered (Figure 10-5). Towels should be handy for removing the lubricant. A cotton sheet between the plastic surface of the table and the athlete is required to absorb perspiration and for the athlete's comfort. The surface of the plastic material is generally too cool for comfort. Pillows should be available to support the athlete.

Lubricant. Some type of lubricant should be used in almost all massage movements to overcome friction and avoid irritations by ensuring smooth contact of hands and skin. If the athlete's skin is too oily, it may be desirable to wash the skin first.

The lubricant should be of a type that is absorbed slightly by the skin but does not make it so slippery that the clinician finds it difficult to perform the required strokes. A light oil is recommended for lubrication. One that works well is a combination of one part beeswax to three parts coconut oil. These ingredients should be melted to-

gether and allowed to cool (Figure 10-6). It is best to use oil in situations in which (1) the clinician's or athlete's skin is too dry, (2) a cast has recently been removed, (3) scar tissue is present, or (4) there is excess hair. Some types of oil that may be used are olive oil, mineral oil, cocoa butter, or hydrolanolin. The "warm creams" or analgesic creams are skin irritants and if used in conjunction with massage may cause a burn, depending on the skin type of the athlete. These are also thought to cause blood to come to the surface of the skin, moving away from the muscles, which is exactly the opposite of what we are trying to accomplish through the massage techniques.

Alcohol may be used to remove the lubricant after massage. It is suggested that alcohol be placed in the clinician's hands before application to avoid the dramatic temperature drop that occurs when alcohol is applied directly to the athlete.

Sometimes unscented powder should be used if the clinician's hands tend to perspire, or it may be used to prevent skin irritation. Lubricant is not desired, nor should it be used, when applying friction movements since a firm contact between the skin and hands of clinician must take place.

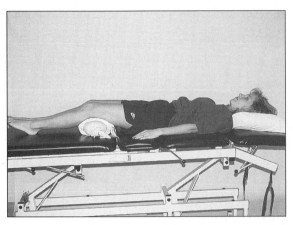

Figure 10-7   Athlete supine with pillow under head and knees.

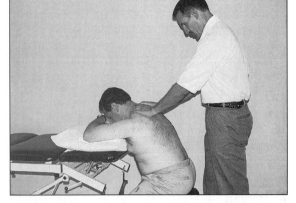

Figure 10-8   Athlete resting in a chair, facing table and leaning forward, is supported by pillows on the table. Forearms and hands are on the table for additional support. The athletic trainer stands behind the athlete.

Preparation of the Athlete

The position of the athlete is probably the most important aspect of ensuring a beneficial relaxation of the muscles from massage. The athlete should be in a relaxed, comfortable position. Lying down, when possible, is most beneficial to the athlete, and this also permits gravity to assist in the venous flow of the blood.

The part involved in treatment must be adequately supported. It may be elevated, depending on the pathology. When the athlete is being treated in the prone position, for massage of the neck, shoulders, back, buttocks, or back of the legs, a pillow or roll should be placed under the abdomen. Another pillow should be placed under the ankles so that the knees are slightly flexed (see Figure 10-5). If the athlete is in the supine position, small pillows should be placed under the head and under the knees (Figure 10-7).

Sometimes the prone position will be too painful for an athlete to assume for massaging a shoulder, upper back, or neck. A position that may be more comfortable is sitting in a chair, facing the table, while leaning forward and supported by pillows on the table. Forearms and hands are on the table for additional support (Figure 10-8). The ath-

letic trainer can administer the massage while standing behind the athlete (Figure 10-8).

The athlete should be appropriately draped before beginning massage. Some athletes are more shy than others and would be uncomfortable if they were required to expose parts of their body with other individuals around.

The body areas not being treated should be covered to prevent the athlete from being chilled (see Figure 10-5). Clothing should be removed from the part being treated. Towels should cover any clothes near the area being treated to protect them from the lubricant (see Figure 10-5).

SPECIFIC MASSAGE TECHNIQUES

Hoffa Massage

Albert Hoffa's text, published in 1900, provides the basis for the various massage techniques that have developed over the years.[27] Hoffa massage is essentially the classical massage technique that uses a variety of superficial strokes, including *effleurage*,

petrissage   Massage technique that is a kneading manipulation. Consists of repeatedly grasping and releasing the tissue with one or both hands or parts thereof, in a lifting, rolling, or pressing movement. The outside characteristic of this movement as contrasted to stroking movements is that the pressure is applied intermittently.

tapotment   A percussion massage; any series of brisk blows following each other in a rapid alternating fashion: hacking, cupping, slapping, beating, tapping, and pinchment. It is used when stimulation is the objective.

vibration   A shaking massage technique; a fine tremulous movement made by the hand or fingers placed firmly against a part that will cause the part to vibrate. Often used for a soothing effect; may be stimulating when more energy is applied.

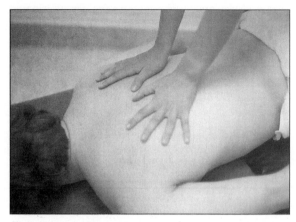

Figure 10-9   The stroke is performed with the heel of the hand, fingers slightly bent and thumbs spread.

petrissage, tapotment, and **vibration**. While some clinicians consider this technique to be mechanical, the strokes may be lighter and more superficial, thus making them more reflexive in nature. This technique opens the door for more mechanical techniques that are directed toward underlying tissues.

Effleurage.   This massage maneuver glides over the skin lightly without attempting to move the deep muscle masses. The main physiologic effect occurs when stroking is begun at the peripheral areas and moves toward the heart. The return flow of the venous and lymphatic systems is probably helped by this process. Circulation to the skin surface is also increased by stroking; the success is traced to the increased rate of metabolic exchange in the peripheral areas.

The primary purpose of effleurage is to accustom the athlete to the physical contact of the clinician. Lubricant should be used liberally with effleurage. Initially, effleurage serves to evenly distribute the lubricant. It also allows sensitive fingers to search for areas of muscle spasm or soreness and to locate trigger points and pressure points that

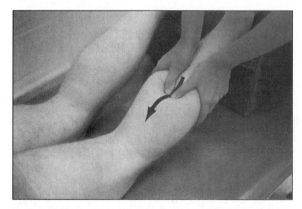

Figure 10-10   The kneading stroke is directed toward the heart, and contact should be maintained with the athlete.

can help determine the type of procedures to be used during the massage.

At the start of the massage, the stroke should be performed with a light pressure, coming from the flat of the hand with fingers slightly bent and thumbs spread (Figure 10-9). Once the unidirectional flow is established, going either centripetally or centrifugally, it should be continued throughout the treatment. Movement of the stroke should be toward the heart, and contact should be maintained with the athlete at all times to enhance relaxation (Figure 10-10).

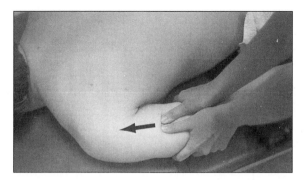

Figure 10-11   Deep stroking massage.

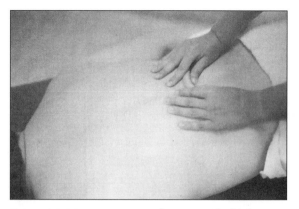

Figure 10-12   Petrissage application on the back.

Deep stroking massage is also a form of effleurage, except it is given with more pressure to produce a mechanical effect as well as a reflexing effect (Figure 10-11). Every massage begins and ends with effleurage. Stroking should also be used between other techniques. Stroking relaxes, decreases the defensive tension against harder massage techniques, and has a generally mentally soothing effect.

Petrissage.   Petrissage consists of kneading manipulations that press and roll the muscles under the fingers or hands. There is no gliding over the skin, except between progressions from one area to another, so only a minimal amount of lubricant is required in petrissage. The muscles are gently squeezed, lifted, and relaxed. The hands may remain stationary or may travel slowly along the length of the muscle or limb. The purpose of petrissage is to increase venous and lymphatic return and to press metabolic waste products out of affected areas through intensive, vigorous action. This form of massage can also break up adhesions between the skin and underlying tissue, loosen adherent fibrous tissue, and increase elasticity of the skin.

Petrissage can be described as a kneading technique. It involves repeated grasping, application of pressure, releasing in a lifting or rolling motion, then moving an adjacent area (Figure 10-12). Smaller muscles may be kneaded with one hand (Figure 10-13). Larger muscles, such as the hamstrings or muscle groups, will require the use of both hands (Figure 10-14). When kneading, the hands

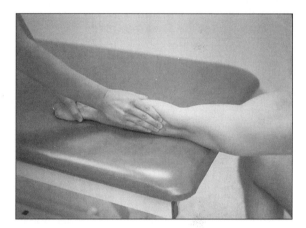

Figure 10-13   Petrissage kneading with one hand.

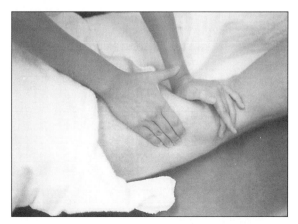

Figure 10-14   Petrissage kneading with both hands.

■ **Clinical Decision-Making** *Exercise 10-1*

....

A track athlete comes into the training room complaining about a "knot" that is palpable in the gastrocnemius. She explains that several months earlier she had suffered a muscle strain in that same muscle and she now feels that she can't stretch out the muscle and that "it is always tight." What can the athletic trainer do to get rid of the knot?

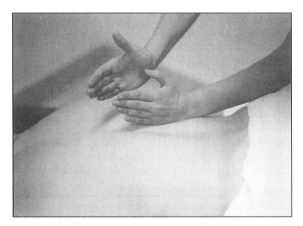

Figure 10-15 Percussion stroke of striking with the ulnar border of the hand.

should move from the distal to the proximal point of the muscle insertion, grasping parallel to or at right angles to the muscle fibers (see Figure 10-10).

Tapotment or Percussion. Percussion movements are a series of brisk blows, administered with relaxed hands and following each other in rapid alternating movements. This technique has a penetrating effect that is used to stimulate subcutaneous structures. Percussion is often used to increase circulation or to get a more active flow of blood. Peripheral nerve endings are stimulated so that they convey impulses more strongly with the use of percussion techniques. No lubricant is needed with tapotment.

Types of percussion techniques are hacking—alternate striking of athlete with the ulnar border of the hand (Figure 10-15); slapping—alternate slapping with fingers (Figure 10-16); beating—half-closed fist using the hypothenar eminence of the hand (Figure 10-17); tapping with the tips of the fingers (Figure 10-18); and clapping or cupping using fingers, thumb, and palm together to form a concave surface (Figure 10-19). Clapping or cupping is used primarily in postural drainage.

Vibration. Vibration technique is a fine tremulous movement, made by the hand or fingers placed firmly against a part; this causes the part to vibrate. The hands should remain in contact with the athlete, and a rhythmical trembling movement will come from the whole forearm, through the elbow (Figure 10-20).

Vibration is a technique that is most often used by physical therapists in treating patients who require a chest massage technique called *postural drainage*. The

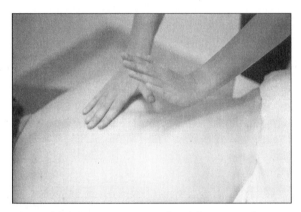

Figure 10-16 Percussion stroke of slapping with fingers.

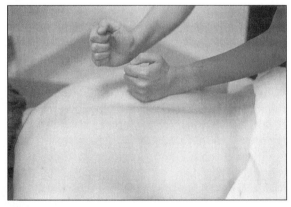

Figure 10-17 Percussion stroke of half-closed fist using hypothenar eminence.

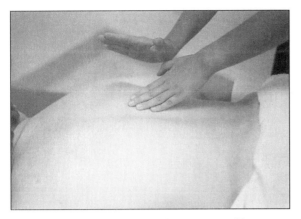

Figure 10-18   Percussion stroke using tips of fingers.

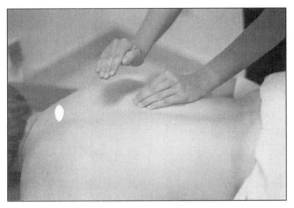

Figure 10-19   Percussion stroke of cupping using fingers, thumb, and palm together.

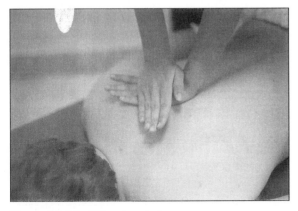

Figure 10-20   Vibration stroke.

> **friction massage**   A technique that affects fibrositic adhesions in tendon, muscle, or ligament. It is performed by small circular movements that penetrate into the depth of a muscle, not by moving the finger on the skin, but by moving the tissues under the skin.

technique is used to assist the patient clearing fluid from the lungs. Individuals who have cystic fibrosis are most likely to require postural drainage.

Routine.   The following is an example of a massage progression or routine:

1. Superficial stroking
2. Deep stroking
3. Kneading
4. Optional friction or tapotment
5. Deep stroking
6. Superficial stroking

The various individual classic massage techniques alone, however, do not make for a good massage. A proper program, intensity, tempo, and rhythm, as well as the proper starting, climax, and closing of the massage, are all important too. The form of the massage depends on the individual requirements of the athlete.

Clinical Applications for Hoffa Massage. The areas of treatment that we will most often see athletes for are muscle, tendon, and joint conditions. Adhesions, muscle spasm, myositis, bursitis, fibrositis, tendinitis or tenosynovitis, and postural strain of the back all generally fall into this category.

Areas of concern that indicate that you should not treat an athlete with massage include arteriosclerosis, thrombosis or embolism, severe varicose veins, acute phlebitis, cellulitis, synovitis, abscesses, skin injections, and cancers. Acute inflammatory conditions of the skin, soft tissues, or joints are also contraindications.

Friction Massage

James Cyriax and Gillean Russell[16] have used a technique called **friction massage** to affect musculoskeletal structures of ligament, tendon, and muscle to provide therapeutic movement over a

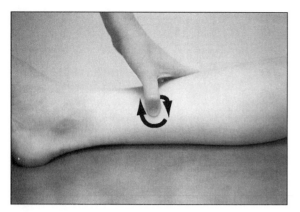

Figure 10-21 Thumb movement in a circle on an acupressure point.

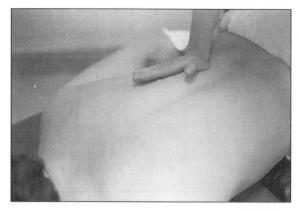

Figure 10-22 Superficial friction applied to the back by using the heel of the hand.

small area. The purposes for friction movements are to loosen adherent fibrous tissue (scar), aid in the absorption of local edema or effusions, and reduce local muscular spasm. Inflammation around joints is softened and more readily broken down so that the formation of adhesions is prevented. Another purpose is to provide deep pressure over trigger points to produce reflex effects. This technique is performed by the tips of the fingers, the thumb, or the heel of the hand, according to the area to be covered, making small circular movements (Figure 10-21). The superficial tissues are moved over the underlying structures by keeping the hand or fingers in firm contact with the skin (Figure 10-22).

Transverse friction massage is a technique for treating chronic tendon inflammations.[16] Inflammation is an important part of the healing process. It must occur before the healing process can advance to the fibroblastic stage. In chronic inflammations, however, the inflammatory process "gets stuck" and never really accomplishes what it is supposed to. The purpose of transverse friction massage is to try and increase the inflammation to a point where the inflammatory process is complete and the injury can progress to the later stages of the healing process. This technique is used most often in chronic overuse problems, such as lateral or medial humeral epicondylitis, "jumper's knee," rotator

■ Analogy *10-3*

There is an old saying that sometimes things have to get worse before they get better. Such is the case with transverse friction massage used to "jump start" the inflammatory process in cases of chronic inflammation. This massage technique is used specifically to make inflammation worse such that this process can go ahead and accomplish what it needs to so that healing can proceed to the subsequent stage.

cuff (supraspinatus) tendinitis, and iliotibial band friction syndrome.

The technique involves placing the tendon on a slight stretch. Massage is done using the thumb or index finger to exert intense pressure in a direction perpendicular to the direction of the fibers being massaged (Figure 10-23). The massage should last for 7 to 10 minutes and should be done every other day. It should be emphasized that transverse friction massage is a painful technique and the athletic trainer should explain this to the athlete before beginning the massage. Since transverse friction massage is a painful technique, it may help to apply ice to the treatment area prior to massage for analgesic purposes.

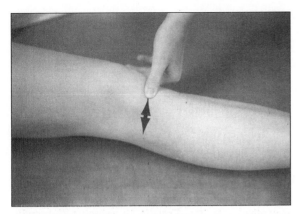

Figure 10-23   Transverse tendon friction massage on the patellar tendon.

Bindegewebsmassage   Reflex some massage; uses a pulling stroke across connective tissue to effect change.

Connective Tissue Massage

Connective tissue massage (**Bindegewebsmassage**) was developed by Elizabeth Dicke, a German physical therapist who suffered from decreased circulation in her right lower extremity for which amputation was advised. In trying to relieve her lower back pain, she massaged the area with pulling strokes. She found that with the continued stroking there was a relaxation of the muscular tension and a prickling warmth in the area. She continued the technique on herself, and after 3 months, she had no low back pain, and she had restored circulation to her right leg.

Connective tissue massage is a stroking technique carried out in the layers of connective tissue on the body surface. This stimulates the nerve endings of the autonomic nervous system.[28] Afferent impulses travel to the spinal cord and the brain, and this causes a change in reaction susceptibility.[43]

Connective tissue is an organ of metabolism; therefore, abnormal tension in one part of the tissue is reflected in other parts.[28] All pathologic changes involve an inflammatory reaction in the affected part. One of the changes caused by inflammatory reaction is accumulation of fluid in the affected area. The area where these changes can most readily be detected is on the body surface. These changes are often seen as flattened areas or depressed bands that may be surrounded by elevated areas. The flat areas are the areas of main response, and the connective tissue is tight, resisting pulling in any direction with movement.

The technique of connective tissue massage is not used as much in the United States as it is in European countries, especially Germany. As more results are seen, especially in the treatment of diseases associated with the pathology of circulation, this technique should become more widely accepted and used in this country.

Position of the Athlete and the Athletic Trainer.   The athlete is usually in the sitting position for a connective tissue massage. Occasionally athletes may be treated in a sidelying or prone position when they cannot be treated in a sitting position. The athletic trainer should be in a position, seated or standing, that provides good body mechanics, is comfortable, and avoids fatigue.

Application technique.   The basic stroke of pulling is performed with the tips, or pads, of the middle and ring fingers of either hand. Fingernails must be very short. The stroking technique is characterized by a tangential pull on the skin and subcutaneous tissues away from the fascia with the fingers. This technique should cause a sharp pain in the tissue. The stroke is a pull, not a push of the tissue. No lubricant is used. All treatments are started by the basic strokes from the coccyx to the first lumbar vertebra. Treatments last about 15 to 25 minutes. After 15 treatments, which are carried out two to three times per week, there should be a rest period of at least 4 weeks.

Other Considerations.   Before any logical plan for treatment can be made, it is important to determine where any alterations in the optimum function of connective tissue have taken place, where the changes started, and if possible, the cause of the alteration.

Evaluation is a most important part of an effective connective tissue massage program. The technique of stroking with two fingers of one hand along each side of the vertebral column will give much information about the sensory changes that are caused by alterations in the tension of surface tissues.

Clinical applications for connective tissue massage. There are numerous arterial and venous disorders that may respond to connective tissue massage. Specific disabilities include (1) scars on the skin; (2) fractures and arthritis in the bones and joints; (3) lower back pain and torticollis in the muscles; (4) varicose symptoms, thrombophlebitis (subacute), hemorrhoids, and edema in the blood and lymph; and (5) Raynaud's disease, intermittent claudication, frostbite, and trophic changes in the circulatory system. Connective tissue massage can also be used for myocardial dysfunctions, respiratory disturbances, intestinal disorders, ulcers, hepatitis, infections of the ovaries and uterus (subacute), amenorrhea, dysmenorrhea, genital infantilism, multiple sclerosis, Parkinson's disease, headaches, migraines, and allergies. Connective tissue massage is recommended to help in the process of revascularization following orthopedic complications such as fractures, dislocations, and sprains. Contraindications to connective tissue massage include tuberculosis, tumors, and mental illnesses that result from psychological dependence.

Connective tissue massage must be learned and performed initially under the direct supervision of someone who has been taught these highly specialized techniques. More detailed information about connective tissue massage can be found listed in the bibliography.[19, 37, 57]

Acupressure and Myofascial Trigger Point Massage

Acupressure is a type of massage based on the ancient Chinese art of acupuncture. Acupuncture, along with herbal medicine, composes traditional Chinese medicine. Only recently has the amount of research, publication, and interest in acupuncture in Western medical literature increased dramatically.

---

acupressure The technique of using finger pressure over acupuncture points to decrease pain.

The Chinese make no distinction between arteries, veins, or nerves when explaining the functions of the body.[38] They concentrate instead on an elaborate system of forces whose interplay is thought to regulate all bodily functions. The traditional, philosophical Chinese explanation has little correlation with the more scientifically oriented Western concepts of medicine, which rely heavily on anatomic and physiologic principles. Consequently, utilization of acupuncture as a therapeutic technique in Western medical practice has encountered considerable skepticism.

The Chinese believe that an essential life force known as Qi (pronounced *che*) exists in everyone and controls all aspects of life. Qi is governed by the interplay of two opposing forces, the yang (positive) forces and the yin (negative) forces. Disease and pain result from some imbalance between the two.[39] The yin and yang flow through passageways or lines within the body called *jing* by the Chinese and known as *meridians* in the West. The twelve meridians within the body are named according to the part of the body with which they are associated. The meridians on one side of the body are duplicated by those on the other; however, two additional meridians exist that cannot be paired.[40]

1. Lung (L)
2. Large Intestine (LI)
3. Stomach (ST)
4. Spleen (SP)
5. Heart (H)
6. Small intestine (SI)
7. Urinary bladder (UB)
8. Kidney (K)
9. Pericardium (P)
10. Triple warmet (TW)
11. Gall bladder (GB)
12. Liver (LIV)
13. Governing vessel (GV)*
14. Conception vessel (CV)*

*Not paired

Along these meridians lie the acupuncture points that are associated with each particular meridian. These points are named according to the meridian on which they lie. Whenever there is pain or illness, certain points on the surface of the body become tender.[39] When pain is eliminated or the disease is cured, these tender points seem to disappear.[2] According to acupuncture theory, stimulation of specific points through needling can dramatically reduce pain in areas of the body known to be associated with a particular point. Thousands of acupuncture points have been identified by the Chinese. In the Nei Ching,[30] a classical text on Chinese medicine, 365 points that lie on the meridians have been enumerated. Additional acupuncture points have been identified on the auricle as well as the hand.

There is some evidence for the actual physical existence of these points.[61] The electrical resistance of the skin at certain points corresponding to the acupuncture points is lower than that of the surrounding skin, especially when a disease state is present. Examining acupuncture points by sectioning indicated increased nerve endings at these points. Russian investigators have reportedly discovered differences in skin temperature at these points. Despite this evidence, there is no definite physical attribute of all acupuncture points, nor is there a thoroughly demonstrated mode of action for the technique. Whatever the explanation, it appears that the locations and effects of stimulating specific acupuncture points for the relief of pain were determined empirically.[42]

Myofascial Trigger Points.   In Western medicine, the counterpart of the acupuncture point is the trigger point. Myofascial trigger points may be found in skeletal muscle and tendons, in myofascia, in ligaments and capsules surrounding joints, in periosteum, and in the skin.[51] Myofascial trigger points may activate and become painful due to some trauma to the muscle occurring either from direct trauma or from overuse that results in some inflammatory response.[59] Like acupuncture points, pain is usually referred to areas that follow a specific pattern associated with a particular point. Stimulation of these points has also been demonstrated to result in a relief of pain.[22]

■ **Clinical Decision-Making**   *Exercise 10-2*

A female athlete is complaining of painful menstrual cramps during practice. She is in such discomfort that she is incapable of continuing with the practice session. Is there anything that the athletic trainer can do to immediately relieve her cramps?

■ **Clinical Decision-Making**   *Exercise 10-3*

An athlete is complaining of pain in the middle of the upper back between the "shoulder blades" that seems to radiate to the left shoulder. What is causing this pain, and what techniques can the athletic trainer use to eliminate this problem?

Acupuncture and myofascial trigger points are not necessarily one and the same. However, a study by Melzack, Fox, and Stillwell[42] attempted to develop a correlation coefficient between acupuncture and trigger points on the basis of two criteria: spatial distribution and associated pain patterns. They found a remarkably high correlation coefficient of .84, which suggested that acupuncture and trigger points used for pain relief, although discovered independently, labeled by totally different methods, and derived from such historically different concepts of medicine, represent a similar phenomenon and may be explained by the same underlying neural mechanisms.[42]

Physiologic explanations of the effectiveness of massaging acupressure and myofascial trigger points may likely be attributed to some interaction of the various mechanisms of pain modulation discussed in Chapter 3.[2] There is considerable evidence that intense, low-frequency stimulation of these points triggers the release of β-endorphin.[48,50,57]

Acupressure Massage Techniques.   By using acupuncture charts (Figure 10-24) or trigger point charts[59] specific points are selected, which are

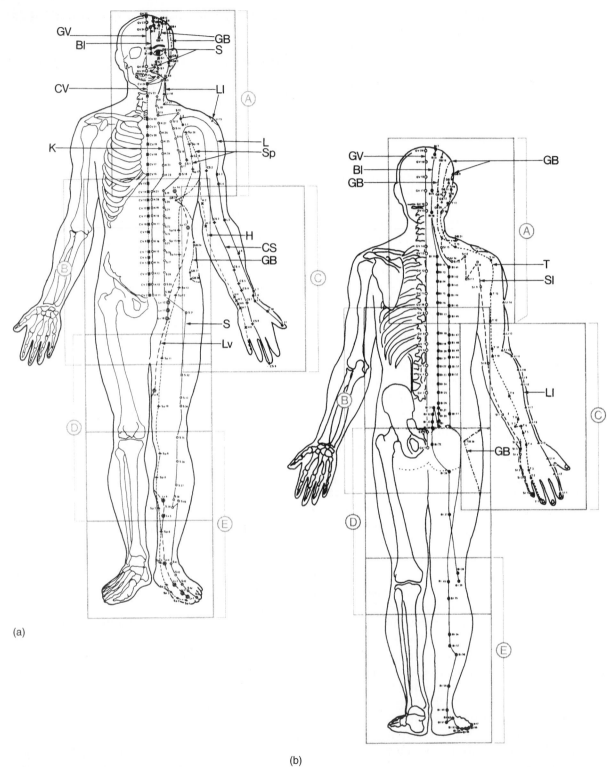

Figure 10-24 Acupuncture point charts should be used to locate specific points. (a) Anterior, (b) posterior, (c) lateral.

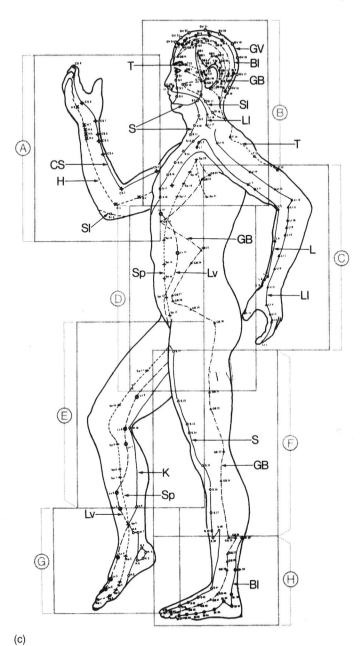

(c)

Figure 10-24 Continued

described in the literature as having some relationship to the area of pain. The charts provide the athletic trainer with a general idea of where these points are located. Two techniques may be used to specifically locate acupressure and myofascial trigger points. Since it is known that electrical impedance is reduced at these points, an ohmmeter may be used to locate the points. Perhaps the easiest technique is simply to palpate the area until either a small fibrous nodule or a strip of tense muscle tissue that is tender to the touch is felt.[10,13,14]

Once the point is located, massage is begun using the index or middle fingers, the thumb, or perhaps the elbow. Small friction-like circular motions are used on the point (see Figure 10-21). The amount of pressure applied to these acupressure points should be determined by athlete tolerance; however, it must be intense and will likely be painful to the athlete. Generally, the more pressure the athlete can tolerate, the more effective the treatment.

Effective treatment times range from 1 to 5 minutes at a single point per treatment. It may be necessary to massage several points during the treatment to obtain the greatest effects. If this is the case, it is best to work distal points first and to move proximally.

During the massage, the athlete will report a dulling or numbing effect and will frequently indicate that the pain diminishes or subsides totally during the massage. The lingering effects of acupressure massage vary tremendously from athlete to athlete. The effects may last for only a few minutes in some but may persist in others for several hours.

Myofascial Release

Myofascial release is a term that refers to a group of techniques used for the purpose of relieving soft tissue from the abnormal grip of tight fascia.[31] It is essentially a form of stretching that has been reported to have significant impact in treating a variety of conditions. Some specialized training is necessary for the athletic trainer to understand specific techniques of myofascial release[3] in addition to an in-depth understanding of the fascial system.

Fascia is a type of connective tissue that surrounds muscles, tendons, nerves, bones, and organs.

> **myofascial release** A group of techniques used to relieve soft tissue from the abnormal grip of tight fascia.

It is essentially continuous from head to toe and is interconnected in various sheaths or planes. Fascia is composed primarily of collagen along with some elastic fibers. During movement, the fascia must stretch and move freely. If there is damage to the fascia owing to injury, disease, or inflammation, it will not only affect local adjacent structures but may also affect areas far removed from the site of injury.[54] Thus, it may be necessary to release tightness in both the area of injury as well as in distant areas.[31] It will tend to soften and release in response to gentle pressure over a relatively long period of time.[31]

Myofascial release has also been referred to as soft-tissue mobilization, although technically, all forms of massage involve mobilization of soft tissue.[54] Soft-tissue mobilization should not be confused with joint mobilization, although it must be emphasized that the two are closely related. Joint mobilization is used to restore normal joint arthrokinematics, and specific rules exist regarding direction of movement and joint position based on the shape of the articulating surfaces. Myofascial restrictions are considerably more unpredictable and may occur in many different planes and directions. Myofascial treatment is based on localizing the restriction and moving into the direction of the restriction, regardless of whether that follows the arthrokinematics of a nearby joint.[12] Thus, myofascial manipulation is considerably more subjective and relies heavily on the experience of the clinician.

Myofascial manipulation focuses on large treatment areas, while joint mobilization focuses on a specific joint. Releasing myofascial restrictions over a large treatment area can have significant impact on joint mobility.[23] Once a myofascial restriction is located, the massage should be directly through the restriction. The progression of the technique is from superficial to deep. Once more superficial restrictions are released, the deep restrictions can be located and released without causing any damage to superficial tissues. Joint mobilization should follow

■ **Clinical Decision-Making** *Exercise 10-4*

A basketball player has a chronic case of patellar tendinitis. The athletic trainer has taken usual anti-inflammatory measures (i.e., rest, medications, etc.) in treating the problem, but it has not improved. Suggest an alternative treatment for chronic inflammation.

myofascial release and will likely be more effective once soft-tissue restrictions are eliminated.

As the extensibility is improved in the myofascia, elongation and stretching of the musculotendinous unit should be incorporated.[44] In addition, strengthening exercises are recommended to enhance neuromuscular re-education, which helps promote new, more efficient movement patterns. As freedom of movement improves, postural re-education may help to ensure the maintenance of the less restricted movement patterns.

Generally, acute cases tend to resolve in just a few treatments. The longer a condition has been present, the longer it will take to resolve. Occasionally, dramatic results will occur immediately after treatment. It is usually recommended that treatment should be done at least three times per week.[13]

Treatment Considerations.

Protecting the hands. The hands are certainly the primary treatment modality in all forms of massage. Certainly, in myofascial release they are constantly subjected to stress and strain, and consideration must be given to protection of the athletic trainer's hands. It is essential to avoid constant hyperextension or hyperflexion of any joints, which may lead to hypermobility. If it is necessary to work in deeper tissues where more force is necessary, then the fist or elbow may be substituted for the thumb and fingers.[12]

Use of lubricant. It is necessary to use a small amount of lubricant, particularly if large areas are to be treated using long stroking movements. Enough lubricant should be used to allow for traction while reducing painful friction without allowing slipping of the hands on the skin.[12]

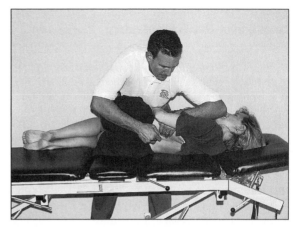

Figure 10-25 Myofascial release is a mild combination of pressure and stretch used to free soft-tissue restrictions.

Rolfing A system devised to correct inefficient structure by balancing the body within a gravitational field through a technique involving manual soft-tissue manipulation.

Positioning of the athlete. As with the other forms of massage, it is critical to appropriately position the athlete such that the effects of the treatment may be maximized. Pillows or towel rolls may be a great aid in establishing an effective treatment position even before the hands contact the athlete (Figure 10-25). The athletic trainer should make certain that good body mechanics and positioning are considered to protect the athletic trainer as well as the athlete.

Rolfing®

Rolfing, also referred to as *structural integration*, is a system devised by Ida Rolf that is used to correct inefficient structure or to "integrate structure."[6] The goal of this technique is to balance the body within a gravitational field through a technique involving manual soft-tissue manipulation.[12] The basic principle of treatment is that if balanced movement is essential at a particular joint, yet nearby tissue is restrained, both the tissue and the

■ **Clinical Decision-Making** *Exercise 10-5*

....

A swimmer wants the athletic trainer to give her a full body massage after a particularly difficult workout. She says that a massage will help her to get rid of the lactic acid in her muscles. How should the athletic trainer respond to this request?

joint will relocate to a position that accomplishes a more appropriate equilibrium.[32,49]

Rolfing is a standardized approach that is administered without regard to symptoms or specific pathologies. The technique involves 10 hour-long sessions, each of which emphasizes some aspect of posture, with the massage directed toward the myofascia. The 10 sessions include

1. Respiration
2. Balance under the body (legs and feet)
3. Sagital plane balance—lateral line from front to back
4. Balance left to right—base of body to midline
5. Pelvic balance—rectus abdominis and psoas
6. Weight transfer from head to feet—sacrum
7. Relationship of head to rest of body—occiput and atlas
8. and 9. Upper half of the body to lower half of the body relationship
10. Balance throughout the system

Once these ten treatments are completed, advanced sessions may be performed in addition to periodic "tune-up" sessions.

A major aspect of this treatment approach is to integrate the structural with the psychological. An emotional state may be seen as the projection of structural imbalances. The easiest and most efficient method for changing the physical body is through direct intervention in the body. Changing the structural imbalances can alter the psychological component.[49]

Trager®

Developed by Milton Trager, **Tragering** combines mechanical soft-tissue mobilization and neurophysiological re-education.[58] Unlike Rolfing, Trager has

■ **TABLE 10-1** Summary of Indications and Contraindications for Therapeutic Sports Massage

....

INDICATIONS	CONTRAINDICATIONS
Increase coordination	Arteriosclerosis
Decrease pain	Thrombosis
Decrease neuromuscular excitibility	Embolism
Stimulate circulation	Severe varicose veins
Facilitate healing	Acute phlebitis
Restore joint mobility	Cellulitis
Remove lactic acid	Synovitis
Alleviate muscle cramps	Abscesses
Increase blood flow	Skin infections
Increase venous return	Cancers
Retard muscle atrophy	Acute inflammatory
Increase range of motion	conditions
Edema	Pregnancy
Myofascial trigger points	
Stretching scar tissue	
Adhesions	
Muscle spasm	
Myositis	
Bursitis	
Fibrositis	
Tendinitis	
Revascularization	
Raynaud's disease	
Intermittent claudication	
Dysmenorrhea	
Headaches	
Migraines	

....

Trager A technique that attempts to establish neuromuscular control so that more normal movement patterns can be routinely performed.

....

no standardized protocols or procedures. The Trager system uses gentle, passive, rocking oscillations of a body part. This is essentially a mobilization technique emphasizing traction and rotation as a relaxation technique to encourage the athlete to relinquish control. This relaxation technique is followed by a series of active movements designed to alter the athlete's neurophysiological control of movement, thus providing a basis for maintaining these changes. This technique does not attempt to make mechanical changes in the soft tissues, but it attempts to establish neuromuscular control so that more normal movement patterns can be routinely performed. Essentially, it uses the nervous system to make changes rather than making mechanical changes in the tissues themselves.

Summary

1. Massage, as we know it today, is an improved and more scientific version of the various procedures that go back for thousands of years to the Greeks, Egyptians, and others.
2. Massage is the mechanical stimulation of tissue by means of rhythmically applied pressure and stretching. It allows the athletic trainer, as a health care provider, to assist an athlete to overcome pain and to relax through the application of the therapeutic massage techniques.
3. Massage has effects on the circulation, the lymphatic system, the nervous system, the muscles, myofascia, the skin, scar tissue, psychologic responses, relaxation feelings, and pain.
4. Hoffa massage is the classic form of massage and uses strokes that include effleurage, petrissage, percussion or tapotment, and vibration.
5. Friction massage is used to increase the inflammatory response, particularly in cases of chronic tendinitis or tenosynovitis.
6. Massage of acupuncture and trigger points is used to reduce pain and irritation in anatomical areas known to be associated with specific points.
7. Connective tissue massage is a reflex zone massage. It is a relatively new form of treatment in this country and has its best effects on circulatory pathologies.
8. Myofascial release is a massage technique used for the purpose of relieving soft tissue from the abnormal grip of tight fascia.
9. Rolfing is a system devised to correct inefficient structure by balancing the body within a gravitational field through a technique involving manual soft tissue manipulation.
10. Trager attempts to establish neuromuscular control so that more normal movement patterns can be routinely performed.

Review Questions

1. Discuss the evolution of massage as a treatment modality.
2. What are the physiologic effects of sports massage?
3. What are the reflexive effects of massage on pain, circulation, and metabolism?
4. What are the mechanical effects of massage on muscle and skin?
5. What psychological benefits can come with massage?
6. What are the various considerations for setting up equipment and preparing an athlete for massage?
7. What are the various stroking techniques used in traditional Hoffa massage?
8. What are the clinical applications for using friction massage?
9. What is connective tissue massage most often used for?
10. What is the difference between acupuncture points and myofascial trigger points?
11. How can myofascial release be used to restore normal functional movement patterns?

Self-Test Questions

T/F

1. Massage will increase blood and lymphatic flow.
2. The "uncorking effect" states massage on a limb with edema should begin distally.
3. Direction of stroking usually follows muscle fibers.

Multiple Choice

4. Which type of massage "kneads" tissue by lifting, rolling, or pressing intermittently?
   a. effleurage
   b. petrissage
   c. tapotment
   d. vibration
5. Pain relief is one of the reflexive effects of massage. What are the other two effects?
   a. increased muscle elasticity and decreased adhesions
   b. increased muscle elasticity and elongated fascia
   c. decreased circulation and metabolism
   d. increased circulation and metabolism
6. Which type of massage does NOT require lubricant?
   a. petrissage
   b. effleurage
   c. Hoffa
   d. friction
7. Acupressure massage technique requires the therapist to identify trigger points and then apply _____ .
   a. pressure
   b. Bindegewebsmassage
   c. friction
   d. lubricant
8. Which of the following massage techniques is designed to balance the body by manipulating soft tissue?
   a. Hoffa
   b. Trager
   c. Rolfing
   d. acupuncture
9. Which of the following is a contraindication to massage?
   a. acute inflammatory conditions
   b. edema
   c. Raynaud's disease
   d. tendonitis
10. Superficial stroking may be utilized at the _____ .
   a. beginning of the massage
   b. end of the massage
   c. both A and B
   d. neither A nor B

Solutions to Clinical Decision-Making Exercises

10-1 The athletic trainer may choose to use a petrissage technique, which involves a deep kneading technique. Petrissage is often used to break up adhesions in the underlying muscle and also to assist the lymphatic system in removing waste from the area.

10-2 Acupressure massage to several acupuncture points may help eliminate her cramps in a few minutes by massaging one or several points. The tender points are located 2 inches to the right of L2, 2 inches bilateral to T10, and bi-laterally over the first sacral openings. Using a circular massage of these points can potentially eliminate the cramps for several hours.

10-3 It is likely that the athlete has a myofascial trigger point in the rhomboids. The athletic trainer could try several different techniques that have proven to be effective, including circular pressure massage, a spray-and-stretch technique (Chapter 4), or a combination of ultrasound and electrical stimulation (Chapter 5).

10-4 A transverse friction massage may help to "jump start" the inflammatory process, thus allowing the healing process to progress to the latter stages. It should be explained that the treatment will be somewhat painful and that the problem should actually get worse before it gets better.

10-5 The athletic trainer should point out that massage post exercise has not been demonstrated to effectively remove lactic acid. The athletic trainer should also inform the athlete that if there is a specific problem that can be helped by incorporating massage, then he/she will be glad to do so. However, the policy is generally not to provide full body massage for relaxation purposes.

References

1. Archer, PA: *Massage for sports health care professionals,* Champaign, Ill., 1999, Human Kinetics.
2. Baldry, PE: *Acupuncture, trigger points and musculoskeletal pain,* London, 1993, Churchill Livingstone.
3. Barnes, J: Five years of myofascial release, *Phys Ther Forum* 6(37):12–14, 1987.
4. Barr, J, and Taslitz, N: Influence of back massage on autonomic functions, *Phys Ther* 50:1679–1691, 1970.
5. Bell, GW: Aquatic sports massage therapy, *Clinics in Sports Medicine* 18(2):427–435, 1999.
6. Bernau-Eigen, M: Rolfing: a somatic approach to the integration of human structures, *Nurse Practitioner Forum* 9(4):235–242, 1998.
7. Birukov, A: Training massage during contemporary sports loads, *Soviet Sports Review* 22:42–44, 1987.
8. Boone, T, Cooper R, and Thompson, W: A physiologic evaluation of the sports massage, *Athletic Training* 26(1): 51–54, 1991.
9. Braverman, DI, and Schulman, RA: Massage techniques in rehabilitation medicine, *Physical Medicine & Rehabilitation Clinics of North America* 10(3):631–649, 1999.
10. Brickey, R, and Yao, J: *Acupuncture and transcutaneous electrical stimulation techniques, course manual in acutherapy post graduate seminars,* Raleigh, N.C., 1978.
11. Cafarelli, E: Vibratory massage and short-term recovery from muscular fatigue, *Inter J Sports Med* 11:474, 1990.
12. Cantu, R, and Grodin, A: *Myofascial manipulation: theory and clinical applications,* Gaithersburg, Md., 1992, Aspen Publications.
13. Castel, J: *Pain management with acupuncture and transcutaneous electrical nerve stimulation techniques and photo stimulation (Laser),* course manual, 1982.
14. Cheng, R, and Pomerantz, B: Electroacupuncture analgesia could be mediated by at least two pain relieving mechanisms: endorphin and non-endorphin systems, *Life Sci.* 25:1957–1962, 1979.
15. Crosman, L, Chateauvert, S, and Weisberg, J: The effects of massage to the hamstring muscle group on range of motion, *J Ortho Sport Phys Ther* 6:168, 1984.
16. Cyriax, J, and Russell, G: *Textbook of orthopedic medicine,* vol II, ed 10, Baltimore, 1980, Williams & Wilkins.
17. Dubrovsky, V: Changes in muscle and venous blood flow after massage, *Soviet Sports Review* 18:134–135, 1983.
18. Ebel, A, and Wisham, L: Effect of massage on muscle temperature and radiosodium clearance, *Arch Phys Med* 33:399–405, 1952.
19. Ebner, M: *Connective tissue manipulations,* Malibar, Fla., 1985, RE Krieger.
20. Elkins, E: Effects of various procedures on flow of lymph, *Arch Phys Med* 34:31–39, 1953.
21. Ernst, E: Does post-exercise massage treatment reduce delayed onset muscle soreness? A systematic review, *British Journal of Sports Medicine* 32(3):212–214, 1998.
22. Fox, E, and Melzack, R: Transcutaneous electrical stimulation and acupuncture: comparison of treatment for low back pain, *Pain* 2:357–373, 1976.
23. Gordon, P: *Myofascial reorganization,* Brookline, Mass., 1988, The Gordon Group.
24. Harmer, P: The effect of preperformance massage on stride frequency in sprinters, *Athletic Training* 26(1):55–59, 1991.
25. Head H: *Die Sensibilitatorungen der Haut bei viszeral Erkran Kungen,* Berlin, 1898.
26. Hemmings, B, Smith, M, Graydon, J, and Dyson, R: Effects of massage on physiological restoration, perceived recovery, and repeated sports performance, *British Journal of Sports Medicine* 34(2):109–114, Apr 2000.
27. Hoffa, A: *Technik der massage,* ed 14, Stutgartt, Germany, 1900, Ferdinand Enke.
28. Holey, EA: Connective tissue massage: a bridge between complementary and orthodox approaches, *Journal of Bodywork & Movement Therapies* 4(1):72–80, 2000.
29. Hungerford, M, and Bornstein, R: Sports Massage, *Sports Med Guide* 4:4–6, 1985.
30. Hwang Ti *Nei Ching (translation),* Berkeley, 1973, University of California Press.
31. Juett, T: Myofascial release—an introduction for the athlete, *Phys. Ther. Forum* 7(41):7–8, 1988.
32. Kallen, B: Deep impact: rolfing is deeper than the deepest massage—and sometimes more painful. Some athletes swear by it anyway, *Men's Fitness* 16(7):96–99, 2000.
33. King, R: *Performance massage,* Champaign, Ill, 1993, Human Kinetics.

34. Kopysov, V: Use of vibrational massage in regulating the pre-competition condition of weight lifters, *Soviet Sports Review* 14:82–84, 1979.

35. Kuprian, W: Massage. In Kuprian, W, editor: *Phys Ther for sports*, Philadelphia, 1981, WB Saunders.

36. Longworth, J: Psychophysiological effects of slow stroke back massage in normotensive females, *Adv Nurs Science* 10:44–61, 1982.

37. Licht, S: *Massage, manipulation and traction*, New Haven, 1960, Elizabeth Licht.

38. Man, P, and Chen, C: Acupuncture anesthesia—a new theory and clinical study, *Curr. Ther. Res.* 14:390–394, 1972.

39. Manaka, Y: On certain electrical phenomena for the interpretation of Chi in Chinese literature, *Am. J. Chin. Med.* 3:71–74, 1975.

40. Mann, F: *Acupuncture: the ancient Chinese art of healing and how it works scientifically*, New York, 1973, Random House.

41. Martin, NA, Zoeller, RF, and Robertson, RJ: The comparative effect of sports massage, active recovery, and rest on promoting blood lactate clearing after supramaximal leg exercise, *Journal of Athletic Training* 33(1):30–35, 1998.

42. Melzack, R, Stillwell, D, Fox, E: Trigger points and acupuncture points for pain: correlations and implications, *Pain* 3:3–23, 1977.

43. Mennell, J: *Physical treatment*, ed 5, Philadelphia, 1968, Blakiston Co.

44. Mock, LE: Myofascial release treatment of specific muscles of the upper extremity (levels 3 and 4): part 4, *Clinical Bulletin of Myofascial Therapy* 3(1):71–93, 1998.

45. Morelli, M, Seaborne, PT, and Sullivan SJ: Changes in H-reflex amplitude during massage of triceps surae in healthy subjects, *J Ortho Sports Phys Ther* 12(2): 55–59, 1990.

46. Patino, O, Novick, C, Merlo, A, and Benaim, F: Massage in hypertrophic scars, *Journal of Burn Care & Rehabilitation* 20(3):268–271, 1999.

47. Pemberton, R: The physiologic influence of massage. In Mock, HE, Pemberton, R, and Coulter, JS, editors: *Principles and practices of physical therapy,* vol. I, Hagerstown, Md., 1939, WF Prior.

48. Prentice, W: The use of electroacutherapy in the treatment of inversion ankle sprains, *J. Nat. Athl. Train. Assoc.* 17(1): 15–21, 1982.

49. Rolf, I: *Rolfing: the integration of human structures,* Rochester, Vermont, 1977, Healing Arts Press.

50. Sjolund, B, and Eriksson, M: Electroacupuncture and endogenous morphines, *Lancet* 2:1085, 1976.

51. Stone, JA: Prevention and rehabilitation. Myofascial techniques: trigger-point therapy, *Athletic Therapy Today* 5(3):54–55, 2000.

52. Stone, JA: Prevention and rehabilitation. The rationale for therapeutic massage, *Athletic Therapy Today* 4(4):26, 1999.

53. Stone, JA: Massage as a therapeutic modality-technique, *Athletic Therapy Today* 4(5):51–52, Sept 1999.

54. Stone, JA: Myofascial release, *Athletic Therapy Today* 5(4):34–35, July 2000.

55. Sullivan, S: Effects of massage on alpha motorneuron excitability, *Phys Ther* 71:555, 1991.

56. Suskind, M, Hajek, N, and Hinds, H: Effects of massage on denervated muscle, *Arch Phys Med* 27:133–135, 1946.

57. Tappan, F: *Healing massage techniques: holistic, classic, and emerging methods,* East Norwalk, Conn., 1988, Appleton & Lange.

58. Trager, M: Trager psychophysical integration and mentastics, *Trager Journal* 5:10, 1982.

59. Travell, J, and Simons, D: *Myofascial pain and dysfunction: the trigger point manual,* Baltimore, 1983, Williams & Wilkins.

60. Vaughn, B, Miller, K, and Fink, D: *Massage for sports health care,* Champaign, Ill., 1998, Human Kinetics.

61. Wei, L: Scientific advances in Chinese medicine, *Am. Chin. Med.* 7:53–75, 1979.

62. Wood, E, and Becker, P: *Beard's massage,* Philadelphia, 1981, WB Saunders.

63. Wyper, D, and McNiven, D: Effects of some physiotherapeutic agents on skeletal muscle blood flow, *Phys Ther* 62:83–85, 1976.

Suggested Readings

Barnes, M, Personius, W, and Gronlund, R: An efficacy study on the effect on myofascial release treatment technique on obtaining pelvic symmetry, *Phys Ther* 19(1):56, 1994

Bean B, Henderson, H, and Martinsen, M: Massage: how to do it and what it can do for you, *Scholastic Coach* 52(5): 10–11, 1982.

Beard, G: A history of massage technique, *Phys Ther Rev* 32: 613–624, 1952.

Beard, G, and Wood, E: *Massage: principles and techniques,* Philadelphia, 1964, WB Saunders.

Beck, M: *Theory and practice of therapeutic massage,* Albany, N.Y., 1994, Malidy Publishing.

Breakey, B: An overlooked therapy you can use ad lib, *RN* 45:7, 1982.

Chamberlain, G: Cyriax's friction massage: a review, *J. Orthop. Sports Phys. Ther.* 4(1):16–22, 1982.

Cyriax, J: *Textbook of orthopedic medicine,* vol I, ed 8, New York, 1982, Macmillan.

Day, J, Mason, P, and Chesrow, S: Effect of massage on serum level of β-endorphin and β-lipotrophin in healthy adults, *Phys Ther* 67:926–930, 1987.

Ebner, M: Connective tissue massage, *Physiotherapy* 64: 208–210, 1978.

Ehrett, S: Craniosacral therapy and myofascial release in entry-level physical therapy curricula, *Phys Ther* 68(4):534–540, 1988.

Ernst, E, Matra, A, and Magyarosy, I: Massages cause changes in blood fluidity, *Physiotherapy* 73:43–45, 1987.

Fritz, S: *Fundamentals of therapeutic massage*, St. Louis, 1995, Mosby.

Goats, G: Massage—the scientific basis of an ancient art: part 1—the techniques, *British J Sports Med* 28(3):149–152, 1994.

Goldberg, J, Seaborne, D, and Sullivan, S: The effect of therapeutic massage on H-reflex amplitude in persons with a spinal cord injury, *Phys Ther* 74(8):728–737, 1994.

Hall, D: A practical guide to the art of massage, *Runner's World*, 14(10):5–59, 1979.

Hammer, W: The use of transverse friction massage in the management of chronic bursitis of the hip or shoulder, *J Manipulative Physiological Therapeutics* 16(2):107–111, 1993.

Hanten, W, and Chandler, S: Effects of myofascial release leg pull and sagittal plane isometric contract-relax techniques on passive straight-leg raise angle, *JOSPT* 20(3):138–144, 1994.

Hollis, M: *Massage for athletic trainers*, Oxford, England, 1987, Blackwell.

Hovind, H, and Neilson, S: Effect of massage on blood flow in skeletal muscle, *Scand J Rehab Med* 6:74–77, 1974.

Kewley, M: What you should know about massage, *International Swimmer*, September: 29–30, 1982.

Kirshbaum, M: Using massage in the relief of lymphoedema, *Professional Nurse* 11(4):230–232, 1996.

Malkin, K: Use of massage in clinical practice, *British J Nursing* 3(6):292–294, 1994.

Manheim, C, and Lavett, D: *The myofascial release manual*, Thorofare, N.J., 1989, Slack Publishing.

Martin, D: Massage, *Jogger* 10(5):8–15, 1978.

McConnell, A: Practical massage, *Nursing Times* 91(36): S 2–14, 1995.

McKeechie, A: Anxiety states; a preliminary report on the value of connective tissue massage, *J Psychosomatic Res* 27(2): 125–129, 1983.

Meagher, J, and Boughton, P: *Sportsmassage*, New York, 1980, Doubleday.

Morelli, M, Seaborne, D, and Sullivan, S: H-reflex modulation during manual muscle massage of human triceps surae, *Arch Phys Med Rehab* 72(11):915–999, 1991.

Morelli, M, Seaborne, PT, Sullivan, SJ: H-reflex modulation during massage of triceps surae in healthy subjects, *Arch Phys Med Rehab* 72:915, 1991.

Newman, T, Martin, D, and Wilson, L: Massage effects on muscular endurance, *J Ath Train* 31 supp:S-18, 1996.

Pellecchia, G, Hamel, H, and Behnke, P: Treatment of infrapatellar tendinitis: a combination of modalities and transverse friction massage versus iontophoresis, *J Sport Rehab* 3(2):135–145, 1994.

Phaigh, R, and Perry, P: *Athletic massage*, New York, 1984, Simon & Schuster.

Pope, M, Phillips, R, and Haugh, L: A prospective randomized three-week trial of spinal manipulation, transcutaneous muscle stimulation, massage and corset in the treatment of subacute low back pain, *Spine* 19(22):2571–2577, 1994.

Rogoff, J: *Manipulation, traction and massage*, ed 2, Baltimore, 1980, Williams & Wilkins.

Ryan, J: The neglected art of massage, *Phys Sports Med* 18(12):25, 1980.

Smith, L, Keating, M, and Holbert, D: The effects of athletic massage on delayed onset muscle soreness, creatine kinase, and neutrophil count: a preliminary report, *JOSPT* 19(2): 93–99, 1994.

Stamford, B: Massage for athletes, *Phys Sports Med* 13(10): 178, 1985.

Steward, B, Woodman, R, and Hurlburt, D: Fabricating a splint for deep friction massage, *JOSPT* 21(3):172–175, 1995.

Sucher, B: Myofascial manipulative release of carpal tunnel syndrome: documentation with magnetic resonance imaging, *J Amer Osteopathic Assn* 93(12):1273–1278, 1993.

Sucher, B: Myofascial release of carpal tunnel syndrome, *J Amer Osteopathic Assn* 93(1):92–94, 100–101, 1993.

Tappan, F: *Healing massage techniques: a study of eastern and western methods*, Reston, Va., 1978, Reston Publishing.

Tiidus, P, and Shoemaker, J: Effleurage massage, muscle blood flow and long-term post-exercise strength recovery, *Inter J Sports Med* 16(7):478–483, 1995.

Trevelyan, J: Massage, *Nursing Times* 89(19):45–47, 1993.

van Schie, T: Connective tissue massage for reflex sympathetic dystrophy: a case study, *New Zealand J Physiotherapy* 21(2):26, 1993.

Wakim, KG, Martin, GM, and Terrier, JC: The effects of massage in normal and paralyzed extremities, *Arch Phys Med* 30:135–144, 1949.

Weber, M, Servedio, F, and Woodall, W: The effects of three modalities on delayed onset muscle soreness, *JOSPT* 20(5):236–242, 1994.

Wiktorrson-Moeller, M, Oberg, B, and Ekstrand, J: Effects of warming up, massage and stretching on range of motion and muscle strength in the lower extremity, *Am J Sports Med* 11:249–251, 1983.

Yates, J: *Physiological effects of therapeutic massage and their application to treatment*, British Columbia, 1989, Massage Athletic Trainers Association.

CHAPTER 11

Intermittent Compression Devices

Daniel N. Hooker

Study Resources

Refer to the lab exercises in the accompanying Laboratory Manual, as well as eSims which simulates the athletic training certification exam at www.mhhe.com/esims. Also, check out the competency information found at www.mhhe.com/prentice11e. For more online study resources, visit our Health and Human Performance Website at www.mhhe.com/hhp/.

Following completion of this chapter, the student athletic trainer will be able to

- Appraise the effectiveness of external compression on the accumulation and the reabsorption of edema after an athletic injury.

- Explain the setup procedures for intermittent external compression.

- Recognize the effects that changing a parameter might have on edema reduction.

- Review the clinical applications for using intermittent compression devices.

---

edema The presence of abnormal amounts of fluid in the extracellular tissue spaces of the body.

joint swelling Accumulation of blood and joint fluid within the joint capsule.

lymphedema Swelling of subcutaneous tissues as a result of accumulation of excessive lymph fluid.

Edema accumulation after athletic trauma is one of the clinical signs to which considerable attention is directed in first aid and therapeutic rehabilitation programs. **Edema** is defined as the presence of abnormal amounts of fluid in the extracellular tissue spaces of the body. Intermittent compression is one of the clinical modalities that is used to help reduce the accumulation of edema.

There are two distinct kinds of tissue swelling that are usually associated with injury. **Joint swelling**, marked by the presence of blood and joint fluid accumulated within the joint capsule, is one kind. This type of swelling occurs immediately following injury to a joint. Joint swelling is usually contained by the joint capsule and will have the appearance and feel of a water balloon. If pressure is placed on the swelling, the fluid moves but immediately returns when the pressure is released.

Lymphedema is the other variety of swelling encountered in athletic injuries. This type of

lymph   A transparent slightly yellow liquid found in the lymphatic vessels.

Types of swelling

- Joint swelling
- Lymphedema

swelling in the subcutaneous tissues results from an excessive accumulation of **lymph** and usually occurs over several hours following the injury. Intermittent compression can be used with both varieties, but it is usually more successful with pitting edema. The lymphatic system is the primary body system that deals with these injury induced changes.

THE LYMPHATIC SYSTEM

Purposes of the Lymphatic System

The lymphatic system has four major purposes:
1. The fluid in the interstitial spaces is continuously circulating. As plasma and plasma proteins escape from the small blood vessels, they are picked up by the lymphatic system and returned to the blood circulation.
2. The lymphatic system acts as a safety valve for fluid overload and helps keep edema from forming. As the interstitial fluid increases, the interstitial fluid pressure increases, which causes an increase in the local lymph flow. The local lymphatic system can be overwhelmed by sudden local increases in the interstitial fluid, and pitting edema will be the result.[33]
3. The homeostasis of the extracellular environment is maintained by the lymphatic system. The lymphatic system removes excess protein molecules and waste from the interstitial fluid. The large protein molecules and fluids that cannot re-enter the circulatory vessels gain entry back into the

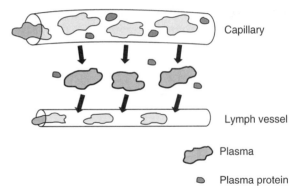

Figure 11-1   Plasma proteins outside the capillaries attract fluid to the intercellular space, leading to an abnormal "wet state" in the intercellular spaces. Plasma is absorbed back into the lymphatic spaces and away from the injured area.

endothelial cell   Cells that line the cavities of vessels.

fibrils   Connective tissue fibers supporting the lymphatic capillaries.

blood circulation through the terminal lymphatics.
4. The lymphatic system also cleanses the interstitial fluid and provides a blockade to the spread of infection or malignant cells in the lymph nodes. The lymph nodes' ability is not clearly understood and is highly variable.[16]

Structure of the Lymphatic System

The lymphatic system is a closed vascular system of **endothelial cell** lined tubes that parallel the arterial and nervous systems. The lymphatic capillaries are made of single layered endothelial cells with **fibrils** radiating from the junctions of the endothelial cells (Figure 11-1). These fibrils support the lymphatic capillaries and anchor them to the surrounding connective tissue. The capillary is surrounded by the interstitial fluid and tissues. These lymphatic capillaries are called the terminal lymphatics, and they provide the entry way into the lymphatic system for the excess interstitial fluid and plasma proteins.

These lymphatic capillaries join together in a network of lymphatic vessels that eventually lead to larger collecting vessels in the extremities. The collecting vessels connect with the thoracic duct or the right lymphatic duct, which join the venous system in the left and right cervical area. As the lymph flows centrally up the system, the lymph moves through one or more lymph nodes. These nodes remove the foreign substances and are the primary area of lymphocytic activity.[16]

Peripheral Lymphatic Structure and Function

Deep and superficial lymphatic collecting systems are found in the extremities. The terminal lymphatics in the skin and subcutaneous tissue drain into the superficial branches. Lymph channels in the fascial and bony layers drain into the deep branches.

In the superficial branches, the dermis is packed with two types of lymphatic channels. The channels closer to the surface have no valves, while those lying under the dermis and in the subcutaneous tissue do have valves. The valves are located approximately a centimeter apart and are similar in construction to the valves in veins. These structures prevent the backflow of lymph when pressure is applied. As with the blood vessels, the lymph system is concentrated on the medial side of the limbs.[16]

As the lymphatic system changes from the entry channels to the collecting channels, the lymphatic vessel changes to look similar to venous tissue. These vessels have smooth muscle and appear to have innervation from the sympathetic nervous system.

As the fluid or tissues move in the interstitial spaces, they push or pull on the fibrils supporting the terminal lymphatics (Figure 11-2). This activity forces the endothelial cells to gap apart at their junctions, creating an opening in the terminal lymphatics for the entry of interstitial fluid, cellular waste, large protein molecules, plasma proteins, extracellular particles, and cells into the lymphatic channels.

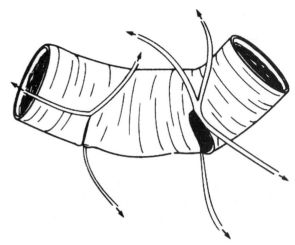

Figure 11-2 Lymphatic capillary with pore open to allow movement of plasma protein out of the intercellular space. As the intercellular fluid accumulates, the fibrils radiating from the seams in the lymphatic capillary pull the seam open to create a pore large enough for plasma proteins to enter.

These junctions are constantly being pushed and pulled open and are then allowed to close, depending on the local activity. Once the interstitial fluid and proteins enter these channels, they become lymph. Terminal lymphatics in inflamed areas are dilated, and an increased number of gaps in the capillary are present (see Figure 11-2).[11,16,20,41,42]

If no tissue activity or interstitial volume increase takes place, these endothelial junctions remain closed. The interstitial fluid, however, can still enter the terminal lymphatics by moving across the endothelial cell or by being transported across in a vesicle or cell organelle. This permeability would be similar to the small blood vessels or capillaries (see Figure 11-1).

Muscle activity, active and passive movements, elevated positions, respiration, and blood vessel pulsation all aid in the movement of lymph by compressing the lymphatic vessels. This allows gravity to pull the lymph down the channels. The valves help by maintaining a unidirectional flow of lymph in response to pressure. The collecting lymph channels all have smooth muscle in their

■ Analogy   *11-1*

The lymphatic system functions in a manner similar to a water drainage system in the mountains. Water flows into small mountain streams, and as gravity pulls the water down the mountain, it collects in progressively larger streams and tributaries until it eventually flows into a raging river (the venous system) in the valley.

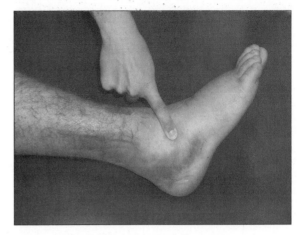

Figure 11-3   Ankle with pitting edema. Finger pressure squeezes fluid out of the intercellular space; an indentation is left when the pressure is removed.

walls. These muscles can provide contractible activity that would promote lymph flow. These muscles have a natural firing frequency that stimulates a rhythmic pumping action. There are also studies that indicate increased lymph flow during heating of animal limbs.

INJURY EDEMA

Following a closed injury, changes in and around the site of the injury occur that have an impact on the accumulation of extracellular fluid and proteins in the local interstitial spaces. The direct effects of the injury include cell death, bleeding, the release of chemical mediators to initiate and guide the healing process, and changes in local tissue electric currents. As discussed in Chapter 2, the first stage of the healing process is inflammation and it is characterized by local redness, heat, swelling, pain. In addition, loss of function frequently occurs.

Formation of Pitting Edema

These changes are brought about by changes in the local circulation. Local edema is formed by the plasma, plasma proteins, and cell debris from the damaged cells all moving into the interstitial spaces. This sudden volume change is compounded by the intact local circulatory responses to the chemical mediators of the inflammatory process. The hormones released by the injured cells stimulate the small anterioles, capillaries, and venules to vasodialate enlarging the size of the vascular pool. This causes the local blood flow to slow down, and

■ Movement of lymph results from

- Muscle activity
- Active and passive motion
- Elevation
- Respiration
- Contraction of vessels

the pressure within the blood vessels increases. The endothelial cells in the blood vessel walls then separate or become more loosely bound to their neighboring cell. The permeability of the vessel increases, allowing more plasma, plasma proteins, and leukocytes to escape into the local area. The increase in the plasma proteins in the interstitial spaces causes the osmotic pressure to push more plasma into the area forming an inflammatory exudate. This exudate forms too quickly for the lymphatic system to maintain the local equilibrium, and pitting edema is formed (Figure 11-3). This small increase in the plasma protein in the intercellular spaces causes an increase in the intercellular fluid volume by several hundred percent.[1,2,3,7,15,21,42,43]

This fluid in the form of a gel is trapped by both collagen fibers and proteoglycan molecules. The gel prevents the free flow of fluid as seen in the pitting edema   A type of swelling that leaves a pit-like depression when the skin is compressed.

joint fluid example. Clinically, this state is recognized as **pitting edema**. After finger pressure on the swollen part is released, a slight pit is left at the finger's previous location. Fluid is squeezed out of the intercellular space, and time is needed for the fluid to move slowly back into that space (see Figure 11-3).

Formation of Lymphedema

As the intercellular fluid volume increases, the lymph begins to flow. If the edema causes an overdistention of the lymph capillaries, the entry pores become ineffective, and lymphedema results. Constriction of lymph capillaries or larger lymphatic vessels from increased pressure will also discourage lymph flow and cause intercellular fluid to increase.[1,2,3,7,15,21,42,43]

Using computerized tomography cross-sectional images, Airaksinen et al. reported a 23% increase in the subcutaneous tissue, thickened skin, and muscular atrophy in athletes following lower leg fracture and casting. They reported an 8% edema decrease in the subcutaneous compartment after intermittent compression. The mean area of the subfascial compartment remained the same, but the density of the muscle tissue increased after treatment. This study indicates that injury edema will follow the path of least resistance and that tissues that have the least natural pressure exerted on them will demonstrate the greatest accumulation of extra fluid. The skin and subcutaneous tissue appear to be the major site for pitting edema; the deep muscle and connective tissue have enough pressure to inhibit major accumulations in the deeper tissues.[3]

Clinical measurement of edema is reasonably accurate and correlates very well with both CT scan and volumetric measures. The standard clinical circumferential measurement of limb and joint are adequate to determine the treatment effects.[3,5]

■ **Clinical Decision-Making**   *Exercise 11-1*

An athlete comes into the training room with an extremely swollen knee that she says has been like that for 2 days. How can the athletic trainer determine whether she has joint swelling or pitting lymphedema?

The Negative Effects of Edema Accumulation

Edema compounds the extent of an injury by causing the secondary hypoxic cellular death in the tissues surrounding the injured area. The edema increases the distance nutrients, and oxygen must travel to nourish the remaining cells. This in turn adds to the injury debris in the damaged area and causes further edema to accumulate perpetuating this cycle.[9]

Other ill effects of edema include the physical separation of torn tissue ends, pain, and restricted joint range of motion. Recovery times become more prolonged. If the edema persists, further problems with extremity function can occur including infection, muscle atrophy, joint contractures, interstitial fibrosis, and reflex sympathetic dystrophy.[7,9,13]

TREATMENT OF EDEMA

Good immediate first aid following injury, as discussed in Chapter 2, can minimize edema (Figure 11-4). The use of ice, compression, electricity, elevation, and early gentle motion retards the accumulation of fluid and keeps the lymphatic system operating at an optimum level. Any treatment that encourages lymph flow will decrease plasma protein content in the intercellular spaces and therefore decrease edema in that part. The standard methods of treatment in most clinical settings include elevation, compression, and muscular contraction.

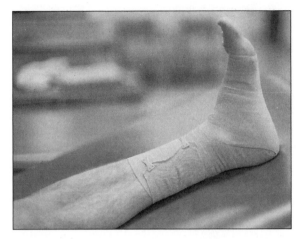

Figure 11-4   Ankle with elastic wrap compression in an elevated position.

Elevation

The force of gravity can be used to augment normal lymph flow. The swollen part can be elevated so that gravity does not resist the flow of lymph but encourages its movement. Elevation of the injured swollen part above heart level is all that is necessary. The higher the elevation, the greater the effect on the lymph flow.[31,34]

In an uninjured population, placing their legs in an elevated position significantly decreased ankle volume after twenty minutes, while the dependent position significantly increased ankle volumes. These findings could be expected to be the same in injured subjects, but the dependent position may markedly increase volume while the elevated position may decrease volumes less well because of the injury to the tissue. In studies using postacute ankle sprain edema, elevation alone provided a significant post-treatment reduction in ankle volume.[5,24,31,34]

Compression

Rhythmic internal compression provided by muscle contraction will also squeeze the lymph through the lymph vessels, improving its flow back to the vascular system. This muscle contraction

endothelial-derived relaxing factor   Relaxes smooth muscle and stimulates blood flow rates in veins.

can be accomplished through isometric or active exercise or through electrically induced muscle contraction. Several authors also advocate the use of noncontractible electric current for edema control and reduction. (See Chapter 8 for a discussion of electrical therapy for edema control.) When elevation is combined with muscle contraction, lymph flow is benefited.[4,6,12]

External pressure can also be used to increase lymph flow. Massage, elastic compression, and intermittent pressure devices are the most often used external pressure devices. This external compression not only moves the lymph along but also may spread the intercellular edema over a larger area, enabling more lymph capillaries to become involved in removing the plasma proteins and water. External pressure from horseshoe, pads, and elastic wraps are also helpful in minimizing the accumulation or re-accumulation of edema in the injured area.[9,41,42,43]

Weight-Bearing Exercise

Gardner has proposed that weight-bearing activities activate a powerful venous pump.[15] The pump consists of the venae comitantes of the lateral plantar artery. It is emptied immediately upon weight bearing and flattening of the plantar arch. Because this emptying occurs so rapidly, it is believed that this process is mediated by the release of an **endothelial-derived relaxing factor** (EDRF) and is not related to muscular activity of the limb. The EDRF is liberated by sudden pressure changes, and it diffuses locally. Its major action is to relax the smooth muscle and stimulate blood flow rates in the veins.[18]

This phenomena may explain the rapid decrease in edema that occurs when athletes switch

■ **Edema is best treated with**
....

- Elevation
- Compression
- Weight-bearing exercise
- Cryotherapy

from a non-weight-bearing gait to a weight-bearing gait. Using this venous pump on lower leg edema is a reason to include early weight bearing in a variety of injury treatment protocols.

Cryotherapy

Using an intermittent compression device to decrease postacute injury edema has recently been shown to have a good effect. The addition of cryotherapy to the intermittent compression has shown the best results in the reduction of postacute injury edema.[1,2,3,5,19,20,24,29,35,36,44]

INTERMITTENT COMPRESSION TREATMENT PARAMETERS

There are three parameters available for adjustment when using most intermittent pressure devices: inflation pressure, on/off time sequence, and total treatment time (Figure 11-5). There are also intermittent pressure devices with multiple compartments that inflate distal to proximal, with gradual reduced pressure in each compartment. These devices try to mimic the massage strokes used in edema removal.[19,20,24,39] Reduction in postacute injury edema does not require this graded sequential action, nor is postinjury edema reduction significantly enhanced by these devices.[24,39] All intermittent compression devices seem to have similar influences on edema.

Little research has been done comparing adjustments of these parameters with volumetric results. Empiricism and clinical trials have been used to design the established protocols.

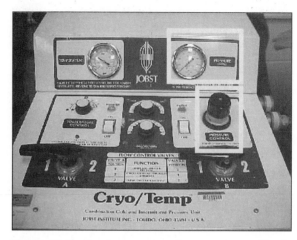

Figure 11-5   Pressure gauge and pressure control knob for an intermittent compression unit.

■ **Treatment parameters**
....

- Inflation pressure
- On/off times
- Total treatment time

Inflation Pressure

Pressure settings have been loosely correlated with blood pressure and athlete comfort to arrive at the therapeutic pressure. A pressure approximating the athlete's diastolic blood pressure has been used in most treatment protocols. The arterial capillary pressures are approximately 30 mm Hg, and any pressure that exceeds this should encourage reabsorption of the edema and movement of the lymph. Maximum pressure should correspond to the diastolic blood pressure. Higher pressure would shut off arterial blood flow and create a potentially uncomfortable tissue response as a result of low blood flow.[1,2,3,11,13,21,22]

More may not necessarily be better. Enough pressure is needed to squeeze the lymphatic vessels and force the lymph to move. This should be accomplished with relatively low pressures of 30 to 40 mm Hg. The other mechanism in operation is the force of the

■ **Clinical Decision-Making**   *Exercise 11-2*

....

An athlete has swelling in the knee joint from a sprain of the anterior cruciate ligament. What treatment techniques should the athletic trainer use on day 2 post injury to help eliminate swelling?

....

- Pressure should be about the same as diastolic blood pressure

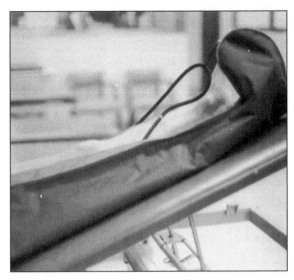

Figure 11-6   Uninflated compression appliance applied to an athlete's leg in an elevated position.

hydrostatic pressure, and pressure in the range of 40 to 50 mm Hg should suffice to raise the interstitial fluid pressure higher than the blood vessel pressures.[13,21,22] Inflation pressure of 30 to 60 mm Hg is recommended for the upper extremity, and 40 to 80 mm Hg is recommended for the lower extremity.

On/Off Sequence

On- and off-time sequences are even more variable, with some protocols calling for a sequence of 30 seconds on, 30 seconds off; 1 minute on, 2 minutes off; while others reverse this to 2 minutes on, 1 minute off. Others use a 4 minutes on to 1 minute off ratio. If lymphatic massage is the primary vehicle used in this therapy, shorter on/off time sequences may have an advantage. The hydrostatic pressure vehicle would require the longer-on times. These time periods are not research-based, and the athletic trainer is left to his or her own empirical judgment as to the optimum time sequence for each athlete. Athlete comfort should be a primary deciding factor here.

Total Treatment Time

Total treatment times have some basis in research, but again this is convenience or empirically based in many instances. Most of the protocols for primary lymphedema call for long 3- to 4-hour treatments. This time frame has been effective in many athletes.[1,2,3,5,12,13,19,20,22,24,29,31,32,35,36,39,44]

Researchers have shown a marked increase in lymph flow on initiation of massage; this flow decreases over a 10-minute period and stops when the massage is discontinued.[28,34] Clinical studies show significant gains in limb volume reduction after 30 minutes of compression.[1,2,3,5,12,24,29,35,36,44] In most situations, a 10- to 30-minute treatment seems adequate unless the edema is overwhelming in volume or is resistant to the treatment. More treatment times per day may also be an advantage in controlling and reducing edema from various musculosketal injuries.

EQUIPMENT SETUP AND INSTRUCTIONS

Treating an athlete with an intermittent compression device is relatively simple. The athlete should have the appropriate-sized compression appliance fitted on the extremity in an elevated position (Figure 11-6). The compression sleeves come as either

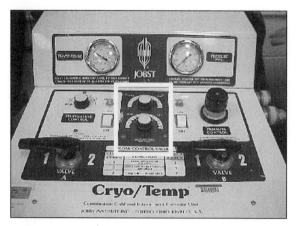

Figure 11-7 Time setting control knobs for on and off cycles of an intermittent compression unit. This illustrates the setting at the beginning of the treatment when the appliance is uninflated. The off-time knob is increased when the proper inflation pressure is reached.

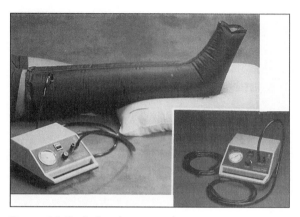

Figure 11-8 Inflated pressure sleeve.

■ **Clinical Decision-Making**   *Exercise 11-3*

....

An athlete comes into the training room 3 days postinversion ankle sprain, which happened at an away contest. He now shows signs of pitting lymphedema, and the athletic trainer decides to use an intermittent compression device to help reduce the edema. What would be the appropriate treatment parameters?

---

half-leg, full-leg, full-arm, or half-arm. The deflated compression sleeve is connected to the compression unit via a rubber hose and connecting valve.

Once the machine has been turned on, the three parameters may be adjusted: on/off time, inflation pressure, and treatment time. The on time should be adjusted between 30 and 120 seconds (Figure 11-7). The off time is left at 0 until the sleeve is inflated and the treatment pressure is reached and then may be adjusted between 0 and 120 seconds. When the unit cycles off, the patient should be instructed to move the extremity. A 30-seconds-on, 30-seconds-off setting seems to be both effective and comfortable for the athlete. Some compression devices will slowly reach the target pressure, while others respond more rapidly. It is important that the on and off times take the machine characteristics into account.

When using electrical stimulation in combination with compression, always adjust the current intensity with the sleeve fully pressurized, since this may affect electrode contact and current density (Figure 11-8).

The treatment should last between 20 and 30 minutes. Athletes do not seem to comfortably tolerate treatments lasting longer than 30 minutes. On completion of the treatment time, the extremity should be measured to see if the desired results have been achieved. The part should be wrapped with elastic compression wraps to help maintain the reduction. If the edema is not reduced, another treatment may be needed after a short recovery time. If not contraindicated, weight bearing should be encouraged to stimulate the venous pump.

COLD AND COMPRESSION COMBINATION

Some manufacturers have coupled intermittent pressure with a coolant (either water or Freon). These devices have the advantage of cooling the injured part as well as compressing it. The Jobst Cry-

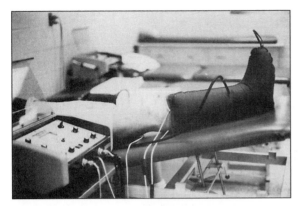

Figure 11-9   Intermittent compression used in combination with electrical stimulating currents to reduce edema.

otemp is a controlled cold/compression unit that has a temperature adjustment ranging between 10° C to 25° C. Cooling is accomplished by circulating cold water through the sleeve. The Cryo-Cuff (see Chapter 4) and another newer device called the PolarCare Cub make use of a combination of cold and compression, and they provide an inexpensive means of treating postsurgical edema.

The combination of cold and compression has been shown to be clinically effective in treating some edema conditions.[5,12,21,24,29,35,36] A study comparing a technique using an intermittent compression unit, cold, and elevation with one using an elastic wrap, cold, and elevation showed that the use of the cold-compression device was more effective in edema reduction.[5]

Compression and Electrical Stimulating Currents

Intermittent compression may also be used in conjunction with a low-frequency pulsed or surging electrical stimulating current set up to produce muscle pumping contractions. The combination of these two modalities should facilitate resorption of injury by-products by the lymphatic system (Figure 11-9).[12]

■ **Clinical Decision-Making**   *Exercise 11-4*

The athletic trainer is treating a swollen ankle with intermittent compression and wants to know whether using electrical-stimulating current or cold or a combination of the two will be more effective in treating lymphedema.

SEQUENTIAL COMPRESSION PUMPS

Intermittent compression pumps have incorporated sequentially inflated, multiple-compartment designs for some time.[16,17,29] Recently, these designs have also included a programmable gradient design (Figure 11-10). Sequential pumps were designed to incorporate the massage effect of a distal-to-proximal pressure with a gradual decrease in the pressure gradient.[20]

The highest pressure is in the distal sleeve and, according to the manufacturer's recommendation, is determined by the mean value of systolic to diastolic pressure at the outset of a specifically determined 48-hour protocol whose purpose is to determine the effectiveness of the device in individual cases.[20] The middle cell is set 20 mm lower than the distal cell, and the proximal cell pressure is reduced an additional 20 mm.

The length of each pressure cycle is 120 seconds. The distal cell is pressurized initially and continues pressurization for 90 seconds. Twenty seconds later, the middle cell is inflated, and after another 20 seconds, the proximal cell inflates. A final 30-second period allows pressure in all three cells to return to 0, after which the cycle repeats itself.

Only a few studies have shown the efficacy of using decreasing pressure in a distal-to-proximal direction relative to previously existing compression sleeves.[15,16] In a study comparing sequential compression and cold and compression, Lemly found both effective in reducing edema but no significant difference between the devices.[24]

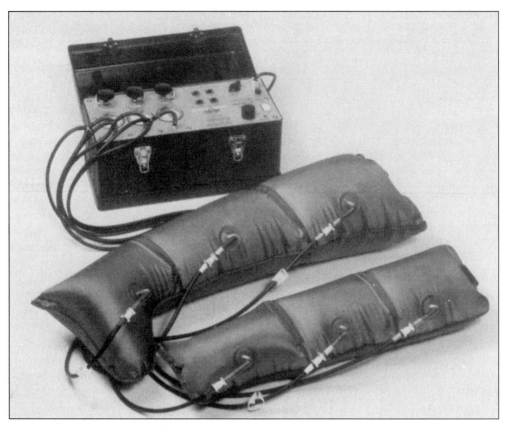

Figure 11-10 Gradient sequential pressure system.
(Courtesy Wright Linear Pump)

CLINICAL APPLICATIONS FOR INTERMITTENT COMPRESSION

Intermittent compression has been recommended for treating lymphedema;[32] traumatic edema that occurs following injury to soft tissue; chronic edema that occurs in athletes with certain types of neurological diseases due to an inability to move a limb; stasis ulcers that develop with the presence of fluid in the interstitial spaces for long periods of time;[27] swelling that occurs with limb amputation;[30] athletes on dialysis due to renal insufficiency, which tends to develop edema in the extremities and hypothesion; athletes with arterial insufficiency, such as in cases of intermittent claudications to increase venous return;[17] edema and contractures in the hand that result from stroke or surgery; and to stimulate proteoglycan synthesis in human cartilage.[23,38] It has also been used postoperatively to reduce the possibility of developing a deep vein thrombosis resulting from inactivity and coagulation[8,26] and to facilitate wound healing following surgery by reducing swelling.[28]

The athletic trainer should avoid using intermittent compression in athletes with known deep vein thrombosis, local superficial infection, congestive heart failure, acute pulmonary edema, and displaced fractures.[14] (Table 11-1).

■ TABLE 11-1   Summary of Indications and Contraindications for Intermittent Compression

INDICATIONS	CONTRAINDICATIONS
Lymphedema	Deep vein thrombosis
Traumatic edema	Local superficial infection
Chronic edema	Congestive heart failure
Stasis ulcers	Acute pulmonary edema
Intermittent claudications	Displaced fractures
Facilitate wound healing following surgery	Cancer

■ Clinical Decision-Making   *Exercise 11-5*

A student athletic trainer is providing initial first aid care to an athlete who has a grade 1 ankle sprain. He asks his supervising athletic trainer if it is ok to use the intermittent compression unit instead of an elastic wrap. How should the supervising athletic trainer respond?

Summary

1. Edema following injury or surgery can be effectively managed using a compression pump program.
2. Lymphedema is swelling in the subcutaneous tissues that results from an excessive accumulation of lymph and usually occurs over several hours following the injury.
3. Muscle activity, active and passive movements, elevated positions, respiration, and blood vessel pulsation all aid in the movement of lymph by compressing the lymphatic vessels and allowing gravity to pull the lymph down the channels.
4. The use of ice, compression, electricity, elevation, and early gentle motion retards the accumulation of fluid and keeps the lympatic system operating at an optimum level.
5. Three parameters may be adjusted when using most intermittent pressure devices: inflation pressure, on/off time sequence, and total treatment time. Adjustments in these parameters should be made using athlete comfort as the primary guide.
6. The combination of cold and compression has been shown to be clinically effective in treating some edema conditions.
7. Sequential compression pumps were designed to incorporate the massage effect of a distal-to-proximal pressure with a gradual decrease in the pressure gradient.

Reveiw Questions

1. What are the various types of edema that can accumulate following athletic trauma?
2. Explain the purpose, structure, and function of the lymphatic system.
3. What is lymphedema?
4. What can be done to facilitate the reabsorption of lymphedema into the lymphatic system?
5. What are the effects of external compression on the accumulation and the reabsorption of edema following an athletic injury?
6. What are the three treatment parameters that should be considered when using intermittent compression?
7. How can intermittent compression be used effectively in combination with other modalities?
8. Are there any clinical advantages to using sequential compression pumps?
9. What are the clinical applications for using intermittent compression devices?

Self-Test Questions

T/F

1. One of the roles of the lymphatic system is to remove excess proteins from interstitial fluid.
2. The lymphatic system runs parallel to the arterial system.
3. None of the lymphatic vessels has muscular linings.

Multiple Choice

4. Excessive accumulation of lymph fluid in subcutaneous tissues is called _____ .
   a. edema
   b. lymphedema
   c. joint swelling
   d. pitting edema
5. Lymph is composed of _____ .
   a. endothelial cells and fibrils
   b. a transparent, slightly yellow liquid found in lymphatic vessels
   c. the fluid in extracellular space
   d. blood and joint fluid in the joint
6. Which of the following are responsible for lymph movement?
   a. muscle activity
   b. active and passive movements
   c. elevated positions
   d. all of the above
7. At what minimum setting should the pressure be when using intermittent compression devices?
   a. greater than or equal to 30 mm Hg
   b. greater than or equal to 100 mm Hg
   c. approximately systolic pressure
   d. approximately diastolic pressure
8. How long should most intermittent compression treatments last, bearing in mind athlete comfort?
   a. 5–10 minutes
   b. 10–20 minutes
   c. 20–30 minutes
   d. over an hour
9. What may be combined with compression treatment?
   a. cold, via a cold/compression unit
   b. electrical stimulating current
   c. neither A nor B
   d. both A and B
10. Which of the following is NOT a contraindication to intermittent compression?
    a. intermittent claudication
    b. deep vein thrombosis
    c. displaced fracture
    d. local superficial infection

Solutions to Clinical Decision-Making Exercises

11-1 Joint swelling is usually contained in the joint capsule and feels very much like a water balloon. The fluid is easily moved around by simply applying pressure on one side of the joint. Lymphedema occurs in the subcutaneous tissues and has more of a gel-like feeling to it and leaves an indentation after finger pressure is removed.

11-2 The athletic trainer should include cold, elevation, compression, using an intermittent compression unit, and some weight-bearing exercise to facilitate venous and lymphatic drainage.

11-3 The compression boot should be applied with the inflation pressure set at about 60 mmHg, the on/off time at 30 secs on 30 secs off, and a total treatment time of 20 minutes initially. The on/off times and total treatment time can be increased over the next several days as can be tolerated.

11-4 Using electrical stimulating currents to induce muscle pumping contractions should facilitate removal of edema. Also, it is well documented that using cold in conjunction with compression is clinically effective in treating cases of lymphedema.

11-5 It will be ok to use the intermittent compression unit as long as it also provides cold and the part can still be elevated. It is perhaps a better choice to use an elastic compression wrap if the intermittent compression unit cannot keep the injured part cold during initial management.

References

1. Airaksinen, O: Changes in post-traumatic ankle joint mobility, pain and edema following intermittent pneumatic compression therapy, *Arch Phys Med Rehab* 70: 341–344, 1989.
2. Airaksinen, O: Treatment of post-traumatic edema in lower legs using intermittent pneumatic compression, *Scand J Rebah Med* 20: 25–28, 1988.
3. Airaksinen, O: Intermittent pneumatic compression therapy in post-traumatic lower limb edema: computed tomography and clinical measurements, *Arch Phys Med Rehab* 72: 667–670, 1991.
4. Angus, J, Prentice, W, and Hooker, D: A comparison of two intermittent external compression devices and their effect on post acute ankle edema, *J Ath Train* 29(2): 179, 1994.
5. Brewer, K, Prentice, W, and Hooker, D: *The effects of intermittent compression and cold on reducing edema in post-acute ankle sprains.* Unpublished master's thesis, University of North Carolina, Chapel Hill, N.C., 1990.
6. Brown, S: Ankle edema and galvanic muscle stimulation, *Phys Sports Med* 9:137, 1981.
7. Carriere, B: Edema—its development and treatment using lymph drainage massage, *Clin Manag Phys Ther* 8(5): 19–21, 1988.
8. Clark, W: Pneumatic compression of the calf and post operative deep vein thrombosis, *Lancet* 2:5, 1974.
9. Duffley, H, and Knight, K: Ankle compression variability using elastic wrap, elastic wrap with a horseshoe, edema II boot and air stirrup brace, *Ath Train* 24:320–323, 1989.
10. Elkins, E, Herrick, J, and Grindley, J: Effect of various procedures on the flow of lymph, *Arch Phys Med Rehab* 34:31–39, 1953.
11. Evans, P: The healing process at the cellular level: a review, *Physiotherapy* 66:256–259, 1980.
12. Flicker, M: *An analysis of cold intermittent compression with simultaneous treatment of electrical stimulation in the reduction of post acute ankle lymphaedema.* Unpublished master's thesis, University of North Carolina, Chapel Hill, N.C., May 1993.
13. Foldi, E, Foldi, M, and Weissleder, H: Conservative treatment of lymphoedema of the limbs, *Angiology* 171–180, 1985.
14. Fond, D, and Hecox, B: Intermittent pneumatic compression. In Hecox, B, Mehreteab, T, and Weisberg, J: *Physical agents: a comprehensive text for physical athlete*, Norwalk, Conn., 1994, Appleton & Lang.
15. Gardner, A: Reduction of post-traumatic swelling and compartment pressure by impulse compression of the foot, *JBJS* 72-B: 810–815, 1990.
16. Gnepp, D: Lymphatics. In Staub, N, and Taylor, A, editors: *Edema*, Raven Press, New York, 1984, 263–298.
17. Henry, J, and Windos, T: Compensation of arterial insufficiency by augmenting the circulation with intermittent compression of the limbs, *Am Heart J* 70(1):77–88, 1965.
18. Hurley, J: Inflammation. In Staub, N, and Taylor, A, editors: *Edema*, Raven Press, New York, 1984, 463–488.
19. Kim-Sing, C, and Basco, V: Postmastectomy lymphedema treated with the Wright Linear Pump, *Can J. Surg.* 30(5):368–370, 1987.
20. Klein, M, Alexander, M, and Wright, J: Treatment of lower extremity lymphedema with the Wright Linear Pump: a statistical analysis of a clinical trial, *Arch Phys Med Rehab* 69:202–206, 1988.
21. Kobi, P, and Denegar, C: Traumatic edema and the lymphatic system, *Ath Train* 18:339–341, 1983.
22. Kruse, R, Kruse, A, and Britton, R: Physical therapy for the athlete with peripheral edema: procedures for management, *Phys Ther Rev* 80:29–33, 1960.
23. Lafeber, F: Intermittent hydrostatic compressive force stimulates exclusively the proteoglycan synthesis of osteoarthritic human cartilage, *British J Rheumatology* 31(7):437–442, 1992.
24. Lemley, T, Prentice, W, and Hooker, D: A comparison of two intermittent compression devices on pitting ankle edema, *J Ath Train* 28(2):156–157, 1993.
25. Liu, N, and Olszewski, W: The influence of local hyperthermia on lymphedema and lymphedematous skin of the human leg, *Lymphology* 26:28–37, 1993.
26. Matzdorff, A, and Green, D: Deep vein thrombosis and pulmonary embolism: prevention, diagnosis, and treatment, *Geriatrics* 47(8):48–52, 55–57, 62–63, 1992.
27. McCulloch, J: Intermittent compression for the treatment of a chronic stasis ulceration: a case report, *Phys Ther* 61:1452–1453, 1981.
28. Pflug, J: Intermittent compression: a new principle in the treatment of wounds, *Lancet* 2(3):15, 1974.
29. Quillen, W, and Rouiller, L: Initial management of acute ankle sprains with rapid pulsed pneumatic compression and cold, *JOSPT* 4:39–43, 1982.
30. Redford, J: Experiences in the use of a pneumatic stump shrinker, *Inter Clin Inform Bull Prosth Orthot* 12:1, 1973.
31. Rucinski, T, Hooker, D, and Prentice, W: The effects of intermittent compression on edema in post-acute ankle sprains, *JOSPT* 14 (2):65–69, 1991.

32. Sanderson, R, and Fletcher, W: Conservative management of primary lymphedema, *Northwest Med* 64:584–588, 1965.

33. Seki, K: Lymph flow in human leg, *Lymphology* 12:2–3, 1979.

34. Sims, D: Effects of positioning on ankle edema, *JOSPT* 8:30–33, 1986.

35. Sloan, J, Giddings, P, and Hain, R: Effects of cold and compression on edema, *Phys Sports Med* 16(8):116–120, 1988.

36. Starkey, J: Treatment of ankle sprains by simultaneous use of intermittent compression and ice packs, *Am J Sports Med* 4:442–444, 1976.

37. Stillwell, G: Further studies on the treatment of lymphedema, *Arch Phys Med Rehab* 38:435–441, 1957.

38. van Veen, S, Hagen, J, and van Ginkel, F: Intermittent compression stimulates cartilage mineralization, *Bone* 17(5):461–465, 1995.

39. Wakim, K: Influence of centripetal rhythmic compression on localized edema of an extremity, *Arch Phys Med Rehab* 36:98–103, 1955.

40. Wilkerson, J: Contrast baths and pressure treatment for ankle sprains, *Phys Sports Med* 7:143, 1979.

41. Wilkerson, J: Treatment of ankle sprains with external compression and early mobilization, *Phys Sports Med* 13(6):83–90, 1985.

42. Wilkerson, J: External compression for controlling traumatic edema, *Phys Sports Med* 13(6):97–106, 1985.

43. Wilkerson, J: Treatment of the inversion ankle sprain through synchronous application of focal compression and cold, *Ath Train* 26:220–237, 1991.

44. Winsor, T, and Selle, W: The effect of venous compression on the circulation of the extremities, *Arch Phys Med Rehab* 34:559–565, 1953.

Suggested Readings

Capper, C: Product focus: External pneumatic compression therapy for DVI prophylaxis, *British Journal of Nursing* 7(14):851–852, 854, 1998.

Chleboun, GS, Howell, IN, Baker, HL, Ballard, TN, Graham, JL, Hallman, HL, Perkins, LE, Schauss, JH, and Conatser, RR: Intermittent pneumatic compression effect on eccentric exercise-induced swelling, stiffness, and strength loss, *Archives of Physical Medicine & Rehabilitation* 76(8):744–749, 1995.

Christen, Y, and Reymond, M: Hemodynamic effects of intermittent pneumatic compression of the lower limbs during laparoscopic cholecystectomy, *Amer J Surgery* 170(4): 395–398, 1995.

Coogan, C: Venous leg ulcers and intermittent pneumatic compression therapy . . . "Care of venous leg ulcers". *Ostomy Wound Management* 45(11):5, 1999.

DePrete, A, Cogliano, T, and Agostinucci, J: The effect of circumferential pressure on upper motoneuron reflex excitability in healthy subjects, *Phys Ther* 74(5) supp: S70, 1994.

Elliot, CG, Dudney, TM, Egger, M, Orme JF, Clemmer, TP, Horn, SD, Weaver, L, Handrahan, D, Thomas, F, Merrell, S, Kitterman, N, and Yeates, S: Calf-thigh sequential pneumatic compression compared with plantar venous pneumatic compression to prevent deep-vein thrombosis after non-lower extremity trauma, *Journal of Trauma-Injury Infection & Critical Care* 47(1):25–32, 1999.

Gilbart, MK, Ogilvie-Harris, DJ, Broadhurst, C, and Clarfield, M: Anterior tibial compartment pressures during intermittent sequential pneumatic compression therapy, *American Journal of Sports Medicine* 23(6):769–772, 1995.

Hamzeh, M, Lonsdale, R, and Pratt, D: A new device producing ambulatory intermittent pneumatic compression suitable for the treatment of lower limb edema: a preliminary report, *J Med Engin Technology* 17(3):110–113, 1993.

Hofman D: Intermittent compression treatment for venous leg ulcers, *J Wound Care* 4(4):163–165, 1995.

Jacobs, M: Leg volume changes with EPIC and posturing in dependent pregnancy edema: external pneumatic intermittent compression, *Nursing Res* 35(2):86–89, 1986.

Jwama, H, Suzuki, M, Hojo, M, Kaneda, M, and Akutsu, I: Intermittent pneumatic compression on the calf improves peripheral circulation of the leg, *Journal of Critical Care* 15(1):18–21, 2000.

Kraemer, W, Bush, J, and Wickham, R: Influence of compression therapy on symptoms following soft tissue injury from maximal eccentric exercise, *Journal of Orthopedic and Sports Physical Therapy* 31(6)282–290, 2001.

Lachmann, E, Rook, J, and Tunkel, R: Complications associated with intermittent pneumatic compression, *Arch Phys Med Rehab* 73(5):482–485, 1992.

Majkowski, R, and Atkins, R: Treatment of fixed flexion deformities of the knee in rheumatoid arthritis using the Flowtron intermittent compression stocking, *British J Rheumatology* 31(1):41–43, 1992.

McCulloch, J: Physical modalities in wound management: ultrasound, vasopneumatic devices and hydrotherapy, *Ostomy Wound Manag* 41(5):30–32, 34, 36–37, 1995.

Murphy, K: The combination of ice and intermittent compression system in the treatment of soft tissue injuries, *Physiotherapy* 74(1):41, 1988.

Smith, P: The use of intermittent compression in treatment of fixed flexion deformities of the knee, *Physiotherapy* 75(8):494, 1989.

Tsang, K, Hertel, J, and Denegar, C: The effects of elevation and intermittent compression on the volume of injured ankles, *Journal of Athletic Training* 36(2 supp): S-50, 2001.

Wicker, P: Clinical feature supplement. Intermittent pneumatic compression therapy for deep vein thrombosis prophylaxis, *British Journal of Theatre Nursing* 9(3):108, 1999.

Yates, P, Cornwell, J, and Scott, G: Treatment of haemophilic flexion deformities using the Flowtron intermittent compression system, *British J Haematology* 82(2):384–387, 1992.

CHAPTER 12

Spinal Traction

Daniel N. Hooker

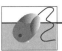

Study Resources

Refer to the lab exercises in the accompanying Laboratory Manual, as well as eSims which simulates the athletic training certification exam at www.mhhe.com/esims. Also, check out the competency information found at www.mhhe.com/prentice11e. For more online study resources, visit our Health and Human Performance Website at www.mhhe.com/hhp/.

Following completion of this chapter, the student athletic trainer will be able to

- Analyze the effects and therapeutic value of traction on bone, muscle, ligaments, joint structures, nerve, blood vessels, and intervertebral disk.

- Evaluate the clinical advantages of using positional lumbar traction and inversion traction.

- Describe the clinical applications for using manual lumbar traction techniques, including level-specific manual traction and unilateral leg pull manual traction.

- Explain the setup procedures and treatment parameter considerations for using mechanical lumbar traction.

- Articulate the advantages of using a manual traction technique for the cervical spine.

- Demonstrate the setup procedure for mechanical traction techniques for the cervical spine.

traction   Drawing tension applied to a body segment.

Traction has been used since ancient times in the treatment of painful spinal conditions. **Traction** is defined as the process of drawing or pulling apart of a body segment.[4] In sports medicine, traction may be performed *mechanically*, using a traction machine or ropes and pulleys to apply a traction force, or it may be performed *manually* by an athletic trainer who understands the appropriate positions and intensities of the force being applied to the joints of the spine or the extremities. Some of the concepts of traction discussed in this chapter are generalizable to the treatment of the extremities; however, this discussion has been aimed specifically at cervical and lumbar spinal traction.

Techniques of manual therapy are rapidly gaining popularity as a treatment modality among athletic trainers. In addition, the availability of new traction equipment for use in both the clinic and the home have renewed the interest in and acceptance of traction for both preventative and therapeutic treatment programs. Thus, some knowledge of traction techniques is essential for the athletic trainer.

PHYSICAL EFFECTS OF TRACTION

Effects of Traction on Spinal Movement

Traction encourages movement of the spine both overall and between each individual spinal segment.[2] Changes in overall spinal length and the amount of separation or space between each vertebra have been shown in studies of both the lumbar and the cervical spine (Figure 12-1).[1,6,20,24,30,31,36,38]

The amount of movement varies according to the position of the spine, the amount of force, and the length of time the force is applied. Separations of 1 to 2 mm per intervertebral space have been reported. This change is very transient and the spine quickly returns to the previous intervertebral space relationships when traction is released and the erect posture is assumed.[10,19,24,31] Decreases in pain, paresthesia, or tingling while traction is applied may be caused by the physical separation of the vertebral segments and the resultant decrease in pressure on sensitive structures. If these changes occur while the athlete is being treated with traction, the prognosis for the athlete is good, and traction should be continued as part of the treatment plan.[2,5,30] Any lasting therapeutic changes must be assumed to occur from adjustments or adaptations of the structures around the vertebrae in response to the traction.

Effects on Bone

Bone changes, according to **Wolff's law**, usually occur in response to compressive or distractive loads. Traction would place a distractive load on each of the vertebrae affected by the traction load. Although bone tissue adapts relatively quickly, bony changes do not occur fast enough to cause the symptomatic changes that occur with traction application. An intermittent traction with a rhythmic on- and off-load cycle not only provides distraction load but also promotes movement. The major effect of traction on the bone may come from the increase in spinal movement that reverses any immobiliza-

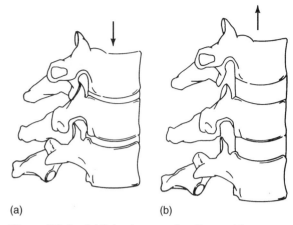

(a)   (b)

Figure 12-1 (a) Spine in normal resting position. (b) Spine under traction load with overall increase in length and overall increased separation between each vertebra.

tion-related bone weakness by increasing or maintaining bone density.

Effects on Ligaments

The ligamentous structures of the spinal column will be stretched by traction. Structural changes of the ligaments occur relatively slowly in response to mechanical stresses because ligaments have **viscoelastic properties** that allow them to resist shear forces and to return to their original form following the removal of a deforming load.[2,5,29]

With rapid loading, the ligaments become stiffer or resistant to changes in length and will be able to absorb a high load or force before failure occurs. With this type of loading, overstress could produce a significant injury.[5]

Slow loading rates will allow the ligament to lengthen as it absorbs the force of the load. Overstress can still produce injury but it will not be as severe as in the high loading rates. The amount of **ligament deformation** accompanying a low rate of loading will be higher than in rapid loading situations. Loading should be applied slowly and comfortably.[5] The ligament deformation will allow the spinal vertebrae to move apart.

- Ligaments may be progressivly stretched with traction

In ligaments shortened or contracted by an injury or a long-term postural problem, traction is important in restoring normal length. The traction force provides the stress that encourages the ligament to make adaptive changes in length and strength. The traction force in this instance would have to be heavy enough to stimulate adaptive changes but not heavy enough to overwhelm the ligament. In acute severely sprained ligaments, a traction force may overwhelm the ligament and have a negative effect on the healing process. Traction treatment should be a part of an overall treatment program that includes strengthening and flexibility exercises.[2]

When they are stretched, the ligaments put pressure on or move other structures within the ligamentous structure (**proprioceptive nerves**) and external to the ligament structure (**disk material, synovial fringes**, vascular structures, nerve roots). This pressure or movement can have a big impact on painful problems if pressure on a sensitive structure (nerve, vessels) is reduced. Activation of the proprioceptive system will also relieve pain by providing a gating effect similar to a transcutaneous electrical nerve stimulation treatment.[2, 8]

Effects on the Disk

The mechanical tension created by the traction has a good effect on **disk protrusions** and disk-related pain. Normally the disk helps to dissipate compressive forces while the spine is in an erect posture (Figure 12-2a).

In the normal disk, internal pressure increases, but the nucleus pulposus (fluidlike center of the fibrocartilaginous vertebral disk) does not move with changes in the weight-bearing forces as the spine moves from flexion to extension.[31] When an injury occurs to the disk structures, and the disk loses its

Wolff's law   Bone remodels itself and provides increased strength along the lines of the mechanical forces placed on it.

viscoelastic properties   The property of a material to show sensitivity to rate of loading.

ligament deformation   Lengthening distortion of ligament caused by traction loading.

proprioceptive nervous system   System of nerves that provides information on joint movement, pressure, and muscle tension.

disk material   Cartilaginous material from vertebral body surfaces, disk nucleus, or annulus fibrosus.

synovial fringes   Folds of synovial tissue that move in and out of the joint space.

disk protrusion   The abnormal projection of the disk nucleus through some or all of the annular rings.

disk nucleus   The protein polysaccharide gel that is contained between the cartilaginous end plates of the vertebrae and the annulus fibrosus.

annulus fibrosus   The interlacing cross-fibers of fibroelastic tissue that are attached to adjacent vertebral bodies that contain the nucleus pulposus.

normal fullness, the vertebrae can move closer together. The annular fibers bulge just as an underinflated car tire bulges when compared with a normally inflated one[31] (Figure 12-2b).

If the disk is damaged and movement occurs in a weight-bearing position, the disk nucleus will shift according to fluid-dynamic principles. Pressure on one side squeezes the nucleus in the opposite direction (Figure 12-2c). If tears develop in the annular fibers, the nucleus will tend to take the path of least resistance and move in this direction (Figure 12-2d).

Traction that increases the separation of the vertebral bodies decreases the central pressure in the disk space and encourages the **disk nucleus** to return to a central position. The mechanical tension of the **annulus fibrosus** and ligaments surrounding

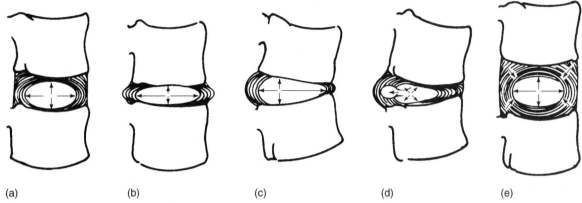

(a)　　　　　　(b)　　　　　　(c)　　　　　　(d)　　　　　　(e)

Figure 12-2 Fluid dynamics of the intervertebral disk. (a) Normal disk in noncompressed position; internal pressure, indicated by arrows, is exerted relatively equally in all directions. The internal annular fibers contain the nuclear materials. (b) Sitting or standing with compression of an injured disk causes the nucleus to become flatter. Pressure in this instance still remains relatively equal in all directions. (c) In an injured disk, movement in the weight-bearing position causes a horizontal shift in the nuclear material. If this was forward bending, the bulge to the left would take place at the posterior annular fibers while the anterior annular fibers would be slackened and narrow. (d) Weakness of the annular wall would allow the nuclear material to create a herniation and possibly put pressure on sensitive structures in the area. (e) When placed under traction, the intervertebral space expands, lowering the disk pressure. The taut annulus creates a centripetally directed force. Both these factors encourage the nuclear material to move and decrease the herniation and its effects.

• Traction will return disk nucleus to a central position

the disk also tends to force the nuclear material and cartilage fragments toward the center.[2,8,12,19,25,29,31]

Movement of these materials relieves pain and symptoms if they are compressing nervous or vascular structures. Decreasing the compressive forces also allows for better fluid interchange within the disk and spinal canal.[2,8] The reduction in **disk herniation** is unstable, and tends to return when compressive forces return[24,25] (Figure 12-2d and e).

The positive effect of traction in this instance may be destroyed by allowing the athlete to sit after treatment. Minimizing compressive forces after treatment may be equally as important to the treatment's success as the traction.[2] The sitting posture increases the disk pressure, causing the nucleus to

■ Analogy　*12-1*

The nuleus within the vertebral disk is like a piece of candy that has a liquid center. If you squeeze the candy, the liquid center is forced to move in the opposite direction away from the pressure. If you pull on the top and bottom of the piece of candy, the liquid center will move back toward the center. Traction can effect movement of the nucleus away from the nerve root, thus decreasing pressure.

follow the path of least resistance and a return of the disk herniation.

Effects on Articular Facet Joints

The articular joints of the spine (**facet joints**) can be affected by traction, primarily through increased separation of the joint surfaces. **Meniscoid structures**, synovial fringes, or osteochondral fragments (calcified bone chips) impinged between joint sur-

- Traction can stretch paraspinal muscles

faces are released, and a dramatic reduction in symptoms is noticed when joint surfaces are separated. Increased joint separation decompresses the articular cartilage, allowing the synovial fluid exchange to nourish the cartilage. The separation may also decrease the rate of degenerative changes from osteoarthritis. Increased proprioceptive discharge from the facet joint structures provides some decrease in pain perception.[2,5,10,25]

Effects on the Muscular System

The vertebral muscles can be effectively stretched by traction, provided that the positions of the spine during traction are selected to optimize the stretch of particular muscle groups. The initial stretch should come from body positioning, and the addition of traction will then provide some additional stretch. EMG recordings of the spinal erector muscles during traction showed some decrease in EMG activity in most athletes, indicating a muscular relaxation.[11,28] This effect can be enhanced by palpating the erector muscles and focusing the athlete's attention on relaxing them. The muscular stretch would lengthen tight muscle structures or create relaxation of contraction allowing better muscular blood flow and would also activate muscle proprioceptors, providing even more of a gating influence on the pain. All these properties lead to a decrease in muscular irritation.[2,10,11,14,23,27]

Effects on the Nerves

The nerve is the structure at which traction's effects are most often directed. Pressure on nerves or roots from bulging disk material, irritated facet joints, bony spurs, or narrowed foramen size causes the neurologic malfunctioning often associated with spinal pain. Tingling is usually the first clinical sign

disk herniation   The protrusion of the nucleus pulposus through a defect in the annulus fibrosus.

facet joints   Articular joints of the spine.

meniscoid structures   A cartilage tip found on the synovial fringes of some facet joints

anoxia   Reduction of oxygen in body tissues below physiologic levels.

fibrosis   The formation of fibrous tissue in the injury repair process.

- Traction can relieve pressure on a nerve root

indicating that there is pressure on a nerve structure. If the pressure is not relieved or if damage of the nerve as a result of trauma or **anoxia** has resulted in inflammation, the tingling may not respond to traction.[10,12,20,30,31,36,39]

Unrelieved pressure on a nerve will cause slowing and eventual loss of impulse conduction. The signs of motor weakness, numbness, and loss of reflex become progressively more apparent and are indicative of nerve degeneration. Pain, tenderness, and muscular spasm are also associated with continued pressure on the nerve.

Anything that decreases the pressure on the nerve increases the blood's circulation to the nerve, decreasing edema, and allowing the nerve to return to normal functioning. Some degenerative changes are reversible, depending on the amount of degeneration and the amount of **fibrosis** that occurs during the repair process.[2,10,20,36,39]

Effects on the Entire Body Part

The previous discussion outlined the effect of traction on the major systems involved in spine-related pain and dysfunction. The complexity and interrelationships among these systems make determining specific causes of pain and dysfunction very difficult. Traction is not specific to one system but has an effect on each system, and collectively the effect can be very good. Traction can affect the pathologic process in any of the systems, and then all the structures involved can begin to normalize. Traction should not stand alone as a treatment but should be considered as part of an overall treatment plan, and each component of any spine-related dysfunction should be treated with other appropriate modalities.[1,2,5,8,23,30,31,32,36]

TRACTION TREATMENT TECHNIQUES

The literature on traction and its clinical effectiveness is somewhat limited.[6,8,12,25,31,37,38,45] Most of the clinical studies go into great depth about the pathology being treated, but unfortunately they provide only a cursory description of the traction setup, making duplication of the traction method difficult.[37]

The following discussion of specific traction setups is organized according to lumbar and cervical traction. Each of these areas will contain discussions of postural, manual, and machine-assisted traction. The traction setups mentioned in this chapter should be used as starting points in a treatment plan. The parameters of time, position, and traction force should be adapted to the athlete, rather than forcing the athlete to adapt to a predetermined traction setup.

The treatment plan should include the clinical criteria for judging the success and continued use of traction. Positive changes should occur within 5 to 8 treatment days if traction is going to be successful; for example, if an athlete has a positive straight leg raise sign (i.e., pain in the back with a passive straight leg raise), this is a measurable clinical criterion that can be used to judge the treatment's success. If the straight leg raise test is positive at 20 degrees of hip flexion before and after traction, and after successive treatments the straight leg raise test is positive at increasing degrees of hip flexion, then the treatment can be considered successful.[26]

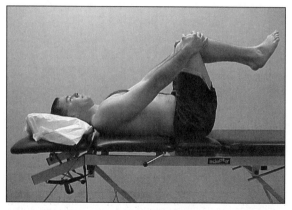

(a)

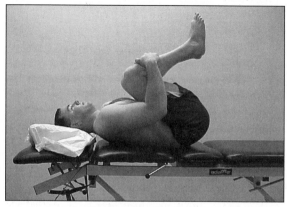

(b)

Figure 12-3 Positional traction: knees to chest posture can be used to increase the size of the lumbar intervertebral foramen bilaterally, (a) Beginning position (b) Terminal Position

LUMBAR POSITIONAL TRACTION

Spinal **nerve root impingement**, from a variety of causes ranging from disk herniation or prolapse to **spondylolisthesis**, is the leading diagnosis for which lumbar traction is prescribed. Traction has also been used to treat joint hypomobility, arthritic conditions of the facet joints, mechanically produced muscle spasm, and joint pain.[2,11,12,30,31,39,40,45]

Normal spinal mechanics allow movements to occur that narrow or enlarge the intervertebral

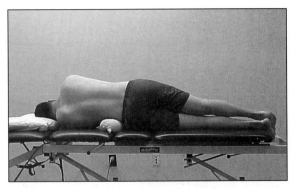

Figure 12-4   Positional traction: athlete positioned sidelying with a blanket roll between the iliac crest and the lower border of the rib cage. This increases the intervertebral foramen size of the left side of the lumbar spine.

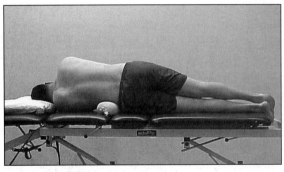

(a)

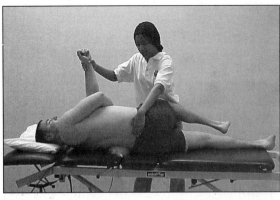

(b)

Figure 12-5   Positional traction: maximum opening of the intervertebral foramen of the left side of the athlete's lumbar spine is achieved by flexing the upper hip and knee and rotating the athlete's shoulders so he is looking over the left shoulder (left rotation).

nerve root impingement   Abnormal encroachment of some body tissue into the space occupied by the nerve root.

spondylolisthesis   Forward displacement of one vertebra over another.

unilateral foramen opening   Enlargement of the foramen on one side of a vertebral segment.

• Traction is most often used to treat nerve root impingement

foramina. If the athlete is placed in the supine position with hips and knees flexed, the lumbar spine bends forward and the spinous processes separate. This movement increases the size of the intervertebral foramen bilaterally (Figure 12-3). The flexed postures used to treat low back pain are examples of this positional traction.

The greatest **unilateral foramen opening** occurs by positioning the athlete sidelying with a pillow or blanket roll between the iliac crest and the lower border of the rib cage. The side on which increased foramen opening is desired should be superior. The roll should be close to the level of the spine where the traction separation is desired. The spine side bends around the roll (Figure 12-4). The athlete's hips and knees are then flexed until the lumbar spine is in a forward-bent position (Figure 12-5a). This accentuates the opening of a foramen. Maximal opening can be achieved by adding trunk rotation toward the side of the superior shoulder[31,36,38,39] (Figure 12-5).

Positional traction is normally used when the athlete is on a very restricted activity program

■ **Clinical Decision-Making** *Exercise 12-1*

An athlete walks into the training room complaining of acute low back pain. She is very guarded and is leaning to the right, away from her left side, which she says is most painful. What can the athletic trainer do to make the athlete more comfortable immediately?

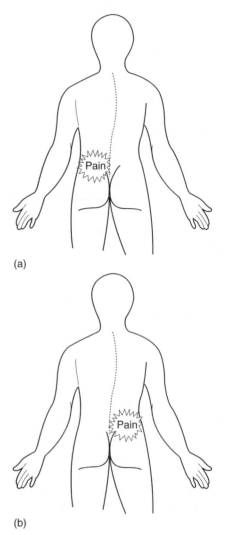

(a)

(b)

Figure 12-6 (a) Athlete leaning away from the painful side. The athlete's left side should be placed up while sidelying over a blanket roll to open up the upper foramen or the nerve roots away from the lateral herniation or both. (b) Athlete leaning toward the painful side. The athlete's left side should be placed up while sidelying over a blanket roll to pull the nerve roots away from a medial herniation.

because of low back pain. The positions are used on a trial and error basis to determine maximum comfort and to attempt to relieve pressure on nerve roots.

The results of the athlete evaluation should be used to determine whether the painful side should be up or down when using the sidelying positional traction technique. Protective scoliosis is the most obvious sign that will help determine athlete position. If the athlete leans away from the painful side, the painful side should be up (Figure 12-6a); if the athlete leans toward the painful side, the painful side should be down (Figure 12-6b).

It is hoped that the athlete will describe excellent results following an initial treatment, but it is not uncommon to complain of increases in pain. This would mean that the treatment position should be changed.

The location of the pressure from the disk herniation was previously believed to cause these signs. Further research suggests that hand dominance may be more of a factor than herniation location in producing this scoliosis. However, the athlete may be more compliant with the treatment regimen if simple mechanical explanations, such as pushing the herniation back into place, are used.[33]

Athletes with these symptoms may also be good candidates for unilateral traction[2,5,30,31,35,36] (see Figure 12-13, pp. 308). Facet irritation is capable of causing similar scoliotic curves; in most instances, the scoliosis is convex toward the painful side.

■ **Clinical Decision-Making**   *Exercise 12-2*

An athlete has been diagnosed with a prolapsed disk at L4, which is impinging the nerve root on the left side. What specific positional traction technique should the athletic trainer recommend to make the athlete most comfortable at home?

Inversion Traction

Inversion traction, another positional traction, is being used for prevention and treatment of back problems.[13] Specialized equipment or simply hanging upside down from a chinning bar will place a person in the inverted position. The spinal column is lengthened because of the stretch provided by the weight of the trunk. The force of the trunk in this position is usually calculated to be approximately 40% of body weight (Figure 12-7).[16]

When the person is comfortable and able to relax, the length of the spinal column will increase. These length changes will coincide with decreases in spinal muscle activity.[1,2,6,7,18,21,22,28]

No research-supported protocols exist for this method of traction, although a slow progression of time in the inverted position seems to be best. One study suggests the electromyographic activity decreases after 70 seconds in the inverted position. If the athlete is comfortable completely inverted, 70 seconds may be used as a minimum treatment time. The inverted position may be repeated 2 or 3 times at a treatment session, with a 2 to 3 minute rest between bouts. Longer treatment times may also enhance results. Maximum treatment times range from 10 to 30 minutes. Setup procedures are equipment-dependent, and the manufacturer's protocols should be followed and modified as necessary to meet the needs of the athlete.[1,2,3,9,28]

Blood pressure should be monitored while the athlete is in the inverted position. If a rise of 20 mm mercury above the resting diastolic pressure is found, the athletic trainer should stop the treatment for that session.[2,3,28]

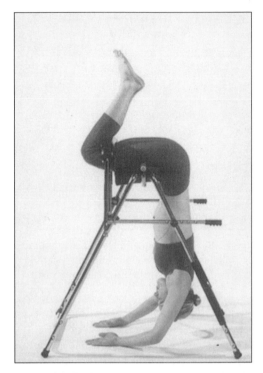

Figure 12-7   Inversion traction apparatus. (Courtesy Invertrac)

■ **Clinical Decision-Making**   *Exercise 12-3*

A gymnast asks the athletic trainer if it is ok for her to hang upside down by her knees from the uneven parallel bars because this seems to help her stretch her low back. Is there any precaution that must be taken?

Contraindications include hypertensive (140/90) individuals and anyone with heart disease or glaucoma. Athletes with sinus problems, diabetes, thyroid conditions, asthma, migraine headaches, detached retinas, or hiatal hernias should consult their physicians before treatment is initiated. Recent surgery or musculoskeletal problems may require modification of the inversion apparatus. In addition, meals or snacks should not be

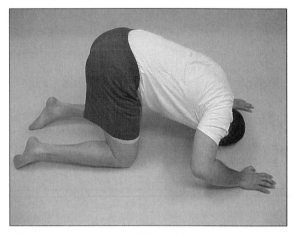

Figure 12-8 Inversion tolerance test position. Any vertigo, dizziness, or nausea may indicate that this athlete is a poor candidate for inversion treatment.

eaten during the hour before treatment to keep the athlete comfortable.

One method of testing the athlete's tolerance to the inverted position is to have the athlete assume the hand-knee position and put his or her head on the floor, holding that position for 60 seconds. Any vertigo, dizziness, or nausea may indicate that this athlete is a poor candidate for inversion and that the treatment progression should be very slow[1,2,3,6,7,9,18,21,22,28] (Figure 12-8).

MANUAL LUMBAR TRACTION

Manual lumbar traction is used for lumbar spine problems to test the athlete's tolerance to traction, to arrive at the most comfortable treatment setup, to make the traction as specific to one vertebral level as possible, and to provide the specificity needed for a traction mobilization of the spine. If the athlete's back pain is diminished by having the athletic trainer flex the athlete's hips and knees to 90 degrees each and apply enough pressure under the calves to lift his/her buttocks off the table, then the athlete is a good candidate for spine 90-90 degree traction. The disadvantage is that maintaining the large forces necessary for separation of the lumbar vertebrae for a period of time is difficult and energy-consuming for the athletic trainer.[2,35,36]

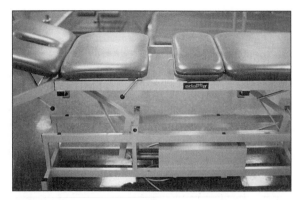

Figure 12-9 Split table with movable section to decrease frictional forces.

Having a split table will eliminate most of the friction between the athlete's body segments and the treatment table and is essential for effective delivery of manual lumbar traction[2,5,24,36,39] (Figure 12-9). The athletic trainer's effort does not cause separation of the vertebral segments unless the frictional forces are overcome first.

Level-Specific Manual Traction

To make the traction specific to a vertebral level, the athlete is positioned sidelying on the split table. For traction specific to L3–4, L4–5, and L5–S1 levels, the athlete's upper leg is used as a lever, and the lumbar spine is flexed until motion of the spinous process just below that level is felt (Figure 12-10). The athlete's trunk is then rotated toward the upper shoulder until the spinous process just above the desired level is felt (Figure 12-11).

If lumbar levels T12, L1, L1–2, and L2–3 are to be given specific traction, the athlete is again positioned sidelying. These levels require positioning in reverse order from the lower levels. First the trunk is rotated (see Figure 12-11), then the lumbar spine is flexed[2,5] (see Figure 12-10).

In both instances the rotation and flexion tighten and lock joint structures in which these motions have taken place, leaving the desired segment with more movement available than the upper or lower levels. When traction is applied, greater movement of the desired level occurs while move-

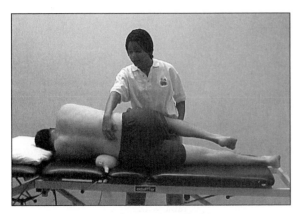

Figure 12-10 Positioning the athlete for maximum effect at a specific level. The lumbar spine is flexed, using the athlete's upper leg as a lever. The athletic trainer palpates the interspinous area between two spinous processes. The upper spinous process is the one at which maximum effect is desired. When the lumbar spine flexes and the athletic trainer feels the motion of the lower spinous process with the palpating hand, the foot is placed against the opposite leg so that further flexion is not allowed.

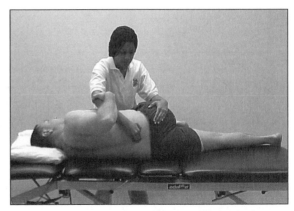

Figure 12-12 Manual lumbar traction with maximum effect at a specific level. The athletic trainer has positioned the athlete for maximum effect and is palpating the interspinous area between the two spinous processes where maximum traction effect is desired. The athletic trainer then places his or her chest against the anterior superior iliac spine and the athlete's upper hip. The split table is released and the athletic trainer leans toward the athlete's feet, using enough force to cause a palpable separation of the spinous processes at the desired level.

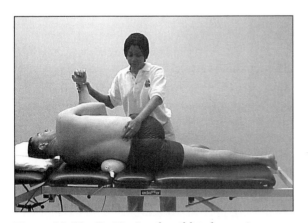

Figure 12-11 Positioning the athlete for maximum effect at a specific level. The athlete's trunk is rotated by the athletic trainer until motion of the upper spinous process is felt by the athletic trainer. Trunk rotation should be passively produced by the sports therapist positioning the athlete's upper arm with hand on the rib cage, and pulling on the athlete's lower arm, creating trunk rotation toward the upper arm. In this case it is rotation to the left.

ment at other levels is minimized because of the joint locking created by the preliminary positioning.

The split table is then released, and the athletic trainer palpates the spinous processes of the selected intervertebral level, places his or her chest against the anteriorsuperior iliac spine of the athlete's upper hip, and leans toward the athlete's feet. Enough force is used to cause a palpable separation of the spinous processes (Figure 12-12). Intermittent movement is most easily accomplished, while sustained traction becomes physically more difficult.[2,5]

Unilateral Leg Pull Manual Traction

Unilateral leg pull manual traction has been used in the treatment of hip joint problems or difficult lateral shift corrections. A thoracic countertraction harness is used to secure the athlete to the table. The athletic trainer grabs the athlete's ankle and brings the athlete's hip into 30-degree flexion, 30-degree abduction, and full external rotation. A

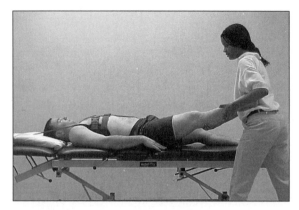

Figure 12-13 Unilateral leg pull traction. With the athlete secured to the table with a thoracic countertraction harness, the athletic trainer brings the athlete's hip into 30-degree flexion, 30-degree abduction, and maximum external rotation. A steady pull is then applied.

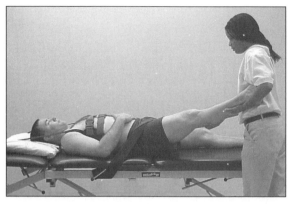

Figure 12-14 Unilateral leg pull traction for sacroiliac joint problems. A strap is placed through the groin and secured to the table. The athletic trainer brings the athlete's hip into 30-degree flexion and 15-degree abduction, and then applies a traction force to the leg.

steady pull is applied until a noticeable distraction is felt[5] (Figure 12-13).

In suspected sacroiliac joint problems, a similar setup can be used. A banana strap is placed through the groin on the side to be stretched. This strap will secure the athlete in position. The athletic trainer grabs the athlete's ankle, brings his or her hip into 30-degree flexion and 15-degree abduction, and then applies a sustained or intermittent pull to create a mobilizing effect on the sacroiliac joint[5] (Figure 12-14).

As a preliminary to mechanical traction, manual traction is helpful in determining what degree of lumbar flexion, extension, or sidebending is most comfortable and will also give an indication of the treatment's success. The most comfortable position is usually the best therapeutic position.[5,35,38]

Athlete comfort may have a bigger impact on the traction's results than the angle of pull, the force used, the mode, or the duration of the treatment. The inability of the athlete to relax in any traction setup will affect the traction's ability to cause a separation of the vertebrae. The lack of vertebral separation would minimize some of the traction's therapeutic benefits.[5,35,38]

MECHANICAL LUMBAR TRACTION

When using mechanical lumbar traction, the athletic trainer will have to select and adjust the following parameters of the traction equipment and athlete position:

1. Body position: prone, supine, hip position, bilateral or unilateral direction of pull
2. Force used
3. Intermittent traction: traction time and rest time
4. Sustained traction
5. Duration of treatment
6. Progressive steps
7. Regressive steps

The research on mechanical lumbar traction gives us a strong protocol for using traction to decrease disk protrusion and nerve root symptoms. The protocols for use in other pathologies are not supported by research, but clinical empiricism and inference from some of the research give a good working protocol. The athletic trainer will need to match the traction treatment to the athlete's symptoms and make adjustments based on the clinical results.[5,12,29,35,42]

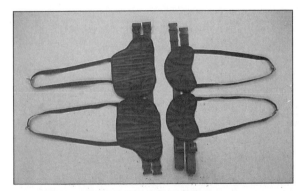

Figure 12-15   Vinyl-backed traction harness.

Equipment and SetUp

A split table or other mechanism to eliminate friction between body segments and the table surface is a prerequisite to effective lumbar traction. Otherwise, most of the force applied would be spent overcoming the coefficient of friction[1,2,5,17,24,36,39,42] (see Figure 12-9).

A nonslip traction harness is needed to transfer the traction force comfortably to the athlete and to stabilize the trunk while the lumbar spine is placed under traction. A harness lined with a vinyl material is best because it adheres to the athlete's skin and does not slip like the cotton-lined harness. Clothing between the harness and the skin will also promote slipping. The vinyl-sided harness does not have to be as constricting as the cotton-backed harness to prevent slippage, thus increasing the athlete's comfort[5,36,39] (Figure 12-15).

The harness can be applied when the athlete is standing next to the traction table prior to treatment. The pelvic harness is applied so the contact pads and upper belt are at or just above the level of the iliac crest (Figure 12-16).

Shirts should never be tucked under the pelvic harness because some of the tractive force would be dissipated pulling on the shirt material. The contact pads should be adjusted so that the harness loops will provide a posteriorly directed pull, encouraging lumbar flexion (Figure 12-17). The harness firmly adheres to the athlete's hips.[5,36,39]

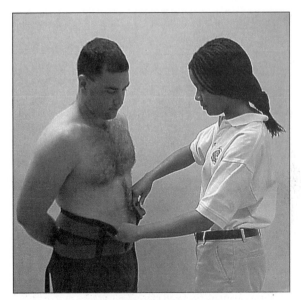

Figure 12-16   Pelvic harness for mechanical lumbar traction. The contact pads are applied so that the upper belt is at or just above the level of the iliac crest.

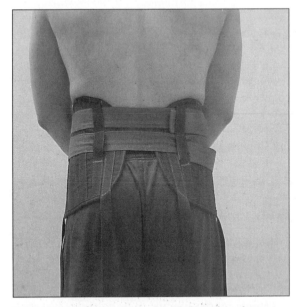

Figure 12-17   The traction straps from the pelvic harness should bracket the athlete's buttocks if a lumbar flexion pull is desired. If a straight pull is desired, the pelvic harness should be adjusted so that the straps bracket the athlete's lateral hip area.

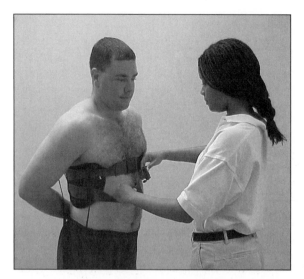

Figure 12-18   Thoracic countertraction harness. Rib pads are positioned over the lower rib cage.

The rib belt is then applied in a similar manner with the rib pads positioned over the lower rib cage in a comfortable manner. The rib belt is then snugged up, and the athlete is positioned on the table[5,36,39] (Figure 12-18).

The standing application of the traction harness is easier and more effective if the athlete is to be placed in prone position for treatment[5,36,39] (Figure 12-19). The traction harness can also be applied by laying it out on the traction table and having the athlete lie down on top of it. The pads are then adjusted and the belts tightened with the athlete lying down.

Body Positioning

Body position has been reported to have a big impact on traction results, but this has been empirically derived rather than research supported. The athletic trainer needs a good understanding of the mechanics of the lumbar spine to make decisions about position that will best affect an athlete's symptoms.[2,5,25,31,36,39]

Generally, the neutral spinal position allows for the largest intervertebral foramen opening, and it is

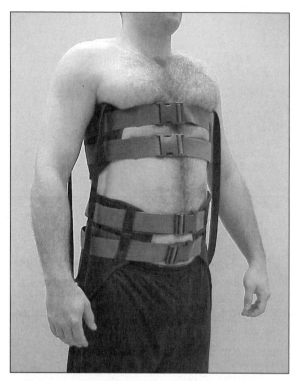

Figure 12-19   Applying the pelvic and thoracic harnesses may be easier if done while the athlete is standing.

usually the position of choice whether the athlete is prone or supine. Extension beyond neutral lumbar spine causes the bony elements of the foramen to create a narrower opening. Lumbar spinal flexion beyond neutral causes the ligamentum flavum and other soft tissues to constrict the foramen's opening[35,38] (Figure 12-20).

Saunders[39,36] recommends the prone position with a normal to slightly flattened lumbar lordosis (an abnormal anterior curve) as the position of choice in disk protrusions. The amount of lordosis may be controlled by using pillows under the abdomen. The prone position also allows the easy application of other modalities to the painful area and an easier assessment of the amount of spinous process separations[5,36,39] (Figure 12-21).

In traction applied to an athlete in the supine position, hip position was found to affect vertebral

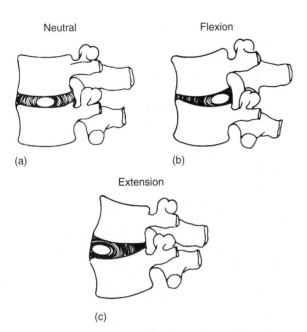

Figure 12-20   (a) Neutral lumbar spine position allows for the largest intervertebral foramen opening before traction is applied. (b) Flexion, while it may tend to increase the posterior opening, puts pressure on the disk nucleus to move posterior. Other soft tissue may also close the foramen opening. (c) Extension beyond neutral tends to close the foramen down as the bony arches come closer together.

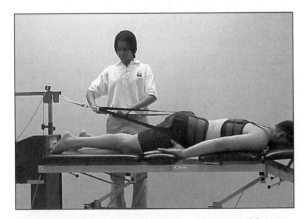

Figure 12-21   Mechanical lumbar traction: athlete in the prone position with a pillow under the abdomen to help control lumbar spine extension.

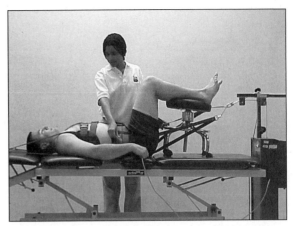

Figure 12-22   Mechanical lumbar traction: athlete in the supine position with hips flexed to approximately 90 degrees.

■ **Clinical Decision-Making**   *Exercise 12-4*

The athletic trainer has decided to treat an athlete with signs and symptoms of a disk protrusion using mechanical traction. What treatment parameters will likely be most effective in treating this problem?

separation. As hip flexion increased from 0 to 90 degrees, traction produced a greater posterior intervertebral space separation[39] (Figure 12-22).

Unilateral pelvic traction has also been recommended when a stronger force is desired on one side of the spine. Athletes with protective scoliosis, unilateral joint dysfunction, or unilateral lumbar muscle spasm with scoliosis may do quite well with this approach. Only one side of the pelvic harness is hooked to the traction device to accomplish this technique[36] (Figure 12-23).

In athletes with protective scoliosis, when the athlete leans away from the painful side, the traction should be applied on the painful side. When the athlete leans toward the painful side, the traction should be applied on the nonpainful side (see Figure 12-6).

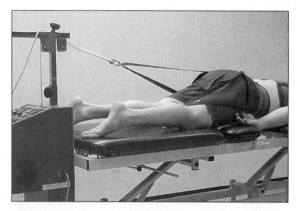

Figure 12-23   Mechanical lumbar traction with a unilateral pull: only one of the pelvic straps is hooked to the traction device.

In athletes with scoliosis caused by muscle spasm, the traction force should be applied from the side with the muscle spasm (Figure 12-24). In unilateral facet joint dysfunction, the traction should be applied from the side of most complaint.[38]

Overall, athlete positioning for traction should be varied according to an athlete's needs and comfort. Experimentation with positioning is encouraged so that the traction's effect on the athlete will be maximized. Athlete comfort is far more important than relative position in making athlete position decisions. If the athlete cannot relax, the traction will not be successful in causing vertebral separation.[5,36,39]

Traction Force

Several researchers have indicated that no lumbar vertebral separation will occur with traction forces less than one quarter of the athlete's body weight. The traction force necessary to cause effective vertebral separation will range between 65 and 200 pounds.[1,2,24,25,36,39] This force does not have to be used on the first treatment, and progressive steps both during and between treatments are often necessary to comfortably reach these therapeutic loads. A force equal to half the athlete's body weight is a

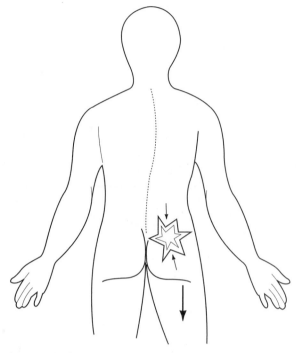

Figure 12-24   In an athlete with scoliosis caused by muscle spasm (right), the unilateral traction force should be applied using only the right pelvic strap.

good guideline to use in selecting a force high enough to cause vertebral separation. These high weight levels pose no danger, since cadaver research indicates a force of 440 pounds or greater is necessary to cause damage to the lumbar spine components[24,25] (Figure 12-25). The athletic trainer should continually make the appropriate adjustment in traction force until satisfactory results are achieved.[39]

Caution must be used when using traction of the lumbar spine, because there is a tendency for the nucleus pulposus gel to imbibe fluid from the vertebral body, thus increasing pressure within the disk. This happens in a very short period of time. When pressure is released and weight is applied to the disk, this excess fluid increases pressure on the annulus and exacerbates the athlete's symptoms.

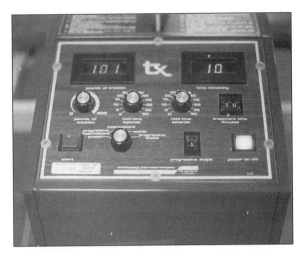

Figure 12-25 Traction device set for traction with 100 pounds of static traction for 10 minutes with 6 progressive steps.

Therefore, it is recommended that during an initial treatment with lumbar traction, a maximum of 30 pounds be used to determine whether traction will have a negative effect on the symptoms.[10]

The research has been aimed at forces necessary to cause vertebral separation. Traction certainly has effects that are not associated with vertebral separation, and if these effects are desired, less force may be necessary to get them.

Intermittent versus Sustained Traction

Good results have been reported with both intermittent and sustained traction. In most cases of lumbar disk problems, sustained traction seems to be the treatment of choice. Partial reduction in disk protrusions was observed in 4 minutes of sustained traction.[24,25,30,36,39] Good results were also reported using intermittent traction in the treatment of ruptured intervertebral disk.[11]

Separation of the posterior intervertebral space was noted with a 10-second-hold intermittent traction.[34] Posterior intervertebral separations using 100 pounds of force were similar when intermittent and sustained traction modes were compared.[25] The electromyographic activity of the sacrospinalis musculature showed similar patterns when sustained and intermittent traction were compared.[11]

Sustained traction is favored in treating intervertebral disk herniation because sustained traction allows more time with the disk uncompressed to cause the disk nuclear material to move centripetally and reduce the disk herniation's pressure on nerve structures. When used for this purpose, sustained traction may be superior to intermittent traction.[5,36,39]

In deciding on sustained versus intermittent traction, the athletic trainer should follow the guidelines for treating diagnosed disk herniations with sustained traction, while most other traction-appropriate diagnoses may be treated with intermittent traction. Intermittent traction, in any case, is usually more comfortable when using higher forces, and increased comfort will be one of the primary considerations because there is no conclusive evidence supporting the choice of one method over the other.[1,2,5,12,25,34,36,39]

The timing of the traction and rest phases of intermittent traction has not been researched. Short (less than 10 seconds) traction phases will cause only minimal interspace separation but will activate joint and muscle receptors and create facet joint movements.[5,8] Longer (more than 10 seconds) traction phases will tend to stretch the ligamentous and muscular tissues long enough to overcome their resistance to movement and create a longer lasting mechanical separation. When using high traction forces, the comfort of the athlete may dictate the adjustment of the traction time. Longer total treatment time will also be tolerated with intermittent traction.[5,8,10,25,36]

Rest phase times should be relatively short but should also be comfort-oriented. The rest time should be adjusted to allow the athlete to recover and feel relaxed before the next traction cycle. The athletic trainer should monitor the traction athlete frequently to adjust traction and rest time to maintain the athlete in a relaxed comfortable state.

Duration of Treatment

The total treatment times of sustained traction and intermittent traction are only partially research-based. With sustained traction, Mathews[24] found reduction in disk protrusion after 4 minutes with further reduction at 20 minutes. Complete reduction in protrusions was seen at 38 minutes. Other researchers found no difference in separation of the cervical spine when times of 7, 30, and 60 seconds were compared.[8,24,25]

When dealing with suspected disk protrusions, the total treatment time should be relatively short. As the disk space widens, the pressure inside the disk decreases, and the disk nucleus will move centripetally. The projected time for pressure within a disk to equalize is 8 to 10 minutes. At this point, the nuclear material is no longer moving centripetally. With longer time in this position, osmotic forces will equalize the pressure within the disk with that of the surrounding tissue. When the pressure equalization occurs, the traction effect on the protrusion is lost. The intradiskal pressure may increase when the traction is released if the traction stays on too long. This increased pressure would result in increased symptoms. This situation has not been reported when treatment times are kept at 10 minutes or less.[36,39] If this reaction does occur, shorter treatment times or long-hold (60 seconds' traction, 10 to 20 seconds' rest) intermittent traction may be necessary to control the symptoms.

Some sources advocate traction times of up to 30 minutes.[5,24,25] The contradiction in philosophy may be because of pathology or the individual anatomy of each athlete. However, an adverse reaction to traction (i.e., a dramatic increase in symptoms when the traction is released) is something the athletic trainer should avoid.

Total treatment time for sustained traction when treating disk-related symptoms should start at less than 10 minutes. If the treatment is successful in reducing symptoms, the time should be left at 10 minutes or less. If the treatment is partially successful or unsuccessful in relieving symptoms, the

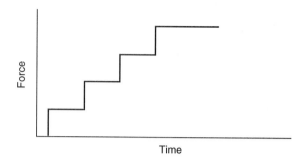

Figure 12-26 Progressive steps for lumbar traction of X pounds. Four steps are used: the first is 1/4 X pounds, the second 2/4 X, and so on. Each lasts for an equal time.

athletic trainer may increase the time gradually over several treatments to 30 minutes.

Progressive and Regressive Steps

Some traction equipment is built with progressive and regressive modes. The machine will progressively increase the traction force in a preselected number of steps. A gradual increase in pressure lets athletes accommodate slowly to the traction and helps them stay relaxed. A gradual progression of force also allows the athletic trainer to release the split table after the slack in the system has been taken up by several progressions[2,5,32] (Figure 12-26). Regressive steps do just the opposite and allow the athlete to come down gradually from the high loads. Again, athlete comfort is the primary consideration because no research supports any protocol[2,5,32] (Figure 12-27).

Some equipment has the capability to be programmed for progressive and regressive steps and also to have minimum traction forces, allowing a sustained force with intermittent peaks[2,5,32] (Figure 12-28). To achieve these kinds of traction set ups with a machine that is not programmable, manual operation and timing will be necessary.

Throughout the discussion on lumbar traction, athlete comfort comes up again and again in regard to the parameters of the treatment setup. One of the

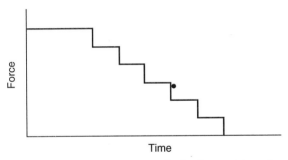

Figure 12-27 Regressive steps for lumbar traction of X pounds. Six equal regressive steps are used: the first drops the traction force from X to 5/6 X, the second to 4/6 X, and so on. Each lasts for an equal time.

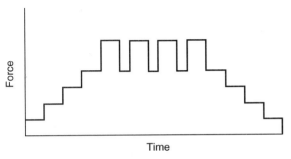

Figure 12-28 Progressive and regressive steps with a minimum sustained traction force.

primary keys to successful traction treatment is relaxation of the athlete. The use of appropriate modalities before and during the traction treatment will add to the total effectiveness of the treatment plan. Bracing or appropriate exercise after traction may also enhance the results and prolong the benefits gained. Better technology and more research will help refine traction and provide better results from this type of treatment.

MANUAL CERVICAL TRACTION

The objectives for using traction in the cervical region do not vary much from the objectives for using traction in the lumbar region. Reasonable objectives for cervical traction include stretch of the muscles and joint structures of the vertebral column, enlargement of the intervertebral spaces and foramina, centripetally directed forces on the disk and soft tissue around the disk, mobilization of vertebral joints, increases and changes in joint proprioception, relief of compressive effects of normal posture, and improvement in arterial venous and lymphatic flow.[5,10,15,25,35,40,43,44] In the sports medicine setting, diagnoses and symptoms requiring traction are found infrequently.[30] These diagnoses are more typically found in older populations.

In most cases involving sprains and strains, simple manual traction used to produce a rhythmic longitudinal movement will be very successful in helping decrease pain, muscle spasm, stiffness, and inflamation, and also in reducing joint compressive forces. Manual traction is infinitely more adaptable than mechanical traction, and changes in the direction, force, duration of the traction, and athlete position can be made instantaneously as the athletic trainer senses relaxation or resistance.[1,2,5,8,25]

The athlete's head and neck are supported by the athletic trainer. The hand should cradle the neck and provide adequate grip for the effective transfer of the traction force to the mastoid processes. One hand should be placed under the athlete's neck with the thenar eminence (base of the thumb) in contact with one mastoid process and the fingers cradling the neck reaching across toward the other mastoid process[2] (Figure 12-29a).

The athletic trainer then provides a gentle (less than 20 pounds) pull in a cephalic direction. Intervertebral separation is not desired because of the damage to the ligaments or capsule. A head halter or similar harness may be used to deliver the force also (Figure 12-29b).

The force should be intermittent, with the traction time between 3 and 10 seconds. The rest time may be very brief, but the tractive force should be released almost completely. The total treatment time should be between 3 and 10 minutes.[1,2,5,8]

When pain is limiting or affecting movement, a bout of traction should be followed by a reassessment of the painful motion to determine increases or

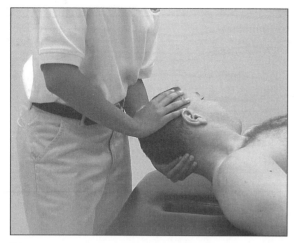

(a)

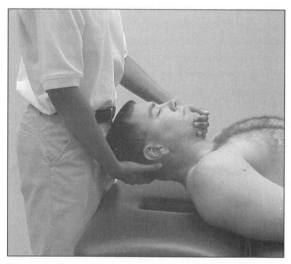

(b)

Figure 12-29 Manual cervical traction: (a) athlete in the supine position with the athletic trainer's fingertips and thenar eminence contacting the mastoid process of the athlete's skull. (b) Traction is applied with both hands.

decreases in pain or motion. Successive bouts of traction can be used as long as the symptoms are improving. When the symptoms stabilize or are worse on the reassessment, the traction should be discontinued.[5]

A variety of athlete head and neck positions can be used in cervical traction. Different head and

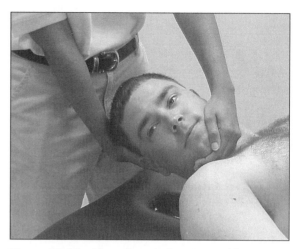

Figure 12-30 Manual cervical traction: athlete is positioned with neck in flexion and with some neck rotation to the right. Laterally flexed positions may also be used.

neck positions will place some vertebral structures under more tension than others. Good knowledge of cervical kinesiology and biomechanics and good knowledge and skill in joint mobilization are required before the athletic trainer should experiment with extensive position changes[2,5,8] (Figure 12-30).

At the completion of the traction treatment, in cases of strain or sprain, protection of the neck with a soft collar is often desirable to prevent extremes of motion, minimize compressive forces, and encourage muscle relaxation. Instructions in sleeping positions and regular support postures are also important in caring for athletes with cervical problems.[2,5]

MECHANICAL CERVICAL TRACTION

The literature does provide a relatively clear protocol to use in trying to achieve vertebral separation using a mechanical traction apparatus. The athlete should be supine or long-sitting with the neck flexed between 20 and 30 degrees (Figure 12-31). A sitting posture can be used, but is clinically more

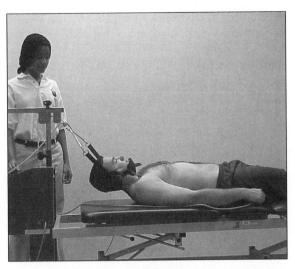

Figure 12-31   Mechanical cervical traction: athlete in the supine position with traction harness placed so that maximum pull is exerted on the occiput and the athlete is in a position of approximately 20 to 30 degrees of neck flexion.

■ **Clinical Decision-Making**   *Exercise 12-5*

....

In treating an athlete who is complaining of cervical neck pain, the athletic trainer is trying to decide whether to use a manual cervical traction technique or mechanical traction. Which would you recommend?

---

cumbersome and is not supported by the research as an optimal position of cervical traction.[41]

The traction harness must be arranged comfortably so that the majority of pull is placed on the occiput rather than the chin (see Figure 12-31). Some cervical traction harnesses do not have a chin-piece. These harnesses may have an advantage, provided that the traction force is effectively transferred to the structures of the cervical spine.[8,10]

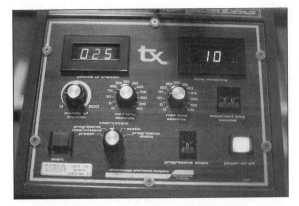

Figure 12-32   Control panel of traction machine with parameters adjusted for intermittent cervical traction.

A traction force above 20 pounds, applied intermittently for a minimum of 7 seconds traction time and with adequate rest time for recovery is recommended (see Figure 12-32). This traction should be continued over 20 to 25 minutes. Higher forces up to 50 pounds may produce increased separation, but the other parameters should remain the same. The average separation at the posterior vertebral area is 1 to 1.5 mm per space, while the anterior vertebral area separates approximately 0.4 mm per space. Greater separations are expected in the younger population than in the older population. Within 20 to 25 minutes from the time traction is stopped and normal sitting or standing postures are resumed, the vertebral separation returns to its previous heights. The upper cervical segments do not separate as easily as lower cervical segments.[8,10,25] The addition of pain-reducing and heating modalities will add to the benefits gained by the traction.[1,2,5,10,25]

CLINICAL APPLICATIONS FOR USING TRACTION

As discussed throughout this chapter, there are a number of conditions for which spinal traction may be useful, including cases where there is impingement on a nerve root resulting from disk

■ **TABLE 12-1** Summary of Indications and Contraindications for Spinal Traction

INDICATIONS	CONTRAINDICATIONS
Impingement on a nerve root	Acute sprains or strains
Disk herniation	Acute inflammation
Spondylolisthesis	Fractures
Narrowing within the intervertebral foramen	Vertebral joint instability
Osteophyte formation	Any condition in which movement exacerbates the existing problem
Degenerative joint diseases	Tumors
Subacute pain	Bone diseases
Joint hypomobility	Osteoporosis
Discogenic pain	Infections in bones or joints
Muscle spasm or guarding	Vascular conditions
Muscle strain	Pregnant females
Spinal ligament or connective tissue contractures	Cardiac or pulmonary problems
Improvement in arterial, venous, and lymphatic flow	

herniation, spondylolisthesis, narrowing within the intervertebral foramen, or osteophyte formation; degenerative joint diseases or subacute pain; joint hypomobility; discogenic pain; and muscle spasm (Table 12-1).

Traction, except as a light mobilization, is contraindicated in acute sprains or strains (first 3 to 5 days), in acute inflammation, or in any conditions in which movement is undesirable or exacerbates the existing problem. In cases of vertebral joint instability, traction may perpetuate the instability or cause further strain. Certainly the serious problems associated with tumors, bone diseases, osteoporosis, and infections in bones or joints are also contraindications. Athletes that can potentially experience problems relating to the fitting of a harness such as those with vascular conditions, pregnant females, or those with cardiac or pulmonary problems should also avoid traction.

Summary

1. Traction has been used to treat a variety of cervical and lumbar spine problems.
2. The effect of traction on each system involved in the complex anatomic makeup of the spine needs to be considered when selecting traction as a part of a therapeutic treatment plan.
3. The traction protocol should be set up to manage a particular problem rather than applied in the same manner regardless of the athlete or pathology.
4. Traction is a flexible modality with an infinite number of variations available. This flexibility should allow sports therapists to adjust their protocols to match the athlete's symptoms and diagnosis.
5. Traction is capable of producing a separation of vertebral bodies; a centripetal force on the soft tissues surrounding the vertebrae; a mobilization of vertebral joints; a change in proprioceptive discharge of the spinal complex; a stretch of connective tissue; a stretch of muscle tissue; an improvement in arterial, venous, and lymphatic flow; and a lessening of the compressive effects of posture. Any of these effects can change the symptoms of the athlete under treatment and help to normalize the athlete's lumbar or cervical spine.
6. Traction techniques in the lumbar region include positional traction; inversion traction; manual traction, which may be done using either level specific or unilateral leg pull techniques; and mechanical traction.
7. Cervical traction is used less frequently than lumbar traction. Cervical traction techniques include manual traction and mechanical traction.

Review Questions

1. What is traction, and how may it be performed by the athletic trainer?
2. What are the physical effects and therapeutic value of spinal traction on bone, muscle, ligaments, facet joints, nerve, blood vessels, and intervertebral disks?
3. What are the clinical advantages of using positional lumbar traction and inversion traction?
4. What are the clinical applications for using manual lumbar traction techniques, including level-specific manual traction and unilateral leg pull manual traction?
5. What are the setup procedures and treatment parameter considerations for using mechanical lumbar traction?
6. What are the advantages of using a manual traction technique of the cervical spine?
7. What are the setup procedures for mechanical traction techniques for the cervical spine?

 ## Self-Test Questions

T/F
1. The goal of traction is to encourage movement of the spine and decrease the athlete's symptoms.
2. Ligament deformation due to traction should occur during slow loading.
3. Traction may only be applied with a machine.

Multiple Choice
4. Traction may help reduce disk herniation. In this condition the _____ protrudes.
   a. annulus fibrosus
   b. nucleus pulposus
   c. disk material
   d. synovial fringe
5. Traction has effects on
   a. articular facet joints
   b. paraspinal muscles
   c. nerve roots
   d. all of the above
6. What is the most common problem traction is used to treat?
   a. spondylolisthesis
   b. fibrosis
   c. nerve root impingement
   d. none of the above

7. Which of the following is NOT a contraindication to traction?
   a. muscle strain
   b. acute inflammation
   c. fractures
   d. vertebral joint instability
8. How long should intermittent manual cervical traction be applied?
   a. less than 30 seconds
   b. 1–2 minutes
   c. 3–10 minutes
   d. 10–15 minutes
9. If traction treatments are resulting in no change in symptoms or a worsening of symptoms, the treatments should be _____ .
   a. done more often
   b. continued 1 more week
   c. performed in a different position
   d. discontinued
10. What is the appropriate range of force to be used on an athlete while performing mechanical lumbar traction?
   a. 0–50 pounds
   b. 65–200 pounds
   c. 200–300 pounds
   d. as great as the athlete can tolerate

Solutions to Clinical Decision-Making Exercises

12-1 The athletic trainer should have the athlete lie on the treatment table on her right side with the left side up, supported with a pillow under the right hip. This position a traction technique should help immediately.

12-2 The athlete should lie on the right side with a towel rolled up and placed under the right side as near to the appropriate segment as possible creating side bending to the right. The knees should be flexed until the spine is bent forward. Finally, the trunk should rotate to the left.

12-3 The athletic trainer should check to make sure that the gymnast does not have a history of hypertension. Then, an inversion tolerance test should be used to make certain that there is not a significant increase in diastolic blood pressure, and that there is no dizziness or vertigo or nausea from being in this position.

12-4 It is recommended that the athletic trainer begin treatments by using sustained traction for a short treatment time of less than 10 minutes at a traction force that would be slightly more than one quarter of that athlete's body weight. Treatment time and traction force may be increased as tolerated. If sustained traction exacerbates symptoms, intermittent traction may be used for about 15 minutes initially.

12-5 Manual traction is considerably more adaptable than mechanical traction, and changes in the direction, force, duration of the traction, and athlete position can be made instantaneously as the athletic trainer senses relaxation or resistance on the part of the athlete.

References

1. Bridger, R: Effect of lumbar traction on stature, *Spine* 15: 522–524, 1990.
2. Burkhardt, S: Course notes, cervical and lumbar traction seminar, Morgantown, W. Va., 1983.
3. Cooperman, J, and Scheid, D: Guidelines for the use of inversion, *Clin. Manage* 4(1): 6, 1984.
4. *Dorland's illustrated medical dictionary*, ed 24, Philadelphia, 1965, WB Saunders.
5. Erhard, R: Course notes, cervical and lumbar traction seminar, Morgantown, W. Va., 1983.
6. Gianakopoulos, G: Inversion devices: their role in producing lumbar distraction, *Arch Phys Med Rehabil* 68: 100–102, 1985.
7. Goldman, R: The effects of oscillating inversion on systemic blood pressure pulse, intraocular pressure and central retinal arterial pressure, *Physician SportsMedicine* 13(3): 93–96, 1985.
8. Grieve, G: Neck traction, *Physiotherapy* 6: 260–265, 1982.
9. Gudenhoven, R: Gravitational lumbar traction, *Arch Phys Med Rehab* 59: 510–512, 1978.
10. Harris, P: Cervical traction: review of the literature and treatment guidelines, *Phys Ther* 57: 910–914, 1977.
11. Hood, C: Comparison of EMG activity in normal lumbar sacrospinalis musculature during continuous and intermittent pelvic traction, *JOSPT* 2:137–141, 1981.
12. Hood, L, and Chrisman D: Intermittent pelvic traction in the treatment of the ruptured intervertebral disk, *Phys Ther* 48: 2 1–30, 1968.
13. Houlding, M: Clinical perspective. Inversion traction: a clinical appraisal, *New Zealand Journal of Physiotherapy*, 26(2):23–4, 1998.
14. Jett, D: Effect of intermittent, supine cervical traction on the myoelectric activity of the upper trapezius muscle in subjects with neck pain, *Phys Ther* 65: 1173–1176, 1985.
15. Katavich, L: Neural mechanisms underlying manual cervical traction, *Journal of Manual & Manipulative Therapy*, 7(1):20–5, 1999.
16. Klatz, R: Effects of gravity inversion on hypertensive subjects, *Physician and Sports Medicine* 13(3): 85–89, 1985.
17. KeKosz, U: Cervical and lumbopelvic traction, *Post Grad Med* 80(8): 187–194, 1986.
18. Kent, B: Anatomy of the trunk, part I, *Phys Ther* 54: 722–744, 1974.
19. Kent, B: Anatomy of the trunk, part II, *Phys Ther* 54: 850–859, 1974.
20. Krause, M, Refshauge, KM, Dessen, M, and Boland, R: Lumbar spine traction: evaluation of effects and recommended application for treatment, *Manual therapy* 5(2), May 2000.
21. LaBan, M: Intermittent traction: a progenetor of lumbar radicular pain, *Arch Phys Med Rehab* 73: 295–296, 1992.
22. LeMarr, J: Cardiorespiratory responses to inversion, *Physician SportsMedicine* 11(11): 51–57, 1983.
23. Letchuman, R, and Deusinger, R: Comparison of sacrospinalis myoelectric activity and pain levels in athletes undergoing static and intermittent lumbar traction, *Spine* 18: 1261–1365, 1993.

24. Mathews, J: Dynamic discography: a study of lumbar traction, *Ann. Phys. Med.* 9: 275–279, 1968.

25. Mathews, J: The effects of spinal traction, *Physiotherapy* 58: 64–66, 1972.

26. Meszaros, TF, Olson, R, and Kulig. K: Effect of 10%, 30%, and 60% body weight traction on the straight leg raise test of symptomatic patients with low back pain, *Journal of Orthopedic and Sports Physical Therapy*, 30(10): 595–601, 2000.

27. Murphy, M: Effects of cervical traction on muscle activity, *JOSPT* 13: 220–225, 1991.

28. Nosse, L: Inverted spinal traction, *Arch. Phys. Med. Rehabil.* 59: 367–370, 1978.

29. O'Donoghue, D: *Treatment of injuries to athletes*, ed. 3, Philadelphia, 1978, WB Saunders.

30. Onel, D: Computed tomographic investigation of the effects of traction on lumbar disc herniations, *Spine* 14: 82–90, 1989.

31. Paris, S: Course notes: basic course in spinal mobilization, Atlanta, Ga., 1977.

32. Petulla, L: Clinical observations with respect to progressive/regressive traction, *JOSPT* 7: 261–263, 1986.

33. Porter, R, and Miller, C: Back pain and trunk list, *Spine* 11: 596–600, 1986.

34. Reilly, J: Pelvic femoral position on vertebral separation produced by lumbar traction, *Phys Ther* 59: 282–286, 1979.

35. Roaf, R: A study of the mechanics of spinal injuries, *J. Bone Joint Surg.* 42B: 810–819, 1960.

36. Saunders, D: Lumbar traction, *JOSPT* 1: 36–45, 1979.

37. Saunders, HD: The controversy over traction for neck and low back pain. *Physiotherapy* 84(6):285–288, 1998.

38. Saunders, D: Unilateral lumbar traction, *Phys Ther* 61: 221–225, 1981.

39. Saunders, D: Use of spinal traction in the treatment of neck and back conditions, *Clin Orthop* 179: 31–38, 1983.

40. Sood, N: Prone Cervical Traction, *Clin Manage Phys Ther* 7(6): 37, 1987.

41. Stoddard, A: Traction for cervical nerve root irritation, *Physiotherapy* 40: 48–49, 1954.

42. Strapp, EJ: Lumbar traction: suggestions for treatment parameters 9–11, *Sports Medicine Update* 13(4): 1998.

43. Varma, S: The role of traction in cervical spondylosis, *Physiotherapy* 59: 248–249, 1973.

44. Walker, G: Goodley polyaxial cervical traction: a new approach to a traditional treatment, *Phys Ther* 66: 1255–1259, 1986.

45. Weinert, A, Rizzo TD: Non-operative management of multilevel lumbar disk herniations in an adolescent athlete, *Mayo Clin Proc* 67: 137–141, 1992.

Suggested Readings

Alice, M, Wong, M, and Chaupeng, I: The traction angle and cervical intervertebral seperation, *Spine* 12(2): 136, 1992.

Beurskens, A, De Vet, H, and Koke, A: Efficacy of traction for non-specific low back pain; a randomised clinical trial, *Lancet* 346(8990):1596–1600, 1995.

Beurskens, A, Van der Heijden, G, and De Vet, H: The efficacy of traction for lumbar back pain: design of a randomized clinical trial, *J Manipulative & Physiological Ther* 18(3): 141–147, 1995.

Creighton, D: Positional distraction, a radiological confirmation, *J Manual & Manipulative Therapy* 1(3):83–86, 1993.

Gilworth, G: Cervical traction with active rotation, *Physiotherapy.* 77(11):782–784, 1991.

Hariman, D: The efficacy of cervical extension-compression traction combined with diversified manipulation and drop table adjustments in the rehabilitation of cervical lordosis: a pilot study, *J Manipulative Physiological Ther* 18(5): 323–325, 1995.

Letchuman, R, and Deusinger, R: Comparison of sacrospinalis myoelectric activity and pain levels in athletes undergoing static and intermittent lumbar traction, *Spine* 18(10): 1361–1365, 1993.

Ljunggren, A Walker, L, and Weber, H: Manual traction vs. isometric exercise in athletes with herniated intervertebral lumbar disks, *Physiotherapy Theory Practice* 8:207, 1992.

Nanno, M: Effects of intermittent cervical traction on muscle pain. Flowmetric and electromyographic studies of the cervical paraspinal muscles, *J Nippon Medical School* 61(2):137–147, 1994.

Pal, B, Magnion, P, and Hossian, M: A controlled trial of continuous lumbar traction in the treatment of back pain and sciatica, *Br J Rheumat* 25: 181, 1989.

Pellecchia, G: Lumbar traction: a review of the literature (review), *JOSPT* 20(5):262–267, 1994.

Pio, A, Rendina, M, and Benazzo, F: The statics of cervical traction, *J Spinal Disorders* 7(4):337–342, 1994.

Terahata, N, Ishihara, H, and Ohshima, H: Effects of axial traction stress on solute transport and proteoglycan synthesis in the porcine intervertebral disc in vitro, *European Spine Journal* 3(6):325–330, 1994.

Tesio, L, and Merlo, A: Autotraction versus passive traction: an open controlled study in lumbar disc herniation, *Arch Phys Med Rehab* 74(8):871–876, 1993.

Trudel, G: Autotraction, *Arch Phys Med Rehab* 75(2):234–235, 1994.

Van de Heijden, G, Beurskens, A, and Koes, B: The efficacy of traction for back and neck pain: a systematic, blinded review of randomized clinical trial methods, *Phys Ther* 75(2):93–104, 1995.

Wong, A, Leong, C, and Chen, C: The traction angle and cervical intervertebral separation, *Spine* 17(2):136–138, 1992.

PART FIVE

Other Modalities

CHAPTER 13

Biofeedback

William E. Prentice

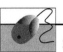

Study Resources

Refer to the lab exercises in the accompanying Laboratory Manual, as well as eSims which simulates the athletic training certification exam at www.mhhe.com/esims. Also, check out the competition information found at www.mhhe.com/prentice11e. For more online study resources, visit our Health and Human Performance Website at www.mhhe.com/hhp/.

Following completion of this chapter, the student athletic trainer will be able to

- Define biofeedback and identify its uses in a clinical setting.

- Contrast the various types of biofeedback instruments.

- Explain physiologically how the electrical activity generated by a muscle contraction can be measured using biofeedback.

- Break down how the electrical activity picked up by the electrodes is amplified, processed, and converted to meaningful information by the biofeedback unit.

- Differentiate between visual and auditory feedback.

- Outline the equipment setup and clinical applications for biofeedback.

---

biofeedback Information provided from some measuring instrument about a specific biologic function.

Biofeedback is a modality that seems to be gaining popularity among athletic trainers. It is a therapeutic procedure that uses electronic or electromechanical instruments to accurately measure, process, and feed back reinforcing information via auditory or visual signals.[26] In clinical practice, it is used to help the athlete develop greater voluntary control in terms of either neuromuscular relaxation or muscle re-education following injury.

ELECTROMYOGRAPHY AND BIOFEEDBACK

Electromyography (EMG) is a clinical technique that involves recording of the electrical activity generated in a muscle for diagnostic purposes. It involves a sophisticated electrodiagnostic study performed in an EMG laboratory that uses either surface or needle electrodes for measuring not only electrical activity in muscle but also various aspects of nerve conduction. An *electromyogram* is a graphic representation of those electrical currents associated with muscle action. While electromyography is widely used, particularly by physical therapists in the diagnosis of a variety of neuromuscular disorders, it is not commonly used in sports medicine except for research purposes. Certainly, electromyography would not be considered a therapeutic modality. The small portable biofeedback units that will be discussed in this chapter also measure electrical activity in the muscle and are in fact small electromyographs. The discussion in this chapter will be limited to the information on electromyography necessary for the athletic trainer to understand to be able to effectively incorporate biofeedback techniques into clinical practice.

THE ROLE OF BIOFEEDBACK

The term *biofeedback* should be familiar because all athletic trainers routinely serve as instruments of biofeedback when teaching a therapeutic exercise or in coaching a movement pattern. Using feedback can help the athlete to regain function of a muscle that may have been lost or forgotten following injury.[12] Using techniques such as having the athlete stand in front of a mirror when performing an exercise is a form of visual feedback. Having an athlete feel the vastus medialis contract is a form of manual feedback. These techniques can be routinely used by the injured athletes in their "home" rehabilitation plans.

Feedback includes information related to the sensations associated with movement itself as well as information related to the result of the action relative to some goal or objective. Feedback refers to the intrinsic information inherent to movement, including kinesthetic, visual, cutaneous, vestibular, and auditory signals collectively termed as response-produced feedback. But it also refers to extrinsic information or some knowledge of results that is presented verbally, mechanically, or electronically to indicate the outcome of some movement performance. Therefore, feedback is ongoing, in a temporal sense, occurring before, during, and after any motor or movement task. Feedback from

■ **Clinical Decision-Making** *Exercise 13-1*

The athletic trainer is beginning rehabilitation day 1 post-op following ACL reconstruction. The athlete is having a difficult time firing the VMO. Unfortunately, the one biofeedback unit in the athletic training room is broken. What can the athletic trainer do to help the athlete regain voluntary control of the VMO?

some measuring instrument that provides moment-to-moment information about a biologic function is referred to as biofeedback.[22]

Perhaps the biggest advantage of biofeedback is that it provides the athlete with a chance to make appropriate small changes in performance that are immediately noted and rewarded so that eventually larger changes or improvements in performance can be accomplished. The goal is to train athletes to perceive these changes without the use of the measuring instrument so that they can practice by themselves. Therefore, the athlete learns early in the rehabilitation process to do something for himself or herself and not to totally rely on the athletic trainer. This will help him or her to build confidence and increase feelings of self-efficacy. Treatments using biofeedback would be useful particularly in athletes who have difficulty in perceiving the initial small correct responses, or who may have a faulty perception of what they are doing. It is hoped that the rehabilitating athlete will be motivated and encouraged by seeing early signs of slight progress, thus to some extent relieving feelings of helplessness and reducing injury-related stress.[22]

To process feedback information, the athlete makes use of a complicated series of interrelated feedback loops involving very complex anatomical and neurophysiological components.[34] The primary focus in this text will be oriented toward how biofeedback may best be incorporated in a treatment program.

BIOFEEDBACK INSTRUMENTATION

Biofeedback instruments are designed to monitor some physiologic event, objectively quantify these monitorings, and then interpret the measurements as meaningful information.[27] There are several different types of biofeedback modalities available for use in rehabilitation. These biofeedback units cannot directly measure a physiologic event. Instead they record some aspect that is highly correlated with the physiologic event. Thus, the biofeedback reading should be taken as a convenient indication of a physiological process but not confused with the physiological process itself.[27]

The most commonly used instruments include those that record peripheral skin temperatures, indicating the extent of vasoconstriction or vasodilation; finger phototransmission units (photoplethysmograph), which also measure vasoconstriction and vasodilation; units that record skin conductance activity, indicating sweat gland activity; and units that measure electromyographic activity (EMG), indicating amount of electrical activity during muscle contraction. Additionally, there are other types of biofeedback units available, including electroencephalographs (EEG), pressure transducers, and electrogoniometers.

Peripheral Skin Temperature

Peripheral skin temperature is an indirect measure of the diameter of peripheral blood vessels. As vessels dilate, more warm blood is delivered to a particular area, thus increasing the temperature in that area. This effect is easily seen in the fingers and toes where the surrounding tissue warms and cools rapidly. Variations in skin temperature seem to be correlated with affective states with a decrease occurring in response to stress or fear. Temperature changes are usually measured in degrees Fahrenheit.[27]

Finger Phototransmission

The degree of peripheral vasoconstriction can also be measured indirectly using a photoplethysmograph. This instrument monitors the amount of light that can pass through a finger or toe, reflect off a bone

Biofeedback instruments measure

- Peripheral skin temperature
- Finger phototransmission
- Skin conductance activity
- Electromyographic activity

and pass back through the soft tissue to a light sensor. As the volume of blood in a given area increases, the amount of light detected by the sensor decreases, thus giving some indication of blood volume. Only changes in blood volume can be detected, since there are no standardized units of measure. These instruments are used most often to monitor pulse.[17]

Skin Conductance Activity

Sweat gland activity can be indirectly measured by determining electrodermal activity, most commonly referred to as the *galvanic skin response*. Sweat contains salt, which increases electrical conductivity; thus, sweaty skin is more conductive than dry skin. This instrument applies a very small electrical voltage to the skin, usually on the palmar surface of the hand or the volar surface of the fingers where there are a lot of sweat glands, and measures the impedance of the electrical current in microhm units. Measuring skin conductance is a technique useful in objectively assessing psychophysiological arousal and is most often used in lie detector testing.[27]

ELECTROMYOGRAPHIC BIOFEEDBACK

Electromyographic biofeedback is certainly the most typically used of all the biofeedback modalities in a clinical setting. Muscle contraction results from the more or less synchronous contraction of individual muscle fibers that compose a muscle. Individual muscle fibers are innervated by nerves that collectively comprise a motor unit. The axon of that motor unit conducts an action potential to the neuromuscular junction where a neurotransmitter substance (acetylcholine) is released. As this neurotransmitter binds to receptor sites on the

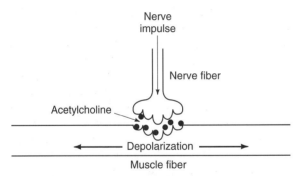

Nerve impulse

Nerve fiber

Acetylcholine

Depolarization

Muscle fiber

Figure 13-1   The nerve fiber conducts an impulse to the neuromuscular junction where acetylcholine binds to receptor sites on the sarcolemma inducing a depolarization of the muscle fiber, which creates movement of ions and thus an electrochemical gradient around the muscle fiber.

sarcolemma, depolarization of that muscle fiber occurs moving in both directions along the muscle fiber, creating movement of ions and thus an electrochemical gradient around the muscle fiber. Changes in potential difference or voltage associated with depolarization can be detected by an electrode placed in close proximity (Figure 13-1).

Motor Unit Recruitment

The amount of tension developed in a muscle is determined by the number of active motor units. As more motor units are recruited and as the frequency of discharge increases, muscle tension increases.

The pattern of motor unit recruitment varies, depending on the inherent properties of specific motorneurons, the force required during the activity, and the speed of contraction. Smaller motor units are recruited first and are somewhat limited in their ability to generate tension. Larger motor units generate greater tension since more muscle fibers are recruited.

Motor units are recruited based on the force required in an activity and not based on the type of contraction performed. Thus, the firing rate and recruitment of the motor units is dependent on the external force required. The speed of contraction also influences motor unit recruitment. Fast contractions tend to excite larger motor units and depress the smaller motor units.

• electromyograph measures electrical activity of muscle and not muscle contraction

Measuring Electrical Activity

Despite the fact that biofeedback is used to determine muscle activity, it does not measure muscle contraction directly. Instead, it measures electrical activity associated with muscle contraction. Movement of ions across the membrane creates a depolarization of the muscle membranes, resulting in a reversal in polarity, followed by repolarization. The various stages of membrane activity generate a triphasic electrical signal.[4] Electrical activity of the muscle is measured in volts, or more precisely, microvolts (1 volt = 1,000,000 microvolts).

Measurement of electrical activity is made in standard quantitative units. Monitoring is useful in detecting changes in electrical activity, although changes cannot be quantified. The advantage of measurement over monitoring is that an objective scale is used on which comparisons can be made between different individuals, occasions, and instruments. Measurement allows procedures to be replicated.

Unfortunately, with biofeedback units there is no universally accepted standardized measurement scale. Each brand of biofeedback unit serves as its own reference standard. Different brands of biofeedback equipment may give different readings for the same degree of muscle contraction. Consequently, biofeedback readings can only be compared when the same equipment is used for all readings.[27]

The biofeedback unit receives small amounts of electrical energy generated during muscle contraction through some type of electrode. It then separates or filters this electrical energy from other extraneous electrical activity on the skin and amplifies the electrical energy. The amplified electrical activity is then converted to some type of information that has meaning to the user. Figure 13-2a is a diagram of the various components of a biofeedback unit.

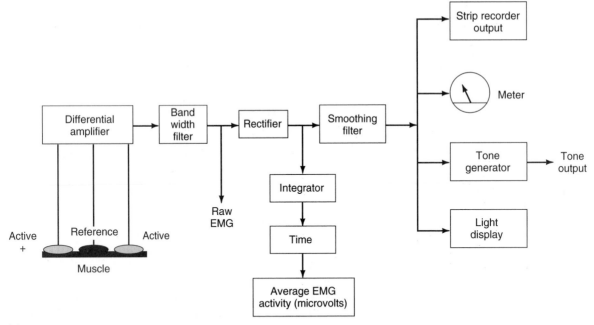

(a)

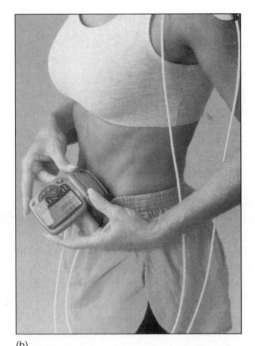

(b)

Figure 13-2 (a) The anatomy of a typical biofeedback unit. (b) Biofeedback unit.
(Courtesy EMG Retrainer)

Separation and Amplification of Electrical Activity

Once the electrodes detect the electrical activity, the extraneous electrical activity or **"noise"** must be eliminated before the electrical activity is amplified and subsequently objectified. This is accomplished by using two **active electrodes** and a single ground or **reference electrode** in a **bipolar arrangement** to create three separate pathways from the skin to the biofeedback unit (Figure 13-3). The active electrodes should be placed in close proximity to one another, while the reference electrode may be placed anywhere on the body. Typically in biofeedback, the reference electrode is placed between the two active electrodes.

The active electrodes pick up electrical activity from motor units firing in the muscles beneath the electrodes. The magnitude of the small voltages detected by each active electrode will differ with respect to the reference electrode creating two separate signals. These two signals are then fed to a **differential amplifier** that subtracts the signal from one active electrode from the other active elec-

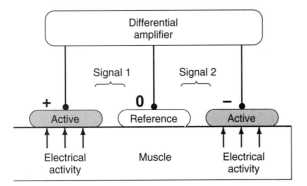

Figure 13-3   The differential amplifier monitors the two separate signals from the active electrodes and amplifies the difference, thus eliminating extraneous noise.

trode. This in effect cancels out or rejects any components that the two signals coming from the active electrodes have in common, thus amplifying the difference between the signals. The differential amplifier uses the reference electrode to compare the signals of the two active or recording electrodes (Figure 13-3).

There will always be some degree of extraneous electrical activity created by power lines, motors, lights, appliances, etc., which is picked up by the body and is eventually detected by the surface electrodes on the skin. Assuming that this extraneous "noise" is detected equally by both active electrodes, the differential amplifier will subtract the noise detected by one active electrode from the noise detected by the other active electrode, leaving only the true difference between the active electrodes. The ability of the differential amplifier to eliminate the common noise between the active electrodes is called the **common mode rejection ratio (CMRR)**.

External noise can be further reduced by using **filters** that essentially make the amplifier more sensitive to some incoming frequencies and less sensitive to others. Therefore, the amplifier will pick up signals only at those frequencies produced by electrical activity in the muscle within a specific frequency range or **bandwidth**. In general, the wider the bandwidth, the higher the noise readings.

noise   Extraneous electrical activity that may be produced by any source other than the contracting muscle.

active electrode   An electrode attached directly to the skin over a muscle that picks up the electrical activity produced by a muscle contraction.

reference electrode   Also referred to as the ground electrode, it serves as a point of reference to compare the electrical activity recorded by the active electrodes.

bipolar arrangement   Two active recording electrodes placed in close proximity to one another.

differential amplifier   Monitors the two separate signals from the active electrodes and amplifies the difference, thus eliminating extraneous noise.

common mode rejection ratio (CMRR)   The ability of the differential amplifier to eliminate the common noise between the active electrodes.

filters   Help to reduce external noise that essentially makes the amplifier more sensitive to some incoming frequencies and less sensitive to others.

bandwidth   A specific frequency range in which the amplifier will pick up signals produced by electrical activity in the muscle.

■ **Clinical Decision-Making**   *Exercise 13-2*

What are the three most important considerations for the athletic trainer who is trying to make a decision regarding the correct placement of electrodes?

It must be noted that the athletic trainer is interested in measuring the electrical activity within the muscle. An excessive external noise that is not eliminated by the biofeedback instrument will mask true electrical activity and will significantly decrease the reliability of the information being generated by that device.

raw A form in which the electrical activity produced by muscle contraction may be displayed and/or recorded before the signal is processed.

rectification A signal processing technique that changes the deflection of the waveform from the negative pole to the positive pole, essentially creating a pulsed direct current.

smoothing A signal processing technique that eliminates the high frequency fluctuations that are produced with a changing electrical signal.

integration A signal processing technique that measures the area under the curve for a specified period of time, thus forming the basis for quantification of electrical activity.

Converting Electrical Activity to Meaningful Information

After amplification and filtering, the electrical signal is indicative of the true electrical activity within the muscles being monitored. This is referred to as **"raw"** activity. Raw activity is an alternating voltage, which means that the direction or polarity is constantly reversing (Figure 13-4a). The amplitude of the oscillations increases to a maximum then diminishes. Biofeedback measures the overall increase and decrease in electrical activity. To obtain this measurement, the deflection toward the negative pole must be flipped upward toward the positive pole; otherwise the sum total of their deflections would cancel out one another (Figure 13-4b). This process is referred to as **rectification**, which essentially creates a pulsed direct current (DC).

    Processing the Electrical Signal. The rectified signal can be **smoothed** and **integrated**. Smoothing the signal means eliminating the peaks and valleys or eliminating the high-frequency fluctuations that are produced with a changing electrical signal (Figure 13-4c). Once the signal has been smoothed, the signal may be integrated by measuring the area under the curve for a specified period of time. Integration forms the basis for quantification of electrical activity (Figure 13-4d).

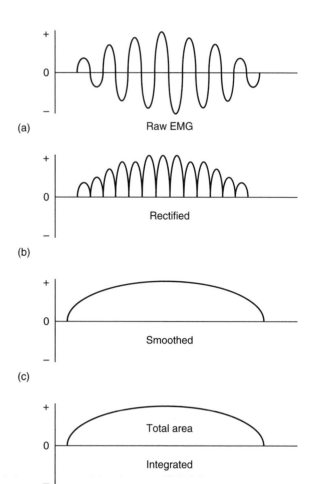

Figure 13-4 Processing an electrical signal involves taking (a) raw activity and then (b) rectifying, (c) smoothing, and (d) integrating it so that the information can be presented in some meaningful format.

Providing Summary Information

Some of the newer and somewhat more expensive biofeedback units have the capability of providing the user with a variety of information that summarizes or even compares the athlete's performance during treatment sessions. Descriptive statistical information relative to performance may be calculated if desired and compared with performance during previous treatment sessions to give

■ Analogy   *13-1*

Coaches routinely use verbal and visual feedback to provide information to the athlete about a specific performance technique or skill. For example, on occasion a video camera may be used so that the athlete can see visually for herself how to alter her body mechanics to produce a more effective performance. Similarly, the athletic trainer may use visual or auditory biofeedback to let the athlete know when she is contracting a muscle at the correct moment or at an appropriate intensity level.

■ Analogy   *13-2*

Taking raw activity and turning it into meaningful information is much like writing a research paper. You begin by taking notes on a particular topic from a variety of sources and scribbling them down on a piece of paper. Then you begin to format and integrate all of the information into a rough draft. Then you work to smooth out the rough spots before turning in that project in a form that it makes sense to whoever is reading it. The reader then interprets the information within the paper to see if it is useful.

the athletic trainer some indication of the progress being made by the athlete. The units provide objective feedback to the athlete, which can certainly serve as a source of motivation throughout the rehabilitative process.

EQUIPMENT SETUP

It is imperative that the athletic trainer have some understanding of how biofeedback units monitor and record the electrical activity being produced in a muscle before attempting to set up and use the biofeedback unit in treatment of an athlete. Specific treatment protocols involve skin preparation, application of electrodes, selection of feedback or output modes, and selection of sensitivity settings—all of which have been previously discussed. Once these are complete, the athletic trainer should

• Most biofeedback units use surface electrodes

choose to have the athlete sitting, lying, or occasionally standing in a comfortable position, depending on the treatment objectives. Generally, the athletic trainer should begin with easier tasks and progressively make the activities more difficult. Teaching the athlete how to appropriately use the biofeedback unit and briefly explaining what is being measured are essential. In most cases, it is recommended that the athletic trainer attach the biofeedback unit to himself and then demonstrate to the athlete exactly what is to be done during the treatment.[20]

Skin Preparation

Prior to attachment of the surface electrodes, the skin must be appropriately prepared by removing oil and dead skin along with excessive hair from the surface to reduce skin impedance. Scrubbing with an alcohol-soaked prep pad is recommended.[36] However, if the skin is cleaned until it becomes irritated, it may interfere with biofeedback recording.

Electrodes

Type.   Skin surface electrodes are most often used in biofeedback. Fine-wire, indwelling electrodes may also be used, which permit localized, highly accurate measurement of electrical activity. However, these electrodes must be inserted percutaneously and thus are relatively impractical in a clinical setting.

Various types of surface electrodes are available for use with biofeedback units. Electrodes are most often made of stainless steel or nickel-plated brass recessed in a plastic holder. These less expensive electrodes are effective in biofeedback applications. More expensive electrodes made of gold or silver/silver chloride have also been used.[36]

■ **Clinical Decision-Making** *Exercise 13-3*

There are two biofeedback units made by different manufacturers available for use in the training room. The athletic trainer has been using the same unit to work on muscle strengthening with an injured athlete throughout his rehabilitation process. Unfortunately, that generator has broken, and he is forced to use the other one. Can comparisons be made from one unit to another?

Some surface electrodes are permanently attached to cable wires while others may snap onto the wire. Some biofeedback units include a set of three electrodes preplaced on a velcro band that may be easily attached to the skin.

Size. The size of the electrodes may range between 4 mm in diameter for recording small muscle activity and 12.5 mm for use with larger muscle groups. Increasing the size of the electrode will not cause an increase in the amplitude of the signal.[20]

Disposable versus Nondisposable. Regardless of whether electrodes are disposable or nondisposable, some type of conducting gel, paste, or cream with high salt content is necessary to establish a highly conductive connection with the skin. Disposable electrodes come with the appropriate amount of gel and an adhesive ring already applied so that the electrode can be easily connected to the skin. Nondisposable electrodes need to have a double-sided adhesive ring applied. Then enough conducting gel must be added such that it is level with the surface of the adhesive ring before the electrode is applied to the skin.

Electrode Placement. The electrodes should be placed as near to the muscle being monitored as possible to minimize recording extraneous electrical activity. They should be secured with the body part in the position in which it will be monitored so that movement of the skin will not alter the positioning of the electrodes over a particular muscle[36] (Figure 13-5). The electrodes should be parallel to the direction of the muscle fibers to ensure

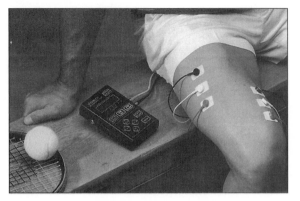

Figure 13-5 The biofeedback unit is connected via a series of electrodes to the skin over the contracting muscle.

Raw activity may be

• Rectified
• Smoothed
• Integrated

that a better sample of muscle activity is monitored while reducing extraneous electrical activity.

Spacing of the electrodes is also a critical consideration. Electrodes generally detect measurable signals from a distance equal to that of the interelectrode spacing. Therefore, as the distance between the electrodes increases, the biofeedback signal will include electrical activity not only from muscles directly under the electrodes but also from other nearby muscles.[4]

Displaying Biofeedback Information

At this point it is necessary to take the biofeedback signal and display this information in a form that has some meaning. Biofeedback units generally provide either visual or auditory feedback relative to the quantity of electrical activity. Some biofeedback units can provide both visual and auditory feedback depending on the output mode selected.

Visual Feedback. Raw activity is usually displayed visually on an oscilloscope. On most biofeedback units, integrated activity is visually

• Biofeedback information may be visual or auditory or both

signal gain   Determines the signal sensitivity. If a high gain is chosen, the biofeedback unit will have a high sensitivity for the muscle activity signal.

presented either as a line traveling across a monitor, as a light or series of lights that go on and off, or as a bar graph that changes dimension—all of which change in response to the incoming integrated signal. Some of the newer biofeedback units have incorporated video games as part of their visual feedback system. If a biofeedback unit uses some type of meter, it may either be calibrated in objective units, such as microvolts, or it may simply give some relative scale of measure.[36]

Meters may also be either analog or digital. Analog meters have a continuous scale and a needle that indicates the level of electrical activity within a particular range. Digital meters display only a number. They are very simple and easy to read. However, the disadvantage of a digital meter is that it is more difficult to tell where in a given range the signal falls.

Audio Feedback.   On some biofeedback units, raw activity can be listened to and is one type of audio feedback. The majority of biofeedback units have audio feedback that produces some tone, buzzing, beeping, or clicking. An increase in the pitch of a tone, buzz, or beep, or an increase in the frequency of clicking indicates an increase in the level of electrical activity. This would be most useful for individuals who need to strengthen muscle contractions. Conversely, decreases in pitch or frequency indicating a decrease in electrical activity would be most useful in teaching athletes to relax.

Setting Sensitivity.   Signal sensitivity or **signal gain** may be set by the athletic trainer on many biofeedback units. If a high gain is chosen, the biofeedback unit will have a high sensitivity for the muscle activity signal. Sensitivity may be set at 1 uV, 10 uV, or 100 uV. A 1-uV setting is sensitive enough to detect the smallest amounts of electrical activity and thus has the highest signal

■ **Clinical Decision-Making**   *Exercise 13-4*

The athletic trainer is using a biofeedback unit for muscle re-education of the hamstrings following knee surgery. The athlete wants to know how the biofeedback unit is going to measure his muscle contraction. How should the athletic trainer respond?

gain. High-sensitivity levels should be used during relaxation training. Comparatively lower sensitivity levels would be more useful in muscle re-education during which the athlete may produce several hundred microvolts of electrical activity. Generally, when adjusting the sensitivity range, it should be set at the lowest level that does not elicit feedback at rest.

CLINICAL APPLICATIONS FOR BIOFEEDBACK

There are a number of clinical conditions for which biofeedback would be useful as a therapeutic modality. The primary applications for using biofeedback include muscle re-education, which involves regaining neuromuscular control and/or increasing strength of a muscle; relaxation of muscle spasm or muscle guarding; and pain reduction.

Muscle Re-Education

The goal in muscle re-education is to provide feedback that will re-establish neuromuscular control or promote the ability of a muscle or group of muscles to contract. It may also be used to regain normal agonist/antagonist muscle action and for postural control retraining. Biofeedback is used to indicate the electrical activity associated with that muscle contraction.[16]

When biofeedback is being used to elicit a muscle contraction, the sensitivity setting should be chosen by having the athlete perform a maximum isometric contraction of the target muscle. Then the gain should be adjusted such that the athlete will be able to achieve the maximum on about two-thirds of the muscle contractions. If the athlete cannot produce a muscle contraction, the athletic trainer should attempt to facilitate a contraction by stroking or tapping the target muscle. It is also helpful to have the athlete look at the muscle when trying to contract. It may be necessary to move the active electrodes to the contralateral limb and have the athlete practice the "muscle" contraction you hope to achieve on the opposite side.

The athlete should maximally contract the target muscle isometrically for 6 to 10 seconds. During this contraction, the visual or auditory feedback should be at a maximum and should be closely monitored by both the athletic trainer and the athlete. Between each contraction the athlete should be instructed to completely relax the muscle such that the feedback mode returns to baseline or zero prior to initiating another contraction. A period of 5 to 10 minutes working with a single muscle or muscle group is most desirable since longer periods tend to produce fatigue and boredom, neither of which is conducive to optimal learning.[19]

As increases in electrical activity occur, the athlete should develop the ability to rapidly activate motor units. This can be accomplished by setting the sensitivity level to 60 to 80% of maximum isometric activity and instructing the athlete to reach that level as many times as possible during a given time period (i.e., 10 or 30 seconds). Again, total relaxation must occur between contractions.

For the athlete, it is essential that the treatment be functionally relevant. Attention to mobility and muscle power cannot be neglected in favor of biofeedback therapy.[19] The athletic trainer should have the athlete perform functional movements while simultaneously observing body mechanics

---

muscle guarding   A protective response in muscle that results from pain or fear of movement.

■ **Clinical Decision-Making**   *Exercise 13-5*

The athletic trainer wishes to use a biofeedback unit to help an injured athlete learn to relax muscle guarding in the low back following a contusion. Should the athletic trainer use a high-sensitivity or low-sensitivity setting and why?

■ **Analogy**   *13-3*

Recruiting motor units to produce tension in a muscle is like playing tug-of-war. If two people begin pulling on a rope from either end and gradually additional people begin to grab hold and tug on that rope at each end, the rope gets tighter and tighter. As more and more motor units are recruited, the tension in a muscle will continue to increase.

---

and the related electrical activity. Then recommendations can be made as to how movements can be altered to elicit normal responses.[8] Biofeedback is useful in athletes who perform poorly on manual muscle tests. If the athlete can only elicit a fair, trace or zero grade, then biofeedback should be incorporated. Stronger muscles should generally be given resistive exercises rather than biofeedback,[19] although biofeedback has been recommended for increasing the strength of healthy muscle.[10,19]

Relaxation of Muscle Guarding

Often in a clinical setting, athletes demonstrate a protective response in muscle that results from pain or fear of movement that is most accurately described as **muscle guarding**. Muscle guarding must be differentiated from those neuromuscular problems arising from central nervous system deficits that result in a clinical condition known as muscle spasticity. For the athletic trainer treating athletes exhibiting muscle guarding, the goal is to induce relaxation of the muscle by reducing electrical activity through the use of biofeedback.[19]

Since muscle guarding most often involves fear of pain that may result when the muscle moves, perhaps the most important goal in treatment is to modulate pain. This is best accomplished through the use of other modalities such as ice or electrical stimulation.

Biofeedback treatments should be designed so that the athlete experiences success from the first treatment. The athlete is now attempting to reduce the visual or auditory feedback to zero. Initially, positioning of the athlete in a comfortable relaxed position is critical to reduction in muscle guarding. A high-sensitivity setting should be selected so that any electrical activity in the muscle will be easily detected.

During relaxation training, the athlete should be given verbal cues that will enhance relaxation of individual muscles, muscle groups, or body segments. For example, with individual muscles or small muscle groups, the athlete may be instructed to contract then relax a specific muscle or to imagine a feeling of warmth within the muscle. For larger muscle groups, using mental imagery or deep breathing exercises may be useful.

As relaxation progresses, the spacing between the electrodes should be increased. Also, the sensitivity setting should move from low to high. Both of these changes will require the athlete to relax more muscles, thus achieving greater relaxation. The athlete must then apply this newly learned relaxation technique in different positions that are potentially more uncomfortable. Again, the goal is to eliminate muscle guarding during functional activities.[19]

Pain Reduction

A number of therapeutic modalities discussed in this text are used for the purpose of reducing or modulating pain. As mentioned in the section on muscle guarding, biofeedback can be used to relax muscles

■ **TABLE 13-1**   Summary of Indications and Contraindications for Biofeedback

INDICATIONS

Muscle re-education
Regaining neuromuscular control
Increasing isometric and isotonic strength of a muscle
Relaxation of muscle spasm
Decreasing muscle guarding
Pain reduction
Psychological relaxation

CONTRAINDICATIONS

Any musculoskeletal condition in which a muscular contraction might potentially exacerbate that condition.

■ **Clinical Decision-Making**   *Exercise 13-6*

An athlete has a sprain of a vertebral ligament in the lumbar region of the low back with accompanying muscle guarding. What modalities might potentially be used to reduce and/or eliminate this muscle guarding?

that are tense secondary to fear of pain on movement. If the muscle can be relaxed, then chances are that breaking the "pain-guarding-pain" cycle will also reduce pain. It has been experimentally demonstrated to reduce pain in headaches[2,7,9] and low back pain.[8,25,31] Pain modulation is often associated with techniques of imagery and progressive relaxation.

Treating Neurological Conditions.   Biofeedback has been identified as an effective technique for treating a variety of neurologic conditions, including hemiplegia following stroke,[15,23,29] spinal cord injury,[6,18] spacicity,[1,23] cerebral palsy,[3] facial paralysis,[5] urinary incontinence,[32] and fecal incontinence.[33]

Summary

1. Biofeedback is a therapeutic procedure that uses electronic or electromechanical instruments to accurately measure, process, and feed back reinforcing information via auditory or visual signals.
2. Perhaps the biggest advantage of biofeedback is that it provides the athlete with a chance to make correct small changes in performance that are immediately noted and rewarded so that eventually larger changes or improvements in performance can be accomplished.
3. Several different types of biofeedback modalities are available for use in rehabilitation, with biofeedback being the most widely used in a clinical setting.
4. A biofeedback unit measures the electrical activity produced by depolarization of a muscle fiber as an indicator of the quality of a muscle contraction.
5. The biofeedback unit receives small amounts of electrical energy generated during muscle contraction through active electrodes, then separates or filters extraneous electrical energy via a differential amplifier before it is processed and subsequently converted to some type of information that has meaning to the user.
6. Biofeedback information is displayed either visually, using lights or meters, or auditorily, using tones, beeps, buzzes, or clicks.
7. High-sensitivity levels should be used during relaxation training, while comparatively lower sensitivity levels would be more useful in muscle re-education.
8. In a clinical setting, biofeedback is most typically used for muscle re-education, to decrease muscle guarding, or for pain reduction.

Review Questions

1. What is biofeedback and how can it be used in sports injury rehabilitation?
2. What are the various types of biofeedback instruments that are available to the athletic trainer?
3. How can the electrical activity generated by a muscle contraction be measured using a biofeedback unit?
4. What are the important considerations for attaching biofeedback electrodes?
5. How is the electrical activity picked up by the electrodes amplified, processed, and converted to meaningful information by the biofeedback unit?
6. What are the advantages and disadvantages of using visual and auditory feedback?
7. How should sensitivity settings be changed during relaxation training versus during muscle re-education?
8. What are the most common uses for biofeedback in an athletic training setting?

 ## Self-Test Questions

T/F
1. Biofeedback units measure physiologic processes.
2. The reference electrode has no charge associated with it.
3. A high-signal gain means the biofeedback unit has a low sensitivity for muscle activity.

Multiple Choice
4. Some biofeedback instruments measure peripheral skin temperature. Which of the following do they also measure?
   a. finger phototransmission
   b. skin conductance activity
   c. electromyographic activity
   d. all of the above

5. Biofeedback electrodes should be placed as near to the muscle of interest as possible. They should also be placed _____ to the muscle.
   a. perpendicular
   b. parallel
   c. obliquely
   d. none of the above
6. What is the principle that allows the biofeedback unit to eliminate common noise between active electrodes?
   a. common mode rejection ratio
   b. filtering
   c. rectification
   d. integration
7. Raw EMG must be converted to a visual or audio format. What is the order of that conversion?
   a. integrated, rectified, smoothed
   b. smoothed, rectified, integrated
   c. rectified, smoothed, integrated
   d. rectified, integrated, smoothed
8. The goal of using biofeedback in muscle re-education is to elicit a _____
   a. twitch response
   b. muscle contraction
   c. decrease in pain
   d. relaxation
9. How long should the average biofeedback period for a single muscle be to avoid fatigue and boredom?
   a. 1–2 minutes
   b. 2–5 minutes
   c. 5–10 minutes
   d. 10–15 minutes
10. What factor(s) must be addressed when using biofeedback to relax muscle guarding?
   a. pain
   b. mental imagery
   c. apprehension
   d. all of the above

Solutions to Clinical Decision-Making Exercises

13-1 The athletic trainer can act as a substitute biofeedback unit. The athlete should be instructed to watch the VMO as he or she tries to contract the muscle. This will serve as visual feedback. The athletic trainer can help to facilitate a contraction by tapping or stroking the muscle. Also by maintaining physical contact with the muscle, the athletic trainer, using verbal feedback, can let the athlete know when the muscle is actually contracted.

13-2 They should be placed as close to the muscle as possible to minimize "noise." They should be placed parallel to the direction of the muscle fibers. The spacing should be close enough to monitor activity from a specific muscle. If spaced too far apart, electrical activity from other anatomically close muscles may also be detected.

13-3 With biofeedback units, there is no universally accepted or standardized measurement scale. Different machines are likely to give different readings for the same degree of muscle contraction. Each manufacturer has its own reference standards for its particular unit.

Thus, information provided from these different units cannot be compared.

13-4 Biofeedback units do not directly measure muscle contraction. Instead, they measure only the electrical activity associated with a muscle contraction. Thus, the athlete should understand that the electrical activity infers some information about the quality of a muscle contraction but does not measure the strength of that muscle contraction specifically.

13-5 The athletic trainer should set the signal gain on the biofeedback unit at a high-sensitivity setting whenever the goal is relaxation, while a low-sensitivity setting should be used with muscle re-education.

13-6 There are several modalities that could potentially help reduce muscle guarding including thermotherapy, cryotherapy, and electrical stimulation. A recommendation would be to first use electrical stimulation to break the pain guarding cycle. Once pain has been modulated, a biofeedback unit may be used to help the athlete learn to relax the low back muscles and to keep them relaxed as movement occurs.

References

1. Amato, A, Hermomeyer, C, and Kleinman, K: Use of electromyographic feedback to increase control of spastic muscles, *Phys Ther* 53: 1063, 1973.

2. Arena, J, Bruno, G, and Hannah, S: A comparison of frontal electromyographic biofeedback training, trapezius electromyographic biofeedback training, and progressive muscle relaxation therapy in the treatment of tension headache, *Headache* 35(7):411–419, 1995.

3. Asato, H, Twiggs, D, and Ellison, S: EMG biofeedback training for a mentally retarded individual with cerebral palsy, *Phys Ther* 61:1447–1451, 1981.

4. Basmajian, J: Description and analysis of EMG signal. In Basmajian, J., and Deluca, C, editors: *Muscles alive: their functions revealed by electromyography*, Baltimore, 1985, Williams & Wilkins.

5. Brown, D, Nahai, F, and Wolf, S: Electromyographic feedback in the re-education of facial palsy, *Am J Phys Med* 57:183–190, 1978.

6. Brucker, B, and Bulaeva, N: Biofeedback effect on electromyography responses in athletes with spinal cord injury, *Arch Phy Med Rehab* 77(2):133–137, 1996.

7. Budzynski, D: Biofeedback strategies in headache treatment. In Basmajian J, editor: *Biofeedback: principles and practice for clinicians*, Baltimore, 1989, Williams & Wilkins.

8. Bush, C, Ditto, B, and Feuerstein, M: Controlled evaluation of paraspinal EMG biofeedback in the treatment of chronic low back pain, *Health Psychol* 4:307–321, 1985.

9. Chapman, S: A review and clinical perspective on the use of EMG and thermal biofeedback for chronic headaches, *Pain* 27:1, 1986.

10. Croce, R: The effects of EMG biofeedback on strength acquisition, *Biofeedback Self Regul* 9:395, 1986.

11. Davlin, CD, Holcomb, WR, and Guadagnoli, MA: The effect of hip position and electromyographic biofeedback training on the vastus medialis oblique: vastus lateralis ratio, *Journal of Athletic Training*. 34(4):342–349, 1999.

12. Draper, V: Electromyographic feedback and recovery in quadriceps femoris muscle function following anterior cruciate ligament reconstruction, *Phys Ther* 70:25, 1990.

13. Draper, V, Lyle, L, and Seymour. T: From the field: EMG biofeedback versus electrical stimulation in the recovery of quadriceps surface EMG, *Clinical Kinesiology: Journal of the American Kinesiotherapy Association*, 51(2):28–32, 1997.

14. Draper, V, Lyle, L, and Seymour, T: EMG biofeedback versus electrical stimulation in the recovery of quadriceps surface EMG, Clinical Kinesiology, 51(2):28–32, 1997.

15. Engardt, M: Term effects of auditory feedback training on relearned symmetrical body weight distribution in stroke athletes: a follow-up study, *Scand J Rehab Med* 26(2): 65–69, 1994.

16. Fogel, E: Biofeedback-assisted musculoskeletal therapy and neuromuscular re-education. In Schwartz, MS editor: *Biofeedback: a practitioner's guide*, New York, 1987, Guilford.

17. Jennings, J, Tahmoush, A, and Redmond, D: Non-invasive measurement of peripheral vascular activity. In Martin, I, and Venables, PH, editors: *Techniques in psychophysiology*, New York, 1980, Wiley.

18. Klose, K, Needham, B, and Schmidt, D: An assessment of the contribution of electromyographic biofeedback as a therapy in the physical training of spinal cord injured persons, *Arch Phys Med Rehab* 74(5):453–456, 1993.

19. Krebs, D: Neuromuscular re-education and gait training. In Schwartz, M, editor: *Biofeedback: a practitioner's guide*, New York, 1987, Guilford.

20. LeCraw, D, and Wolf, S: Electromyographic biofeedback (EMGBF) for neuromuscular relaxation and re-education. In Gersh, M, editor: *Electrotherapy in rehabilitation*, Philadelphia, 1992, FA Davis.

21. Linsay, KA: Electromyographic biofeedback. *Athletic Therapy Today* 2(4):49, July 1997.

22. Miller, N: Biomedical foundations for biofeedback as a part of behavioral medicine. In Basmajian, J, editor: *Biofeedback principles and practice for clinicians*, Baltimore, 1989, Williams & Wilkins.

23. Moreland, J, and Thompson, M: Efficacy of EMG biofeedback compared with conventional physical therapy for upper extremity function in athletes following stroke: a research overview and meta-analysis, *Phys Ther* 74(6): 534–543, 1994.

24. Moreland, JD, Thomson, MA, and Fuoco, AR: Electromyographic biofeedback to improve lower extremity function after stroke: a meta-analysis, *Archives of Physical Medicine & Rehabilitation*, 79(2): 134–140, 1998.

25. Nouwen, A, and Bush, C: The relationship between paraspinal EMG and chronic low back pain, *Pain* 20:109–123, 1984.

26. Olson, R: Definitions of Biofeedback. In Schwartz, M, editor: *Biofeedback: a practitioner's guide*, New York, 1987, Guilford.

27. Peek, C: A primer of biofeedback instrumentation. In Schwartz, M, editor: *Biofeedback: a practitioner's guide*, New York, 1987, Guilford.

28. Regenos, E, and Wolf, S: Involuntary single motor unit discharges in spastic muscles during EMG biofeedback training, *Arch Phys Med Rehab* 60:72–73, 1979.

29. Schleenbaker, R, and Mainous, A: Electromyographic biofeedback for neuromuscular reeducation in the hemiplegic stroke athlete: a meta-analysis, *Arch Phys Med Rehab* 74(12):1301–1304, 1993.

30. Shinopulos, NM, and Jacobson, J: Relationship between health promotion lifestyle profiles and patient outcomes of biofeedback therapy for urinary incontinence, *Urologic Nursing* 19(4):249–53, 1999.

31. Studkey, S, Jacobs, A, and Goldfarb, J: EMG biofeedback training, relaxation training, and placebo for the relief of chronic back pain, *Percept Mot Skills* 63:1023, 1986.

32. Sugar, E, and Firlit, C: Urodynamic feedback: a new therapeutic approach to childhood incontinence/infection, *J Urol* 128:1253, 1982.

33. Whitehead, W: Treatment of fecal incontinence in children with spina bifida: comparison of biofeedback and behavior modification, *Arch Phys Med Rehab* 67:218, 1986.

34. Wolf, S, and Binder-Macleod, S: Electromyographic feedback in the physical therapy clinic. In Basmajian, JV, editor: *Biofeedback principles and practice for clinicians*, Baltimore, 1989, Williams & Wilkins.

35. Wolf, S, and Binder-Macleod, S: Neurophysiological factors in electromyographic feedback for neuromotor disturbances. In Basmajian, JV, editor: *Biofeedback principles and practice for clinicians*, Baltimore, 1989, Williams & Wilkins.

36. Wolf, S: Treatment of neuromuscular problems, treatment of musculoskeletal problems. In Sandweiss, J, editor: *Biofeedback review seminars*, Los Angeles, 1982, University of California.

37. Wong, AMK, Lee, M, Chang, WH, and Tang, F: Clinical trial of a cervical traction modality with electromyographic biofeedback, *American Journal of Physical Medicine & Rehabilitation* 76(1):19–25, 1997.

Suggested Readings

Baker, M, Regenos, E, and Wolf, S: Developing strategies for biofeedback: applications in neurologically handicapped athletes, *Phys Ther* 57:402–408, 1977.

Baker, M, Hudson, J, and Wolf, S: "Feedback" cane to improve the hemiplegic patient's gait: suggestion from the field, *Phys Ther* 59:170, 1979.

Balliet, R, Levy, B, and Blood, K: Upper extremity sensory feedback therapy in chronic cerebrovascular accident patients with impaired expressive aphasia and auditory comprehension, *Arch Phys Med Rehabil* 67:304, 1986.

Basmajian, J, and Samson, J: Special review: standardization of methods in single motor unit training, *Am. J. Phys. Med.* 52:250–256, 1973.

Basmajian, J, Kukulka, C, Narayan, M, and Takebe, K: Biofeedback treatment of foot drop after stroke compared with standard rehabilitation technique: effects on voluntary control and strength, *Arch. Phys. Med. Rehabil.* 56:231–236, 1975.

Basmajian, J: Learned control of single motor units. In Beatty, J, and Schwartz, J: editors: *Biofeedback: theory and reorg.*, New York, 1977, Academic Press.

Basmajian, J: *Biofeedback: principles and practice for clinicians*, Baltimore, 1989, Williams & Wilkins.

Basmajian, J, and Blumenthal, R: Electroplacement in electromyographic biofeedback. In Basmajian, JV, editor: *Biofeedback: principles and practice for clinicians*, ed 3, Baltimore, 1989, Williams & Wilkins.

Basmajian, J, Regenos, E, and Baker, M: Rehabilitating stroke athletes with biofeedback, *Geriatrics* 32:85, 1977.

Basmajian, J: Biofeedback in rehabilitation: a review of principles and practices, *Arch Phys Med Rehabil* 62:469, 1981.

Beal, M, Diefenbach, G, and Allen, A: Electromyographic biofeedback in the treatment of voluntary posterior instability of the shoulder, *Am J of Sports Med* 15: 175, 1987.

Bernat, S, Wooldridge, P, and Marecki, M: Biofeedback-assisted relaxation to reduce stress in labor, *J Obstetric, Gynecologic, Neonatal Nursing* (4):295–303, 1992.

Biedermann, H: Comments on the reliability of muscle activity comparisons in EMG biofeedback research with back pain athletes, *Biofeedback Self Regul* 9:451–458, 1984.

Biedermann, H, McGhie, A, and Monga, T: Perceived and actual control in EMG treatment of back pain, *Behav Res Ther.* 25:137–147, 1987.

Bowman, B, Baker, L, and Waters, R: Positional feedback and electrical stimulation: an automated treatment for the hemiplegic wrist, *Arch Phys Med Rehabil* 60:497, 1979.

Brudny, J, Grynbaum, B, and Korein, J: Spasmodic torticollis: treatment by feedback display of EMG, *Archives of Physical Medicine and Rehabilitation* 55:403–408, 1974.

Burke, R: Motor unit recruitment: what are the critical factors? In Desmedt, J, editor: *Progress in clinical neurophysiology*, vol 9, Karger, Basel, 1981.

Burnside, I, Tobias, H, and Bursill, D: Electromyographic feedback in the rehabilitation of stroke athletes: a controlled trial, *Arch Phys Med Rehabil* 63: 217, 1982.

Burnside, I, Tobias, H, and Bursill, D: Electromyographic feedback in the remobilization of stroke athletes: a controlled trial, *Arch Phys Med Rehabil* 63: 1393, 1983.

Carlsson, S: Treatment of temporo-mandibular joint syndrome with biofeedback training, *J Am Dental Assoc* 91, 602–605, 1975.

Christie, D, Dewitt, R, and Kaltenbach, P: Using EMG biofeedback to signal hyperactive children when to relax, *Except. Child.* 50:547–548, 1984.

Cox, R, and Matyas, T: Myoelectric and force feedback in the facilitation of isometric strength training: a controlled comparison, *Psychophysiology* 20:35–44, 1983.

Crow, J, Lincoln, N, and De Weerdt, N: The effectiveness of EMG biofeedback in the treatment of arm function after stroke, *Intern Disability Studies* 11(4):155–160, 1989.

Cummings, M, Wilson, V, and Bird, E: Flexibility development in sprinters using EMG biofeedback and relaxation training, *Biofeedback Self Regul.* 9:395–405, 1984.

Debacher, G: Feedback goniometers for rehabilitation. In Basmajian, J, editor: *Biofeedback: principles and practice for clinicians*, Baltimore, 1983, Williams & Wilkins.

Deluca, C: Apparatus, detection, and recording techniques. In Basmajian, J, and Deluca, C, editors: *Muscles alive: their functions revealed by electromyography*, Baltimore, 1985, Williams & Wilkins.

Draper, V, and Ballard, L: Electrical stimulation versus electromyographic biofeedback in the recovery of quadriceps femoris muscle function following anterior cruciate ligament surgery, *Phys Ther* 71(6):455–464, 1991.

Draper, V: Electromyographic biofeedback and recovery of quadriceps femoris muscle function following anterior cruciate ligament reconstruction, *Phys Ther* 70(1):11–17, 1990.

English, A, and Wolf, S: The motor unit: anatomy and physiology, *Phys Ther* 62:1763, 1982.

Fields, R: Electromyographically triggered electric muscle stimulation for chronic hemiplegia, *Arch. Phys. Med. Rehabil.* 68:407–414, 1987.

Flom, R, Quast, J, and Boller, J: Biofeedback training to overcome post stroke footdrop, *Geriatrics* 31:47–51, 1976.

Flor, H, Haag, G, and Turk, D: Long-term efficacy of EMG biofeedback for chronic rheumatic back pain, *Pain* 27:195–202, 1986.

Flor, H, Haag, G, Turk, D, and Koehler, H: Efficacy of EMG biofeedback, pseudotherapy, and conventional medical treatment for chronic rheumatic back pain, *Pain* 17:21–31, 1983.

Gaarder, K, and Montgomery, P: *Clinical biofeedback: a procedural manual*, Baltimore, 1977, Williams & Wilkins.

Gallego, J, Perez de la Sota, A, and Vardon, G: Electromyographic feedback for learning to activate thoracic inspiratory muscles, *Am J Phys Med Rehab* 70(4):186–190, 1991.

Goodgold, J, and Eberstein, A: *Electrodiagnosis of neuromuscular diseases*, Baltimore, 1972, Williams & Wilkins.

Green, E, Walters, E, and Green, A: Feedback technology for deep relaxation, *Psychophysiology* 6:371–377, 1969.

Hijzen, T, Slangen, J, and van Houweligen, H: Subjective, clinical and EMG effects of biofeedback and splint treatment, *J Oral Rehabil.* 13:529–539, 1986.

Hirasawa, Y, Uchiza, Y, and Kusswetter, W: EMG biofeedback therapy for rupture of the extensor pollicis longus tendon, *Arch Orthop Trauma Surg* 104:342, 1986.

Honer, L, Mohr, T, and Roth, R: Electromyographic biofeedback to dissociate an upper extremity synergy pattern: a case report, *Phys Ther* 62:299–303, 1982.

Howard, P: Use of EMG biofeedback to reeducate the rotator cuff in a case of shoulder impingement, *JOSPT* 23(1):79, 1996.

Ince, L, and Leon, M: Biofeedback treatment of upper extremity dysfunction in Guillain-Barre syndrome, *Arch. Phys. Med. Rehabil.* 67:30–33, 1986.

Ince, L, Leon, M, and Christidis, D: EMG biofeedback with upper extremity musculature for relaxation training: a critical review of the literature, *J. Behav. Ther. Exp. Psychiatry* 16:133–137, 1985.

Ince, K, Leon, M, and Christidis, D: Experimental foundations of EMG biofeedback with the upper extremity: a review of the literature, *Biofeedback Self Regul.* 9:371–383, 1984.

Inglis, J, Donald, M, and Monga, T: Electromyographic biofeedback and physical therapy of the hemiplegic upper limb, *Arch. Phys. Med. Rehabil.* 65:755–759, 1984.

Johnson, H, and Garton, W: Muscle reeducation in hemiplegia by use of electromyographic device, *Arch. Phys. Med. Rehabil.* 54:322–323, 1973.

Johnson, H, and Hockersmith, V: Therapeutic electromyography in chronic back pain. In Basmajian, JV, editor: *Biofeedback: principles and practice for clinicians*, ed 2, Baltimore, 1983, Williams & Wilkins.

Johnson, R, and Lee, K: Myofeedback: a new method of teaching breathing exercise to emphysematous athletes, *Journal of the American Physical Therapy Association* 56, 826–829, 1976.

Kelly, J, Baker, M, and Wolf, S: Procedures for EMG biofeedback training in involved upper extremities of hemiplegic athletes, *Phys Ther* 59:1500, 1979.

King, A, Ahles, T, and Martin J: EMG biofeedback-controlled exercise in chronic arthritic knee pain, *Arch. Phys. Med. Rehabil.* 65:341–343, 1984.

King, T: Biofeedback: a survey regarding current clinical use and content in occupational therapy educational curricula, *Occ Ther J Res* 12(1):50–58, 1992.

Kleppe, D, Groendijk, H, and Huijing, P: Single motor unit control in the human mm. abductor pollicis brevis and mylohyoideus in relation to the number of muscle spindles, *Electromyogr. Clin. Neurophysiol.* 22:21–25, 1982.

Krebs, D: Biofeedback in neuromuscular reeducation and gait training. In Schwartz, M, editor: *Biofeedback: a practitioner's guide*, New York, 1987, Guilford.

Large, R, and Lamb, A: Electromyographic (EMG) feedback in chronic musculoskeletal pain: a controlled trial, *Pain* 17:167–177, 1983.

Large, R: Prediction of treatment response in pain athletes: the illness self-concept repertory grid and EMG feedback, *Pain* 21:279–287, 1985.

Lucca, J, and Recchiuti, S: Effect of electromyographic biofeedback on an isometric strengthening program, *Phys Ther* 63:200–203, 1983.

Mandel, A, Nymark, J, and Balmer, S: Electromyographic versus rhythmic positional biofeedback in computerized gait retraining with stroke athletes, *Arch Phys Med Rehab* 71(9):649–654, 1990.

Marinacci, A, and Horande, M: Electromyogram in neuromuscular reeducation, *Bulletin of the Los Angeles Neurological Society* 25, 57–67, 1960.

Mims, H: Electromyography in clinical practice, *South Med J* 49:804, 1956.

Morasky, R, Reynolds, C, and Clarke, G: Using biofeedback to reduce left arm extensor EMG of string players during musical performance, *Biofeedback Self Regul.* 6:565–572, 1981.

Morris, M, Matyas, T, and Bach, T: Electrogoniometric feedback: its effect on genu recurvatum in stroke, *Arch Phys Med Rehab* 73(12):1147–1154, 1992.

Mulder, T, and Hulstijn, W: Delayed sensory feedback in the learning of a novel motor task, *Psychol. Res.* 47:203–209, 1985.

Mulder, T, Hulstijn, W, and van der Meer, J: EMG feedback and the restoration of motor control: a controlled group study of 12 hemiparetic athletes, *Am. J. Phys. Med.* 65:173–188, 1986.

Nafpliotis, H: EMG feedback to improve ankle dorsiflexion, wrist extension and hand grasp, *Phys Ther* 56:821–825, 1976.

Nouwen, A: EMG biofeedback used to reduce standing levels of paraspinal muscle tension in chronic low back pain, *Pain* 17:353–360, 1983.

Poppen, R, and Maurer, J: Electromyographic analysis of relaxed postures, *Biofeedback Self Regul.* 7:491–498, 1982.

Russell, G, and Woolbridge, C: Correction of a habitual head tilt using biofeedback techniques—a case study, *Physiotherapy Canada* 27:181–184, 1975.

Saunders, J, Cox, D, and Teates, C: Thermal biofeedback in the treatment of intermittent claudication in diabetes: a case study, *Biofeedback Self Regulation* 19(4):337–345, 1994.

Smith, D, and Newman, D: Basic elements of biofeedback therapy for pelvic muscle rehabilitation, *Urologic Nursing* 14(3):130–135, 1994.

Soderback, I, Bengtsson, I, and Ginsburg, E: Video feedback in occupational therapy: its effect in athletes with neglect syndrome, *Arch Phys Med Rehab* 73(12):1140–1146, 1992.

Swaan, D, Van Wiergen, P, and Fokkema, S: Auditory electromyographic feedback therapy to inhibit undesired motor activity, *Arch Phys Med Rehabil* 55:251, 1974.

Winchester, P: Effects of feedback stimulation training and cyclical electrical stimulation on knee extension in hemiparetic athletes, *Phys Ther* 63:1097, 1983.

Wolf, S: *Fallacies of clinical EMG measures from athletes with musculoskeletal and neuromuscular disorders.* Paper presented at the 14th annual meeting of the Biofeedback Society of America, Denver, 1983.

Wolf, S, and Binder-Macleod, S: Electromyographic biofeedback applications to the hemiplegic athlete: changes in lower extremity neuromuscular and functional status, *Phys. Ther* 63:1404–1413, 1983.

Wolf, S, Regenos, E, and Basmajian, J: Developing strategies for biofeedback applications in neurologically handicapped athletes, *Phys Ther* 57, 402–408, 1977.

Wolf, S, Baker, M, and Kelly, J: EMG biofeedback in stroke: a 1-year follow-up on the effect of athlete characteristics, *Arch. Phys. Med. Rehabil.* 61:351–355, 1980.

Wolf, S, Baker, M, and Kelly, J: EMG biofeedback in stroke: effect of athlete characteristics, *Arch. Phys. Med. Rehabil.* 60:96–102, 1979.

Wolf, S: Electromyographic biofeedback in exercise programs, *Phys. Sports. Med.* 8:61–69, 1980.

Wolf, S, and Binder-Macleod, S: Electromyographic biofeedback applications to the hemiplegic athlete: changes in upper extremity neuromuscular and functional status, *Phys Ther* 63:1393, 1983.

Wolf, S, and Hudson, J: Feedback signal based upon force and time delay: modification of the Krusen limb load monitor: suggestion from the field, *Phys Ther* 60: 1289, 1980.

Wolf, S, Edwards, D, and Shutter, L: Concurrent assessment of muscle activity (CAMA): a procedural approach to assess treatment goals, *Phys Ther* 66:218, 1986.

Wolf, S, LeCraw, D, and Barton, L: A comparison of motor copy and targeted feedback training techniques for restitution of upper extremity function among neurologic athletes, *Phys Ther* 69:719, 1989.

Wolf, S, Nacht, M, and Kelly, J: EMG feedback training during dynamic movement for low back pain athletes, *Behav Ther* 13:395, 1982.

Wolf, S: Biofeedback. In Currier, DP, and Nelson, RM, editors: *Clinical electrotherapy,* ed 2, Norwalk, Conn. 1991, Appleton Lange.

Wolf, S: EMG biofeedback application in physical rehabilitation: an overview, *Physiotherapy Canada* 31:65, 1979.

Wolf, S: Essential considerations in the use of EMG biofeedback, *Phys Ther* 58:25, 1978.

Young, M: Electromyographic biofeedback use in the treatment of voluntary posterior dislocation of the shoulder: a case study, *JOSPT* 20(3):173–175, 1994.

CHAPTER 14

Low-Power Lasers

Ethan Saliba and Susan Foreman-Saliba

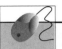

Study Resources

Refer to the lab exercises in the accompanying Laboratory Manual, as well as eSims which simulates the athletic training certification exam at www.mhhe.com/esims. Also, check out the competency information found at www.mhhe.com/prentice11e. For more online study resources, visit our Health and Human Performance Website at www.mhhe.com/hhp/.

Following completion of this chapter, the student athletic trainer will be able to

- Identify the different types of lasers.

- Explain the physical principles used to produce laser light.

- Contrast the characteristics of the helium neon and gallium arsenide low-power lasers.

- Analyze the therapeutic applications of lasers in wound and soft-tissue healing, edema reduction, inflammation, and pain.

- Demonstrate the treatment techniques of low-power lasers.

- Incorporate the safety considerations into the use of lasers.

- Be aware of the precautions and contraindications for low-power lasers.

- *LASER* = Light Amplification for the Stimulated Emission of Radiation

LASER is an acronym that stands for Light Amplification of Stimulated Emission of Radiation. Despite the image presented in science fiction movies, lasers offer valuable applications in the industrial, military, scientific, and medical environments. Einstein, in 1916, was the first to postulate the theorems that conceptualized the development of lasers. The first work with amplified electromagnetic radiation dealt with MASERs: microwave amplification of stimulated emission of radiation. In 1955, Townes and Schawlow showed it was possible to produce stimulated emission of microwaves beyond the optical region of the electromagnetic spectrum. This work with stimulated emission soon extended into the optical region of the electromagnetic spectrum, resulting in the development of devices called optical masers. The first working optical maser was constructed in 1960 by Theodore Maiman when he developed the synthetic ruby laser. Other types of lasers were devised shortly afterward. It was not until 1965 that the term *laser* was substituted for optical masers.[31]

Although lasers are relatively new, they have gone through extensive advances and refinements in a very short time. Lasers have been incorporated into numerous everyday applications that range from audio discs and supermarket scanning to communication and medical applications. This chapter will give an overview of lasers but will deal principally with the application of low-power lasers as they are used in conservative management of medical conditions.

PHYSICS OF THE LASER

Light is a form of electromagnetic energy that has **wavelengths** between 100 and 10,000 nanometers (nm = 10^{-9}) within the electromagnetic spectrum.[31] Visible light ranges from 400 nm (violet) to 700 nm (red). Beyond the red portion of the visual range is the **infrared** and microwave region, and below the violet end are the ultraviolet, x-ray, and gamma and cosmic ray regions (see Figure 1-2). Light energy is transmitted through space as waves that contain tiny "energy packets" called photons. Each **photon** contains a definite amount of energy depending on its wavelength (color).

Basics of the atomic theory are used to explain the principles of laser generation. The atom is the smallest particle of an element that retains all the properties of that element. The atom is divisible into fundamental particles called neutrons, protons, and electrons. Neutrons and positively charged protons are contained in the nucleus of the atom. **Electrons,** which are negatively charged, are equal in number to the protons and orbit the nucleus at distinct energy levels.

If an atom gains or loses an electron, it will become a negatively or positively charged ion respectively. The polarity difference between the positively charged nucleus and negatively charged electrons keeps the electrons orbiting the nucleus at these distinct energy levels. Electrons neither absorb nor radiate energy as long as they are maintained in their distinct orbit. An electron will stay in its lowest energy level **(ground state)** unless it absorbs an adequate amount of energy to move it to

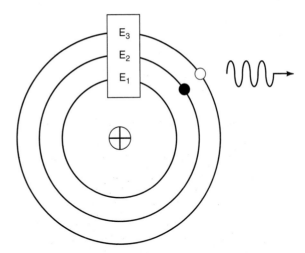

Figure 14-1 When energy is absorbed by an atom, an orbiting electron can become excited to a higher orbit. As the electron drops back to its original level, energy (photon) is released.

laser A device that concentrates high energies into a narrow beam of coherent, monochromatic light (Light Amplification by the Stimulated Emission of Radiation).

wavelength The distance from one peak to the same point on the next peak of an electromagnetic or acoustic wave.

infrared A portion of the electromagnetic spectrum between the visible and microwave regions. Wavelengths range from 780 to 100,000 nm.

photon The basic unit of light; a packet or quanta of light energy.

electron Fundamental particle of matter possessing a negative electrical charge and small mass.

ground state The normal, unexcited state of an atom.

one of its higher orbital levels (Figure 14-1). If an electron changes orbit, it will either gain or lose a distinct amount (quanta) of energy; it cannot exist between orbits.

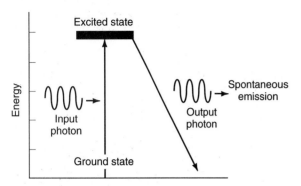

Figure 14-2   Spontaneous emission occurs when a photon changes energy level.

If a photon of adequate energy level collides with an electron of an atom, it will cause the electron to change levels. When this occurs, the atom is said to be in an **excited state.** The atom stays in this excited state only momentarily, and releases an identical photon (energy level) to the one it absorbed, which returns it to a ground state. This process is called **spontaneous emission** (Figure 14-2). Energy levels are particular to the type of atom; therefore, an electron accepts only the precise amount of energy that will move it from one energy level to another. Another means of exciting atoms other than with photon collision is with an electrical discharge. The energy is generated by collision of electrons that are accelerated in an electrical field.[21]

Stimulated Emissions

The concept of **stimulated emission** was postulated by Einstein and is essential to the working principle of lasers. It states that a photon released from an excited atom would stimulate another similarly excited atom to de-excite itself by releasing an identical photon.[31] The triggering photon would continue on its way unchanged and the subsequent photon released would be identical in **frequency,** direction, and phase. These two photons would promote the release of additional identical photons as long as other excited atoms were present. A critical factor for this occurrence is having an environment

excited state   State of an atom that occurs when outside energy causes the atom to contain more energy than normal.

spontaneous emission   When an atom in a high energy state emits a photon and drops to a more stable ground state.

stimulated emission   When a photon interacts with an atom already in a high-energy state and decay of the atomic system occurs, releasing two photons.

frequency   The number of cycles or pulses per second.

population inversion   A condition where more atoms exist in a high-energy, excited state than those atoms that are in a normal ground state; this is required for lasing to occur.

■ Analogy *14-1*

The concept of stimulated emissions is similar to investing money in the stock market (emission chamber). An investor takes some money (photons) and buys 10 shares of a growth stock. In a strong economy, the stock price increases and eventually splits so that the investor now owns 20 shares. The stock price continues to increase and again splits so that the investor now has 40 shares. The stock will continue to grow as long as there is a sufficient number of excited investors (unlimited excited atoms). When the stock portfolio has enough shares, the investor pulls the excess money out of the account (photons are ejected from the chamber).

with unlimited excited atoms, which is termed **population inversion.** Population inversion occurs when there are more atoms in an excited state than in a ground state. It is caused by applying an external power source to the lasing medium. The released photons are identical in phase, direction, and frequency. To contain them, and to generate more photons, mirrors are placed at both ends of the chamber. One mirror is totally reflective while

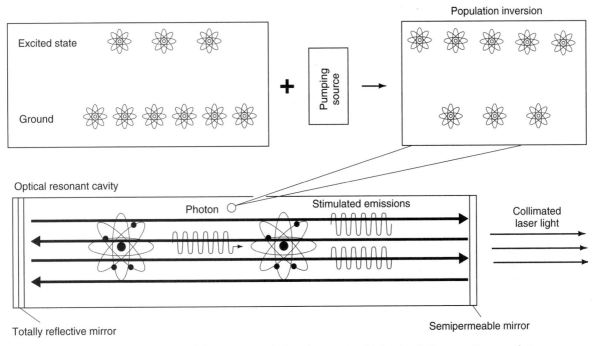

Figure 14-3   Pumping is a process of elevating an orbiting electron to a higher level, thus creating population diversion that is essential for laser operation.

coherence   Property of identical phase and time relationship. All photons of laser light are the same wavelength.

monochromaticity   When a light source produces a single color or wavelength.

collimate   To make parallel.

the other is semipermeable. The photons are reflected within the chamber, which amplifies the light and stimulates the emission of other photons from excited atoms. Eventually, so many photons are stimulated that the chamber cannot contain the energy. When a specific level of energy is attained, photons of a particular wavelength are ejected through the semipermeable mirror. Thus, amplified light through stimulated emissions (laser) is produced (Figure 14-3).

Three properties of laser

- Coherence
- Monochromaticity
- Collimation

The laser light is emitted in an organized manner rather than in a random pattern as from a light bulb. Three properties distinguish the laser from incandescent and fluorescent light sources: **coherence, monochromaticity,** and **collimation.**[31]

Coherence means all photons of light emitted from individual gas molecules are the same wavelength and that the individual light waves are in phase with one another. Normal light, on the other hand, is composed of many wavelengths that superimpose their phases on one another.

Monochromaticity refers to the specificity of light in a single, defined wavelength; if the specificity

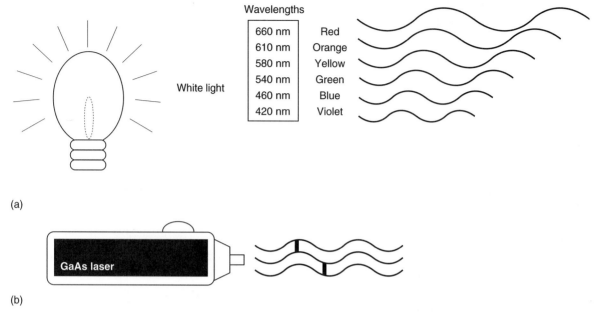

Figure 14-4 (a) White light contains electromagnetic energy of all wavelengths (colors) that are superimposed on each other. (b) Laser light is monochromatic (single wavelength), coherent (in phrase), and collimated (minimal divergence).

....

divergence The bending of light rays away from each other; the spreading of light.

....

is in the visible light spectrum, it is only one color. The laser is one of the few light sources that produces a specific wavelength.

The laser beam is well-collimated—that is, there is minimal **divergence** of the photons.[1] That means the photons move in a parallel fashion, thus concentrating a beam of light (Figure 14-4).

TYPES OF LASERS

Lasers are classified according to the nature of the material placed between two reflecting surfaces. There are potentially thousands of different types of lasers, each with specific wavelengths and unique characteristics depending on the lasing medium utilized. The lasing mediums used to create lasers include the following categories: crystal and glass (solid-state), gas and excimer, semiconductor, liquid dye, and chemical.

- Crystal lasers include the synthetic ruby (aluminum oxide and chromium) and the neodymium, yttrium, aluminum, garnet (Nd:YAG) lasers, among others. Synthetic, rather than natural materials are used to ensure purity of the medium, which is necessary for the physical characteristics of lasers to occur.[16]
- Gas lasers were developed in 1961, shortly after the first ruby laser. The gas lasers developed include the helium neon (HeNe), argon, and carbon dioxide (CO_2) along with numerous others. The HeNe laser is one type of low-power device under investigation in the United States for application in physical medicine.
- Semiconductor or diode lasers were developed in 1962 after the production of gas

■ **Clinical Decision-Making** *Exercise 14-1*

After watching a show on the use of lasers in surgery, an athlete expresses genuine concern to the athletic trainer that using a laser to treat a myofascial trigger point will cause skin burns. What should the athletic trainer explain to the athlete to allay his or her fears?

(HeNe) lasers. The gallium arsenide (GaAs) was the first diode laser developed and is another low-power laser under investigation in the United States for application in physical medicine.
- Liquid lasers are also known as dye lasers because they use organic dyes as the lasing medium. By varying the mixture of the dyes, the wavelengths of the laser can be varied.
- Chemical lasers are usually extremely high powered and are frequently used for military purposes.[21]

Lasers can be categorized as either high- or low-power, depending on the intensity of energy they deliver. High-power lasers are also known as "hot" lasers because of the thermal responses they generate. These are used in the medical realms in numerous areas, including surgical cutting and coagulation, ophthalmological, dermatological, oncological, and vascular specialties. The use of low-power lasers (also known as "cold" or "soft" lasers) for wound healing and pain management is a relatively new area of application in medicine. These lasers produce a maximal output of less than 1 milliwatt (1 mW = 1/1000 watt) in the United States and work by causing photo-chemical, rather than thermal, effects. No tissue warming occurs. The exact distinction of the power output that delineates a low- versus high-power laser varies. Low-power devices are considered to be any laser that does not generate an appreciable thermal response. This category can include lasers capable of producing up to 500 milliwatts of power (up to a Class IV laser).[6]

Types of lasers
- Crystal
- Gas
- Semiconductor
- Liquid
- Chemical

Low-power lasers, which have been studied and used in Europe for the past 25 to 30 years, have been investigated in the United States for the past 15 to 20 years. The potential applications for low-power lasers include treatment of tendon and ligament injury, arthritis, edema reduction, soft tissue injury, ulcer and burn care, scar tissue inhibition, and acutherapy.

LASER GENERATORS

Lasers require the following components to be operational:[21]

1. Power Supply—Lasers use an electrical power supply that can potentially deliver up to 10,000 volts and hundreds of amps.
2. Lasing Medium—This is the material that generates the laser light. It can include any type of matter: gas, solid, or liquid.
3. Pumping Device—*Pumping* is the term used to describe the process of elevating an orbiting electron to a higher, "excited" energy level (see Figure 14-4). This creates the population inversion that is essential for laser operation. The pumping device may be high voltage, photoflash lamps, radio-frequency oscillators or other lasers. The pumping device is very specific to the type of lasing medium being used.
4. Optical Resonant Cavity—This contains the lasing medium. Once population inversion has occurred, this cavity, which contains the reflecting surfaces, directs the beam propagation.

The helium neon (HeNe) and gallium arsenide (GaAs) lasers are the two principle lasers currently under investigation in the United States for conservative management of medical conditions. The following discussion will concentrate on these two laser types.

HeNe Lasers

The HeNe gas laser uses a gas mixture of primarily helium with neon in a pressurized tube. This creates a laser in the red portion of the electromagnetic spectrum with a wavelength of 632.8 nanometers. The power output of the HeNe can vary but typically runs from 1.0 to 10.0 mW, depending on the gas density used. Larger tubes are necessary for higher power outputs, and each requires a precise power drive to operate.[6] Laser output can decrease depending on the care of the equipment, on the number of operating hours, and on whether **fiber optics** are used. For example, rough handling can jar the reflecting surfaces, and a high number of hours in operation or poor fiber optic quality can diminish the laser output. The HeNe laser in the United States delivers a power output of 1 mW through a fiber optic tube in a continuous mode. Although the HeNe laser light is well collimated, the utilization of fiber optics causes a divergence of the beam from 18° to 21°.[6] Fiber optics can decrease the output delivery 50% or more as the light travels from the lasing medium to the tip of the applicator. Fiber optics are used to make the delivery more convenient because the size of the gas tube would make direct application difficult. HeNe lasers up to 6 mW have been manufactured for clinical use in Canada, which has fewer governmental restrictions. These higher output lasers, although still considered low power, allow delivery of desired dosages in reduced time.[7]

Gallium Arsenide Lasers

The gallium arsenide (GaAs) lasers utilize a diode to produce an infrared (invisible) laser at a wavelength of 904 nm. **Diode lasers** are composed of semiconductor silicone materials that are precisely cut and layered. An electrical source is applied to

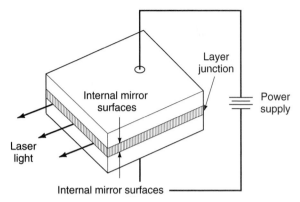

Figure 14-5 A diode is composed of silicone material that is cleaved and layered. The lasting action occurs at the junction of the layers when an electrical source is applied.

fiber optic A solid glass or plastic tube that conducts light along its length.

diode lasers A solid-state/semiconductor used as a lasing medium.

▶ **Most commonly used lasers**

- Helium neon (HeNe)
- Gallium arsenide (GaAs)

each side, and lasing action is produced at the junction of the two materials. The cleaved surfaces function as partially reflecting surfaces that will ultimately produce coherent light[16] (Figure 14-5).

Diode lasers produce a beam that is elliptically shaped so the lasers have a 10° to 35° divergence, despite the fact that no fiber optics are used.[21] The 904 nm laser is delivered in a pulsed mode because of the heat produced at the junction of the diode chips. The GaAs laser manufactured in the United States has a peak power of 2 watts but is delivered in a pulsed mode that decreases the average power to 0.4 mW output if delivered at 1000 hertz (see calculations in "Dosage" section).

The application of additional layers of materials to other types of diodes allows their operation in a continuous mode at room temperature.[21] The continuous mode results in higher average power outputs from the lasers. Higher output diode lasers are manufactured for clinical applications in Canada and include the following:

780 nm wavelength with a 5 mW output, continuous-mode delivery

810 nm wavelength with a 20 mW output, continuous-mode delivery

830 nm wavelength with a 30 mW output, continuous-mode delivery

These diodes are interchangeable in a single base unit.[7]

The laser units available in the United States have the ability to deliver both HeNe and/or GaAs lasers. The same device can both measure electrical impedance and deliver electrical point stimulation. The impedence detector allows hypersensitive or acupuncture points to be located. The point stimulator can be combined with laser application when treating pain. The electrical stimulation is believed to provide spontaneous pain relief whereas the laser provides more latent tissue responses.[8]

TREATEMENT TECHNIQUES

The method of application of laser therapy is relatively simple, but certain principles of dosimetry should be discussed so the clinician can accurately determine the amount of laser energy delivered to the tissues. For general application, only the treatment time and the pulse rate vary. For research purposes, the investigator should measure the exact energy density emitted from the applicator before the treatments. Dosage is the most important variable in laser therapy and may be difficult to determine because of the variables mentioned previously (e.g., hours of operation or condition of the unit).

The laser energy is emitted from a handheld remote applicator. The GaAs laser houses the semi-

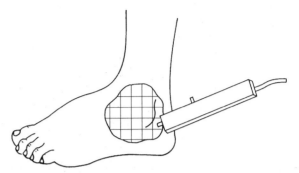

Figure 14-6   Grid application of laser. Laser aperture should be perpendicular to the surface. Lase each square centimeter of the injured area for the specified time. The aperture should be in light contact with the skin.

conductor elements in the tip of the applicator, while the HeNe lasers contain their componentry inside the unit and deliver the laser light to the target area via a fiber optic tube. The fiber optic assembly is fragile and should not be crimped or twisted excessively. The fiber optics used with the HeNe and the elliptical shape of the GaAs laser create beam divergence with both devices. This divergence causes the beam's energy to spread out over a given area so that as the distance from the source increases, the intensity of the beam lessens.

Lasing Techniques

To administer a laser treatment, the tip should be in light contact with the skin and directed perpendicularly to the target tissue while the laser is engaged for the designated time. Commonly, a treatment area is divided into a grid of square centimeters, with each square centimeter stimulated for the specified time. This *gridding technique* is the most frequently utilized method of application and should be used whenever possible. Lines and points should not be drawn on the athlete's skin because this may absorb some of the light energy (Figure 14-6). If open areas are to be treated, a sterilized clear plastic sheet can be placed over the wound to allow surface contact.

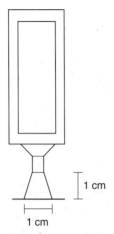

Figure 14-7   Scanning technique. When skin contact cannot be maintained, the remote should be held still in the center of the square centimeter grid at a distance of less than 1 cm. If using the HeNe laser, the red beam should fill a 1 cm² grid.

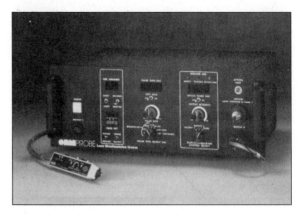

Figure 14-8   Low-power laser. (PhysioTechnology, Ltd. Topeka, KS)

An alternative is a *scanning technique* in which there is no contact between the laser tip and the skin. With this technique, the applicator tip should be held 5 to 10 millimeters from the wound. Since beam divergence occurs, there is a decrease in the amount of energy as the distance from the target increases. The amount of energy lost becomes difficult to quantify accurately if the distance from the target is variable. Therefore, it is not recommended to treat at distances greater than 1 cm. When using a laser tip of 1 mm with 30° of divergence, the red laser beam of the HeNe should fill an area the size of one square centimeter (Figure 14-7). Although the infrared laser is invisible, the same consideration should be given when using the scanning technique. If the laser tip comes into contact with an open wound, the tip should be cleaned thoroughly with a small amount of bleach or other antiseptic agents to prevent cross contamination.

The scanning technique should be differentiated with the *wanding technique* in which a grid area is bathed with the laser in an oscillating fashion for the designated time. As in the scanning technique, the dosimetry is difficult to calculate if a distance of

Lasing techniques

- Gridding
- Scanning
- Wanding

■ Clinical Decision-Making   *Exercise 14-2*

An athletic trainer is treating a postacute inversion ankle sprain with a HeNe laser. How can the athletic trainer ensure that the amount of energy delivered to the injured area is relatively uniform?

less than 1 cm cannot be maintained. The wanding technique is not recommended because of irregularities in the dosages.

Dosage

PhysioTechnology, Ltd. (Topeka, Kan.), is the only manufacturer in the United States that currently produces low-power HeNe and GaAs lasers (Figure 14-8). Table 14-1 describes the contrasting specifications of these lasers. The HeNe laser has a 1.0 mW average power output at the fiber tip and

■ TABLE 14-1   Parameters of Low-Output Lasers

	HELIUM NEON (HeNe)	GALLIUM ARSENIDE (GaAs)
Laser type	Gas	Semiconductor
Wavelength	632.8 nm	904 nm
Pulse rate	Continuous wave	1–1000 Hz
Pulse width	Continuous wave	200 nsec
Peak power	3 mW	2 W
Average power	1.0 mW	.04–0.4 mW
Beam area	0.01 cm	0.07 cm
FDA class	Class II laser	Class I laser

Copied with permission from PhysioTechnology.

continuous wave   An uninterrupted beam of laser light, as opposed to pulsed.

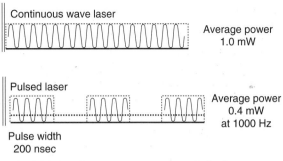

Figure 14-9   Continuous wave versus pulsed energies.

is delivered in the **continuous wave** mode. The GaAs laser has an output of 2 watts (W) but has only a 0.4 mW average power when pulsed at its maximum rate of 1000 Hz. The frequency of the GaAs is variable and the clinician may choose a pulse rate of 1 to 1000 Hz, each with a pulse width of 200 nsec (nanosec = 10^{-9}) (Figure 14-9).

The pulsed modes drastically reduce the amount of energy emitted from the laser. For example, a 2W laser is pulsed at 100 Hz:

$$\text{average power} = \text{pulse rate} \times \text{peak power} \times \text{pulse width}$$
$$= 100\,\text{Hz} \times 2\text{W} \times (2 \times 10^{-7}\,\text{sec})$$
$$= 0.04\,\text{mW}$$

This contrasts the power output of 0.4 mW with the 1000 Hz. Therefore, it can be seen that adjustment of the pulse rate alters the average power, which significantly affects the treatment time if a specified amount of energy is required. In the past it was thought that altering the frequency of the laser would increase its benefits. Recent evidence indicates that the total number of joules is more impor-

tant; therefore, higher pulse rates are recommended to decrease the treatment time required for each stimulation point.[7]

The dosage or energy density of laser is reported in the literature as joules per square centimeter (J/cm^2). One joule is equal to one watt per second. Therefore, dosage is dependent on the following:

1. the output of the laser in mWatts
2. the time of exposure in seconds
3. the beam surface area of the laser in cm^2

Dosage should be accurately calculated to standardize treatments and to establish treatment guidelines for specific injuries. The intention is to deliver a specific number of J/cm^2 or mJ/cm^2. After setting the pulse rate, which determines the average power of the laser, only the treatment time per cm^2 needs to be calculated:[7]

$$T_A = (E/P_{av}) \times A$$
$$T_A = \text{treatment time for a given area}$$
$$E = \text{millijoules of energy per cm}^2$$
$$P_{av} = \text{Average laser power in milliwatts}$$
$$A = \text{beam area in cm}^2$$

For example, to deliver 1 J/cm^2 with a 0.4 mW average power GaAs laser with a 0.07 cm^2 beam area:

$$T_A = (1\,\text{J/cm}^2 / .0004\text{W}) \times 0.07\,\text{cm}^2$$
$$= 175\,\text{seconds or }2{:}55\,\text{minutes}$$

To deliver 50 mJ/cm^2 with the same laser, it would only take 8.75 seconds of stimulation. Charts are available to assist the clinician in calculating the treatment times for a variety of pulse rates. The

■ **TABLE 14-2** Treatment Times for Low-Output Lasers

LASER TYPE	AVERAGE POWER (mW)	Joules per Centimeter Squared (J/cm²)						
		0.05	**0.1**	**0.5**	**1**	**2**	**3**	**4**
HeNe (632.8 nm) Continuous wave	1.0	0.5	1.0	5.0	10.0	20.0	30.0	40.0
GaAs (904 nm) Pulsed at 1000 Hz	0.4	8.8	17.7	88.4	176.7	353.4	530.1	706.9

Copied with permission from PhysioTechnology.

■ **Clinical Decision-Making** *Exercise 14-3*

The athletic trainer is trying to calculate the dosage in J/cm² of a HeNe Laser treatment. What factors will need to be taken into account that collectively determine the correct dosage?

GaAs laser can only be pulsed up to 1000 Hz, resulting in an average energy of 0.4 mW. Therefore, the treatment times may be exceedingly long to deliver the same energy density with a continuous wave laser (Table 14-2).

Depth of Penetration

Any energy applied to the body can be absorbed, reflected, transmitted, and refracted. Biological effects result only from the absorption of energy, and as more energy is absorbed, there is less available for the deeper and adjacent tissues.

Laser light's depth of penetration depends on the type of laser energy delivered. Absorption of HeNe laser energy occurs rapidly in the superficial structures, especially within the first 2 to 5 mm of soft tissue. The response that occurs from absorption is termed the **direct effect**. The **indirect effect** is a lessened response that occurs deeper in the tissues. The normal metabolic processes in the deeper tissues are catalized from the energy absorption in the superficial structures to produce the in-

direct effect The tissue response that occurs from energy absorption.

indirect effect A decreased response that occurs in deeper tissues.

---

direct effect. HeNe laser has an indirect effect on tissues up to 8 to 10 mm.[7]

The GaAs, which has a longer wavelength, is directly absorbed in tissues at depths of 1 to 2 cm and has an indirect effect up to 5 cm (Figure 14-10). Therefore, this laser has better potential for the treatment of deeper soft tissue injuries such as strains, sprains, and contusions. The radius of the energy field expands as the nonabsorbed light is reflected, refracted, and transmitted to adjacent cells as the energy penetrates. The clinician should stimulate each square centimeter of a "grid," although there will be an overlap of areas receiving indirect exposure.

CLINICAL APPLICATIONS FOR LASERS

Since the production of lasers is relatively new, the biological and physiological effects of this concentrated light energy are still being explored. The effects of low-power lasers are subtle, primarily occurring at a cellular level. Various in vitro and animal studies have attempted to elucidate the

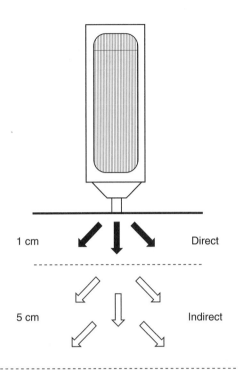

Figure 14-10   Depth of penetration with the GaAs laser. Direct penetration is up to 1 cm with the GaAs laser. The stimulation causes an indirect effect up to 5 cm. Penetration is greatest with skin contact.

interaction of photons with the biological structures. Although there are few controlled clinical studies in the literature, documented case studies and empirical evidence indicate that lasers are effective in reducing pain and aiding wound healing. The exact mechanisms for action are still uncertain, although proposed physiological effects include an acceleration in collagen synthesis, a decrease in microorganisms, an increase in vascularization, reduction of pain, and an anti-inflammatory action.[7]

Low-power lasers are best recognized for increasing the rate of wound and ulcer healing by enhancing cellular metabolism. Results from animal studies have varied as to the benefits on wound healing, perhaps because the types of lasers, dosages, and protocols used have been inconsistent. In humans, improvement of nonhealing wounds indicates promising possibilities for treatment with lasers.

Wound Healing

Early investigations of the effects of low-power laser on biological tissues were limited to in vitro experimentation. Although it was known that high-power lasers could damage and vaporize tissues, little was known about the effect of small dosages on the viability and stability of cellular structures. It was found that low dosages (less than 10 J/cm^2) of radiation from low-output lasers had a stimulatory action on metabolic processes and cell proliferation compared to incandescent or tungsten light.[2]

Mester conducted numerous in vitro experiments with two lasers in the red portion of the visual spectrum: the ruby laser—wavelength of 694.3 nm—and the HeNe laser—wavelength 632.8 nm. Human tissue cultures showed significant increases in fibroblastic proliferation following stimulation by either laser tested.[22] Fibroblasts are the precursor cells to connective tissue structures, such as collagen, epithelial cells, and chondrocytes. When the production of fibroblasts is stimulated, one should expect a subsequent increase in the production of connective tissue. Abergel and associates documented that certain dosages of HeNe and GaAs laser—wavelength 904 nm—caused in vitro human skin fibroblasts to have a threefold increase in procollagen production.[2] This effect was most marked when low-level stimulation (1.94×10^{-7} to 5.84×10^{-6}J/cm^2 of GaAs and dosages of 0.053 to 1.589 J/cm^2 of HeNe) was repeated over 3 to 4 days versus a single exposure. Samples of tissue showed increases in fibroblast and collagenous structures as well as increases in the intracellular material and swollen mitochondria of cells.[22] Furthermore, cells were undamaged in regard to their morphology and structure after exposure to low-power laser.[4]

Analysis of the cellular metabolism, with attention to the activity of DNA and RNA, has been made.[2,22,29] Through radioactive markers, it was suggested that laser stimulation enhances the synthesis of nucleic acids and cell division.[11,22] Abergel reported that laser treated cells had significantly greater amounts of procollagen messenger RNA, further confirming that increased collagen production occurs from modifications at the transcriptional level.[1]

Low-power lasers were used in animal studies to further delineate both the beneficial applications of laser light and its potential harm. In an early study by Mester and his associates, mechanical and burn wounds were made on the backs of mice.[23] Similar wounds on the same animals served as the controls, with the experimental wounds subjected to various doses of ruby laser. Although there were no histological differences among the wounds, the laser wounds healed significantly faster, especially at a dosage of 1 J/cm^2. It was also demonstrated that repeated laser treatments were more effective than a single exposure.

Other researchers investigated the rate of healing and tensile strength of full thickness wounds when exposed to laser irradiation.[2,17,18,19,20,28] There were conflicting reports regarding rates of healing, with some studies showing no change in the rate of wound closure,[17,20,28] and others showing significantly faster wound healing.[2,18,19] Although the experimental results were conflicting, an explanation for the discrepancy may be an indirect systemic effect of laser energy. Mester showed that it was not necessary to irradiate an entire wound to achieve beneficial results, since stimulation of remote areas had similar results.[22] Kana and associates described an increase in the rate of healing of both the irradiated and nonirradiated wounds on the same animal compared to nonirradiated animals.[18] This systemic effect was most marked with the argon laser. Several studies that investigated the rate of healing on living animal tissue used a second, nontreated control wound on the same animal. The rate of healing may have been confounded by this systemic effect. Whether the systemic effect involves a humoral component—a circulating element—producing immunological effects has yet to be determined or identified. Bacteriocidal and lymphocyte stimulation are proposed mechanisms for this phenomenon.

Tensile Strength of Wounds.   The increased tensile strength of lased wounds was confirmed more often.[2,17,18,20,23,28] Wound contraction, collagen synthesis, and increases in tensile strength are fibroblast mediated functions and were demonstrated most markedly in the early phase of wound healing. Wounds were tested at various stages of healing to determine their breaking point and were compared to a control or nonlased wound. Laser-treated wounds had significantly greater tensile strengths, most commonly in the first 10 to 14 days after injury, although they approached the values of the control after that time.[1,20,28] Hypertrophic scars did not result as tissue responses normalized after a 14-day period. HeNe laser of doses ranging from 1.1 to 2.2 J/cm^2 elicited positive results when lased either twice a day or on alternate days. The increased tensile strength corresponds to higher levels of collagen.

Immunological Responses

These early studies led to the hypothesis that laser exposure could enhance healing of skin and connective tissue lesions, but the mechanism was still unclear. Biochemical analysis and radioactive tracers were used to delineate the immunological effects of laser light on human tissue cultures. The laser irradiation caused increased phagocytosis by leukocytes with dosages of .05 joules per square centimeter (J/cm^2).[22] This led to the possibility of a bacteriocidal effect, which was further demonstrated with laser exposures on cell cultures containing Escherichia-coli, a common intestinal bacteria in humans. The ruby laser had an increased effect both on cell replication and on the destruction of bacteria via the phagocytosis of leukocytes.[22,23] Mester also concluded that there were immunological effects with the ruby, HeNe, and argon lasers. Specifically, there was a direct stimulatory influence on the T and B lymphocyte activity, a phenomenon that is specific to laser output and wavelength. HeNe and Argon lasers gave the best results with dosages ranging from 0.5 to 1 J/cm^2.[22] Trelles did similar investigations in vitro and in vivo and reported that laser did not have bacteriocidal effects alone, but when used in conjunction with antibiotics, there were significantly higher bacteriocidal effects compared to controls.[29]

With the confidence that they would cause little or no harm and that they could serve a therapeutic purpose, low-power lasers have been used clinically on human subjects since the 1960s. In Hungary, Mester treated nonhealing ulcers that did not respond to traditional therapy with HeNe and Argon lasers with respective wavelengths of 632.8 and 488 nm.[22] The dosages were varied but had a maximum of 4 J/cm^2. By the time of Mester's publication, 1125 athletes had been treated, of which 875 healed, 160 improved and 85 did not respond. The wounds, which were categorized by etiology, took an average of 12 to 16 weeks to heal. Trelles also showed promising results clinically using the infrared GaAs and HeNe lasers on the healing of ulcers, nonunion fractures, and on herpetic lesions.[29]

Gogia et al., in the United States, treated non-healing wounds with GaAs lasers pulsed at a frequency of 1000 Hz for 10 seconds/cm^2 with a sweeping technique held about 5 mm from the wound surface.[15] This protocol was used in conjunction with daily or twice daily sterile whirlpool treatments and produced satisfactory results, although statistical information was not reported. Empirical evidence by these authors suggested faster healing and cleaner wounds when subjected to GaAs laser treatment three times per week.

Inflammation

Biopsies of experimental wounds were examined for prostaglandin activity to delineate the effect of laser stimulation on the inflammatory process. A decrease in prostaglandin (PGE$_2$) is a proposed mechanism in which laser therapy promotes the reduction of edema. During inflammation, prostaglandins cause vasodilation, which contributes to the flow of plasma into the interstitial tissue. By reducing prostaglandins, the driving force behind edema production is reduced.[7] The prostaglandin E and F contents were examined after treatments with HeNe laser at 1 J/cm^2.[22] In four days, both types of prostaglandins accumulated more than the controls. However, at eight days, the PGE$_2$ levels decreased, while PGF$_{2alpha}$ increased. There was also an increased capillarization during this phase. This data indicates that prostaglandin production is affected by laser stimulation, and

these changes possibly reflect an accelerated resolution of the acute inflammatory process.[22]

Scar Tissue

Macroscopic examination of healed wounds was subjectively described after the laser experiments in most studies. In general, the wounds exposed to laser irradiation had less scar tissue and a better cosmetic appearance. Histological examination showed greater epithelialization and less exudative material.[19]

Studies that utilized burn wounds showed more regular alignment of collagen and smaller scars. Trelles lased third-degree burns on the backs of hairless mice with GaAs and HeNe lasers and showed significantly faster healing in the lased animals.[29] The best results were obtained with the GaAs laser, because of its greater penetration. Trelles found increased circulation with the production of new blood vessels in the center of the wounds compared to the controls. Edges of the wounds maintained viability and contributed to the epithelialization and closure of the burn. Since there was less contracture associated with irradiated wounds, laser treatment has been suggested for burns and wounds on the hands and neck, where contractures and scarring can severely limit function.

Pain

Lasers have also been effective in reducing pain and have been shown to effect peripheral nerve activity. Rochkind and others produced crush injuries in rats and treated experimental animals with 10 J/cm^2 of HeNe laser energy transcutaneously along the sciatic nerve projection.[24] The amplitude of electrically stimulated action potentials was measured along the injured nerve and compared with controls up to one year later. The amplitude of the action potentials was 43% greater after 20 days, which was the duration of laser treatment. By one year, all lased nerves demonstrated equal or higher amplitudes than pre-injury. The controls followed an expected course of recovery and did not reach normal levels even after a year.

The effect of HeNe irradiation on peripheral sensory nerve latency has been investigated on humans by Snyder-Mackler and Bork.[27] This double-blind study showed that exposure of the superficial radial nerve to low dosages of laser resulted in a significantly decreased sensory nerve conduction velocity, which may provide information about the pain-relieving mechanism of lasers. Other explanations for pain relief may be the result of hastened healing, anti-inflammatory action, autonomic nerve influence, and neurohumoral responses (serotonin, norepinephrine) from descending tract inhibition.[7,8]

Chronic pain has been treated with GaAs and HeNe lasers, and positive results have been observed empirically and through clinical research. Walker conducted a double-blind study to document analgesia after exposure to HeNe irradiation in chronic pain athletes compared with sham treatments.[32] When the superficial sites of the radial, median, and saphenous nerves as well as painful areas were exposed to laser irradiation, there were significant decreases in pain and less reliance on medication for pain control. These preliminary studies suggest positive results, although pain modulation is difficult to measure objectively.

Bone Response

Future uses of laser irradiation include the treatment of other connective tissue structures such as bone and articular cartilage. Schultz et al. studied various intensities of Nd:YAG laser on the healing of partial thickness articular cartilage lesions in guinea pigs.[25] During the surgical procedure, the lesions were irradiated for 5 seconds with intensities ranging from 25 to 125 J. After four weeks, the low dosage group (25 J) had chondral proliferation and by six weeks the defect had reconstituted to the level of the surface cartilage. Normal basophilia cells were present with staining, indicating normal cellular structures. The higher dosage groups and controls had little or no evidence of restoration of the lesion with cartilage. Bone healing and fracture consolidation have been investigated by Trelles and

■ **Clinical Decision-Making**   *Exercise 14-4*

An athlete is complaining of pain in the upper back. Following an evaluation, the athletic trainer determines that the pain is radiating from an active trigger point in the upper trapezius. How should this trigger point be treated using a HeNe laser?

Mayayo.[30] An adapter was attached to an intramuscular needle so that the laser energy could be directed deeper to the periosteum. Rabbit tibial fractures showed faster consolidation with HeNe treatment of 2.4 J/cm^2 on alternate days. Histological examination indicated more mature Haversian canals with detached osteocytes in the laser treated bone. There was also a remodeling of the articular line, which is impossible with traditional therapy.[29,30] The use of lasers for the treatment of nonunion fractures has begun in Europe.

SUGGESTED TREATMENT PROTOCOLS

Research suggests some laser densities for treating several clinical models. These average from 0.05 to 0.5 J/cm^2 for acute conditions and range from 0.5 to 3 J/cm^2 for more chronic conditions.[7] The responses of the tissues depend on the dosage delivered, although the type of laser used can also influence the effect. The response obtained with different dosages and with different lasers varies considerably among studies, leaving treatment parameters to be determined largely empirically. In the literature, there seems to be little differentiation when comparing the dosages of HeNe and GaAs lasers, although their depths of penetration differ significantly. The laser units produced in the United States have relatively little average power, so the tendency is to administer dosages in millijoules rather than joules. Three to six treatments may be required before the effectiveness of laser therapy can be determined.

■ **TABLE 14-3**   Suggested Treatment Application

APPLICATION	LASER TYPE	ENERGY DENSITY
TRIGGER POINT		
Superficial	HeNe	1–3 J/cm^2
Deep	GaAs	1– J/cm^2
EDEMA REDUCTION		
Acute	GaAs	0.1–0.2 J/cm^2
Subacute	GaAs	0.2–0.5 J/cm^2
WOUND HEALING (SUPERFICIAL TISSUES)		
Acute	HeNe	0.5–1 J/cm^2
Chronic	HeNe	4 J/cm^2
WOUND HEALING (DEEP TISSUES)		
Acute	GaAs	0.05–0.1 J/cm^2
Chronic	GaAs	0.5–1 J/cm^2
SCAR TISSUE	GaAs	0.5–1 J/cm^2

Copied with permission from PhysioTechnology.

Although higher laser output is recommended to reduce treatment times, overstimulation should be avoided. The Arndt Schultz principle (see Chapter 1) that states more is not necessarily better is applicable with laser therapy. For this reason, laser should be administered at a maximum of once daily per treatment area. When using large dosages, treatment is recommended on alternate days. If the effects of laser plateau, the frequency of treatments should be reduced or the treatments discontinued for one week, at which time the treatment can be reinstated if needed.[29]

Treating Pain

The use of low-power lasers in the treatment of acute and chronic pain can be implemented in various manners. After proper diagnosis of the pain's etiology, the pathology site can be gridded. The entire area of injury should be lased as described previously. Table 14-3 lists some suggested treatment protocols for various clinical conditions. When trigger points are being treated, the probe should be held perpendicular to the skin with light contact. If a specific structure, such as a ligament, is the target tissue, the laser probe should be held in contact with the skin and perpendicular to that structure. When treating a joint, the athlete should be positioned so that the joint is open to allow penetration of the energy to the intra-articular areas.

The treatment of acupuncture and trigger points with laser can be augmented with electrical stimulation for pain management. Reference to charts should be made to determine appropriate acupuncture points. The impedence detector in the laser remote enhances the ability to locate these sites. Points should be treated from distal to proximal for best results.

Occasionally athletes may experience an increase in pain after a laser treatment. This phenomenon is believed to be the initiation of the body's normal responses to pain that have become dormant.[6] Laser has been found to help resolve the condition by enhancing normal physiological processes needed to resolve the injury. As stated previously, several treatments should be administered before deeming the modality ineffective in pain management.

Treatment for Wound Healing

Although ulcerations and open wounds are not common in an athletic training environment, contusions, abrasions, and lacerations can be treated with laser to hasten healing time and decrease infection. The wound should be cleaned appropriately, and all debris and eschar should be removed. Heavy exudate that covers the wound will diminish the laser's penetration; therefore, lasing around the periphery of the wound is recommended. The scanning technique should be utilized over open wounds unless a clear plastic sheet is placed over the wound to allow direct contact. Opaque materials can absorb some of the laser energy and are not recommended. Facial lacerations can be treated with the laser, although care should be taken not to direct the beam into the athlete's eyes. Risk of retinal damage from the low-power lasers used in the United States is low.

Treating Scar Tissue

The laser energy affects only what is metabolically diminished and does not change normal tissue. Hypertrophic scars can be treated with lasers due to the bioinhibitive effects. Bioinhibition requires prolonged treatment times and may be clinically impractical because of the low-power output of the lasers used in the United States. Pain and edema associated with pathological scars have been effectively treated with low-power lasers. Thick scars have varied vascularity which makes laser transmission irregular; therefore, it is often recommended to treat the periphery of the scar rather than directly over it.

Treating Edema and Inflammation

The primary action of laser application for control of edema and inflammation is through the interruption of the formation of intermediate subtrates necessary for the production of inflammatory chemical mediators: kinins, histamines, and prostaglandins. Without these chemical mediators, the disruption of the body's homeostatic state is minimized, and the extent of pain and edema is diminished. It is also believed that laser energy can optimize cell membrane permeability, which regulates interstitial osmotic-hydrostatic pressures. Therefore, during tissue trauma, the flux of fluid into the intracellular spaces would be reduced. Laser treatment is usually applied by gridding over the involved areas or by treating related acupuncture points if the area of involvement is generalized.

SAFETY

Few safety considerations are necessary with the low-power laser. But as the variety of lasers has evolved and their uses increased in the United States, it has become necessary to develop national guidelines not only for safety but for therapeutic efficacy. The U.S. Food and Drug Administration's Center for Devices and Radiological Health now regulates the manufacture and sale of lasers in the United States. Laser equipment commonly is grouped into four FDA classes with simplified and well-differentiated safety procedures for each.[26]

Class I, or "exempt" lasers, are considered nonhazardous to the body. All invisible lasers with average power outputs of 1 mW or less are Class I devices. These include the GaAs lasers with wavelengths from 820 to 910 nm.[21] The invisible, infrared lasers should contain an indicator light to identify when the laser is engaged.

Class II, or "low-power" lasers, are hazardous only if a viewer stares continuously into the source. This class includes visible lasers that emit up to 1 mW average power, such as the HeNe laser.

Class III, or moderate-risk lasers, can cause retinal injury within the natural reaction time. The operator and athlete are required to wear protective eyewear. However, these lasers cannot cause serious skin injury, nor can they produce hazardous diffuse reflections from metals or other surfaces under normal use.[26]

Class IV, or high-power lasers, present a high risk of injury and can cause combustion of flammable materials. Other dangers are diffuse reflections that may harm the eyes and cause serious skin injury from direct exposure. These high-power lasers seldom are used outside research laboratories and restricted industrial environments.[26]

The low-power lasers used in treating sports injuries are categorized as Class I and II laser devices and Class III medical devices. Class III medical devices include new or modified devices not equivalent to any marketed before May 28, 1976.[12] To use a low-power laser in the United States on human subjects, a research proposal must be approved by an Institutional Review Board (IRB). The IRB can be established through the manufacturer, a university, or a hospital to obtain an Investigational Device Exemption (IDE). By requiring documentation of the results and side effects of lasers, the FDA regulations serve to generate scientific data to determine safety and efficacy of the device in question.

■ Clinical Decision-Making   *Exercise 14-5*

How can the athletic trainer treat a new abrasion using a laser to facilitate healing time and lessen infection?

Treatment Precautions and Considerations

There have been no ill effects reported from laser treatments for wound healing.[5] More controlled clinical data are needed to determine efficacy and to establish dosimetry that elicits reproducible responses. The impressions of low-power lasers are that they have a biostimulative effect on impaired tissues unless higher dosages, in excess of 8 to 10 J/cm^2, are administered.[1] This effect does not influence normal tissue. Beyond these ranges, a bioinhibitive effect may occur.

The applications of the low-power laser in an athletic training environment are potentially unlimited. Its applications can include wound healing properties on lacerations, abrasions, or infections. Clean procedures should be maintained to prevent cross contamination of the laser tip. Because the depth of penetration of the infrared laser is about 5 cm, other soft tissue injuries can be treated effectively by laser irradiation. Sprains, strains, and contusions have been observed by the authors to have faster healing rates with less pain. Acupuncture and superficial nerve sites also can be lased or combined with electrical stimulation to treat painful conditions.

Lasers deliver nonionizing radiation so no mutagenic effects on DNA and no damage to the cells or cell membranes have been found.[7] No deleterious effects have been reported after low-power laser exposure, including carcinogenic responses unless applied to already cancerous cells. Tumorous cells may proliferate when stimulated.[13]

Some suggestions on laser use:
- Laser should not be used over cancerous growths.
- It is better to underexpose than to overexpose. If clinical results plateau, a reduction in

■ TABLE 14-4   Summary of Indications and Contraindications for Using Low-Power Laser

INDICATIONS	CONTRAINDICATIONS
Facilitate wound healing	Cancerous tumors
Pain reduction	Directly over eyes
Increasing the tensile strength of a scar	Pregnancy
Decreasing scar tissue	
Decreasing inflammation	
Bone healing and fracture consolidation	

dosage or treatment frequency may facilitate results.
- Avoid direct exposure into the eyes because of possible retinal burns. If lasing for extended periods as with wound healing, safety glasses are recommended to avoid exposure from reflection.
- Although no adverse reactions have been documented, the use of laser during the first trimester of pregnancy is not recommended.
- A low percentage of athletes, especially with chronic pain, may experience a syncopy episode during the laser treatment. Symptoms usually subside within minutes. If symptoms exceed five minutes, no further treatments should be given.

CONCLUSION

The use of low-power lasers appears to have nothing but positive effects: this in itself should create a state of professional caution in deeming it a panacea modality. Currently, with these power outputs, lasers are recognized as insignificant risk devices. However, low-power lasers have not been granted recognition by the Food and Drug Administration as being a safe or effective modality. Although many empirical and clinical findings show promising results, more controlled studies are essential to determine the types of lasers and dosages that are required to attain reproducible results.

Summary

1. The first working laser was the ruby laser developed in 1960 and was initially called an optical maser.

2. Visible light wavelengths range from 400 to 700 nanometers. Light is transmitted through space in waves and is comprised of photons emitted at distinct energy levels.

3. An atom is excited when energy is applied and raises an orbiting electron to a higher orbit. When the electron returns to its original orbit, it releases energy in the form of a photon, a process called spontaneous emission.

4. Stimulated emission occurs when the photon is released from an excited atom and promotes the release of an identical photon to be released from a similarly excited atom.

5. For lasers to operate, a medium of excited atoms must be generated. This is termed *population inversion* and results when an external energy source (pumping device) is applied to the medium.

6. Characteristics of laser light vary from conventional light sources in three manners: laser light is monochromic (single color or wavelength), coherent (in phase), and collimated (minimal divergence).

7. Laser can be thermal (hot) or nonthermal (low-power, soft or cold). The categories of lasers include solid state (crystal or glass), gas, semiconductor, dye, or chemical lasers.

8. Helium neon, HeNe (gas) and gallium arsenide, GaAs (semiconductor) lasers are two low-power lasers being investigated by the FDA for application in physical medicine. These low-power lasers are currently being used in the United States and other countries for wound and soft-tissue healing and pain relief.

9. HeNe lasers deliver a characteristic red beam with a wavelength of 632.8 nm. The laser is delivered in a continuous wave and has a direct penetration of 2 to 5 mm and indirect penetration of 10 to 15 mm.

10. GaAs lasers are invisible and have a wavelength of 904 nm. They are delivered in a pulse mode and have an average power output of 0.4 milliwatts. This laser has a direct penetration of 1 to 2 cm and an indirect penetration to 5 cm.

11. The proposed therapeutic applications of lasers in physical medicine include acceleration of collagen synthesis, decrease in microorganisms, increase in vascularization, and reduction of pain and inflammation.

12. The technique of laser application is ideally done with gentle contact with the skin surface and should be perpendicular to the target surface. Dosage appears to be the critical factor in eliciting the desired response, but exact dosimetry has not been determined. Dosage fluctuates by varying the pulse frequency and the treatment times.

13. The laser is applied by developing an imaginary grid over the target area. The grid is comprised of 1-cm squares, and the laser is applied to each square for a pre-determined time. Trigger or acupuncture points are also treated for painful conditions.

14. The FDA considers low-power lasers as low-risk investigational devices. For use in the United States, they require an IRB approval and informed consent prior to their use.

15. Although no deleterious effects have been reported, certain precautions and contraindications exist. Contraindications include lasing over cancerous tissue, directly into the eyes, and during the first trimester of pregnancy. Occasionally, pain may initially increase when laser treatments begin but does not indicate cessation of treatment. A low percentage of athletes have experienced a syncope episode during laser treatment, but this is usually self-resolving. If symptoms persist for longer than five minutes, future laser treatments are not advised.

16. Future research for determining efficacy and treatment parameters is critically needed to substantiate the application of low-power lasers in physical medicine.

Review Questions

1. What does the acronym LASER stand for?
2. How does the laser use the concept of stimulated emission to produce a laser beam?
3. What are the characteristics of the helium neon and gallium arsenide low-power lasers?
4. What are the various therapeutic applications of lasers in wound and soft tissue healing, edema reduction, inflammation, and pain reduction?

5. What are the scanning and gridding techniques of application of the laser?
6. What seems to be the most critical treatment parameter in eliciting a desired response?
7. What are the treatment precautions and contraindications for low-power lasers?
8. Where does the low-power laser stand in terms of FDA approval as a therapeutic modality?

 ## Self-Test Questions

T/F
1. An atom containing more energy than normal is considered to be in an excited state.
2. HeNe and AuAg lasers are the most common.
3. Tissue responses occurring from absorption of the laser are direct effects.

Multiple Choice
4. Which of the following is NOT a property of lasers?
   a. monochromaticity
   b. coherence
   c. divergence
   d. collimation
5. _____ lasers may be used for wound healing and pain management.
   a. High-power
   b. Low-power
   c. Hot
   d. Chemical
6. Wounds treated with low-power lasers were shown to have what?
   a. increased tensile strength
   b. increased collagen synthesis
   c. both A and B
   d. neither A nor B

7. How are lasers thought to influence the inflammatory process?
   a. decrease prostaglandin production
   b. increase lymphocyte activity
   c. realign collagen
   d. increase metabolism
8. What type of laser application technique consists of holding the applicator over each square cm for the appropriate period of time?
   a. dosimetry
   b. wanding
   c. scanning
   d. gridding
9. Which of the following is a contraindication for low-power lasers?
   a. bone fracture
   b. cancerous tumors
   c. inflammation
   d. wounds
10. What energy density range is used in therapeutic applications?
   a. 0.05-4 mJ/cm^2
   b. 0.05-4 J/cm^2
   c. 5-15 mJ/cm^2
   d. 5-15 J/cm^2

Solutions to Clinical Decision-Making Exercises

14-1 It should be made clear that the type of laser being used in surgery is different from the one that is going to be used in treating the athlete's trigger point. The surgical techniques require a "hot" laser, whereas the athletic trainer will be using a cold laser. The athlete will feel nothing during the treatment and there will be no burns or any other residual indication from the laser treatment.

14-2 The athletic trainer should use a gridding technique in which there is contact between the tip of the laser and the skin. Moving the laser at a uniform speed over the predetermined grid area can help to ensure reasonably even coverage.

14-3 Dosage is dependent on the beam surface area of the laser in cm², the time of exposure in seconds, and the output of the laser in mW.

14-4 The athletic trainer should use a gridding laser technique with the probe held perpendicular to the skin with light contact. The energy density should be set at 3 J/cm². The laser treatment can be combined with electrical stimulation using low-frequency (1 to 5 Hz), high-intensity current to produce pain modulation via the release of β-endorphin.

14-5 First the wound should be cleaned appropriately and debrided as necessary. A scanning lasing technique with no direct contact should be done around the periphery of the abrasion. It is recommended that a HeNe laser be used at an energy density of 0.5 to 1 J/cm².

References

1. Abergel, R: *Biochemical Mechanisms of Wound and Tissue Healing With Lasers.* Second Canadian Low Power Medical Laser Conference, March 1987.

2. Abergel, R, Lyons, R, and Castel, J: Biostimulation of wound healing by lasers: experimental approaches in animal models and in fibroblast cultures, *J Dermatol Surg Oncol* 13:127–133, 1987.

3. Bartlett, WP, Quillen, WS, and Gonzalez, JL: Effect of gallium aluminum arsenide triple-diode laser on median nerve latency in human subjects, *Journal of Sport Rehabilitation* 8(2):99–108, 1999.

4. Bostara, M, Jucca, A, and Olliaro, P: In vitro fibroblast and dermis fibroblast activation by laser irradiation at low energy, *Dermatologica* 168:157–162, 1984.

5. Castel, J: *Laser Biophysics.* Second Canadian Low Power Medical Laser Conference, Ontario, Canada, March 1987.

6. Castel, M: Personal communication, MEDELCO, Downsview, Ontario, March, 1989.

7. Castel, M: *A clinical guide to low-power laser therapy*, Downsview, 1985, Ontario, PhysioTechnology Ltd.

8. Cheng, R: *Combination Laser/Electrotherapy in Pain Management.* Second Canadian Low Power Laser Conference, Ontario, Canada, March, 1987.

9. de Bie, RA, de Vet, HCW, Lenssen, TF, van den Wildenberg, FAJM, Kootstra, G and Knipschild, PG: Low-level laser therapy in ankle sprains: a randomized clinical trial, *Archives of Physical Medicine and Rehabilitation* 79(11): 1415–1420, 1998.

10. DeSimone, NA, Christiansen, C, and Dore, D: Bactericidal effect of 95mW Helium-Neon and Indium-gallium-aluminum-phosphate laser irradiation at exposure times of 30, 60, and 120 secs on photosensitized staphylococcus aureus and psuedomonas aeruginoas in vitro, *Phys Ther* 79(9):839–846, 1999.

11. Enwemeka, C: Laser biostimulation of healing wounds: specific effects and mechanisms of action, *JOSPT* 9:333–338, 1988.

12. Fact Sheet: Laser Biostimulation. Center of Devices and Radiological Health, FDA, Rockville, Md., 1984.

13. Farnham, J: Personal communication. Center of Devices and Radiological Health, FDA, Rockville, Md., March, 1989.

15. Gogia, P, Hurt, B, and Zirn, T: Wound management with whirlpool and infrared cold laser treatment, *Phys Ther* 68:1239–1242, 1988.

16. Hallmark, C, Horn, D: Lasers—the light fantastic, ed 2, Blue Ridge Summit, Pa., 1987, TAB Books.

17. Hunter, S, Leonard, L, and Wilson, R: Effects of low energy laser on wound healing in a porcine model, *Lasers Surg Med* 3:285–290, 1984.

18. Kana, J, Hutschenreiter, G, and Haina, D: Effect of low power density laser radiation on healing of open skin wounds in rats, *Arch Surg* 116:293–296, 1981.

19. Longo, L, Evangelista, S, and Tinacci, G: Effect of diode-laser silver arsenide-aluminum (Ga-Al-As) 904 nm on healing of experimental wounds, *Lasers Surg Med* 7:444–447, 1987.

20. Lyons, R, Abergel, R, and White, R: Biostimulation of wound healing in vivo by a Helium Neon Laser, *Ann. Plastic Surgery* 18: 47–77, 1987.

21. McComb, G: *The laser cookbook: 88 practical projects*, Blue Ridge Summit, Pa., 1988, TAB Books.

22. Mester, E, Mester, A, and Mester, A: Biomedical effects of laser application, *Laser Surg Med* 5:31–39, 1985.

23. Mester, E, Spiry, T, and Szende, B: Effect of laser rays on wound healing, *Am. J. Surg.* 122:532–535, 1971.

24. Rochkind, S, Nissan, M, and Barr-Nea, L: Response of peripheral nerve to HeNe Laser: experimental studies, *Lasers Surg Med* 7:441–443, 1987.

25. Schultz, R, Krishnamurthy, S, and Thelmo, W: Effects of varying intensities of laser energy on articular cartilage: a preliminary study, *Lasers Surg Med* 5:577–588, 1985.

26. Sliney, D, and Wolkarsht, M: *Safety with lasers and other optical sources: a comprehensive handbook*, New York, 1980, Plenum Press.

27. Snyder-Mackler, L, and Bork, C: Effect of helium neon laser irradiation on peripheral nerve sensory latency, *Phys Ther* 68:223–225, 1988.

28. Surinchak, J, Alago, M, and Bellamy, R: Effects of low-level energy lasers on the healing of full-thickness skin defects, *Lasers Surg Med* 2:267–274, 1983.

29. Trelles, M: *Medical Applications of Laser Biostimulation: Second Canadian Low power Medical Laser Conference*, Ontario, Canada, March, 1987.

30. Trelles, M, and Mayayo, E: Bone fracture consolidates faster with low power laser, *Lasers Surg Med* 7:36–45, 1987.

31. Van Pelt, W, Stewart, H, and Peterson, R: *Laser fundamentals and experiments*, Rockville, Md., 1970, U.S. Dept. HEW.

32. Walker, J: Relief from chronic pain by low power laser irradiation, *Neuroscience Letters* 43:339–344, 1983.

Suggested Readings

Abergel, R: Biostimulation of procollagen production by low energy lasers in human skin fibroblast culture, *Journal of Investigative Dermatology* 82:395, 1984.

Baxter, G, Bell, A, and Allen, J: Low level laser therapy: current clinical practice in Northern Ireland, *Physiotherapy* 77:171–178, 1991.

Baxter, G: *Therapeutic lasers theory and practice*, New York, 1994, Churchill Livingstone.

Beckerman, H, De Bie, R, and Bouter L: The efficacy of laser therapy for musculoskeletal and skin disorders: a criteria-based meta-analysis of randomized clinical trials, *Phys Ther* 72(7):483–491, 1992.

Bolton, P, Young, S, and Dyson, M: Macrophage response to laser therapy: a dose response study, *Laser Ther* 2:101–106, 1990.

Bolton, P, Young, S, and Dyson, M: Macrophage responsiveness to laser therapy with varying power and energy densities, *Laser Ther* 3:105–112, 1991.

Braverman, B, McCarthy, R, and Ivankovich, A: Effect on helium neon and infrared laser irradiation on wound healing in rabbits, *Lasers Surg Med* 9:50–58, 1989.

Crous, L, and Malherbe, C: Laser and ultraviolet light irradiation in the treatment of chronic ulcers, *Physiotherapy* 44:73–77, 1988.

Cummings, J: The effect of low energy (HeNe) laser irradiation on healing dermal wounds in an animal model, *Phys Ther* 65:737, 1985.

Dreyfuss, P, and Stratton, S: The low-energy laser, electroacuscope, and neuroprobe: treatment options remain controversial, *Phys Sportsmedicine* 21(8):47–50, 55–57, 1993.

Dyson, M, and Young, S: Effects of laser therapy on wound contraction and cellularity in mice, *Lasers Surg Med* 1:125, 1986.

Gogia, P, and Marquez, R: Effects of helium-neon laser on wound healing, *Ostomy Wound Management* 38(6):33, 36, 38–41, 1992.

Hayashi, K, Markel, M, and Thabit, G: The effect of nonablative laser energy on joint capsular properties: an in vitro mechanical study using a rabbit model, *Amer J Sports Med* 23(4):482–487, 1995.

Herbert, K, Bhusate, L, and Scott, D: Effect of laser light at 820 nm on adinosine nucleotide levels in human lymphocytes, *Lasers in the Life Sciences* 3:37–45, 1989.

Karu, T, Tiphlova, S, and Samokhina, M: Effects of near infrared laser and superluminous diode irradiation on escherichia coli division rate, *IEEE J Quantum Electronics* 26:2162–2165, 1990.

Kramer, J, and Sandrin, M: Effect of low-power laser and white light on sensory conduction rate of the superficial radial nerve, *Physiotherapy Canada* 45(3):165–170, 1993.

Laakso, L, Richardson, C, and Cramond, T: Factors affecting Low Level Laser Therapy, *Aust J Physiotherapy* 39(2):95–99, 1993.

Lam, T, Abergerl, R, and Meeker, C: Biostimulation of human skin fibroblasts: low energy lasers selectively enhance collagen synthesis, *Laser Surg Med* 3:328, 1984.

Lundeberg, T, Haker, E, and Thomas, M: Effect of laser versus placebo in tennis elbow, *Scand J. Rehabil Med* 19:135–138, 1987.

Lyons, R, Abergel, R, and White, R: Biostimulation of wound healing in vivo by a helium neon laser, *Ann Plas Surg* 18:47–50, 1987.

Malm, M, and Lundeberg, T: Effect of low-power gallium arsenide laser on healing of venous ulcers, *Scand J Reconstructive Hand Surg* 25:249–251, 1991.

Martin, D: An investigation into the effects of low level therapy on arterial blood flow in skeletal muscle, *Physiotherapy* 81(9):562, 1995.

McMeeken, J, and Stillman, B: Perceptions of the clinical efficacy of laser therapy, *Aust J Physiotherapy* 39(2):101–106, 1993.

Mester, E, and Jaszsagi-Nagy, E: The effects of laser radiation on wound healing and collagen synthesis, *Studia Biophysica* 35(3):227, 1973.

Nussbaum, E, Biemann, I, and Mustard, B: Comparison of ultrasound/ultraviolet-C and laser for treatment of pressure ulcers in athletes with spinal cord injury, *Phys Ther* 74(9):812–823, 1994.

Palmgren, N, Dahlin, J, and Beck, H: Low level laser therapy of infected abdominal wounds after surgery, *Lasers Surg Med Supp* 3:11, 1991.

Rockhind, S, Russo, M, and Nissan, M: Systemic effect of low-power laser on the peripheral and central nervous system, cutaneous wounds, and burns, *Lasers Surg Med* 9:174–182, 1989.

Saperia, D, Glassberg, E, and Lyons, R: Stimulation of collagen synthesis in human fibroblast cultures, *Laser in the Life Sciences* 1:61–77, 1986.

Vasseljen, O: Low-level laser versus traditional physiotherapy in the treatment of tennis elbow, *Physiotherapy* 78(5):329–334, 1992.

Waylonis, G, Wilke, S, and O'Toole, D: Chronic myofascial pain: management by low-output helium-neon laser therapy, *Arch Pays Med Rehab* 69(12):1017–1020, 1988.

Young, S: Macrophage responsivity to light therapy, *Lasers Surg Med* 9:497–505, 1989.

Young, S, Dyson, M, and Bolton, P: *Effect of light on calcium uptake by macrophages.* Presented at the Fourth International Biotherapy Association Seminar on Laser Biostimulation, Guy's Hospital, London, 1991.

CHAPTER 15

....

Ultraviolet Therapy

J. Marc Davis

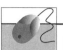

Study Resources

Refer to the lab exercises in the accompanying Laboratory Manual, as well as eSims which simulates the athletic training certification exam at www.mhhe.com/esims. Also, check out the competency information found at www.mhhe.com/prentice11e. For more online study resources, visit our Health and Human Performance Website at www.mhhe.com/hhp/.

Following completion of this chapter, the student athletic trainer will be able to

- Describe the position of ultraviolet radiation (UVR) in the electromagnetic spectrum and the relationship of UVR to other forms of electromagnetic energy.

- Explain how UVR raises energy levels within irradiated objects.

- Articulate the effect of UVR on individual cells and human tissue and explain the tanning process.

- Recognize the effect of long-term exposure to UVR and the effect of UVR on the eyes.

- Demonstrate the physical setup and procedures for operating a UVR device, including safety precautions, the skin test, the inverse square law, and the cosine law.

- Illustrate various clinical uses of UVR.

Ultraviolet radiation (UVR) is one of the oldest medical modalities. The physicians of ancient Egypt and Greece attributed many healing powers to sunlight, and in fact, life itself would not be possible without the interaction of solar UVR and plant photosynthesis. Before this century, the sun was the only satisfactory source of UVR, but now a wide selection of UVR generators is available.

This chapter serves to familiarize the student athletic trainer with the properties of UVR, to explain how UVR affects human tissue, and to explore different UVR treatment apparatus and techniques. Subsequently, the athletic trainer should be able to understand why UVR therapy can be effective in treating certain maladies, and therefore be able to correctly choose UVR therapy when it is the appropriate treatment for a given problem, even though ultraviolet therapy is rarely used in a sports medicine setting.

ULTRAVIOLET RADIATION

Ultraviolet radiation (UVR) is the portion of the electromagnetic spectrum that ranges from 2000 to 4000 Å and is bordered below 2000 Å by x-ray and above 4000 Å by visible light (see Figure 1-2). The UVR portion of the electromagnetic spectrum is further divided into three sections: UV-A, UV-B, and UV-C (Table 15-1). UV-C (also called short-wave UV, extreme UV, and far UV) ranges from

■ **TABLE 15-1** Ultraviolet radiation (2000–4000 Å)

TYPE	RANGE	NAME	EFFECTS
UV-A	3200–4000 Å	Near ultraviolet	No harmful effects
UV-B	2900–3200 Å	Middle ultraviolet	Sunburn
UV-C	2000–2900 Å	Far ultraviolet	Bacteriocidal

- Athletic trainers use UV-B and UV-C

2000 to 2900 Å and is bactericidal.[28,34] UV-B (called middle UV and the sunburn spectrum) ranges from 2900 to 3200 Å and is associated with sunburn and age-related skin changes.[27-34] UV-A (near UV) ranges from 3200 to 4000 Å. Until recently, little or no physiologic effect was attributed to UV-A , but recent research and clinical use of UV-A are showing possible benefits and hazards for UV-A exposure. The UVR apparatus most likely to be encountered by the athletic trainer in a sports medicine setting would generate UVR in the UV-B or UV-C range, or in both ranges.[13]

The beneficial effects of UVR as a treatment modality are mediated by its limited absorption. UVR is absorbed within the first 1 to 2 mm of human skin and most of the physiologic effects are superficial.[8] Therefore, the most effective use of UVR therapy is in the treatment of various skin disorders such as acne and psoriasis.[5,12,16]

EFFECT ON CELLS

UVR is a form of electromagnetic energy. As indicated in Chapter 1, according to the Arndt-Schultz principle when ultraviolet light contacts any surface, skin included, it must be either reflected or absorbed and transmitted. According to the cosine

DNA Deoxyribonucleic acid—the substance found in the chromosomes of the cell nucleus that carries the genetic code of the cell.

RNA Ribonucleic acid—an acid found in the cell cytoplasm and nucleolus; it is intimately involved in protein synthesis.

law, if UVR strikes the skin at a 90-degree angle, 90% to 95% of the energy will be absorbed. Most will be absorbed within the epidermis of the skin (80% to 90%) while the rest will reach the dermis.[8] As the UVR is absorbed within the tissue, it causes the energy level of exposed atoms to increase. These atoms will quickly return to their normal energy state; however, the presence of excess energy causes chemical excitation within the cells of the exposed tissue. This chemical excitation is the cause of the various effects of UVR on living cells and tissue. Even a single exposure to UVR will cause chemical excitation within exposed cells, which leads to physiologic changes within these cells.

These physiologic changes are the result of a photochemical event that is the end product of the UVR-induced chemical excitation. This photochemical event results in an alteration of cell biochemistry and cellular metabolism. The synthesis of **DNA** and **RNA** is affected, leading to alterations in protein and enzyme production. As a consequence, cell protein structure can be altered, and this alteration of cellular protein and DNA may leave the cell inactive or dead.[28-33]

Fortunately, defenses have evolved that protect microorganisms and cells that are exposed to a constant barrage of UVR from the sun. The damaged cells may be restored by enzymatic action or by simple deterioration of the damaged portion, the damaged segment may be replaced by normal material, or it may be bypassed when the cell reproduces.[28] DNA synthesis within cells of the human epidermis is suppressed for 24 to 48 hours following exposure to UVR in the range of 2500 to 2700 Å and is then followed by a period of increased DNA synthesis.[28,33]

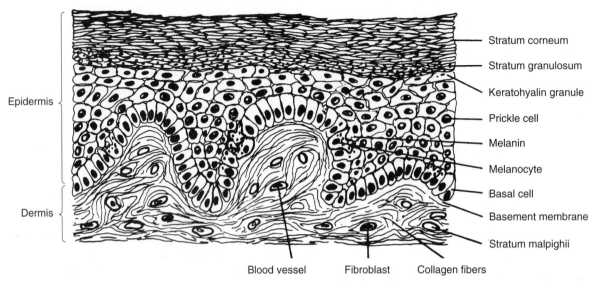

Figure 15-1   A cross section of the skin showing the dermis and epidermis layers.

EFFECT ON NORMAL HUMAN TISSUE

Short-Term Effect On Skin

Normal human skin consists of two layers, the superficial epidermis and the underlying dermis (Figure 15-1). The epidermis is avascular and composed mostly of well-organized layers of **keratinocytes.** These produce **keratin,** the fibrous protective protein of the skin. The keratinocytes are produced from cells of the basal layer of the epidermis and then move upward through the epidermis. The dermis is divided into two layers, the papillary layer that contains a rich blood supply, and the reticular layer that is composed of heavy connective tissue and contains fibroblasts, histiocytes, and most cells.

Erythema.   When human skin is exposed to UVR, the individual cells react as previously described. However, the skin is a protective organ covering the entire human exterior, and it will respond in a generalized manner over the entire area that is irradiated. This generalized response culminates in the development of an acute inflammatory reac-

keratinocytes   A cell that produces keratin.

keratin   The fibrous protein that forms the chemical basis of the epidermis.

erythema   A redness of the skin caused by capillary dilation.

pigmentation   Tanning of the skin from sun exposure.

tion. The end results of an active inflammation within the skin are **erythema** (the reddening of the skin associated with sunburn), **pigmentation** (tanning), and increased epidermal thickness.[8,17,28,33]

Inflammation.   Inflammation is the response of any human tissue, skin included, to an irritating or injurious substance or event. In the case of UVR exposure the irritating substances are the end products of the previously described photochemical event and may include damaged DNA, RNA, and cell proteins. The inflammatory process removes these injurious and irritating substances from the skin. Since the appearance of these irritating sub-

hyperplasia   An increase in the size of a tissue; in the skin, an increased thickness of the epidermis.

photosensitization   A process in which a person becomes overly sensitive to UVR.

stances does not occur immediately following UVR exposure, the inflammatory response is delayed. Normally, it begins several hours after irradiation and peaks 8 to 24 hours following exposure.[28]

This inflammatory response is characterized by local vasodilation and increased capillary permeability. Theoretically, this is caused by (1) the absorption of UVR by keratinocytes, leading to the release of substances that diffuse to the papillary dermis and cause vasodilation; or (2) the absorption of UVR by mast cells in the dermis that in turn release histamine, resulting in vasodilation.[8,17,28] Erythema is caused by this vasodilation and the subsequent increase of blood within the dermis. The increased capillary permeability permits certain proteins to move from the capillaries and into the dermis. This results in a change in osmotic pressure; consequently water is drawn into the area and edema occurs. Leukocytes, lymphocytes, and monocytes pass into the dermis and to a small degree into the epidermis. These cells phagocytize (consume or engulf) dead cells and other debris. At 24 hours, the inflammatory process is completed, and at 30 hours the rebuilding begins. The reparative process is characterized by increased activity of the keratinocytes and results in a thickening of the epidermis **(hyperplasia)**.[28] This is protective; areas covered with a thick epidermis, such as the soles of the feet, do not sunburn.

Photosensitization.   The acute effects of UVR exposure can be exacerbated if certain chemicals or medications are present on the skin or in the body. **Photosensitization** is a process in which a person becomes overly sensitive to UVR as a result of the excitation of a chemical by UVR exposure.[8] Any person taking a photosensitizing medication is very susceptible to the effects of UVR and should be

■ **TABLE 15-2**   List of Photosensitizing Agents

ANTIBACTERIAL AND MICROBIAL AGENTS

Tetracyclines—a group of broad spectrum antibiotics
Sulfonamides—a group of synthetic antimicrobial drugs
Griseofulvin (Fulvicin, Grifulvin, Grisactin)—an antibiotic with an additional antifungal action

THIAZIDE DIURETICS A group of drugs that act on the kidney to increase sodium and water in the urine

Chlorothiazide (Diuril)
Hydrochlorothiazide (Hydrodiuril, Oretic, Esidrix)
Methychlorothiazide (Enduron)

OTHER MEDICATIONS

Phenothiazines (Thorazine)—widely used tranquilizers
Psoralens—a group of dermal pigmenting agents
Sulfonylureas (Dymelor, Diabinese)
Diphenhydramine (Benadryl)—an antihistamine

MISCELLANEOUS

Sunscreens
Tar
Oral contraceptives
Certain cosmetics[8,27,28]

melanin   A group of dark brown or black pigments that occur naturally in the eye, skin, hair, and other animal tissues.

treated accordingly. It should be noted that such an adverse reaction can occur even after limited exposure to natural sunlight. A list of common photosensitizing agents appears in Table 15-2.

Tanning

Tanning reflects the increase of pigmentation within the skin and is a protective mechanism activated by UVR exposure. An increase of **melanin**,

Phases of tanning

- Immediate
- Delayed

the pigment responsible for darkening, within the skin causes the tan (see Figure 15-1). The melanin functions as a biologic filter of UVR by scattering the radiation, by absorbing the UVR, and by dissipating the absorbed energy as heat.[33] The process of tanning is divided into two phases: immediate tanning and delayed tanning.

Immediate tanning appears most often in darkly pigmented individuals and occurs immediately following UVR exposure. Immediate tanning represents the darkening of melanosomes already present in the skin. It begins to fade 1 hour after exposure and is hardly noticeable 3 to 8 hours later.[28,33] Delayed tanning is the result of the formation of new pigment (melanin) through the process of melanogenesis. The process is initiated by production of erythema (sunburn) within the skin. Melanogenesis occurs within the melanocytes of the basal layer of the epidermis (see Figure 15-1), and the end products of this process are melanosomes, or new pigment granules. These melanosomes are transferred from the melanocytes via nerve cells to nearby keratinocytes. As the keratinocytes gradually move outward to the skin's surface, the new pigment also migrates to the periphery. Delayed tanning usually becomes apparent 72 hours after UVR exposure.

Human skin color is a baseline that is influenced by various environmental factors (exposure to solar radiation, occupation, leisure activities) and the genetically determined level of melanin within the skin.[8,34] Individuals of all races have the same number of melanocytes per unit area, but darker individuals are able to produce greater amounts of melanin.[7]

Long-Term Effect on Skin. The most serious effects of long-term UVR exposure are premature aging of the skin and skin cancer.[20,30,31] Lightly pigmented individuals are more susceptible

■ **Clinical Decision-Making** *Exercise 15-1*

It has been suggested that an athlete use ultraviolet radiation to clear up a fungal infection on his feet. The athlete tells the athletic trainer that he is worried that repeated exposure to ultraviolet light might predispose him to developing skin cancer. How can the athletic trainer minimize his fear?

Cancers of the skin

- Basal cell carcinoma
- Equamous cell carcinoma
- Malignant melanoma

to these maladies. Premature aging of the skin is characterized by dryness, cracking, and a decrease in the elasticity of the skin, and it results from a change in the epidermis called solar elastosis. An alteration in the skin's elastic fibers causes solar elastosis and has been tentatively linked to UVR-induced DNA damage.[28]

Skin cancer is the most common malignant tumor found in humans and has been epidemiologically and clinically associated with solar UVR.[1,28,30,34] Damage to DNA is suspected as the cause of skin cancer, but the exact cause is yet unknown. The major types of skin cancer are basal cell carcinoma, which rarely metastasizes (spreads to other areas), squamous cell carcinoma, which metastasizes in 5% of all cases, and malignant melanoma, which metastasizes in a majority of cases.[28,30] Fortunately, the rate of cure exceeds 95% with early detection and treatment.

EFFECT ON EYES

For centuries it has been known that sunlight can have an adverse effect on vision. Snow blindness, the result of solar UVR being reflected from the snow to the unprotected eyes of winter outdoor en-

photokeratitis   An inflammation of the eyes caused by exposure to UVR.

thusiasts, was first described in 375 BC.[33] UVR exposure of the eyes causes an acute inflammation called **photokeratitis.** It is a delayed reaction occurring from 6 to 24 hours after exposure, but occasionally it develops within 30 minutes. Conjunctivitis (inflammation of the mucous membrane that lines the inside of the eyelid) develops, accompanied by erythema of adjacent facial skin, and the injured person reports the sensation of a foreign body on the eye. Photophobia, increased tear production, and spasm of the ocular muscles may occur.[28,34] The acute reaction lasts from 6 to 24 hours, and all symptoms will generally clear by 48 hours with few residual effects. The eye, unlike the skin, does not develop a tolerance to UVR. The development of cataracts has been attributed to UVR, especially in wavelengths of greater than 2900 Å.[32,34]

SYSTEMIC EFFECTS

The only systemic effect that can be objectively attributed to UVR (the only positive effect in general, for that matter) is the photosynthesis of vitamin D following irradiation of the skin by UVR in the UV-B range.[19,32] The process is activated when the skin is irradiated by UVR at approximately 300 A wavelength. This activates a complicated biochemical pathway that travels from the skin to the liver and kidney and results in vitamin D being delivered to bones, to the intestines, to various organs, and to muscles. Vitamin D is responsible for regulating calcium and phosphorus, and after UVR exposure the absorption of these elements increases within the intestines and results in increased amounts of calcium and phosphorus within the blood. Consequently, UVR can be used as a treatment for disorders of calcium and phosphorus metabolism, such as rickets and tetany. Presently, the treatment of choice for such problems is dietary supplementation; however, if this is not effective, UVR is an acceptable alternative.

- Systemic effect of UVR is photosynthesis of Vitamin D

UVR generators

- Carbon arc lamp
- Xenon compact arc lamp
- Fluorescent ultraviolet lamp (backlight)
- Mercury arc lamp

ULTRAVIOLET GENERATORS

Since the beginning of this century many types of UVR generators have been developed, including the carbon arc lamp, the fluorescent lamp, the xenon compact arc lamp, and the mercury arc lamps. Of these, the mercury arc lamps are the most common and they have been found to be safe, effective, and easy to operate.

Carbon Arc Lamp

The carbon arc lamp is composed of two carbon electrodes that consist of carbon and certain inorganic salts and metals. Initially, the two electrodes are in contact when the current is applied and then are moved slightly apart, causing the current to arc across this small gap. As the salts and metals within the electrodes become heated, UVR is emitted, the majority between 3500 and 4000 Å. The electrode gradually burns, and so the lamp will deteriorate and the electrodes must be replaced. This burning is noisy, causes an unpleasant odor, and the device requires a high electrical input.

Xenon Compact Arc Lamp

The xenon compact arc lamp is composed of xenon gas enclosed in a vessel in which it is compressed to 20 times atmospheric pressure. An electric arc is passed through the gas, causing increased temperature. When the gas is heated to 6000° C (10,832° F), the atoms become incandescent and emit infrared, visible, and ultraviolet light waves. Most of the UVR is in the range of 3200 to 4000 Å. Caution must be exercised when using a device with gas under such high pressure because rupture of the containing vessel could endanger the athlete and operator.

Fluorescent Ultraviolet Lamp (Blacklight)

The fluorescent ultraviolet lamp or "blacklight" is actually a low-pressure mercury lamp. It consists of a tube of UV-transmitting glass that is coated with phosphors. The phosphors are fluorescing substances that absorb the UVR and then re-emit it at a longer wavelength. Most of the UVR-emitted ranges are from 3000 to 4000 Å, within the high UV-B and entire UV-A range.[32] These lamps are low-powered and generally used in multiples. These lamps are used where exposure of several people simultaneously is desired.

Mercury Arc Lamp

The mercury arc lamps are divided into two categories, low-pressure and high-pressure mercury arcs. Both consist of mercury (a heavy metal in a liquid state) contained in a quartz envelope. When an electric arc is passed through the envelope, the mercury becomes vaporized and at 8000° C (14,432° F), the atoms become incandescent and emit ultraviolet, infrared, and visible light. In the low-pressure lamp, also called the cold quartz lamp, the temperature of the mercury electrons is greater than the mercury vapor and the temperature of the quartz envelope is about 60° C—hot but not dangerous. The UVR spectrum produced by low-pressure lamps is limited to 1849 Å and 2537 Å. The 1849 Å wavelength is blocked by the quartz envelope or it would combine with oxygen and produce ozone; 95% of the UVR produced by these lamps is the 2537 Å wavelength, which is highly germicidal. The low-pressure mercury arc

• Mercury arc lamp is most commonly used in sports medicine

lamp does not require a warm-up or cool-down period, and it is used mainly where the bactericidal effect of UVR is desired.

A high-pressure mercury arc occurs when the mercury vapor temperature equals the mercury electron temperature and the pressure within the envelope reaches one atmosphere or more.[31] The quartz envelopes of these lamps becomes quite hot and may be cooled by a water jacket or circulating air; subsequently, these are called hot quartz lamps. The UVR spectrum produced peaks at 2537, 2800, 2967, 3025, 3130, and 3660 Å.[8,17,32,33] The 2537 Å wavelength is absorbed by the increased density of the mercury vapor and does not pass from the lamp. Most of the UVR produced falls within the UV-B range. These lamps require a warm-up period before reaching peak efficiency, and a cool-down period after the current is stopped before the lamp can be restarted. The high-pressure mercury arc lamps are mainly used to produce erythema and the accompanying photochemical reactions.

The mercury arc lamps are the most likely kind of UVR lamp to be used in a sports medicine setting, and generally the lamps will be either a standing model or a hand-held model. The standing model consists of a mercury arc lamp surrounded by a reflector. The opening below the lamp and reflector can be closed by the use of shutters. The lamp, re-

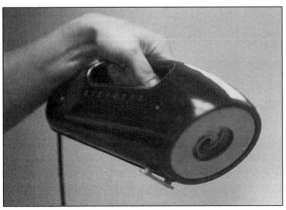

(a)

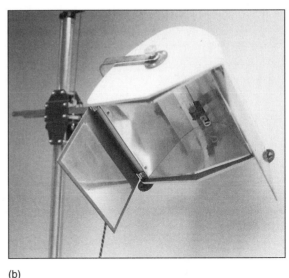

(b)

Figure 15-2   (a) A hand-held cold quartz ultraviolet lamp. (b) A standing hot quartz ultraviolet lamp. Note the open shutters.

flector, and shutters are supported by a column and the height of the column is adjustable. At the base of the column is a housing that contains the electrical controls contained within the configuration of the unit (Figure 15-2). The hand-held unit is used for very local treatments and produces the bactericidal spectral bond of 2536 Å. It is very effective for treating local skin infections and, with the addition of a special lens, is used for diagnostic purposes.

TECHNIQUES OF APPLICATION

Before operation of any UVR generator, athletic trainers must thoroughly familiarize themselves with the equipment; the operation manual must be understood and available if needed. Faulty operation of the equipment can endanger both the athlete and the operator.[21] The lamp and reflector must be kept clean by wiping with gauze and methyl alcohol or by following the manufacturer's instructions. The quality of UVR is greatly diminished by dirty lamps and reflectors. The entire device must be completely inspected prior to use to ensure safe operation.

minimal erythemal dose   The amount of time of exposure to UVR necessary to cause a faint erythema 24 hours after exposure.

Determining the Minimal Erythemal Dose (Skin Test)

The effectiveness of the apparatus must be determined before UVR therapy can begin. The lamps in these devices deteriorate over time, and accumulation of dirt and other residues on the lamp and reflector can also alter the effect of the UVR. Two lamps of the same model may have two differing effects, depending on the age of the lamp and its condition. The effectiveness of the lamp is assessed by determining the skin sensitivity to UVR of the athlete to be treated. This sensitivity is measured by the **minimal erythemal dose.** The minimal erythemal dose is the exposure time needed to produce a faint erythema of the skin 24 hours after exposure.[8,30] Prior to testing, the athlete should be questioned regarding photosensitizing drugs and the

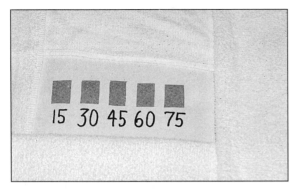

Figure 15-3 The ultraviolet skin test. The athlete's back is draped and has been sequentially exposed to ultraviolet radiation for 15, 30, 45, 60, and 75 seconds.

area of skin to be tested should be cleaned. The area of the test should have pigmentation similar to the area to be treated. The forearm is a common choice for the test site.

For the skin test, the athlete should be positioned comfortably, and eye protection must be provided the athlete and the athletic trainer. The goggles must fit snugly, since UVR can be reflected behind the lens of ordinary sunglasses. The athlete may be instructed to close his or her eyes as an added precaution. The athlete is draped except for the test site; a good quality bed sheet or bath towel provides an adequate barrier to UVR. A piece of typing paper with five cutouts 1 inch square and 1 inch apart is placed over the test site (Figure 15-3). If necessary the lamp is warmed up with the protective shutters closed. The lamp is positioned over the athlete with care being taken to adjust the height of the lamp from the athlete to the same level as for treatment. With the lamp in position, the shutters are opened and the cutouts covered at 15-second intervals so that the five portions of the skin will be exposed for 15, 30, 45, 60, and 75 seconds. The athlete returns in 24 hours and a visual inspection determines the minimal erythemal dose. This information is used as the basis for determining treatment time.[4]

Areas tested that reveal no erythema 24 hours after testing have received a suberythemal dose, whereas those demonstrating erythema at 24 hours have received the minimal erythemal dose. At

■ Analogy 15-1

Doing a skin test to determine a minimal erythemal dose is like going to the beach and trying to figure out how long you can stay in the sun without getting red. Of course, the presence of clouds or rain or the time of day can greatly influence how long it takes you to begin to burn. Likewise, there are differences in UV generators as well and thus a skin test is necessary to achieve the correct amount of exposure without burning the skin.

48 hours, if erythema is still present, a first-degree erythemal dose has been given, and a second-degree erythemal dose has been given if erythema persists from 48 to 72 hours. If the erythema lasts past 72 hours after testing, then a third-degree erythemal dose has been given. The third-degree erythemal dose is pathologic and causes destruction of the skin. Second-degree and third-degree doses are seldom used except in the case of stubborn skin infections, and when they are used, the skin surrounding the area of treatment should be well protected from exposure. First-degree and second-degree doses can be estimated; first-degree erythemal doses approximately correspond to 2.5 times the minimal erythemal dose and second-degree doses correspond to 5 times the minimal erythemal dose.[8,22]

Since human skin adapts to UVR exposure, the minimal erythemal dose will gradually increase with repeated treatments. Therefore, it is necessary to gradually increase exposure time to achieve the same reaction. Once the treatment time has been determined, it is increased 5 seconds per treatment with the height of the lamp remaining constant. Conversely, treatment time should be reduced 5 seconds for each day missed or it should be set back to the original minimal erythemal dose.

Positioning the Lamp

To give consistent treatments, the operator needs to be aware of the two laws of physics, previously discussed in Chapter 1, which apply directly to UVR treatments: the inverse square law and the cosine

■ **Clinical Decision-Making**   *Exercise 15-3*

The athletic trainer is treating an athlete who has a mild case of acne on his upper back. The athletic trainer is trying to determine a minimal erythemal dose. At 24 hours following exposure the areas exposed for 45, 60, and 75 seconds are red. At 48 hours, only the areas exposed for 60 and 75 seconds are still red. What would be considered a second-degree erythemal dose?

law. The inverse square law states that the strength of radiation of light from a point source varies inversely with the square of the distance from the source.[6,8,32] Therefore, if the lamp is set closer to the athlete than during the skin test, a stronger dose is given; if it is set further away, a weaker dose is given. The distance of the lamp from the athlete must be kept constant if the intensity of the treatments is to be equal. The height of the lamp is generally standardized at each clinic, usually ranging from 24 to 40 inches.[7] My preference is to set the height of the lamp at 30 inches.

The cosine law states that for maximum absorption of radiant energy, the source must be perpendicular to the absorbing surface (the athlete being the absorbing surface).[8,32] A deviation of 10 degrees causes no major alteration in the amount of energy absorbed. Therefore, care should be taken in positioning the lamp and athlete during testing and treatment.

Treatment Technique

Once the minimal erythemal dose has been established, treatment can commence. As with the skin test, the treatment area should be warm and should provide maximum privacy since the athlete may be partially or fully disrobed. Goggles, stopwatch, measuring tape, and draping must be readily available. The athlete should be carefully draped so that areas not to receive UVR exposure are protected. Besides the eyes, the nipples and genitalia should be protected. It should be taken into account that UVR

■ **Laws that apply to UVR**

• Cosine law
• Inverse square law

can be reflected from white linen and shiny equipment surfaces. If needed, the UVR apparatus should be warmed up with the protective shutter in place. The athlete and athletic trainer are ready to begin treatment when the athlete is comfortable, properly draped, and has his or her eyes protected. The lamp is positioned at proper height and angle, and the operator has his or her goggles in place and stopwatch ready. Treatment commences when the operator simultaneously opens the shutters and activates the stopwatch. At the end of the predetermined treatment time, the shutters are closed, the lamp is extinguished, and the athlete is allowed to remove the goggles and dress. Accurate records noting the height of the lamp, time of exposure, and condition of the area treated must be kept. Also, the same lamp should be used for subsequent treatments since lamp deterioration causes differing intensities from UVR sources of even the same manufacturer's model.

Consistency is crucial if safe and effective UVR treatments are to be given.[21] The setup of the athlete and equipment should not vary without adequate reason. Usually the only variable is the length of treatment (exposure) and that is determined by and based on the skin test, the treatment prescription, the lesion to be treated, and the progression of treatment. If the length of treatment is in doubt, it is always best to yield to brevity rather than to endanger an athlete.

CLINICAL APPLICATIONS FOR ULTRAVIOLET THERAPY

UVR therapy may be used to obtain one or more of the following effects: increased vitamin D production, stimulation of the skin, sterilization, tanning, hyperplasia, and exfoliation (peeling).[32] The use of UVR is indicated for treatment of infectious and noninfectious skin diseases and for the excitation of calcium metabolism.[8] The development of antibiotics and other medications has greatly reduced the clinical use of UVR since these drugs are very effective and simple to employ in the treatment of disease. Today the most common use of UVR is in the treatment of dermatologic conditions such as psoriasis and acne and hard-to-cure infectious skin conditions such as pressure sores.[14,15,26] The protocol for treating certain maladies with UVR follows.

Skin Lesions

UVR may be used successfully to treat the following skin lesions: acne (general body irradiation may help, minimal erythemal dose applied three times per week); septic wounds (local second-degree erythemal response, repeated every 3 days); aseptic wounds (suberythemal dose applied every 3 days[3,8,20,25,30]); folliculitis (suberythemal dose applied every 3 days until clear); pityriasis rosea (general body irradiation, minimal erythemal dose applied three times per week[18]); tinea capitis (local first-degree erythemal reaction, repeated when initial response clears).

Psoriasis

The Goekerman technique developed in 1925 is still widely used.[35] This consists of applying a crude tar ointment (2% to 5%) over the patches of psoriasis the night prior to treatment. The next morning the tar is removed, except for a thin film, and the area is irradiated with a UV-B source at minimal erythemal dosage.[3,8] The exposure time is gradually increased, and the treatment is usually carried out for several weeks. In the past decade, a UV-A source and the photosensitizing drug psoralen have been used to treat psoriasis.[12] This technique is called PUVA therapy.

Puva Therapy. A treatment for psoriasis that consists of ingestion of oral methoxsalen, a psoralen, and exposure of the affected site to a UV-A light source. The methoxsalen increases the athlete's sensitivity to UVR, and in the presence of UV-A, it binds with DNA and inhibits DNA synthesis.[9] Unfortunately, several studies point to an increased risk of developing skin cancer following PUVA therapy, and problems with the safety of the UV-A sources have been uncovered.[2,9,10,29] Still, in selected cases PUVA therapy is considered by the American Academy of Dermatology to be safe, but its use should be limited to physicians with training in photochemotherapy.[2]

Disturbances of Calcium and Phosphorus Absorption

Conditions such as osteomalacia (rickets) and tetany can be treated with irradiation by a UV-B source. These disturbances of absorption are caused by a vitamin D deficiency. As previously discussed, vitamin D is produced following irradiation of the skin. Whole body irradiation is indicated if diet and oral supplementation of calcium and phosphorus do not produce improvement.[19,32]

Pressure Sores

Unlike most infectious skin disorders, pressure sores do not respond readily to antibiotic therapy. Irradiation of the lesion by low-pressure mercury or cold quartz lamp, which produces UVR of the bactericidal 2537 Å wavelength, can be an effective means of treating this problem. The hand-held lamps are most useful since they can be used to produce a very localized reaction. Exposure time should be sufficient to produce a second-degree or third-degree erythemal dose response.[8,11,32] Care must be taken to protect the surrounding skin.

Sterilization

Bacteria are destroyed when exposed to UVR in the range of 2500 to 2700 Å. This technique has been used to sterilize the air in operating rooms and to sterilize water. The technique is quite safe if human exposure to the UVR source is kept to a minimum.

Diagnosis

A UVR source fitted with a special filter, a Wood's filter, can be used to aid in the diagnosis of certain skin disorders. The filter blocks all the UVR except that in

■ **TABLE 15-3**   Summary of Indications and Contraindications for Ultraviolet Therapy

INDICATIONS	CONTRAINDICATIONS
Acne	Porphyrias
Aseptic wounds	Pellagra
Folliculitis	Lupus erythematosus
Pityriasis rosea	Sarcoidosis
Tinea capitum	Xeroderma pigmentosum
Septic wounds	Acute psoriasis
Sinusitis	Acute eczema
Psoriasis	Herpes simplex
Pressure sores	Renal and hepatic insufficiencies
Osteomalacia	Diabetes
Diagnosis of skin disorders	Hyperthyroidism
Increased vitamin D production	Generalized dermatitis
Sterilization	Advanced arteriosclerosis
Tanning	Active and progressive pulmonary tuberculosis[3,8,20,24,25,32]
Hyperplasia	
Exfoliation	

the range of 3600 to 3700 Å. This wavelength is most effective in causing exposed areas to fluoresce. The test is performed in a darkened room, and since all animal tissues fluoresce, the exposure to the filtered UVR will cause the exposed tissue to appear a specific color.[32] However, if an infection is present, the color of the area will correspond to the fluorescence of the infecting organism rather than the expected normal color. This abnormal coloration can be evaluated and a tentative diagnosis made.

USING ULTRAVIOLET THERAPY IN ATHLETIC TRAINING

The use of UVR therapy in athletic training has been limited. Many indications for its use, such as acne, skin infections, and fungal infections, are adequately treated with medication. Other problems, such as pressure sores and vitamin D deficiency, are seldom found among an athletic population. This does not mean that UVR should be excluded from the clinic; it most certainly has beneficial effects that could be used by athletic trainers. But considering the small number of potential uses and the limited budgetary resources most athletic trainers have available, UVR equipment will remain a low-priority item.

However, the population of the United States is gradually growing older and more active. Clinical patients are no longer limited to the college football star or the Olympic hopeful. Today sports medicine clinics are treating patients ranging from prepubescent marathoners to 70-year-old triathletes. As the number and age of active persons increases, so will the variety of problems to be treated. At present there is some inconclusive evidence that UVR can aid in the reduction of blood pressure, help to relieve asthma, cause a reduction in blood cholesterol, and aid in reducing the severity of upper respiratory infections.[18] The average patient being seen in a sports medicine clinic is generally not a world-class athlete but perhaps a 50-year-old executive who is emerging from 25 years of sedentary living. UVR might be a helpful part of this patient's treatment; as research continues, UVR may once again become a favored and useful treatment just as it was earlier in this century.

Summary

1. UVR is that portion of the electromagnetic spectrum that ranges from 2000 to 4000 Å.
2. Exposure to UVR causes a photochemical reaction within living cells and can cause alterations of DNA and cell proteins.
3. The irradiation of human skin causes an acute inflammation that is characterized by an erythema, increased pigmentation, and hyperplasia.
4. The effects of long-term exposure to UVR are premature aging of the skin and skin cancer.
5. The eye is extremely sensitive to UVR and will develop photokeratitis following exposure.
6. Many types of equipment are manufactured that produce UVR, but the majority used clinically are of the low- and high-pressure mercury arc lamp variety.

Review Questions

1. What is the position of ultraviolet radiation (UVR) in the electromagnetic spectrum and the relationship of UVR to other forms of electromagnetic energy?
2. How does UVR raise energy levels within irradiated objects?
3. What are the effects of UVR on individual cells and human tissue and explain the tanning process?
4. What are the effects of long-term exposure to UVR and the effect of UVR on the eyes?
5. What are the procedures for operating a UVR device, including safety precautions, the skin test, the inverse square law, and the cosine law?
6. What are the various clinical applications of UVR?
7. What are the treatment precautions when using UVR?
8. What are the potential uses for UVR in sports medicine?

Self-Test Questions

T/F
1. Athletic trainers use UV-A and UV-B.
2. The minimum SPF recommended is 15.
3. Only the athlete must wear safety goggles during UVR therapy.

Multiple Choice
4. What the the short-term effect(s) of UVR on the skin?
   a. erythema and pigmentation
   b. inflammation and hyperplasia
   c. both A and B
   d. neither A nor B
5. Which of the following is NOT a type of skin cancer?
   a. squamous cell carcinoma
   b. basal cell carcinoma
   c. malignant melanoma
   d. epidermal melanoma
6. Which type of UV generator is most common in sports medicine?
   a. carbon arc lamp
   b. mercury arc lamp
   c. xenon arc lamp
   d. fluorescent UV lamp

7. Which law states that the UV lamp must be perpendicular to the skin to maximize absorption?
   a. cosine law
   b. inverse square law
   c. Angstrom's law
   d. Wolff's law
8. What must be determined prior to UV treatment?
   a. skin type
   b. minimum SPF needed
   c. UV range required
   d. minimal erythemal dose
9. What is a current common use for UVR?
   a. treating dermatologic conditions
   b. antibacterial effects
   c. vitamin D deficiency
   d. generalized dermatitis
10. What could occur if eye protection is not worn during UVR treatment?
    a. melanin pigmentation
    b. photosensitization
    c. photokeratitis
    d. pupil dilation

Solutions to Clinical Decision-Making Exercises

15-1 The athletic trainer should explain to the athlete that the length of time that he will be exposed to the UV radiation is minimal and that, despite the fact that he will have several treatments, the total exposure is certainly not enough to worry about this causing skin cancer.

15-2 The best type of UV generator to purchase in this particular situation is a mercury arc lamp. Most of the UVR produced is within the UV-B range, is highly germicidal, and is most effective in treating bacterial infection. Another advantage of the mercury arc lamp is that it does not require a warm-up or cool-down period.

15-3 It is first necessary to determine how long the athlete can be exposed to the sun before the skin begins to turn red. If that happens at about 10 minutes of exposure, then a sunscreen with an SPF of 15 should provide enough protection. However, since the athlete will be sweating and possibly toweling off, it would likely be wise to recommend an SPF of 20.

References

1. Bergner, T, and Przybilla, B: Malignant melanoma in association with phototherapy, *Dermatology* 184(1):59–61, 1992.
2. Bickford, E: Risks associated with the use of UV-A irradiators, *Photochem. Photobiol.* 30(2):199–202, 1979.
3. Burdick Corp.: *Burdick syllabus*, ed 7, Milton, Wis., 1969.
4. Downer, A: *Physical therapy procedures*, ed 3, Springfield, 1981, Charles C Thomas.
5. Gilmour, J, Vestey, J, and Norval, M: The effect of UV therapy on immune function in athletes with psoriasis, *Brit J Dermat* 129(1):28–38, 1993.
6. Goats, G: Appropriate use of the inverse square law, *Physiotherapy* 74(1):8, 1988.
7. Goldman, L: *Introduction to modern phototherapy*, Springfield, 1978, Charles C Thomas.
8. Griffin, J, and Karsalis, T: *Physical agents for physical athletic trainers*, ed 2, Springfield, 1982, Charles C Thomas.
9. Hall, L: Current status of oral PUVA therapy for psoriasis, *J. Am. Acad. Dermatol.* 1(2):106–107, 1979.
10. Harbor, L: PUVA therapy status, *J. Am. Acad. Dermatol.* 1(2):150, 1979.
11. High, A, and High, J: Treatment of infected skin wounds using ultra-violet radiation—an in-vitro study, *Physiotherapy* 69(10):359–360, 1983.
12. Hudson-Peacock, M, Diffey, B, and Farr, P: Photoprotective action of emollients in ultraviolet therapy of psoriasis, *Brit J Dermat* 130(3):361–365, 1994.
13. Kitchen, S, Partridge, and C: A review of ultraviolet radiation therapy, *Physiotherapy* 77(6):423–432, 1991.
14. Kloth, L: Physical modalities in wound management: UVC, therapeutic heating and electrical stimulation, *Ostomy Wound Management* 41(5):18–20, 22–24, 26–27, 1995.
15. Kowalzick, L, Kleinheinz, A, and Weichenthal, M: Low dose versus medium dose UV-A1 treatment in severe atopic eczema, *Acta Dermato-Venereologica* 75(1):43–45, 1995.
16. Kottke, F: *Krusen's handbook of physical medicine and rehabilitation*, ed 3, Philadelphia, 1983, WB Saunders.
17. Kovacs, R: *Light therapy*, Springfield, 1950, Charles C Thomas.

18. Leenutaphong, V, and Jiamton, S: UVB phototherapy for pityriasis rosea: a bilateral comparison study, *J. Am. Acad. Dermatol.* 33(6):996–999, 1995.

19. Lemke, E: The influence of UV irradiation on vitamin D metabolism in children with chronic renal diseases, *Int Urology Nephrology* 25(6):595–601, 1993.

20. Lewis, G: *Practical dermatology*, Philadelphia, 1967, WB Saunders.

21. Low, J, Bazin, S, and Docker, M: Guidelines for the safe use of ultraviolet therapy equipment, *Physiotherapy* 80(2):89–90, 1994.

22. Low, J: Quantifying the erythema due to UVR, *Physiotherapy* 72(1):60–64, 1986.

23. Lowe, N: Home ultraviolet phototherapy, *Seminars in Dermatology* 11(4):284–286, 1992.

24. Mayer, E: *Clinical application of sunlight and artificial radiation*, Baltimore, 1926, Williams & Wilkins.

25. Mayer, E: *The curative value of light*, New York, 1932, D Appleton.

26. Owoeye, I, and Adeyemi-Doro, H: The therapeutic effect of ultra-violet irradiation on traumatic open wounds: an experimental investigation, *J Nigeria Society Physio* 13(1):33–44, 1995.

27. Parish, P: *The doctors and athletes handbook of medicines and drugs*, New York, 1980, Alfred A Knopf, Inc.

28. Parrish, J: *UV-A biological effects of ultraviolet radiation*, New York, 1979, Plenum.

29. Pittekow, M: Skin cancer in athletes with psoriasis treated with coal tar, *Arch. Dermatol.* 117:465–468, 1981.

30. Rook, A: *Textbook of dermatology*, Oxford, 1979, Blackwell.

31. Stewart, W: *Dermatology: diagnosis and treatment of cutaneous disorders*, St. Louis, 1978, Mosby.

32. Stillwell, G: *Therapeutic electricity and ultraviolet radiation*, Baltimore, 1983, Williams & Wilkins.

33. Urbach, F: *The biologic effects of ultraviolet radiation*, London, 1969, Pergamon.

34. U.S. Dept. of HEW, Public Health Service: *Occupational exposure to ultraviolet radiation*, Washington, D.C., 1972, National Institute for Occupational Safety and Health, HSM73-1 1009.

35. Williams, R: PUVA therapy vs. Goeckerman therapy in the treatment of psoriasis: a pilot study, *Physiotherapy Canada* 37(6):361–366, 1985.

Suggested Readings

Bryant, B: Treatment of psoriasis, *Am. J. Hosp. Pharm.* 37:814–820, 1980.

Cerio, R, and Low, J: Successful treatment by general ultra-violet radiation of pruritus due to biliary cirrhosis, *Physiotherapy* 73(12):689, 1987.

Challner, A, Corless, D, and Davis, J.: Personnel monitoring exposure to ultraviolet radiation, *Clin Exp Dermat* 1:175–179, 1976.

Challner, A, and Duffey, B: Problems associated with ultraviolet dosimetry in the photochemotherapy of psoriasis, *Br. J. Dermatol.* 97:643–648, 1977.

Collins, P, and Ferguson, J: Narrow-band UVB (TL-01) phototherapy: an effective preventative treatment for the photodermatoses, *Brit J Dermatology* 132(6):956–963, 1995.

Corless, D, and Gupta, S: Response of plasma 25 hydroxyvitamin D to ultraviolet irradiation in long stay geriatric athletes, *Lancet* 2 23:649–651, 1978.

Dietzel, F: Effects of non-ionizing electromagnetic radiation on the development and intrauterine implantation of the rat. In Tyler, AE, editor: Biological effects of nomonizing radiation, *Ann. N.Y. Acad. Sci.* 247:367, 1975.

Diffey, B: Ultraviolet radiation and skin cancer: are physioathletic trainers at risk? *Physiotherapy* 75(10):615–616, 1989.

Dootson, G, Norris, P, and Gibson C: The practice of ultraviolet phototherapy in the United Kingdom, *Brit J Dermat* 131(6):873–877, 1994.

Everett, M, Olson, R, and Sayer, R: Ultraviolet erythema, *Arch. Dermatol.* 92:713, 1975.

Fischer, T: Comparative treatment of psoriasis with UV-light trioxsalen plus UV-light and coal tar plus UV-light, *Acta Derm. Venereol.* 57:345–350, 1977.

Fitzpatrick, T, Pathak, A, and Magnus, I: Abnormal reactions of man to light, *Ann. Rev. Med.* 14:195, 1963.

Giese, A, editor: *Photophysiology*, vol. IV, New York, 1968, Academic Press.

Giese, A, editor: *Photophysiology*, vol. V, New York, 1970, Academic Press.

Giese, A, editor: *Photophysiology*, vol. VII, New York, 1972, Academic Press.

Gordon, M, editor: *Pigment cell biology*, New York, 1959, Academic Press.

Green, C, Diffey, B, and Hawk, J: Ultraviolet radiation in the treatment of skin disease, *Physics Medicine Biology* 37(1):1–20, 1992.

Grynbaum, B: Prevention of ultraviolet induced erythema, *Arch. Phys. Med. Rehabil.* 31:587–592, 1950.

Hardie, R, Hunter, J: Psoriasis, *Br. J. Hosp. Med.* 20:13–23, 1978.

Holick, M, and Clark, M: The photogenesis and metabolism of vitamin D, *Fed. Proc.* 37 # 12:2567–2574, 1978.

Hollaender, A, editor: *Radiation biology*, vol. II, New York, 1955, McGraw-Hill.

Holti, G: Measurements of the vascular responses in skin at various time intervals after damage with histamine and ultraviolet radiation, *Clin. Sci.* 14:143–155 1955.

Jarratt, M, and Knox, J: Photodynamic action: theory and applications, *Prog. Dermatol.* 8:1, 1974.

Jekler, J: Phototherapy of atopic dermatitis with ultraviolet radiation, *Acta Dermato-Venereologica* 171:1–37, 1992.

Jekler, J, Bergbrant, I, and Faergemann, J: The in vivo effect of UVB radiation on skin bacteria in athletes with atopic dermatitis, *Acta Dermato-Venereologica* 72(1):33–36, 1992.

Kelner, A: Photoreactivation of ultraviolet irradiated eschericoli, with special reference to the dose reduction principal and to ultraviolet induced mutation, *J. Bacteriol.* 58:11–22, 1949.

Lebwohl, M, and Martinez, J: Effects of topical preparations on the erythemogenicity of UVB: implications for psoriasis phototherapy, *J Amer Acad Dermat* 32(3):469–471, 1995.

Licht, S, editor: *Therapeutic electricity and ultraviolet radiation*, ed 2, New Haven, 1967.

Lynch, W: Clinical results of photochemotherapy, *Cutis*, 20:477–480, 1977.

MacKinnon, J, and Cleek, P: The penetration of ultraviolet light through transparent dressings: a case report, *Phys Ther* 64(2):204, 1984.

Macleod, M, and Blacklock, N: UVL induced changes in calcium absorption and excretion and in serum vitamin D^3 levels measured in black skinned and caucasian males, *J.R. Nav. Med. Serv.* 65:75–78,1979.

Marisco, A: Ultraviolet light and tar in the Goeckermann treatment of psoriasis, *Arch. Dermatol.* 112:1249–1250, 1976.

Montagna, W, and Labitz, W, editors: *The epidermis*, New York, 1964, Academic Press.

Morison, W: Controlled study of PUVA and adjunctive therapy in the management of psoriasis, *Br. J. Dermatol.* 98:125–132, 1978.

Moseley, H, Thomas, R, and Young, M: UVB lamps: a burning issue, *Brit J Dermat* 128(6):704–706, 1993.

Nussbaum, E, Biemann, I, and Mustard, B: Comparison of ultrasound/ultraviolet-C and laser for treatment of pressure ulcers in athletes with spinal cord injury, *Phys Ther* 74(9):812–825, 1994.

Ohayashi, T, Yoshimoto, S, and Yasamura, M: Effect of wavelength on the photochemical reaction of ergocalciferol (vitamin D^2) irradiated by monochromatic ultraviolet light, *J. Nutr. Sci. Vitaminol.* 23:281–290, 1977 (in English).

Parrish, J: Photochemotherapy of psoriasis with oral methoxsalen and longwave ultraviolet light, *N. Engl. J. Med.* 291:1207–1222, 1974.

Pathak, M, Harber, J, and Seiji, M: editors: *Sunlight and man*, Tokyo, 1974, U. of Tokyo Press.

Peak, M: Inactivation of transforming DNA by ultraviolet light. II. Protection by histadine, *Mutat. Res.* 20:137–141, 1973.

Roenig, H: Comparison of phototherapy systems for photochemotherapy, *Cutis* 20:485–489, 1977.

Rogers, S: Effect of PUVA on serum 25-OH vitamin D in psoriatics, *Br. Med. J.* 833:34, 1979.

Rolston, K, Gold, M, and Elson M: Ultraviolet—a treatment of pruritus secondary to hyperbilirubinemia, *Dermatology Nursing* 2(1):31–32, 1990.

Salem, L: Theory of photochemical reactions, *Science* 191:822, 1976.

Sams, W, and Winkleman, R: The effect of ultraviolet light on isolated cutaneous blood vessels, *J. Invest. Dermatol.* 53:79–83, 1969.

Sauer, G, editor: *Manual of skin diseases*, ed 3, Philadelphia, 1973, J.B. Lippincott.

Segal, S: PUVA: a caution, *Pediatrics* 62:253, 1978.

Sjovall, P, and Christensen, O: Treatment of chronic hand eczema with UV-B Handylux in the clinic and at home, *Contact Dermatitis* 31(1):5–8, 1994.

Smith, K, Skelton, H, and Yeager, J: Ultraviolet radiation therapy and HIV disease, *J Amer Acad Dermat* 33(5 Pt 1):841–842, 1995.

Sulzberger, W, Wolf, J, and Witten, V: *Dermatology: diagnosis and treatment*, ed 2, Chicago, 1961, Yearbook, pp. 85–96.

Task Force Committee on Photobiology of the National Program for Dermatology, L.C. Harber, Chairman: *Arch. Dermatol.* 109:833–839, 1974.

Taylor, R: Clinical study of ultraviolet in various skin conditions, *Phys Ther* 52:279–282, 1972.

Telles, J, Coakley, C, and Kluger, A. Bureau of Radiological Health. Food and Drug Administration: *Possible hazards from high intensity discharge mercury vapor and metal halide lamps*, Nov. 1977.

Thomsen, D: Phototherapy: treatment with light, *Science News* 105:404, 1974.

Urbach, F, editor: Biological effects of ultraviolet radiation, New York, 1969, Pergamon. UV radiation, *Clin. Exp. Dermatol.* 1:175–179, 1976.

Van Der Leun, J: Theory of ultraviolet erythema, *Photochem. Photobiol.* 4:453–458, 1965.

Van Pelt, W, Payne, W, and Peterson, R: *A review of selected bioeffects thresholds for various spectral ranges of light*, DH EW Publ. no. (FDA) 74–8010.

Weber, G: Combined 8-methoxypsoralen and black light therapy of psoriasis: technique and results, *Br. J. Dermatol.* 90:317–323, 1974.

Wurtman, R: The effects of light on the human body, *Sci. Am.* 233:69, 1975.

Young, P: Turning on light turns off disease, *National Observer*, May 29, 1976.

Locations of the Motor Points

T he illustrations in this appendix show the locations of the motor points located on the extremities and the torso. (Courtesy Mettler Electronics Corporation, 1333 S. Claudina Street, Anaheim, Calif. 92805.)

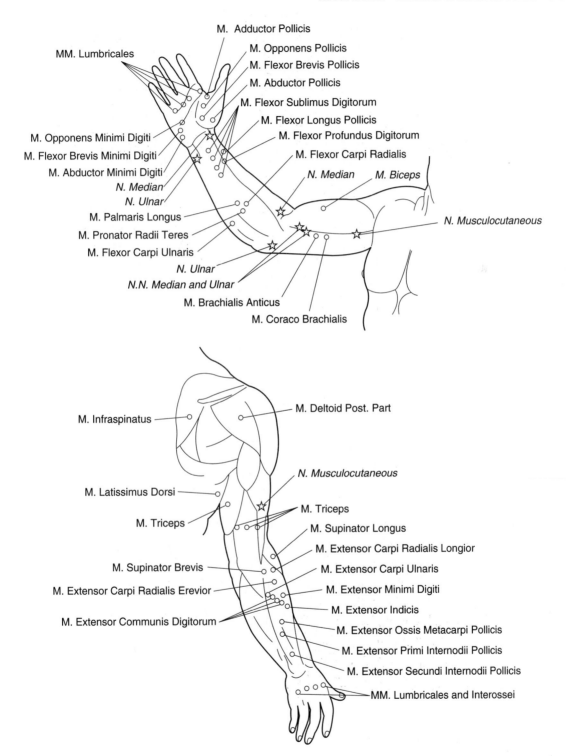

M. Adductor Pollicis

MM. Lumbricales

M. Opponens Pollicis

M. Flexor Brevis Pollicis

M. Abductor Pollicis

M. Flexor Sublimus Digitorum

M. Opponens Minimi Digiti

M. Flexor Longus Pollicis

M. Flexor Brevis Minimi Digiti

M. Flexor Profundus Digitorum

M. Abductor Minimi Digiti

M. Flexor Carpi Radialis

N. Median

N. Median   *M. Biceps*

N. Ulnar

M. Palmaris Longus

M. Pronator Radii Teres

N. Musculocutaneous

M. Flexor Carpi Ulnaris

N. Ulnar

N.N. Median and Ulnar

M. Brachialis Anticus

M. Coraco Brachialis

M. Infraspinatus

M. Deltoid Post. Part

N. Musculocutaneous

M. Latissimus Dorsi

M. Triceps

M. Triceps

M. Supinator Longus

M. Extensor Carpi Radialis Longior

M. Supinator Brevis

M. Extensor Carpi Ulnaris

M. Extensor Carpi Radialis Erevior

M. Extensor Minimi Digiti

M. Extensor Indicis

M. Extensor Communis Digitorum

M. Extensor Ossis Metacarpi Pollicis

M. Extensor Primi Internodii Pollicis

M. Extensor Secundi Internodii Pollicis

MM. Lumbricales and Interossei

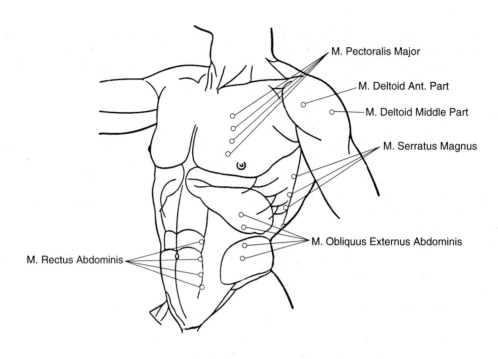

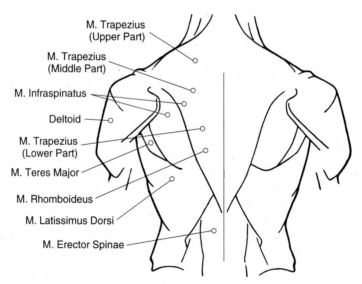

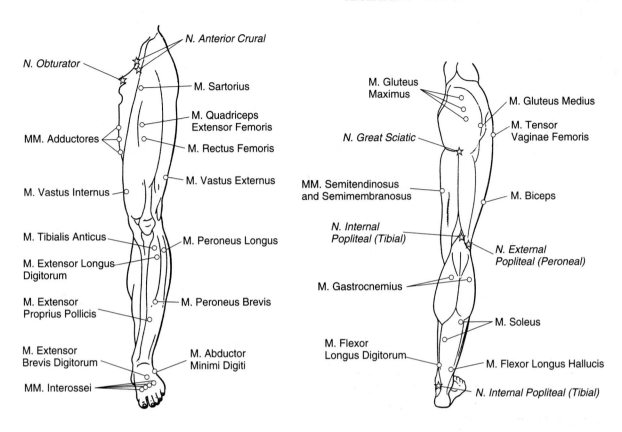

N. Anterior Crural

N. Obturator

M. Sartorius

M. Quadriceps
Extensor Femoris

MM. Adductores

M. Rectus Femoris

M. Vastus Externus

M. Vastus Internus

M. Tibialis Anticus

M. Peroneus Longus

M. Extensor Longus
Digitorum

M. Extensor
Proprius Pollicis

M. Peroneus Brevis

M. Extensor
Brevis Digitorum

M. Abductor
Minimi Digiti

MM. Interossei

M. Gluteus
Maximus

M. Gluteus Medius

M. Tensor
Vaginae Femoris

N. Great Sciatic

MM. Semitendinosus
and Semimembranosus

M. Biceps

N. Internal
Popliteal (Tibial)

N. External
Popliteal (Peroneal)

M. Gastrocnemius

M. Soleus

M. Flexor
Longus Digitorum

M. Flexor Longus Hallucis

N. Internal Popliteal (Tibial)

Index of Equipment Manufacturers and Distributors

T he first part of this index lists the various types of therapeutic modalities and supplies identified by the manufacturers and distributors of the specific product. This is followed by an alphabetical listing of these manufacturers and distributors with addresses, telephone and fax numbers, e-mail addresses, and website addresses, when available. For a continuously updated listing, check the accompanying book website at www.mhhe.com/prentice5e.

Modalities and Supplies by Manufacturer and Distributor

ELECTROTHERAPEUTIC MODALITIES

Electrodes
AliMed Inc
AloeTran Products Inc
American Imex
Amrex Electrotherapy Equipment
Autogenic Systems
Axelgaard Manufacturing Co Ltd
BioMedical Life Systems Inc
Chattanooga Group Inc
Continental SEL Inc
Devco Medical Systems
Electro-Med Health Industries
Electronic Research Devices Corp
ELMED Inc
FES Information Center/
Cleveland FES Center
LSI International

MARKnew Products
McBeth Therapy Co Inc
Med-Fit Systems Inc
Medical Science Products Inc
Mettler Electronics Corp
MultiBiosensors Inc
NeuMed
Noraxon USA Inc
OMS Medical Supplies Inc
Progressive Medical Inc
MA Rallis Corp
Rehabilicare
Rich-Mar Group
SRS Medical Systems Inc
Therapeutic Alliances Inc
Thought Technology Ltd
Vermont Medical Inc

Williams Healthcare Systems
Zimmer Elektomedizin

Electrotherapy Equipment
AliMed Inc
American Imex
Amrex Electrotherapy Equipment
Biomedical Life Systems Inc
Chattanooga Group Inc
Devco Medical Sytems
Dynatronics Corp
ElectroLogic of America Inc
Electro-Med Health Industries
ELMED Inc
FES Information Center/
Cleveland FES Center
GNR Health Systems Inc

Ideal
International Medical Electronics Inc
I-REP Inc
LSI International
MARKnew Products
Martin Medical Equipment Servicing Co
McBeth Therapy Co Inc
Medical Science Products Inc
Med Labs Inc
MED-TECH Equipment
Mettler Electronics Corp
NeuMed
OMS Medical Supplies Inc
Professional Care Systems
Progressive Medical Inc
MA Rallis Corp
Rehabilicare
Rich-Mar Group
Smith & Nephew Inc, Rehabilitation Division
Therapeutic Alliances Inc
Theraquip Inc
Vonco Medical
Williams Healthcare Systems

Galvanic Stimulators

American Imex
Amrex Electrotherapy Inc
BioMedical Life Systems Inc
Devco Medical Systems
Electro-Med Health Industries
ELMED Inc
Medical Science Products Inc
Med Labs Inc
Mettler Electronics Corp
NeuMed
Rehabilicare

Gels/Sprays

AloeTran Products Inc
American Imex
Amrex Electrotherapy Equipment
Axelgaard Manufacturing Co Ltd

BioFreeze/Performance Health Inc
BioMedical Life Systems Inc
Electro-Med Health Industries
Gebauer Co
Kustomer Kinetics
Medical Science Products Inc
MultiBiosensors Inc
NeuMed
Parker Laboratories Inc
Rich-Mar Group
Therapeutic Alliances Inc
Vann Healthcare Systems
Williams Healthcare Systems

Interferential Therapy

American Imex
Amrex Electrotherapy Equipment
BioMedical Life Systems Inc
Devco Medical Systems
Dynatronics Inc
ELMED Inc
LSI International
Medical Science Products Inc
Mettler Electronics Corp
Rehabilicare
Rehab Med + Equip Inc
Rich-Mar Group
Williams Healthcare Systems

Muscle Stimulators

American Imex
Amrex Electrotherapy Equipment
BioMedical Life Systems Inc
Devco Medical Systems
Dynatronics Group
Electro-Logic of America Inc
Electro-Med Health Industries
ELMED Inc
Flaghouse Inc
Gebauer Co
Hill Laboratories Inc
LSI International
MARKnew Products
Medical Science Products Inc

Med Labs Inc
Med-Pro Corp
Mettler Electronics Corp
NeuMed
Progressive Medical Inc
MA Rallis Corp
Rehabilicare
Rich-Mar Group
SRS Medical Systems Inc
Therapeutic Alliances Inc
Williams Healthcare Systems

Neuromuscular Stimulators

American Imex
Amrex Electrotherapy Equipment
BioMedical Life Systems Inc
Chattanooga Group Inc
Devco Medical Systems
Dynatronics Group
ElectroLogic of America
Electro-Med Health Industries
ELMED Inc
FES Information Center/ Cleveland FES Center
Medical Science Products Inc
Med Labs Inc
Med-Pro Corp
Mettler Electronics Corp
NeuMed
MA Rallis Corp
Rehabilicare
Rich-Mar Group
Sigmedics Inc
Therapeutic Alliances Inc

TENS Units

American Imex
Amrex Electrotherapy Equipment
BioMedical Life Systems Inc
Devco Medical Systems
Electro-Med Health Industries
Electronic Research Devices Corp
ELMED Inc
Flaghouse Inc
GNR Health Systems

LSI International
MARKnew Products
Medical Science Products Inc
NeuMed
OMS Medical Supplies Inc
Progressive Medical Inc
MA Rallis Corp
Rehabilicare
Rehab + Equip Inc

**Miscellaneous
Electrotherapeutic Modalities**

American Imex
Amrex Electrotherapy Equipment

Axelgaard Manufacturing Co Ltd
BioMedical Life Systems Inc
Continental SEL Inc
ElectroLogic of America Inc
Electro-Med Health Industries
ELMED Inc
Fabrifoam Products
FES Information Center/
Cleveland FES Center
Ideal
LSI International
Martin Medical Equipment
Servicing Co

The MED Group Inc
Medical Science Products Inc
NeuMed
OMS Medical Supplies Inc
Rehabilicare
Rich-Mar Group
Sammons Preston
Sigmedics Inc
Sports Health
Therapeutic Alliances Inc
Thought Technology Ltd
Vann Healthcare Services

IONTOPHORESIS SYSTEMS

Amrex Electrotherapy Equipment
BioMedical Life Systems Inc
Dynatronics Corp

ELMED Inc
IOMED Inc
LSI International

Medical Science Products Inc
Theraquip Inc
Williams Healthcare Systems

DIATHERMY

Microwave

MED-TECH Equipment
Service Inc
Southwest Technologies Inc

Short Wave

ELMED Inc
I-REP Inc
International Medical
Electronics Ltd

Med-Pro Corp
MED-TECH Equipment
Mettler Electronics Corp
Vonco Medical

COLD THERAPY

Cryotherapy

AliMed Inc
BioFreeze/Performance
Health Inc
Corflex/Medic-Air
Dura-Kold Corp
General Physiotherapy Inc
Grimm Scientific Industries Inc
Kustomer Kinetics Inc
Martin Medical Equipment
Servicing Co

McBeth Therapy Co Inc
Rich-Mar Corp
Sportsware West

Ice Packs, Disposable

Armstrong Medical Industries Inc
Briggs Corp
Fitter International Inc
Gebauer Co
MARKnew Products
Mastex Industries Inc

Micro Bio-Medics Inc
Tempra Technology Inc
Water Gear Inc

Ice Packs, Reusable

Battle Creek Equipment Co
Body Therapeutics
Briggs Corp
Brown Medical Industries
Chattanooga Group Inc
Corflex/Medic-Air

Creations Magiques Inc
Dura-Kold Corp
Dynatronics Corp
Gebauer Co
Mastex Industries Inc
Mettler Electronics Corp
Micro Bio-Medics Inc
OMS Medical Supplies Inc
Pelton Shepherd Industries
pi Professional Therapy
MA Rallis Corp
Rehab Med + Equip Inc
The Saunders Group
Southwest Technologies Inc
Sportsware West

Tempra Technology Inc
Whitehall Manufacturing

Sprays, Vapocoolants

Gebauer Co
Stopain/DRJ Group Inc
Vann Healthcare Services

Miscellaneous Cold Therapy

Aquatica
BioFreeze/Performance Health Inc
Body Therapeutics
Continental SEL Inc
Evans Associates
Fabrifoam Products

Gebauer Co
Grimm Scientific Industries Inc
Hydro Worx International Inc
Kustomer Kinetics Inc
MedPro Corp
Mettler Electronics Corp
North Coast Medical Inc
ORMED
Posey Co
Rich-Mar Group
Southwest Technologies Inc
Sports Health
Sportsware West
Tempra Technologies Inc
Theraquip Inc

THERMOTHERAPY

Heating Pads

Creations Magiques Inc
Mastex Inc
Medical Science Products Inc
Tempra Technologies Inc

Hot Packs

Armstrong Medical Industries Inc
Chattanooga Group Inc
Corflex/Medic-Air
Creations Magiques Inc
Dynatronics Corp
Electro-Med Health Industries
Fitter International
Flaghouse Inc
LSI International
Mastex Industries
Mettler Electronics Corp
Med-Pro Corp
Medical Science Products Inc
OPTP
Pelton Shepherd Industries
pi Professional Therapies
Rehab Med + Equip Inc
Tempra Technologies Inc
Whitehall Manufacturing

Moist Heat Pads

American Imex
Battle Creek Equipment Co
Creations Magiques Inc
LSI International
Mastex Industries
Medical Science Products Inc
Mettler Electronics Group
Pelton Shepherd Industries
The Saunders Group
Southwest Technologies Inc
Tempra Technologies Inc

Parrafin Baths

Chattanooga Group Inc
Comfort House
Ferno Ille, Ferno-Washington Inc
Grimm Scientific Industries
The Hygenic Corp
LSI International
Mastex Industries
Medical Science Products Inc
Med-Pro Corp
Service Engineering Co
Whitehall Manufacturing

Fluidotherapy

Davol Inc
MED-TECH Equipment

Miscellaneous Heat Therapy

AMI Inc
Aquatica
Continental SEL Inc
Corflex/Medic-Air
Fabrifoam Products
Hydro Worx International
Ideal
Martin Medical Equipment
Servicing Co
Mastex Industries Inc
MEDEXPERT
Medical Science Products Inc
North Coast Medical Inc
pi Professional Therapy
Sammons Preston
Tempra Technology Inc
Theraquip

ULTRASOUND

Gels

AloeTran Products Inc
Amrex Electrotherapy
Equipment
Ari-Med Pharmaceuticals
ELMED Inc
General Physiotherapy Inc
Kustomer Kinetics Inc
LSI International
MARKnew Products
Med-Pro Corp
Mettler Electronics Corp
Parker Laboratories Inc
Rich-Mar Corp
Sports Health
Vann Healthcare Services
Williams Healthcare Systems

Ultrasound Equipment

AliMed Inc
AloeTran Products Inc
Amrex Electrotherapy Equipment
Chattanooga Group Inc
Dynatronics Corp
ELMED Inc
GNR Health Systems Inc
Hill Laboratories Co
Ideal
I-REP Inc
LSI International
McBeth Therapy Co Inc
Med-Pro Corp
MED-TECH Equipment Service Inc
Mettler Electronics Corp
Rehab Med + Equip Inc

Rich-Mar Corp
Sports Health
Theraquip Inc
Vonco Medical
Williams Healthcare Systems

Miscellaneous Ultrasound

Amrex Electrotherapy Equipment
Biofreeze/Performance Health Inc
Ideal
Martin Medical Equipment
Servicing Co
Med-Pro Corp
MED-TECH Equipment Service Inc
Rich-Mar Group
Sammons Preston

HYDROTHERAPY

Bathtubs

Arjo Inc
Nor-Am Patient Care Products Ltd
Service Engineering Co

Foot Baths

Aquatica
Arjo Inc
Comfort House
Ferno Ille, Ferno-Washington Inc

Hydrotherapy Equip

AMI Inc
Aquatica
Davol Inc
Ferno Ille, Ferno-Washington Inc
Finis Inc
Flaghouse Inc
Grimm Scientific Industries Inc
HydroWorx International Inc
Kinetic Innovations
MARKnew Products
McBeth Therapy Co Inc

MEDEXPERT
Med-Pro Corp
MED-TECH Equipment
Rehab Med + Equip Inc
Service Engineering Co
Sports Health
Sprint/Rothhammer
International
SwimEx Systems, A Division
of TPI Inc
Therapeutic Systems Inc
Water Gear Inc
Water Wear

Therapeutic Pools

AquaMotion Inc
Ferno Ille, Ferno-Washington Inc
Grimm Scientific Industries Inc
Hydro Worx International Inc
Med-Fit Systems Inc
Rio Plastics Inc
Sprint/Rothhammer
International

SwimEx Systems, A Division
of TPI Inc
Therapeutic Systems Inc

Water Sanitizing Systems

Kustomer Kinetics Inc
Service Engineering Co
Sydsons Medical Inc

Whirlpool Additives

Ferno Ille, Ferno-Washington Inc
Kustomer Kinetics Inc
McBeth Therapy Co Inc
Med-Pro Corp
Service Engineering Co
Theraquip Inc

Whirlpools

AquaMotion Inc
Arjo Inc
Comfort House
Continental SEL Inc
Davol Inc

Ferno Ille, Ferno-Washington Inc
GNR Health Systems Inc
Grimm Scientific Industries Inc
I-REP Inc
Med-Pro Corp
MED-TECH Equipment Service Inc
Micro Bio-Medics Inc
Nor-Am Patient Care Products Ltd
Rio Plastics Inc
SwimEx Systems, A Division
of TPI Inc
Theraquip Inc
Vonco Medical
Whitehall Manufacturing

Miscellaneous Hydrotherapy

AMI Inc
AquaMotion Inc
Aquatica
Aquatic Access Inc
Aquatic Therapy & Rehab
Institute Inc
Barrier Free Lifts Inc
Davol Inc
Hydro Worx International Inc
Kustomer Kinetics Inc
Martin Medical Equipment
Servicing Co

MEDEXPERT
PHD Merchants
Sammons Preston
Service Engineering Co
Sprint/Rothhammer
International
SwimEx Systems, A Division
of TPI Inc
Sydsons Medical Inc
Therapeutic Systems Inc
Water Gear Inc

TRACTION

Ankle

Hill Laboratories Co

Cervical

AliMed Inc
Bodyline Comfort Systems
Core Products International Inc
Florida Manufacturing Corp dba
FlaManCo Intl
Granberg International
Hill Laboratories Co
Lossing Orthopedic Inc
Pneumex Inc
Rehabilicare
The Saunders Group
Shamrock Medical Inc
Therapeutic Dimensions Inc

Leg

Armstrong Medical Industries Inc
Florida Manufacturing Corp dba
FlaManCo Intl
Hill Laboratories Co

Lumbar

BackMaster by Back-Jack Inc
Evans Associates

Florida Manufacturing Corp dba
FlaManCo Intl
Granberg International
Hill Laboratories Co
Lossing Orthopedic Inc
Nada-Chair
Pneumex Inc
Rehabilicare
Serola Biomechanics
The Saunders Group
Shamrock Medical Inc

Pelvic

A2Z Possibilities Inc
Evans Associates
Florida Manufacturing Corp
Hill Laboratories Co
Lossing Orthopedic Inc
Serola Biomechanics

Traction Equipment

AloeTran Products Inc
Chattanooga Group Inc
Dynatronics Corp
Evans Associates
Florida Manufacturing Corp dba
FlaManCo Intl

GNR Health Systems Inc
Granberg International
Hang Ups
Hill Laboratories Co
I-REP Inc
Lossing Orthopedic Inc
MARKnew Products
McBeth Therapy Co Inc
MED-TECH Equipment Service Inc
N-K Products Co
MA Rallis Corp
Rehab Med + Equip Inc
Shamrock Medical Inc
Theraquip Inc
Vonco Medical

Miscellaneous Traction

BackMaster by Back-Jack Inc
Cardon Rehabilitation
Products Inc
Florida Manufacturing Corp dba
FlaManCo Intl
Hill Laboratories Co
Martin Medical Equipment
Servicing Co
The MED Group Inc
MED-TECH Equipment Service Inc

Manufacturers' and Distributors' Addresses

AliMed Inc
297 High St
Dedham, MA 02026
e-mail: info@alimed.com
website: www.alimed.com
800/225-2610
781/329-2900
FAX: 800/437-2966

AloeTran Products Inc
PO Box 337
Farmerville, LA 71241
e-mail: aloetran@bayou.com
800/328-8367
318/368-7266
FAX: 318/368-7270

American Imex
16520 Aston St
Irvine, CA 92714
e-mail: info@americanimex.com
website: www.americanimex.com
800/521-8286
949/553-8885

AMI Inc
PO Box 808
Groton, CT 06340-0808
e-mail: amiaqua@aol.com
800/248-4031
860/536-3735
FAX: 860/536-4362

Amrex Electrotherapy Equipment
641 E Walnut St
Carson, CA 90746
e-mail: amrex@amrex-zetron.com
website: www.amrex-zetron.com
800/221-9069
310/527-6868
FAX: 310/366-7343

AquaMotion Inc
14320 Longs Peak Ct
Longmont, CO 80504
e-mail: aqua@aquamotion.com
website: www.aquamotion.com
800/423-9090
970/535-0308
FAX: 970/535-0336

Aquatica
1273 Lakeside Dr, Ste 3161
Sunnyvale, CA 94086
e-mail: info@aquatica-usa.com
website: www.aquatica-usa.com
888/874-6782
408/736-8833
FAX: 408/736-8843

Aquatic Access Inc
417 Dorsey Way
Louisville, KY 40223
e-mail: info@aquatic-access.com
website: www.aquatic-access.com
800/325-LIFT
502/425-5817
FAX: 502/425-9607

Aquatic Therapy & Rehab Institute Inc
Rte 1, Box 218
Chassell, MI 49916
e-mail: atri@up.net
website: www.atri.org
906/482-9500
FAX: 906/482-4388

Arjo Inc
50 N Gary Ave
Roselle, IL 60172
e-mail: lchevrie@arjousa.com
website: www.arjousa.com
800/323-1245
630/307-6112
FAX: 888/594-ARJO (2756)

Armstrong Medical Industries Inc
575 Knightsbridge Pkwy
PO Box 700
Lincolnshire, IL 60069-0700
e-mail: csr@armstrongmedical.com
website: www.armstrongmedical.com
800/323-4220
847/913-0101
FAX: 847/913-0138

A2Z Possibilities Inc
10 Kyle Rd
Merrimack, NH 03054
800/338-9669
603/598-2860
FAX: 603/598-2860

Autogenic Systems
620 Wheat Ln
Wood Dale, IL 60191
e-mail: autogenics@stoeltingco.com
website: www.stoeltingco.com/autogen
630/860-9700
FAX: 630/860-9775

Axelgaard Manufacturing Co Ltd
1667 S Mission Rd
Fallbrook, CA 92028
e-mail: dnelson@axelgaard.com
888/811-7257
760/723-7554
FAX: 760/723-2356

BackMaster by Back-Jack Inc
10622 Garland Rd
Dallas, TX 75218
website: www.backmaster.com
800/597-5225
214/324-8877
FAX: 214/321-4329

Barrier Free Lifts Inc
9230 Prince William St
Manassas, VA 20110
website: bfl-inc.com
800/582-8732
703/361-6531
FAX: 703/361-7861

Battle Creek Equipment Co
307 W Jackson St
Battle Creek, MI 49017-2385
800/253-0854
616/962-6181
FAX: 616/962-8058

BIOflex Medical Magnetics
3370 NE 5 Ave
Oakland Park, FL 33334
e-mail: bmmi@worldnet.att.net
website: www.bioflexmagnets.com
800/471-7999
954/565-8500
FAX: 954/568-6117

BioMedical Life Systems Inc
2448 Cades Way
Vista, CA 92085
e-mail: sales@bmls.com
website: www.bmls.com
800/726-8367
760/727-5600
FAX: 760/727-4220

Bodyline Comfort Systems
3730 Kori Rd
Jacksonville, FL 32257
e-mail: info@bodyline.com
website: www.bodyline.com
800/874-7715
904/262-4068
FAX: 800/323-2225

Body Therapeutics
29885 Second St, Ste G
Lake Elsinore, CA 92532
e-mail: btwilhelm@juno.com
800/530-3722
909/674-5722
FAX: 909/674-8126

Briggs Corp
PO Box 1698
Des Moines, IA 50306-1698
e-mail: nrodriguez@briggscorp.com
website: www.briggscorp.com
800/247-2343
515/327-6400
FAX: 800/222-1996

Brown Medical Industries
1300 Lundberg Dr W
Spirit Lake, IA 51360
e-mail: beckim@rconnect.com
website: www.brownmed.com
800/843-4395
712/336-4395
FAX: 712/336-2874

**Cardon Rehabilitation
Products Inc**
PO Box 237
Niagra Falls, NY 14304-0237
800/944-7868
FAX: 716/297-0411

Chattanooga Group Inc
4717 Adams Rd
PO Box 489
Hixson, TN 37343
website: www.chattgroup.com
800/592-7329
423/870-2281
FAX: 800/242-8329

Comfort House
189 Frelinghuysen Ave
Newark, NJ 07114
e-mail: sales@comforthouse.com
website: www.comforthouse.com
973/242-8080
FAX: 973/242-0131

Continental SEL Inc
2321 NE 29th Ave
Ocala, FL 34479
e-mail: sales@continentalsel.com
website: www.continentalsel.com
800/826-9946
352/369-4900
FAX: 352/369-4906

**Core Products
International Inc**
808 Prospect Ave
Osceola, WI 54020
e-mail: info@coreproducts.com
website: www.coreproducts.com
800/365-3047
715/294-2050
FAX: 715/294-2622

Corflex/Medic-Air
669 E Industrial Park Dr
Manchester, NH 03109
e-mail: sales@corflex.com
website: www.corflex.com
800/426-7353
603/623-3344
FAX: 603/623-4111

Creations Magiques Inc
3001, Visitation
Joliette, Quebec, Canada J6E 7Y8
e-mail: admin@magicbag.com
website: www.magicbag.com
450/753-3892
FAX: 450/753-4287

Davol Inc
100 Sockanossett Crossroad
Cranston, RI 02920
website: www.davol.com
800/556-6756
401/463-7000
FAX: 401/946-5379

Devco Medical Systems
700 Cornelia
Joliet, IL 60435-5912
e-mail: devcomedsys@mediaone.net
800/317-4500
815/722-0598
FAX: 815/722-9828

Dura-Kold Corp
3525 S Purdue
Oklahoma City, OK 73179
e-mail: durakold@theshop.net
website: www.dura-kold.com
800/541-7199
405/943-8811
FAX: 405/943-9339

Dynatronics Corp
7030 Park Centre Dr
Salt Lake City, UT 84121
e-mail: info@dynatron.com
website: www.dynatronics.com
800/874-6251
801/568-7000
FAX: 801/568-7711

ElectroLogic of America Inc
3035 Dryden Rd
Dayton, OH 45439
e-mail: info@electrologic.com
website: www.electrologic.com
800/758-3460
937/299-7588
FAX: 937/299-7589

Electro-Med Health Industries
11601 Biscayne Blvd, Ste 200A
Miami, FL 33181
e-mail: emhi@bellsouth.net
800/232-3644
305/892-2866
FAX: 305/892-2980

Electronic Research Devices Corp
9220 SW Barbur Blvd, Ste 107
Portland, OR 97219-5433
800/547-0366
503/245-7241
FAX: 503/245-4863

ELMED Inc
60 W Fay Ave
Addison, IL 60101
e-mail: medical@elmed.com
website: www.elmed.com
630/543-2792
FAX: 630/543-2102

Evans Associates
102 Farmstead Cir
Lebanon, PA 17042
800/543-9288
717/228-0442
FAX: 717/228-2043

Fabrifoam Products
900 Springdale Dr
Exton, PA 19341
e-mail: fabrifoam@aol.com or
fabrifaom1 @aol.com
800/577-1077
610/363-1077
FAX: 610/363-1014

Ferno Ille, Ferno-Washington Inc
70 Weil Way
Wilmington, OH 45177-9371
e-mail: gshields@ferno.com
website: www.ferno.com
800/733-3766
937/382-1451
FAX: 937/383-1157

FES Information Center/ Cleveland FES Center
11000 Cedar Ave, Ste 230
Cleveland, OH 44106-3052
e-mail: info@fesc.org
website: www.fesc.org
800/666-2353
216/231-3257
FAX: 216/231-3258

Finis Inc
3941 Holly Dr, Ste F
Tracy, CA 95376
e-mail: info@finis-net.com
website: www.finis-net.com
888/333-4647
209/830-2890
FAX: 209/830-2896

Fitter International Inc
4519 1 St SE
Calgary, Alberta, Canada,
T2G 2L2
e-mail: sales@fitter1.com
website: www.fitter1.com
800/348-8371
403/243-6830
FAX: 403/229-1230

Flaghouse Inc
601 Flaghouse Dr
Hasbrouck Heights, NJ 07604-3116
e-mail: info@flaghouse.com
website: www.flaghouse.com
800/793-7900
201/288-7600
FAX: 800/793-7922

Florida Manufacturing Corp dba FlaManCo Intl
501 Beville Rd
Daytona Beach, FL 32119
e-mail: flamanco@worldnet.att.net
website: flamanco.com
800/447-2372
904/767-2372
FAX: 800/447-6167

Gebauer Co
9410 St Catherine Ave
Cleveland, OH 44104
website: www.gebauerco.com
800/321-9348
216/271-5252
FAX: 216/271-5335

General Physiotherapy Inc
13222 Lakefront Dr
St. Louis, MO 63045-1504
e-mail: jwestphale@g-5.com
website: www.g-5.com
800/237-1832
314/291-1442
FAX: 314/291-1485

GNR Health Systems Inc
3660 NE 42nd Ln
Ocala, FL 34479
e-mail: gnrcatalog@att.net
website: www.ptcatalog.com
800/523-0912
352/622-6434
FAX: 800/523-0914

Granberg International
200 S Garrand Blvd
PO Box 70425
Richmond, CA 94807-0425
e-mail: granberg@aol.com
website: www.granberg.com
800/233-6499
510/237-2099
FAX: 510/237-1667

**Grimm Scientific
Industries Inc**
Newport Pike
PO Box 2143
Marietta, OH 45750
800/223-5395
740/374-3412
FAX: 740/374-5745

Hang Ups
10004 162nd St, Ct E
Puyallup, WA 98375
e-mail: mail@inversiontherapy.com
website: www.inversiontherapy.com
800/847-0143
253/840-5252
FAX: 253/840-5757

Hill Laboratories Co
3 Bacton Hill Rd
PO Box 2028
Frazer, PA 19355
e-mail: info@hillabs.com
website: www.hillabs.com
610/644-2867
FAX: 610/647-6297

HydroWorx International Inc
1961 Fulling Mill Rd
Middletown, PA 17057
website: www.hydroworx.com
800/753-9633
717/985-1723
FAX: 717/985-1913

The Hygenic Corp
1245 Home Ave
Akron, OH 44310-2575
800/321-2135
330/633-8460
FAX: 330/633-9359

Ideal
Rte 1, Box 56
Broseley, MO 63932
e-mail: customers@idealproducts.com
website: www.idealproducts.com
800/321-5490
573/686-0003
FAX: 800/532-4691

**International Medical
Electronics Ltd**
3939 Broadway, Ste 100
Kansas City, MO 64111-2516
800/432-8003
816/931-5358

I-REP Inc
29885 Second St, Ste G
Lake Elsinore, CA 92532
e-mail: btwilhelm@juno.com
800/828-0852
909/674-7628
FAX: 909/674-8126

Kinetic Innovations
PO Box 19066
Omaha, NE 68119
e-mail: bionoprene@aol.com
www.kineticinnovations.com
877/272-2376
712/347-5152
FAX: 712/347-2124

Kustomer Kinetics Inc
1145 Encanto Dr
Arcadia, CA 91007
e-mail: sales@kustomerkinetics.com
website: www.kustomerkinetics.com
800/959-1145
626/445-6161
FAX: 626/445-6162

Lossing Orthopedic Inc
3230 Snelling Ave S
PO Box 6224
Minneapolis, MN 55406-0224
e-mail: lossingo@wavetech.net
800/328-5216
612/724-2669
FAX: 612/724-5089

LSI International
8849 Bond
Overland Park, KS 66214
e-mail: lsiinternational@att.net
website: www.lsiinternationsl.com
800/832-0053
913/894-4493
FAX: 913/894-1980

MARKnew Products
13020 Tom White Way, Ste F
Norwalk, CA 90650
800/404-7376
562/404-2257
FAX: 562/404-2347

**Martin Medical Equipment
Servicing Co**
81 Ward Rd
North Tonawanda, NY 14120
716/694-3542
FAX: 716/694-3610

Mastex Industries Inc
2035 Factory Ln
Petersburg, VA 23803
e-mail: mastex@mindspring.com
800/343-7444
804/732-8300
FAX: 804/732-8395

McBeth Therapy Co Inc
61 Spencer Ave
Lancaster, PA 17603
e-mail: mcbetherco@aol.com
800/346-2171
717/392-1616
FAX: 717/392-7159

MEDEXPERT
1614 MacDade Blvd
Folsom, PA 19033
610/461-7060
FAX: 610/461-7061

Med-Fit Systems Inc
2759 Secret Lake Ln
Fallbrook, CA 92028
e-mail: med-fit@aol.com
website: www.medfitsystems.com
800/831-7665
760/723-9618
FAX: 760/723-5396

The MED Group Inc
3223 S Loop 289, Ste 600
Lubbock, TX 79423
e-mail: sribble@medgroup.com
website: www.medgroup.com
800/825-5633
806/793-8421
FAX: 806/793-6480

Medical Science Products Inc
517 Elm Ridge Ave
PO Box 381
Canal Fulton, OH 44614
e-mail: msp@sssnet.com
website: www.medsciencepro.com
800/456-1971
330/854-4060
FAX: 330/854-1953

Med Labs Inc
28 Vereda Cordillera
Goleta, CA 93117
e-mail: medlabsinc@aol.com
website: hometown.aol.com/
medlabsinc
800/968-2486
805/968-2486
FAX: 805/968-2486

Medline Industries Inc
One Medline Place
Mundelein, IL 60060
website: www.medline.com
800/MEDLINE
847/949-3150
FAX: 847/949-3012

Med-Pro Corp
2A Firwood Rd
Port Washington, NY 11050-1510
800/633-7761
516/944-9613
FAX: 516/767-2672

**MED-TECH Equipment
Service Inc**
216 Hendrickson Mill Rd
Swedesboro, NJ 08085
800/322-2609
609/423-0641
FAX: 609/423-8062

Mettler Electronics Corp
1333 S Claudina St
Anaheim, CA 92805
e-mail: mettlerelec@earthlink.com
website: www.mettlerelec.com
800/854-9305
714/533-2221
FAX: 714/635-7539

Micro Bio-Medics Inc
846 Pelham Pkwy
Pelham Manor, NY 10803
website: www.microbiomedics.com
800/431-2743
914/738-8400
FAX: 914/738-8999

MultiBiosensors Inc
4944 Vista Grande
El Paso, TX 79922
e-mail: multibio@juno.com
800/441-4627
915/581-9684
FAX: 915/772-2034

Nada-Chair
2448 Larpenteur Ave W
St. Paul, MN 55113
e-mail: nadachair@aol.com
website: www.nadachair.com
800/722-2587
651/644-4466
FAX: 651/644-4488

N-K Products Co
29885 Second St, #G
Lake Elsinore, CA 92532
e-mail: btwilhelm@juno.com
800/462-6509
714/545-6509
FAX: 714/545-3618

NeuMed
1590 Reed Rd, Ste 102B
Pennington, NJ 08534
e-mail: sales@neumedinc.com
website: www.neurmedinc.com
800/367-1238
609/896-3444
FAX: 609/896-2798

**Nor-Am Patient Care
Products Ltd**
PO Box 543
Lewiston, NY 14093-0543
e-mail: noram@bserv.com
website: www.nor-am.net
800/387-7103
905/825-0094
FAX: 905/825-0501

Noraxon USA Inc
13430 N Scottsdale Rd, Ste 104
Scottsdale, AZ 85254
e-mail: noraxon@aol.com
website: www.noraxon.com
800/364-8985
480/443-3413
FAX: 480/443-4327

North Coast Medical Inc
18305 Sutter Blvd
Morgan Hill, CA 95037
e-mail: custserv@ncmedical.com
website: www.ncmedical.com
800/821-9319
408/776-5000
FAX: 877/213-9300

OMS Medical Supplies Inc
230 Libbey Pkwy
Weymouth, MA 02189
website: omsmedical.com
800/323-1839
781/331-3370
FAX: 781/335-5779

OPTP
PO Box 47009
Minneapolis, MN 55447-0009
e-mail: optp@worldnet.att.net
website: www.optp.com
800/367-7393
763/553-0452
FAX: 763/553-9355

ORMED
2615 River Rd, Unit 7
Cinnaminson, NJ 08077
website: www.ormedtech.com
800/440-2784

Parker Laboratories Inc
286 Eldridge Rd
Fairfield, NJ 07004
e-mail: parker@parkerlabs.com
website: www.parkerlabs.com
800/631-8888
973/276-9500
FAX: 973/276-9510

Pelton Shepherd Industries
PO Box 30218
Stockton, CA 95213
e-mail: sales@peltonshepherd.com
website: www.peltonshepherd.com
800/BLUEICE
209/983-0893
FAX: 209/983-0260

PHD Merchants
6080 S Jamaica Cir
Englewood, CO 80111-5749
e-mail: info@phdmerchants.com
website: www.phdmerchants.com
800/883-9210
303/741-5875
FAX: 303/770-1266

pi Professional Therapy Products
PO Box 1067
Athens, TN 37371-1067
website: www.pi-ptp.com
888/818-9632
423/744-8000
FAX: 800/842-4156

Pneumex Inc
PO Box 1006
Sandpoint, ID 83864
e-mail: pneumex@micron.net
website: www.pneumex.com
800/447-5792
208/265-4105
FAX: 208/265-9651

Posey Co
5635 Peck Rd
Arcadia, CA 91006
e-mail: custsvc@posey.com
website: www.posey.com
800/447-6739
626/443-3143
FAX: 800/767-3933

Professional Care Systems
PO Box 16650
St. Louis, MO 63105
800/727-0202
FAX: 800/329-1727

Progressive Medical Inc
142 Wetherby Ln
Westerville, OH 43081
800/777-3574
614/794-3300
FAX: 614/794-9582

MA Rallis Corp
2031 Hwy 130
Monmouth Junction, NJ 08852
e-mail: info@rallis.com
website: www.rallis.com
800/852-8898
732/940-0456
FAX: 732/940-0458

Rehabilicare
1811 Old Highway 8
New Brighton, MN 55112
e-mail: info@rehabilicare.com
website: www.rehabilicare.com
800/343-0488
FAX: 800/272-6458

Rehab Med + Equip Inc
PO Box 2238
Collegedale, TN 37315
e-mail: ahughes@rehabmedequip.com
website: rehabmedequip.com
800/358-5588
432/238-7800
FAX: 800/899-9972

Rich-Mar Corp
PO Box 879
Inola, OK 74036
800/762-4665
918/543-2222
FAX: 918/543-3334

Rio Plastics Inc
PO Box 3707
Brownsville, TX 78523
e-mail: info@rioplastics.com
website: www.rioplastics.com
956/831-2715
FAX: 956/831-9851

Sammons Preston
4 Sammons Ct
Bolingbrook, IL 60440
website: sammonspreston.com
800/323-5547
630/226-1300
FAX: 800/547-4333

The Saunders Group
4250 Norex Dr
Chaska, MN 55318
e-mail: sales@thesaundersgroup.com
website: thesaundersgroup.com
800/456-1289
612/368-9214
FAX: 612/368-9249

Serola Biomechanics
4376 Sunset Terr
Loves Park, IL 61111
800/624-0008
815/636-2780
FAX: 815/636-2781

Service Engineering Co
8621 Barefoot Industrial Rd
Raleigh, NC 27613
e-mail: sd1@mindspring.com
website: www.serviceeng.com
800/334-5528
919/783-6116
FAX: 919/782-8234

Shamrock Medical Inc
3620 SE Powell Blvd
Portland, OR 97202
800/231-2225
503/233-5055
FAX: 503/234-6974

Sigmedics Inc
200 Larkin Dr, Ste F
Wheeling, IL 60090-6498
e-mail: fzeiss@ameritech.net
847/279-0390
FAX: 847/279-0393

**Smith and Nephew Inc,
Rehabilitation Division**
One Quality Dr
PO Box 1005
Germantown, WI 53022
website: www.smith-
nephew.com
800/558-8633
414/251-7840
FAX: 800/545-7758

Southwest Technologies Inc
1746 Levee Rd
N Kansas City, MO 64116
e-mail: swtech@tfs.net
800/247-9951
816/221-2442
FAX: 816/221-3995

Sports Health
865 Muirfield Dr
Hanover Park, IL 60103
e-mail: peter_hovoka@
healthgiant.com
website: www.healthgiant.com
800/323-1305
FAX: 800/235-1305

Sportsware West
415 E Figueroa St, Ste A
Santa Barbara, CA 93101
e-mail: cryocup@aol.com
805/962-7454
FAX: 805/966-6585

**Sprint/Rothhammer
International**
PO Box 3840
San Luis Obispo, CA 93403
e-mail: info@sprintaquatics.com
website: www.sprintaquatics.com
800/235-2156
805/541-5330
FAX: 805/541-5339

SRS Medical Systems Inc
14950 NE 95th St
Redmond, WA 98052
e-mail: jstansbury@srsmedical.com
website: www.srsmedical.com
800/345-5642
425/882-1101
FAX: 425/882-1935

Stopain/DRJ Group Inc
2075 Corte Del Nogal, Ste W
Carlsbad, CA 92009
e-mail: stopain@gte.net
website: www.stopain.com
800/201-PAIN
760/602-9474
FAX: 760/602-9479

**SwimEx Systems,
A Division of TPI Inc**
373 Market St
PO Box 328
Warren, RI 02885-0328
e-mail: swimex@tpicomp.com
website: www.swimex.com
800/877-7946
FAX: 401/245-3160

Sydsons Medical Inc
353 McCaffrey St
St Laurent, Quebec, Canada,
H4T 1Z7
e-mail: sydons@vertigo.net
800/731-3212
514/731-3212
FAX: 514/731-5684

Tempra Technology Inc
6140 15th St E
Bradenton, FL 34203
e-mail: ivey@tempratech.com
website: www.tempratech.com
800/867-9189
941/739-8900
FAX: 941/753-6841

Therapeutic Alliances Inc
333 N Broad St
Fairborn, OH 45324
e-mail: taiinfo@aol.com
website: musclepower.com
937/879-0734
FAX: 937/879-5211

Therapeutic Dimensions Inc
PO Box 365
Spokane, WA 99210
800/755-0455
509/235-1685
FAX: 509/235-1687

Therapeutic Systems Inc
800 W State St, Ste 103
Doylestown, PA 18901
800/777-1870
215/340-1155
FAX: 215/340-1138

Theraquip Inc
209-E Creekridge Rd
Greensboro, NC 27406
e-mail: theraquip@aol.com
800/632-1312
336/333-9612
FAX: 336/333-9620

Thought Technology Ltd
2180 Belgrave Ave
Montreal, Quebec, Canada
H4A 2L8
e-mail: mail@thoughttechnology
.com
website: www.thoughttechnology
.com
800/361-3651
514/489-8251
FAX: 514/489-8255

Vann Healthcare Services
1220 N Race St
Glasgow, KY 42141
e-mail: vannhealthcare@
glasgow-ky.com
website: www.vannhealthcare.com
800/869-7651
270/651-7627
FAX: 270/651-9261

Vermont Medical Inc
Industrial Park
PO Box 556
Bellows Falls, VT 05101-0556
e-mail: vermed@sover.net
website: www.vermed.com
800/245-4025

802/463-9976
FAX: 802/463-9318

Vonco Medical
11201 Stemmons Frwy
Dallas, TX 75229
e-mail: voncomed@flash.net
website: www.voncomed.com
800/972-6461
972/247-6155
FAX: 972/247-1815

Water Gear Inc
PO Box 759
Pismo Beach, CA 93448
e-mail: hammer@watergear.com
website: watergear.com
800/794-6432
805/343-1778
FAX: 805/343-6078

WaterWear
PO Box 687
Wilton, NH 03086
e-mail: h2owear@aol.com
website: www.h2owear.com
888/321-7848
603/654-9885
FAX: 603/654-6426

Whitehall Manufacturing
PO Box 3527
City of Industry, CA 91744
e-mail: info@whitehallmfg.com
website: www.whitehallmfg.com
800/782-7706
626/968-6681
FAX: 626/855-4862

Williams Healthcare Systems
158 N Edison Ave
Elgin, IL 60123
e-mail:info@williamshealthcare.com
website: williamshealthcare.com
800/441-4967
847/741-3650
FAX: 847/741-3661

Zimmer Elektromedizin
2691 Richter, Ste 117
Irvine, CA 92606
e-mail: info@zimmerusa.com
website: www.zimmerusa.com
800/327-3576
949/727-3356
FAX: 949/727-2154

Appendix C

Units of Measure

Milliseconds (msec)	$= \frac{1}{1,000}$ of a second
Microseconds (μsec)	$= \frac{1}{1,000,000}$ of a second
Nanosecond (nsec)	$= \frac{1}{1,000,000,000}$ of a second
Milliamp (mamp)	$= \frac{1}{1,000}$ of an amp
Microamp (μamp)	$= \frac{1}{1,000,000}$ of an amp
Angstrom (Å)	$= \frac{1}{10,000,000,000}$ of a meter
Nanometer (nm)	$= \frac{1}{1,000,000,000}$ of a meter
Hertz (Hz)	= 1 cycle per second
Kilohertz (KHz)	= 1,000 cycles per second
Megahertz (MHz)	= 1,000,000 cycles per second

Answers to Self-Quizzes

CHAPTER 1 (16)

1. F	6. A
2. T	7. B
3. T	8. D
4. B	9. C
5. D	10. A

CHAPTER 2 (29-30)

1. T	6. D
2. F	7. C
3. T	8. A
4. B	9. D
5. C	10. A

CHAPTER 3 (50)

1. T	6. A
2. F	7. D
3. T	8. C
4. B	9. D
5. D	10. C

CHAPTER 4 (85-86)

1. F	6. D
2. T	7. B
3. T	8. C
4. C	9. B
5. A	10. A

CHAPTER 5 (129)

1. T	6. C
2. F	7. A
3. F	8. D
4. B	9. C
5. A	10. B

CHAPTER 6 (159-160)

1. T	6. A
2. T	7. D
3. F	8. A
4. C	9. D
5. B	10. B

CHAPTER 7 (187)

1. F	6. A
2. T	7. B
3. T	8. D
4. B	9. D
5. C	10. A

CHAPTER 8 (230)

1. T	6. B
2. F	7. C
3. T	8. A
4. D	9. D
5. B	10. D

CHAPTER 9 (251)

1. F	6. D
2. F	7. C
3. T	8. A
4. B	9. D
5. A	10. C

CHAPTER 10 (278)

1. T	6. D
2. F	7. A
3. T	8. C
4. B	9. A
5. D	10. C

CHAPTER 11 (294)

1. T	6. D
2. T	7. A
3. F	8. C
4. B	9. D
5. B	10. A

CHAPTER 12 (319)

1. T	6. C
2. T	7. A
3. F	8. C
4. B	9. D
5. D	10. B

CHAPTER 13 (336-337)

1. F	6. A
2. T	7. C
3. F	8. B
4. D	9. C
5. B	10. D

CHAPTER 14 (361)

1. T	6. C
2. F	7. A
3. T	8. D
4. C	9. B
5. B	10. B

CHAPTER 15 (376-377)

1. F	6. B
2. T	7. A
3. F	8. D
4. C	9. A
5. D	10. C

Glossary

A

absolute refractory period Brief time period (.5 μsec) after membrane depolarization during which the membrane is incapable of depolarizing again.

absorption Energy that stimulates a particular tissue to perform its normal function.

accommodation Adaptation by the sensory receptors to various stimuli over an extended period of time.

acidic reaction The accumulation of negative ions under the positive pole, which produces hydrochloric acid.

acoustic impedance Determines the amount of ultrasound energy reflected at tissue interfaces.

acoustic microstreaming The unidirectional movement of fluids along the boundaries of cell membranes, resulting from the mechanical pressure wave in an ultrasonic field.

acoustic spectrum The range of frequencies and wavelengths of sound waves.

ACTH Adrenocorticotropic hormone. This hormone stimulates the release of glucocorticoids (cortisol) from the adrenal glands.

action potential A recorded change in electrical potential between the inside and outside of a nerve cell, resulting in muscular contraction.

active electrode Electrode at which greatest current density occurs or the electrode that is used to drive ions into the tissues.

acupressure The technique of using finger pressure over acupuncture points to decrease pain.

acute Pain of sudden onset often associated with physical trauma.

acute injury An injury in which active inflammation is present that includes the classic symptoms of tenderness, swelling, redness, and warmth.

afferent Conduction of a nerve impulse toward an organ.

air space plate A capacitor type electrode in which the plates are separated from the skin by the space in a glass case; used with shortwave diathermy.

alkaline reaction The accumulation of positive ions under the negative electrode, which produces sodium hydroxide.

all-or-none response The depolarization of nerve or muscle membrane is the same once a depolarizing intensity threshold is reached; further increases in intensity do not increase the response. Stimuli at intensities less than threshold do not create a depolarizing effect.

alternating current Current that periodically changes its polarity or direction of flow.

ampere Unit of measure that indicates the rate at which electrical current is flowing.

amplifier A device using electrical components to increase electrical power.

amplitude Describes the magnitude of the vibration in a wave. It is the maximum distance from equilibrium that any particle reaches. It is also referred to as the intensity of current flow as indicated by the height of the waveform from baseline.

analgesia Loss of sensibility to pain.

anesthesia Loss of sensation.

annulus fibrosus The interlacing cross-fibers of fibroelastic tissue that are attached to adjacent vertebral bodies that contain the nucleus pulposus.

anode Positively charged electrode in a direct current system.

anoxia Reduction of oxygen in body tissues below physiologic levels.

applicator The electrode used to transfer energy in microwave diathermy.

Arndt-Schultz principle No reactions or changes can occur in the body if the amount of energy absorbed is not sufficient to stimulate the absorbing tissues.

attenuation A decrease in energy intensity while the ultrasound wave is transmitted through various tissues caused by scattering and dispersion.

average current The amount of current flowing per unit of time.

avulsion fracture A fracture in which a small piece of bone is torn away by an attached tendon or ligament.

B

bacteriostatic A chemical environment in which bacteria is destroyed.

bandwidth A specific frequency range in which the amplifier will pick up signals produced by electrical activity in the muscle.

beam nonuniformity ratio (BNR) Indicates the amount of variability of intensity within the ultrasound beam and is determined by the maximal point intensity of transducer to the average intensity across the transducer surface.

beat Distinct wave pattern created by combining two distinct circuit electrical waves that blend into a gradual rising and falling wave.

β-endorphin A neurohormone derived from proopiomelanocortin (POMC). It is similar in structure and properties to morphine.

Bindegewebsmassage Reflex zone massage; uses a pulling stroke across connective tissue to effect change.

bioelectromagnetics The study of biologic tissues' electrical and magnetic properties.

biofeedback Information provided from some measuring instrument about a specific biologic function.

biphasic current Another name for alternating current, in which the direction of current flow reverses direction.

bipolar arrangement Two active recording electrodes placed in close proximity to one another.

bursts A combined set of three or more pulses; also referred to as packets or envelopes.

C

cable electrodes An inductance type electrode in which the electrodes are coiled around a body part, creating an electromagnetic field.

capacitor electrodes Air space plates or pad electrodes that create a stronger electrical field than a magnetic field.

cathode Negatively charged electrode in a direct current system.

cavitation The formation of gas-filled bubbles that expand and compress because of ultrasonically induced pressure changes in tissue fluids.

central biasing A theory of pain modulation where higher centers, such as the cerebral cortex, influence the perception of and response to pain. Also the use of hyperstimulation—analgesia to bias the central nervous system against transmitting painful stimuli to the sensory recognition area. This occurs through hormonal influences created by brain stem stimulation.

chronaxie The duration of time necessary to cause observable tissue excitation, given a current intensity of two times rheobasic current.

chronic injury An injury in which the normal cellular response in the inflammatory process is altered, replacing leukocytes with macrophages and plasma cells.

chronic pain Pain lasting more than 6 months.

circuit The path of current from a generating source through the various components back to the generating source.

coherence Property of identical phase and time relationship. All photons of laser light are the same wavelength.

collimate To make parallel.

collimated beam A focused, less divergent beam of ultrasound energy produced by a large diameter transducer.

common mode rejection ratio (CMRR) The ability of the differential amplifier to eliminate the common noise between the active electrodes.

compressions Regions of high molecular density (i.e., a great amount of ultrasound energy) within the longitudinal wave.

conductance The ease with which a current flows along a conducting medium.

conduction Heat loss or gain through direct contact.

conductors Materials that permit the free movement of electrons.

congestion Presence of an abnormal amount of blood in the vessels resulting from an increase in blood flow or obstructed venous return.

consensual heat vasodilation Vasodilation and increased blood flow will spread to remote areas, causing increased metabolism in the unheated area.

constructive interference The combined amplitude of two distinct circuits increases the amplitude.

continuous wave An uninterrupted beam of laser light, as opposed to pulsed.

continuous wave ultrasound The sound intensity remains constant throughout the treatment, and the ultrasound energy is being produced 100% of the time.

contrast bath Hot (106° F) and cold (50° F) treatments in a combined sequence to stimulate superficial capillary vasodilation or vasoconstriction.

convection Heat loss or gain through the movement of water molecules across the skin.

conversion Changing from one energy form into another.

cosine law Optimal radiation occurs when the source of radiation is at right angles to the center of the area being radiated.

coulomb Indicates the number of electrons flowing in a current.

coupling medium A substance used to decrease the acoustic impedance at the air-skin interface and thus facilitate the passage of ultrasound energy.

cryokinetics The use of cold and exercise in the treatment of pathology or disease.

cryotherapy The use of cold in the treatment of pathology or diseases.

current The flow of electrons.

current density Amount of current flow per cubic area.

current of injury A bioelectric current produced by any type of cellular trauma that plays a key role in stimulating healing.

D

decay time The time required for a waveform to go from peak amplitude to 0 V.

denervated muscle Muscle that has lost its peripheral nerve supply.

depolarization Process or act of neutralizing the cell membrane's resting potential.

destructive interference Combined amplitude of two distinct circuits decreases the amplitude.

diathermy The application of high-frequency electrical energy that is used to generate heat in body tissue as a result of the tissue to the passage of energy. It may also be used to produce nonthermal effects.

differential amplifier Monitors the two separate signals from the active electrodes and amplifies the difference, thus eliminating extraneous noise.

diode laser A solid-state/semiconductor used as a lasing medium.

dipoles Molecules whose ends carry opposite charges.

direct current Galvanic current that always flows in the same direction and may flow in either a positive or a negative direction.

direct effect The tissue response that occurs from energy absorption.

disk herniation The protrusion of the nucleus pulposus through a defect in the annulus fibrosus.

disk material Cartilaginous material from vertebral body surfaces, disk nucleus, or annulus fibrosus.

disk nucleus The protein polysaccharide gel that is contained between the cartilaginous end plates of the vertebrae and the annulus fibrosus.

disk protrusion The abnormal projection of the disk nucleus through some or all of the annular rings.

divergence The bending of light rays away from each other; the spreading of light.

DNA Deoxyribonucleic acid—the substance found in the chromosomes of the cell nucleus that carries the genetic code of the cell.

drum electrodes Induction electrodes that produce a strong magnetic field. Primarily used with pulsed shortwave diathermy.

duration Sometimes referred to as pulse width. Indicates the length of time the current is flowing.

duty cycle The percentage of time that ultrasound is being generated (pulse duration) over one pulse period, which is also referred to as the mark: space ratio.

dynorphin An endogenous opioid derived from the prohormone prodynorphin.

E

eddy currents Small circular electrical fields induced when a magnetic field is created that result in intramolecular oscillation (vibration) of tissue contents, causing heat generation.

edema Excessive fluid in cells.

effective radiating area The total area of the surface of the transducer that actually produces the sound wave.

efferent Conduction of a nerve impulse away from an organ.

effleurage To stroke; any stroke that glides over the skin without attempting to move the deep muscle masses. The hand is molded to the part, stroking with more or less constant pressure, usually upward. Any degree of pressure may be applied, varying from the lightest possible touch to very deep pressure.

electrets Insulators carrying a permanent charge similar to a permanent magnet.

electrical current The net movement of electrons along a conducting medium.

electrical field The lines of force exerted on charged ions in the tissues by the electrodes that cause charged particles to move from one pole to the other.

electrical impedance The opposition to electron flow in a conducting material.

electrical potential The difference between charged particles at a higher and lower potential.

electrolytes Solutions in which ionic movement occurs.

electromagnetic spectrum The range of frequencies and wavelengths associated with radiant energy.

electromyographic biofeedback A therapeutic procedure that uses electronic or electromechanical instruments to accurately measure, process, and feed back reinforcing information via auditory or visual signals.

electron Fundamental particle of matter possessing a negative electrical charge and very small mass.

electrophoresis The movement of ions in solution.

electropiezo activity Changing electric surface charges of a structure forces the structure to change shape.

endogenous opioids Opiate-like neuroactive peptide substances made by the body.

endorphins Endogenous opioids whose actions have analgesic properties (i.e., β-endorphin).

endothelial cell Cells that line the cavities of vessels.

endothelial-derived relaxing factor Relaxes smooth muscle and stimulates blood flow rates in veins.

enkephalinergic interneurons Neurons with short axons that release enkephalin. They are widespread in the central nervous system and are found in the substantia gelatinosa, nucleus raphe magnus, and periaqueductual grey matter.

erythema A redness of the skin caused by capillary dilation.

excited state State of an atom that occurs when outside energy causes the atom to contain more energy than normal.

F

facet joints Articular joints of the spine.

faradic current An asymmetric biphasic waveform seldom used on modern electrical generators.

Federal Communications Commission (FCC) Federal agency charged with assigning frequencies for all radio transmitters, including diathermies.

fiber optic A solid glass or plastic tube that conducts light along its length.

fibrils Connective tissue fibers supporting the lymphatic capillaries.

fibroplasia The period of scar formation that occurs during the fibroblastic repair phase.

fibrosis The formation of fibrous tissue in the injury repair process.

filter Changes pulsating DC current to smooth DC.

filters Devices that help to reduce external noise that essentially makes the amplifier more sensitive to some incoming frequencies and less sensitive to others.

fluidotherapy A modality of dry heat using a finely divided solid suspended in a stream with the properties of liquid.

fluorescence The capacity of certain substances to radiate when illuminated by a source of a given wavelength; a light of a different wavelength (color) than that of the irradiating source when illuminated by a given wavelength.

focusing Narrowing attention to the appropriate stimuli in the environment.

free nerve endings Receptors that are sensitive to extreme mechanical, chemical, or thermal energy.

frequency The number of cycles or pulses per second.

frequency window selectivity Cellular responses may be triggered by a certain electrical frequency range.

friction massage A technique that affects fibrositic adhesions in tendon, muscle, or ligament. It is performed by small circular movements that penetrate into the depth of a muscle, not by moving the finger on the skin, but by moving the tissues under the skin.

functional electrical stimulation Utilizes multiple channel electrical stimulators to recruit muscles in a programmed sequence that produces a functional movement pattern.

G

gap junctions Specialized junction areas connecting cells of like structure that contain channels for ionic, electrical, and small molecule signaling that passes messages from cell to cell.

glutamate enkephalin Neurotransmitter proteins that block the passage of noxious stimuli from first order to second order afferents. They inhibit the release of substance P and are produced by enkephalinergic neurons.

ground A wire that makes an electrical connection with the earth.

ground-fault interrupters (GFI) A safety device that automatically shuts off current flow and reduces the chances of electrical shock.

ground state The normal, unexcited state of an atom.

H

heterodyne Cyclic rising and falling wave form of interferential current.

high-voltage current Current in which the waveform has an amplitude of greater than 150 V with a relatively short pulse duration.

hot spots Areas at tissue interfaces that may become overheated.

Hubbard tank An immersion tank for the whole body, it may have vertical depth for walking or supine treatment.

hunting response A reflex vasodilation that occurs in response to cold approximately 15 minutes into the treatment. This has been demonstrated to be only an increase in temperature and not necessarily a change in blood flow.

hybrid currents Currents that have waveforms containing parameters that are not classically alternating or direct.

hydrocollator A synthetic hot (170° F) or cold (0° F) gel used as an adjunctive modality to stimulate a rise or fall in tissue temperature.

hydrotherapy Cryotherapy and thermotherapy techniques that use water as the medium for heat transfer.

hyperemia Presence of an increased amount of blood in part of the body.

hyperplasia An increase in the size of a tissue; in the skin, an increased thickness of the epidermis.

I

impedance The resistance of the tissue to the passage of electrical current.

indication The reason to prescribe a remedy or procedure.

indifferent or dispersive electrode Large electrode used to spread out electrical charge and decrease current density at that electrode site.

indirect effect A decreased response that occurs in deeper tissues.

induction electrodes Cable or drum electrodes that create a stronger magnetic field than electrical field.

inflammation A redness of the skin caused by capillary dilations.

infrared The portion of the electromagnetic spectrum associated with thermal changes located adjacent to the red portion of the visible light spectrum.

insulators Materials that resist current flow.

integration A signal processing technique that measures the area under the curve for a specified period of time, thus forming the basis for quantification of electrical activity.

intensity A measure of the rate at which energy is being delivered per unit area.

intermolecular oscillation (vibration) Movement between molecules that produces friction and thus heat.

interneurons Neurons contained entirely in the central nervous system. They have no projections outside the spinal cord. Their function is to serve as relay stations within the central nervous system.

interpulse interval The interruptions between individual pulses or groups of pulses.

intrapulse interval The period of time between individual pulses.

inverse square law The intensity of radiation striking a particular surface varies inversely with the square of the distance from the radiating source.

ion A positively or negatively charged particle.

ion transfer A technique of transporting chemicals across a membrane using an electrical current as a driving force.

ionization A process by which soluble compounds, such as acids, alkaloids, or salts, dissociate or dissolve into ions that are suspended in some type of solution.

iontophoresis Uses continuous direct current to drive ions into the tissues.

J

joint capsule Ligamentous structure that surrounds and encapsulates a joint.

joint swelling Accumulation of blood and joint fluid within the joint capsule.

K

Kehr's sign Referred pain pattern involving pain in the left jaw, shoulder, and arm.

keratin The fibrous protein that forms the chemical basis of the epidermis.

keratinocytes A cell that produces keratin.

L

laser A device that concentrates high energies into a narrow beam of coherent, monochromatic light (Light Amplification by the Stimulated Emission of Radiation).

Law of Grotthus-Draper Energy not absorbed by the tissues must be transmitted.

leukocytes A white blood cell that is the primary effector cell against infection and tissue damage that functions to clean up damaged cells.

ligament deformation Lengthening distortion of ligament caused by traction loading.

longitudinal wave The primary waveform in which ultrasound energy travels in soft tissue, with the molecular displacement along the direction in which the wave travels.

low-voltage current Current in which the waveform has an amplitude of less than 150 V.

lymph A transparent slightly yellow liquid found in the lymphatic vessels.

lymphedema Swelling of subcutaneous tissues as a result of accumulation of excessive lymph fluid.

M

macroshock An electrical shock that can be felt and has a leakage of electrical current of greater than 1 mA.

macrotears Significant damage to soft tissues caused by acute trauma that results in clinical symptoms and functional alterations.

magnetic field Field created when current is passed through a coiled cable that affects surrounding tissues by inducing localized eddy currents, within the tissues.

massage The act of rubbing, kneading, or stroking the superficial parts of the body with the hand or with an instrument for the purpose of modifying nutrition, restoring power of movement, or breaking up adhesions.

maximum voluntary isometric contraction Peak torque produced by a muscular contraction.

medical galvanism Creates either an acidic or alkaline environment that may be of therapeutic value.

melanin A group of dark brown or black pigments that occur naturally in the eye, skin, hair, and other animal tissues.

meniscoid structures A cartilage tip found on the synovial fringes of some facet joints.

metabolites Waste products of metabolism or catabolism.

microcurrent electrical nerve stimulator (MENS) Used primarily in tissue healing, the current intensities are too small to excite peripheral nerves.

microshock An electrical shock that is imperceptible because of a leakage of current of less than 1 mA.

microtears Minor damage to soft tissue most often associated with overuse.

minimal erythemal dose The amount of time of exposure to UVR necessary to cause a faint erythema 24 hours after exposure.

modulation Refers to any alteration in the magnitude or any variation in the duration of an electrical current.

monochromaticity When a light source produces a single color or wavelength.

monophasic current Another name for direct current, in which the direction of current flow remains the same.

mottling A reddening of the skin in a blotchy pattern.

muscle guarding A protective response in muscle that results from pain or fear of movement.

myofascial pain A type of referred pain associated with trigger points.

myofascial release A group of techniques used to relieve soft tissue from the abnormal grip of tight fascia.

N

nerve root impingement Abnormal encroachment of some body tissue into the space occupied by the nerve root.

neuromuscular electrical stimulator (NMES) Also called an electrical muscle stimulator (EMS), it is used to stimulate muscle directly as would be the case with denervated muscle where peripheral nerves are not functioning.

neurotransmitter Substance that passes information between neurons. It is released from one neuron terminal (presynaptic membrane), enters the synaptic cleft, and attaches (binds) to a receptor on the next neuron (postsynaptic membrane). Substance P, enkephalins, serotonin, methionine, acetylcholine, and leucine enkephalin are neurotransmitters.

nociceptive Pain information or signals of pain stimuli.

noise Extraneous electrical activity that may be produced by any source other than the contracting muscle.

norepinephrine A neurotransmitter.

nutrients Essential or nonessential food substance.

O

ohm A unit of measure that indicates resistance to current flow.

Ohm's law The current in an electrical circuit is directly proportional to the voltage and inversely proportional to the resistance.

opiate receptors Neurons that have receptors that bind to opiate substances.

oscillator Used to produce and output a specific waveform, which may be different from that used to power or drive the stimulating unit.

output amplifier Used to magnify or increase the amplitude of the voltage output of the generator and control it at a specific level.

P

pad electrodes Capacitor-type electrode used with shortwave diathermy to create an electrical field.

pain An unpleasant sensory and emotional experience associated with actual or potential tissue damage.

paraffin bath A combined paraffin and mineral oil immersion technique in which the paraffin substance is heated to 126° F for conductive heat gains; commonly used on the hands and feet for distal temperature gains in blood flow and temperature.

parallel circuit A circuit in which two or more routes exist for current to pass between the two terminals.

periaqueductal grey A midbrain structure that plays an important role in descending tracts that inhibit synaptic transmission of noxious input in the dorsal horn.

periosteum A highly vascularized and innervated membrane lining the surface of bone.

petrissage Massage technique that is a kneading manipulation. Consists of repeatedly grasping and releasing the tissue with one or both hands or parts thereof in a lifting, rolling, or pressing movement. The outside characteristic of this movement as contrasted to stroking movements is that the pressure is applied intermittently.

phagocytic cells A cell that has the ability to destroy and ingest cellular debris.

phases That portion of the pulse that rises above or below the baseline for some period of time.

phonophoresis A technique in which ultrasound is used to drive a topical application of a selected medication into the tissues.

photokeratitis An inflammation of the eyes caused by exposure to UVR.

photon The basic unit of light; a packet or quanta of light energy.

photosensitization A process in which a person becomes overly sensitive to UVR.

piezoelectric activity Changing electric surface charges of a structure forces the structure to change shape.

piezoelectric effect When an alternating electrical current generated at the same frequency as the crystal resonance is passed through the piezoelectric crystal, the crystal will expand and contract or vibrate at the frequency of the electrical oscillation, thus generating ultrasound at a desired frequency.

pigmentation Tanning of the skin from sun exposure.

pitting edema A type of swelling that leaves a pitlike depression when the skin is compressed.

population inversion A condition where more atoms exist in a high energy, excited state than those atoms that are in a normal ground state; this is required for lasing to occur.

power The total amount of ultrasound energy in the beam; is expressed in watts.

proprioceptive nervous system System of nerves that provides information on joint movement, pressure, and muscle tension.

prostaglandins Irritants that are synthesized locally during injury in tissue from a fatty acid precursor (arachidonic acid). They act with bradykinin to amplify pain by sensitizing afferent neurons to chemical and mechanical simulation. Aspirin is thought to be capable of interrupting the process. Prostaglandins are powerful vasodilators. They induce erythema, increase leakage of plasma from vessels, and attract leukocytes to an injured area.

pulse An individual waveform.

pulse charge The total amount of electricity being delivered to the athlete during each pulse.

pulse period The combined time of the pulse duration and the interpulse interval.

pulsed-polyphasic current Current that contains three or more grouped phases in a single pulse and that is used in interferential and "Russian" currents.

pulsed shortwave diathermy Created by simply interrupting the output of continuous shortwave diathermy at consistent intervals; it is used primarily for nonthermal effects.

pulsed ultrasound The intensity is periodically interrupted with no ultrasound energy being produced during the off period. When using pulsed ultrasound, the average intensity of the output over time is reduced.

R

radiating pain Pain that moves away from the site of a lesion, usually associated with some pressure in the area of injury.

radiation The process of emitting energy from some source in the form of waves. A method of heat transfer through which heat can be either gained or lost.

ramping Another name for surging modulation, in which the current builds gradually to some maximum amplitude.

raphe nucleus Part of the brain that is known to inhibit pain impulses being transmitted through the ascending system.

rarefactions Regions of lower molecular density (i.e., a small amount of ultrasound energy) within a longitudinal wave.

rate of rise How quickly a waveform reaches its maximum amplitude.

raw A form in which the electrical activity produced by muscle contraction may be displayed or recorded before the signal is processed.

rectification A signal processing technique that changes the deflection of the waveform from the negative pole to the positive pole, essentially creating a pulsed direct current.

rectifier Converts AC current to pulsating DC current.

reference electrode Also referred to as the ground electrode, it serves as a point of reference to compare the electrical activity recorded by the active electrodes.

referred pain (referred myofascial pain) When nociceptive impulses reach the dorsal grey matter, they converge, and their summation can depolarize internuncial neurons over several spinal segments, causing the individual to feel pain in distal areas innervated by these segments.

reflection The bending back of light or sound waves from a surface that they strike.

refraction The change in direction of a sound wave or radiation wave when it passes from one medium or type of tissue to another.

regulator Produces a specific controlled voltage output.

resistance The opposition to electron flow in a conducting material.

resting potential The potential difference between the inside and outside of a membrane.

rheobase The intensity of current necessary to cause observable tissue excitation given a long current duration.

RNA Ribonucleic acid—an acid found in the cell cytoplasm and nucleolus; it is intimately involved in protein synthesis.

Rolfing A system devised to correct inefficient structure by balancing the body within a gravitational field through a technique involving manual soft-tissue manipulation.

Russian current A medium frequency (2000 to 10,000 H$_z$) polyphasic AC wave generated in 50 burst-per-second envelopes.

S

sclerotome A segment of bone innervated by a spinal segment.

series circuit A circuit in which there is only one path for current to get from one terminal to another.

sensitization Prolonged depolarization of nociceptive neurons that results in continuous stimulation. Most sensory receptors are rendered less sensitive after prolonged stimulations. This is not the case with nociceptive neurons.

serotonin A neurotransmitter found in neurons descending in the dorsolateral tract. The dorsolateral tract is thought to play a significant role in pain control. Serotonin is found in the vesicles in nerve endings that bind when released to postsynaptic membranes. Its action is terminated by re-uptake into presynaptic membranes. It is probably involved in both endogenous pain control and opiate analgesia. Increased levels of serotonin in the central nervous system are generally associated with increased analgesia.

signal gain Determines the signal sensitivity. If a high gain is chosen, the biofeedback unit will have a high sensitivity for the muscle activity signal.

smoothing A signal processing technique that eliminates the high-frequency fluctuations that are produced with a changing electrical signal.

specific absorption rate (SAR) Represents the rate of energy absorbed per unit area of tissue mass.

spondylolisthesis Forward displacement of one vertebra over another.

spontaneous emission When an atom in a high-energy state emits a photon and drops to a more stable ground state.

standing wave As the ultrasound energy is reflected at tissue interfaces with different acoustic impedances, the intensity of the energy is increased as the reflected energy meets new energy being transmitted, forming waves of high energy, that can potentially damage surrounding tissues.

stereodynamic interference current Three distinct circuits blending and creating a distinct electrical wave pattern.

stimulated emission When a photon interacts with an atom already in a high-energy state and decay of the atomic system occurs, releasing two photons.

strain-related potentials Tissue-based electric potentials generated in response to strain of the tissue.

strength-duration curve A graphic illustration of the relationship between current intensity and current duration in causing depolarization of a nerve or muscle membrane.

stretching window The time period of vigorous heating when tissues will undergo their greatest extensibility and elongation.

substance P A peptide believed to be the neurotransmitter of small-diameter primary afferent. It is released from both ends of the neuron.

substantia gelatinosa (SG) Lamina II of the dorsal horn of the grey matter. Melzack and Wall proposed that the SG is responsible for closing the gate to painful stimuli.

summation of contractions Shortening of muscle myofilaments caused by increasing the frequency of muscle membrane depolarization.

sun protection factor (SPF) A sunscreen's effectiveness in absorbing the sunburn-inducing radiation.

synovial fringes Folds of synovial tissue that move in and out of the joint space.

T

tapotment A percussion massage; any series of brisk blows following each other in a rapid alternating fashion: hacking, cupping, slapping, beating, tapping, and pinchment. It is used when stimulation is the objective.

tetanization When individual muscle-twitch responses can no longer be distinguished and the responses force maximum shortening of the stimulated muscle fiber.

tetany Muscle condition that is caused by hyperexcitation and results in cramps and spasms.

thermal Pertaining to heat.

thermopane An insulating layer of water next to the skin.

thermotherapy The use of heat in the treatment of pathology or disease.

traction Drawing tension applied to a body segment.

Trager A technique that attempts to establish neuromuscular control so that more normal movement patterns can be routinely performed.

transcutaneous electrical nerve stimulator (TENS) A transcutaneous electrical stimulator used to stimulate peripheral nerves.

transcutaneous electrical stimulator All therapeutic electrical generators regardless of whether they deliver AC, DC, or pulsed currents through electrodes attached to the skin.

transformer Reduces the amount of voltage from the power supply.

transmission The propagation of energy through a particular biologic tissue into deeper tissues.

transverse wave Occurring only in bone, the molecules are displaced perpendicular to the direction in which the ultrasound wave is moving.

trigger point Localized deep tenderness in a palpable firm band of muscle. When stretched, a palpating finger can snap the band like a taut string, which produces local pain, a local twitch of that portion of the muscle, and a jump by the athlete. Sustained pressure on a trigger point reproduces the pattern of referred pain for that site.

twitch muscle contraction A single muscle contraction caused by one depolarization phenomenon.

U

ultrasound A portion of the acoustic spectrum located above audible sound.

ultraviolet The portion of the electromagnetic spectrum associated with chemical changes located adjacent to the violet portion of the visible light spectrum.

unilateral foramen opening Enlargement of the foramen on one side of a vertebral segment.

V

vasconstriction Narrowing of the blood vessels.

vasodilation Dilation of the blood vessels.

vibration A shaking massage technique; a fine tremulous movement made by the hand or fingers placed firmly against a part that will cause the part to vibrate. Often used for a soothing effect; may be stimulating when more energy is applied.

viscoelastic properties The property of a material to show sensitivity to rate of loading.

volt The electromotive force that must be applied to produce a movement of electrons.

voltage The force resulting from an accumulation of electrons at one point in an electrical circuit, usually corresponding to a deficit of electrons at another point in the circuit.

voltage sensitive permeability The quality of some cell membranes that makes them permeable to different ions based on the electric charge of the ions. Nerve and muscle cell membranes allow negatively charged ions into the cell while actively transporting some positively charged ions outside the cell membrane.

W

watt A measure of electrical power. Mathematically, watts = volts × amperes.

waveform The shape of an electrical current as displayed on an oscilloscope.

wavelength The distance from one point in a propagating wave to the same point in the next wave.

Wolff's law Bone remodels itself and provides increased strength along the lines of the mechanical forces placed on it.

Index